D1564476

Rogues,
Rebels,
and
Geniuses

Also by Donald Jack

The Bandy Papers
I. *Three Cheers For Me*
II. *That's Me in the Middle*
III. *It's Me Again*
IV. *Me Bandy, You Cissie*

Plays
Exit Muttering

Nonfiction
Sinc, Betty, and the Morning Man

Rogues, Rebels, and Geniuses

The Story of Canadian Medicine

Donald Jack

1981
Doubleday Canada Limited,
Toronto, Ontario
Doubleday & Company, Inc.,
Garden City, New York

Library of Congress Catalog Card Number 81-43107
Copyright © 1981 by Donald Jack
Forewords copyright © 1981 by Pierre Berton and Martin M. Hoffman
All rights reserved
First Edition

Printed in Canada by the John Deyell Company

Typesetting by ART-U Graphics

Design by Robert Burgess Garbutt

Canadian Cataloguing in Publication Data

Jack, Donald, 1924-
Rogues, rebels and geniuses

Bibliography: p. 650
Includes index.
ISBN 0-385-15575-1

1. Physicians—Canada—Biography. 2. Medicine—
Canada—History. I. Title.

R464.A1J36   610′.92′2   C81-094817-6

The author acknowledges the assistance
of the Canada Council in the completion of this book.

The photograph of William Tolmie is from the book
Physician and Fur Trader, the Diary of William Fraser Tolmie,
published by Mitchell Press, Vancouver, B.C., 1963.

Foreword

by Pierre Berton

This lively work is more than a history of Canadian medicine: in a curious way it is also a history of the Canadian nation. In his monumental examination of the place of doctors in our history, Donald Jack makes it clear that ever since Cartier's day medical men have been bound up in the development of the country—not only as practitioners but also as politicians, explorers, gadflies, soldiers, and community leaders.

We ought to have known this: was not John Christian Schultz, Louis Riel's *bête noire*, a medical man? Wasn't John McLoughlin, the ruler of Rupert's Land, a doctor? Wasn't John Richardson, the Arctic adventurer, a naval surgeon? Wasn't William Warren Baldwin, the Upper Canadian reformist and politician, also a practicing physician? Of course. And how about John A. Macdonald's right-hand man, Charles Tupper? How about John Sebastian Helmcken, British Columbia's great pre-Confederation statesman? How about William "Tiger" Dunlop, the surgeon-turned-journalist-turned-land developer in Upper Canada?

These and many more are chronicled in these pages, warts and all. The eccentrics and iconoclasts are here, too: Dr. James Barry, who was actually a woman; Henry Morgentaler, jailed for his stand on abortion; Morton Shulman, the controversial Toronto coroner, politician and broadcaster.

But nobody can read this book without realizing the enormous contribution to international medicine made by Canadians. Indeed, I can think of no other field which has produced so many men of world stature. The list is imposing: Grenfell, Bethune, Osler, Penfield, Selye, Banting,

Best—not to mention Alan Brown, Marion Hilliard, William R. Beaumont, Allan Roy Dafoe, Clarence Hincks, Gordon Murray, and Robert McClure.

But is it so surprising that a pioneer country should produce such an array of medical frontiersmen? After reading this book, the reader will be inclined, I think, to agree that the land—raw, forbidding, often dangerous—provided the environment in which medical genius flourished. Certainly he cannot finish Donald Jack's spritely account without knowing his own country a little better and feeling a sense of pride in the accomplishments revealed herein.

PIERRE BERTON

Foreword

by Martin M. Hoffman, M.D.

This is no dull, traditional history of Canadian medicine. Instead Donald Jack has given us a series of provocative and candid portraits of Canada's medical pioneers. Readers will be particularly fascinated by the contributions to the science and practice of medicine made by Canadian physicians and surgeons. Many will be surprised by the importance and scope of these contributions.

Medical advances are made in diverse ways. A careful hypothesis may lead to a great discovery; an observation made solely by chance or through coincidence may do the same. An example of the former is Wilder Penfield's brilliantly planned and meticulously performed experiments on the human brain that led to a better understanding of its functional organization and of the common disorder, epilepsy.

Chance, on the other hand, played an important role in what many consider Canada's greatest medical achievement, Frederick Banting's discovery of insulin in 1921. While preparing a lecture on the pancreas, Banting came across a statement in a surgical journal that provoked the idea that led to the cure for diabetes.

It is no accident, however, that *Rogues, Rebels, and Geniuses* is a thoroughly enjoyable and informative work. The author's skill in making the most opaque medical subject transparent ensures that the layperson interested in "Canada, medicine, and Canadian medicine" will read this book with pleasure. The health professional will find in it inspiration and, from the lives described, models to study and imitate.

MARTIN M. HOFFMAN, M.D., Ph.D.,
F.R.C.P.(C.), D.Sc. (Hon.)
Professor of Medicine,
University of British Columbia

Contents

Foreword by Pierre Berton vii
Foreword by Martin Hoffman, M.D. ix

1 Life Blood *1*
2 The Med School of Torture *3*
3 Perspective: From Mummies to Fathers of Science *10*
4 Botchers, Bunglers, and a Genius or Two *22*
5 "Fleglottomy" and Other Emergencies *31*
6 Perspective: From Circulation to Vaccination *39*
7 Pork, Pickles, and Pock-Marks *47*
8 Mercury and Venus *52*
9 The Tiger *59*
10 Maritime Lancets *74*
11 The Forty-Below Execution *85*
12 Forceps and Fisticuffs *94*
13 Perspective: "Oh, I'm an Angel!" *112*
14 One-Eyed MacKay and Others *126*
15 Perspective: The Bloodstained Frock Coat *137*
16 William Osler *147*
17 Osler Abroad *177*
18 A Cheeky Gynecologist *204*
19 Marooned on an Ice Pan *215*
20 The Magnetic Dr. Shepherd *236*
21 Women in Medicine? Certainly Not! *258*
22 King Murrough of Manitoba *280*
23 Two Prairie Surgeons *304*

24 And Four Psychiatrists *318*

25 The Most Famous Woman Doctor of Her Time *342*

26 Establishment Figures *352*

27 War Heroes *368*

28 A Most Unlikely Genius *380*

29 Perspective: The Inside Story *412*

30 The Specialist *423*

31 Jews Were Not Gentlemen *433*

32 The Missionary Position *442*

33 Bethune: All the Rage *464*

34 Dr. Black's Skull *481*

35 That Vicious Power in Women *487*

36 Seagull for Christmas *494*

37 Arctic Blues *509*

38 Perspective: Infection — Quest and Conquest *534*

39 Two Famous Country Doctors *550*

40 Penfield *567*

41 The Rescue Specialist *589*

42 Defiance *598*

43 The Selfish Paragon *618*

44 Blood and Sympathy *623*

Capsule Biographies 629

Notes 645

Bibliography 650

Canadian Faculties of Medicine 654

Index 655

1

Life Blood

T HIS IS THE story of Canada's contribution to the glory of the independent spirit, and to the progress of medicine, as told through the lives of its passionate, crude, roistering, neurotic, brilliant doctors.

A remarkable number of Canadian physicians and surgeons have earned international renown in their time, many of them through qualities of character and personality as well as through scientific ability, the supreme example being William Osler, acknowledged as one of the greatest of all physicians. Among their major achievements are the discovery of insulin, the equally important discoveries on cellular determination of sex, contributions to anesthesia, the work on living fascial grafts, the biological teamwork at the Connaught Laboratories, and a number of other developments from pablum to the G-suit, from the cobalt bomb to the electron microscope. It is the sum total of these and a thousand less widely-known gifts to humanity that have made Canadian medicine internationally respected. The high proportion of works by Canadians in the world's medical libraries attests to its broad and authoritative character: Wood on ophthalmology, Moseley and Harris on orthopedics, Farquharson on clinical endocrinology, Bigelow on surgical hypothermia, McCallum on malaria, Best and Taylor on physiology, Cameron on biochemistry, Rhodes and von Rooyen on virology, Rabinovitch on invertebral disc disease, Quastel on neurochemistry, Constantinides on atherosclerosis, Grant, Friedman, and Barr on anatomy.

The richness of the contribution is suggested by the fact that there is not nearly enough space, even in this fairly comprehensive national portrait gallery, for all of the exceptional medical men and women who worked in their own country, or for the many who contributed to medical science in other countries, such as bacteriologist Roy Vallum of Vancouver, orthopedic surgeon John Scott of Toronto, pediatrician Donald Paterson of Winnipeg, biochemist Earl King of British Columbia, Saskatchewan-trained biophysicist E. J. Baldes, Manitoba pathologist Frank Westbrook, Toronto microscopic anatomist R. R. Bensley, Montreal ophthalmologist Casey Wood, and Acadia University's premed graduate Charles Huggins, who received the Nobel Prize for his work on hormonal therapy in prostate cancer. But then my intention is not to compile a complete textbook of accomplishments as much as to introduce those doctors whose lives most dramatically exemplify the spirit of Canada, medicine, and Canadian medicine.

The many doctors who do appear, in their furs and shirtsleeves, bloodstained frock coats and sterilized gowns, tell an intensely personal story of triumphant response to challenge; triumphant not least because their lives affirm the supreme value of the individual ego.

2

The Med School of Torture

W HEN THEY REACHED the coast of what is now British Columbia, the European explorers encountered a medicine that showed how medicine itself had begun. Sir Francis Drake may have been one of the explorers. If so, he would certainly have come upon a medicine man, dressed, perhaps in an apron with a fringe of deer hoofs and a crown of bear claws, with a magic bone driven through his nose and a charm or rattle in his fist. Drake, that Elizabethan hero or common pirate, may even have seen the medicine man in action, seen him using psychotherapeutic measures, urging the sick patient to respond through autosuggestion, by dancing, rattling and symbolically sucking out the offending affliction through a tube. That medicine man was a shaman, and the shaman went back to prehistory.

When primitive man, shambling homeward through the forest, heard the forest moan, he did not comprehend the cause and effect of the wind in the pines. To him, it was the voice of the spirits of the forest, just as it was the sky-spirit that charged the distant hills with its javelins of light. When he paused to drink at a wayside pool, he would be careful not to lean over the still water, that he might not find himself face to face with the demon of the pool. Home, after feasting in his stone refuge, he might, abruptly engorged with desire, drive off a weaker rival with snarls and bared teeth, and seize and thrust at his momentary mate, to which she might respond with a frenzied matching drive, seeing no continuity between that connection and the birth of another helpless polytheist nine months later.

As time went by it would occur to him that disease must also be the work of a spirit, one that had to be placated or otherwise overcome, the means to which end being shamanism. So the medicine man would be dancing to an ancient choreography, as, dressed up in alarming garb, he cavorted and raved around the patient before finally eliminating the evil spirit of disease through magical cajolery and the vacuum of his mouth.

Studies by anthropologists suggest that the North American Indian came originally from northeastern Siberia. Shamans were still practicing there in 1908. An American anthropological expedition in Siberia at that time noted that, "The spirits enter into any person they may choose and force him to become their servant. Those who become shamans are usually nervous young men subject to hysterical fits..." One shaman of the Tungus tribe, the expedition noted, was sometimes incited by his spirit to slash at himself with a knife. When he was in spiritual ecstasy his wife had to keep sharp implements out of his reach. Another of this particular shaman's peculiarities was that his spirits spoke in the Koryak language, though he himself was of the Tungus tribe and could not normally understand Koryak.

The expedition also reported the claim that some of the Siberian shamans could change their sex when inspired to do so by their spirits. The leader of the expedition was somewhat skeptical about this, however, as no proof was forthcoming.

The shaman or medicine man whom Sir Francis might have encountered would be of a similarly excitable or sensitive nature, inclined to otherworldliness, or to seizures, possibly epileptic. Four centuries later, shaman candidates were just as susceptible. In 1920 a medicine man practicing at Hazelton, B.C., Isaac Tens, described his experience as a trainee shaman. He was thirty years old when, one day, he went up into the hills to gather firewood. A large owl appeared. "The owl took hold of me, caught my face, and tried to lift me up. I lost consciousness. As soon as I came back to my senses I realized that I had fallen into the snow. My head was coated with ice, and some blood was running out of my mouth."

After a subsequent trance he was advised by other shamans that the time had come for him to become a medicine man like them; but he was not willing. Later he was beset by voices, and while the medicine men were trying to fix him up again he went into another trance. "While I remained in this state, I began to sing. A chant was coming out of me without my being able to do anything to stop it. Many things appeared to me presently: huge birds and other animals.... Such visions happen when a man is about to become a halaait; they occur of their own accord. The songs force themselves out complete without any attempt to compose them. But I learned and memorized those songs by repeating them."

Isaac Tens gave up all other work and a year later he accepted his destiny and aspired to become a medicine man, or swanassu. "I had to have dreams before being able to act," he said. "This period lasted a year, in reclusion at my father's house out of touch with other folk excepting the four attendants."

"When later I attended a patient for the first time, on my own, I had a new vision. The halaait doctors were still training me, teaching me. For this reason I was invited to all the swanassu activities. As soon as I was able to go out by myself, I began to diagnose the cases by dreaming, with the help of my instructors. I acquired charms, that is, things I would dream of: the Hoqwest (snare for the bear), Hlorhs (the Moon), and Angohawtu (Sweat-house). And besides I had also dreamed of charms: the Mink...the Otter and Canoe...."

"I acquired charms when I attended a patient. I used a charm and placed it over me first, then over the body of the person from whom I was to extract the disease or illness. It was never an actual object, but only one that had appeared in a dream....Many time [a canoe] appeared to me in my dreams. The canoe sometimes was floating on the water, sometimes on the clouds. When any trouble occurred anywhere, I was able to see my canoe in visions."

His first patient was a woman whose grave illness had resisted the efforts of other medicine men. After asking for a fire to be lit: "As I began to sing over her, many people around me were hitting sticks on boards and beating skin drums for me. My canoe came to me in a dream, and there were many people sitting in it. The canoe itself was the Otter. The woman whom I was doctoring sat with the other inside this Otter canoe. By that time, about twenty other halaaits were present in the house. To them I explained what my vision was, and asked, 'What shall I do? There the woman is sitting in the canoe, and the canoe is the Otter.'

"They answered, 'Try to pull her out.'

"I told them, 'Spread the fire out, into two parts, and make a pathway between them.' I walked up and down this path four times, while the other halaaits kept singing until they were tired. Then I went over to the couch on which the sick woman was lying. There was a great upheaval in the singing and the clapping of drums and the sticks on the boards. I placed my hand on her stomach and moved round her couch, all the while trying to draw the canoe out of her. I managed to pull it up very close to the surface of her chest. I grasped it, drew it out, and put it in my own bosom. This I did."

Two days later the woman was cured and Tens earned great prestige. His fees rose to as high as ten blankets, prepaid, for each patient, though "The fees depended upon the wealth of the family calling for services, also upon the anxiety of the relatives of the sick person."

The shaman, however, had a few anxieties of his own. "Should a halaait or swanassu refuse to doctor a patient," Tens said, "he might be suspected of being himself the cause of the sickness, or of the death should it occur. In this eventuality, the relatives would seek revenge and kill the one suspected. This was the hard law of the country. But the doctors were not known to decline any invitation to serve the people in need."

The business of the canoe sounds highly mysterious to white ears, but it was the psychotherapeutic effect that counted. The patient believed as fervently in the healer as the healer did in himself. The medicine man's self-confidence was further bolstered by the knowledge that a few of the remedies in his deerskin doctor's bag were valid remedies of nature. For sore throat, staghorn sumach. For nervousness, a potion of steeped lady's slippers roots. For swollen glands, high bush cranberries and for swollen feet a poultice of cedar leaves or a mash of cow lily. For bleeding piles, white oak bark steeped and then drunk. For defective hearing, urine from a porcupine bladder dropped into the ear and stoppered with a plug. He also had his own strictly personal aids and implements, their efficacy revealed to him in a dream, or during a trance, by his personal activating spirit: special rattles, bone tubes, soul snatchers; teeth, claws, hooves, tails, and perhaps something small, furry, and alive.

There was a good deal of legitimate trickery in the art of the shaman to convince the dense crowd of relatives, rubberneckers, and the sick, that he was tuned-in to the spirit world. He could put himself into a trance, induce hypnosis or perform magic tricks. One legendary medicine man used sound effects. He "went to the chief, and... cupping his hands over the part of his body in which he felt the pain, the young halaait seemed to extract something from the chief's body, and then went under the smoke hole and blew through his cupped hand as if blowing at something. He blew it through the smoke hole. The people in the house heard something fall on the roof. Then the young halaait told one of his companions, 'Go and see what fell on the roof.' The man went and climbed up on top of the house, and then he came down and into the house to the chief who was now well. He said, 'This is what I found; it is an arrow point.'"

The shaman's art was by no means all tricks and distractions. If he conjured up an arrowhead it was in the justifiable cause of his psychological treatment. As for his ability to throw himself into a trance, it is possible that this was a pathway to genuine mystic power.

The trance ability must certainly have been a considerable asset when it came time for him to be initiated into the profession. This took place at the end of a lengthy apprenticeship. He had first to prepare a suitable habitation for his particular activating spirit (such as the Otter canoe) in order that others might be properly aware of that spirit. The habitation was his own body, which he prepared by starving himself; laying himself open to mystic experience just as the European saints prepared themselves for union with the godhead. "The first movement of the aspirant for medical honors," wrote Dr. Walkem in his book *Stories of Early British Columbia* "is to take to the woods and find some isolated lonely spot, either on some mountain top or by the waters of some lake, where his cries to his 'temenwos' will not be heard by human ears."

Dr. Walkem, however, heard the cries. "When camped on the shores of Lake Buttle some twenty years ago," he wrote in 1914, "I was awakened about two o'clock in the morning by a most plaintive wail, which struck up on my ear from a distance which, I judged, was half a mile away. The wailing continued for fully three hours. I recognized it as the plaintive appeal of the future Medicine Man to his temenwos. My companion, a young Irishman not long out from the 'ould sod' would not agree with me as to the reason or cause of the wail. He insisted that it was a 'banshee' for he had heard the same on the Lakes of Killarney, when he was a boy.... I saw the novitiate the next day. He was almost naked, but stole away into the timber as fast as possible on seeing me.

"For six weeks or more the 'would-be Shaman' wanders sadly through the mountains picking his sustenance from the berries, or edible tubers which everywhere abound. His nights are wholly consumed in the never-ending appeal to the temenwos, or to those spirits, good or evil, which may hear his distressing appeals for recognition.... Privation and lack of food no doubt reduce the Indian novitiate to a condition bordering on hysteria, and when in that condition he is liable to believe that he hears the answer to his plaintive wails for help and recognition. It is at this stage that he determines to return to the homes of his tribe. He is now dangerous—a species of demon, whose hunger must be appeased by flesh."

Just how demonic the novitiate could be was witnessed by a Hudson's Bay factor in the late nineteenth century, while on a visit to Sitka, up the Pacific coast in what was then Russian territory. The Russian governor entertained the Hudson's Bay man with typical slavic lavishness. It was just as well that the vodka flowed, for when the factor was invited to the initiation ceremony he saw a sight to churn the stomach. One of the novitiates was so crazed with hunger that the moment he saw his chance he rushed at several other Indians and attempted to eat them. He had swallowed several mouthfuls of choice flesh before he was seized by other shamans and made ready for the first stage of the ceremony. As the Hudson's Bay representative watched in horror, two sharpened skewers of bone were driven under the muscles of his back. Ropes were attached to the skewers. He was then hoisted upward by the ropes until he was suspended high overhead, his muscles threatening to tear loose at any moment. The other shamans then proceeded to swing him back and forth like a fleshly trapeze, lashing at him every time he swung within reach. Yet the initiate uttered no complaint, possibly because the enormous prestige of the shaman was sufficient compensation for the agony, or more likely because he had eliminated pain from his consciousness in much the same way as an East Indian fakir or yogi is able to do so.

Dr. Walkem was a glutton for vicarious punishment. He accepted an invitation from an Indian chief to attend another such ceremony. He found himself walking through the mouth of a bald eagle. The eagle's glittery-eyed head formed the entrance to the ceremonial chamber. "The planks on which we entered the building filled the place of the lower beak or mandible. We, therefore, came in through the bird's throat."

Inside, he noted a large square opening in the centre of the roof, and up there an arrangement of timbers and a pulley. He soon learned what this apparatus was for.

"We were shown to seats well up from the floor, but commanding a perfect view of the whole inside of the rancherie. At intervals along the front were sentinels encased in a complete suit of feathers, their figures being topped by a mask of a most perfect imitation of the bald-headed eagles, and glittering eyes as already described, as completing the eagle head entrance. I noticed that all the women of the tribe were seated well up from the ground floor, and appeared to me to wear upon their faces an aspect of anxiety, if not of fear."

Soon the Indians started to dance, accompanied by drummers, singers, and rattlers. After a while a deathly hush fell. "Then a noise, with much howling was suddenly heard proceeding from the roof. In a few moments a human body was pushed through the square hole in the roof of the rancherie. As the body dangled inside the skylight, as I will call it, I was able to see that the figure was dependent by four hooks and chains, from the pulley I have already mentioned as being at the end of the four poles, lying across the skylight. It was the body of Johnny Chiceete which was dangling in the upper air. He was hanging suspended by four hooks, one through the muscles of each upper arm, and one through the muscles of each thigh. He was completely naked, with the exception of a loincloth covering made from the inner bark of the cedar.

"His attendants of the roof lowered him slowly to the ground, then back to the roof and down again. This was repeated three times. While going up and down he shouted out some words which I took to be a species of ritual, for at every pause in his speech he was answered by the Shamans on the ground below. They kept walking up and down in line for about twenty feet and back, silent while Johnny Chiceete was speaking, and picking up the words just as Johnny ceased. No sign of Johnny's face told of the horrible torture he must have been enduring. He could not have been more quiet if he had been lowered and raised in a capacious basket.

"At the termination of the third rope, four big powerful members of his tribe rushed out and grasped him by the arms, while the hooks were kept quite taut to prevent his breaking away. Straps were round his arms to give his captors a good firm hold and command of his body. The hooks were then removed, and Johnny sprang to his feet and attempted to break away.

"Many of the audience, fearful he should escape from his captors, began to seek safer positions. Now came the most curious part of the ceremony. Ten Indians came down the circular pathway, naked to the waist. Johnny saw them and began to gnash his teeth in anticipation of a feast, for he was fearfully hungry, having arrived from the mountain a short hour before his appearance on the roof. As Johnny strained like a dog on the leash to get at the first semi-naked Siwash, he seemed more like a wild beast than a human being.

"Gradually he dragged his keepers to his first victim, the Shaman following in the rear with pieces or strips of cotton and Indian Balm. Arriving at the first man, he seized his arm, and bit a large piece out of it, and then passed on toward the next. The Shamans to our surprise called our special attention to the wound in the first man's arm, to show there was no fake about it, I suppose. Then they applied some balm or ointment, and wrapped up the whole in cotton.

"After binding up the wound in the first man's arm, a Shaman slipped a ten-dollar gold piece into the victim's hand, according, as I was afterward told by Mr. Horne, to an arrangement between the victim and Johnny Chiceete's friends. After this performance with his teeth, Mrs. Horne and Mrs. Grant retired from the building. It was too horrible for their sensitive nerves. Mr. Horne, Mr. Grant and I stayed on to see the ceremony through. Johnny completed his round with the hired victims, and just as he finished with the last, he saw a small dog near the platform which he seized with both hands and began to eat alive. He was pushed, with the dog in his hands, toward the entrance and was taken by his friends to a cabin specially prepared for him, where his hook wounds received special attention. All of those who supplied Johnny with arms to bite were rewarded in the same way as the first one was, who by the way was an Indian known to the whites as Siwash George. I only heard the names of three others. They were Three Fingered Jimmy, Saweetlum and Potato Johnny.

"If this represented the ceremony of making an Indian Medicine Man at a time when the province was well settled, what must have been the orgies in connection with the same performance before the whites came."

It is not difficult to guess the reason for such barbaric ceremonies. They were just as much a part of the shaman's training as his tuition in the nature of illness and psychology. The patients needed to feel awe in the presence of the shaman in order to help cure themselves. The shaman's final ordeal did more than anything else to create that awe.

3

Perspective:
From Mummies
to Fathers of Science

A S FOR THE medicine that the white man brought to the New World, though it had sprung from the same superstitious beginnings in prehistory, it had developed with far more power and lasting effect. White medicine had one enormous advantage over the Indian shamanism that it would soon supplant. While the Indians had been passing on their medical lore by word of mouth, their invaders had been writing it all down.

The white man's medicine was decidedly imperfect. Most of his remedies were rubbish, many of his procedures were lethal. When Jacques Cartier stepped ashore on the Labrador coast in 1534, European medicine still rested on the sand of hypothesis rather than on the rock of the experimental method. It had barely begun to solve the mysteries of nature, and its greatest triumph, the human body.

But at least the mistakes of the past had been recorded, put down on paper for others to correct. One of the most ancient samples of medical writing was an Egyptian gynecological papyrus dating back about two thousand years before Christ. Among other topics, it discussed various contraceptive methods, using such materials as honey and crocodile dung, and a preparation of glue for pouring upon the vulva. A bride's ability to conceive was determined by examining her breasts.

Another papyrus, sixty-five feet long, dealt with a great many ills that flesh is heir to. It described all kinds of blemishes, diseases, and pains, and their treatment, from baldness and glaucoma to weals and welts caused by flogging. Similarly a surgical papyrus detailed a fair number of battle wounds and how to deal with them, though the papyrus scribe blithely admitted that most of the cases were hopeless.

The Egyptians found many cases to be hopeless because there was madness in their method. Their medicine was so obsessed with magic that even when a specific treatment was repeatedly observed to produce favourable results, it was exceedingly difficult for Egyptian doctors to come to any valid conclusion, for the results were attributed to the divinities. Even their more respectable remedies, like opium and castor oil, were inextricably bound up with invocations to Re, Osiris, or Nut. So if the patient recovered, it was a Nut who got the credit. The physicians were priests first, and healers only after the deities had been satisfied. In his *Story of Medicine*, Victor Robinson remarks about the surgical papyrus that, "The text is sober, and we are about to be grateful that at last we have an Egyptian document free from demonology, but when we turn the papyrus over and look on the back, we find a magic formula for casting out the winds that carry the plagues, and the last two columns are devoted to the 'incantation of Transforming an Old Man into a Youth of Twenty.'"

The greatest difficulty that faced medical men until quite recently was the hostile attitude, official and public, to the dissection of the dead. Failing to recognize the fundamental importance of anatomy to a proper understanding of sickness and health, even the Imperial Romans were horrified at the idea of bodies being deliberately cut up. Possibly the Egyptians did not share the universal abhorrence of dissection because of their tradition of mummification. Their skill in this art was as remarkable as their pyramid engineering, though even the Egyptians seemed to have had reservations about the propriety of opening up a body. Accordingly a low caste person was employed to make the initial incision. He had to be fleet-footed as well as low class; the moment he made the first cut he was subjected to a ritual volley of stones and curses. But once the deed was done, the embalmers felt free to rinse and scoop with a will, and did so with a consummate skill that inspired Diodorus (an unreliable historian) to write that "the Egyptians, keeping the dead bodies of their ancestors in magnificent houses, so perfectly see the true visage and countenance of those that died many ages before they themselves were born, that in viewing the proportions of every one of them, and the lineaments of their faces, they take as much delight as if they were still living among them."

Herodotus, named the Father of History, provided detailed descriptions of the embalming process. In the most costly method the brain was extracted through the nostrils by means of an iron hook. The abdominal cavity was then cleaned out, rinsed and sweetened, and the viscera repacked in the cavity with binding materials. The body was then soaked in brine for seventy days, and finally coated with gum and wrapped in bandages. A cheaper method was to squirt cedar oil through the rectum, soak the body in brine for seventy days, then allow the cedar oil to flow out, bringing with it the dissolved internal organs.

Herodotus also noted that women of beauty or reputation were kept back from the embalmers until they had been dead for a few days. This rule was applied after one of the embalmers was caught tying a nuptial knot with a newly dead woman.

The ancient Greeks revered Egyptian learning, but far surpassed it in their own work. For Greece was the land of Hippocrates, whose *Oath*, giving medicine its ethical basis, is still recited on the great day when the student receives his doctorate.

Hippocrates watched and learned with a mind cleared of cant and prejudice. He struggled to understand the world as a rational place rather than as a stage for the dramatic interventions of the gods. He refuted the belief, for instance, that the epileptic was possessed by a demon. He founded clinical medicine with his detailed case-histories in the treatise, *Epidemics*. He established new rules of medical conduct. The habit of some of his colleagues of demanding their fees before attending to the patient, caused Hippocrates to wax wrathful. Far better, he said, to reproach the patient after he has been cured than to badger him while he's sick, not least because "some patients, though conscious that their condition is perilous, recover their health simply through their contentment with the goodness of the physician."

The physical appearance of the doctor would also help. "The dignity of a physician requires that he should look healthy, and as plump as nature intended him to be; for the common crowd consider those who are not of this excellent bodily condition to be unable to take care of others. Then he must be clean in person, well dressed, and anointed with sweet-smelling unguents that are not in any way suspicious."

Though Will Durant maintains that Greek medicine shows no essential advance upon the medical and surgical knowledge of Egypt, Hippocrates is still known as the Father of Medicine because he lifted medicine from the airy heights of Mount Olympus and began to rebuild it on the footings of science; founded clinical medicine, and made it work by urging rest, fresh air, proper diet, and physiotherapy on the patient, instead of the violent activity hitherto forced upon him.

Hippocrates' standards in direct observation, unfortunately, were not consistently sustained down the years. Medicine has often wandered down the one-way streets of false speculation. One brilliant but overconfident guide was Galen, who lived in the second century A.D., and whose works, rediscovered in the eleventh century, were to paralyze medicine for hundreds of years.

Galen, the first to make a serious attempt to investigate the functions of the body, was the son of an architect, who gave the boy the name Galen, which meant quiet and peaceable, in the hope "that he would take after his mother." After studying at medical schools in Celicia, Phoenicia,

Palestine, Cyprus, Crete, Greece, and Alexandria, Galen was appointed to a gladiatorial school at Pergamum on the Aegean Sea, which must have given him a fair amount of experience in surgical work. He soon evidenced a gift for healing. In order that the world might appreciate his genius as thoroughly as he did himself, he established a practice in Rome. He already had at least one friend in Imperial circles, for he had once cured the wife of a consul. Another notable case that added to his reputation involved the wife of another aristocrat. She suffered from insomnia, and her problem had baffled many physicians, until Galen succeeded in establishing the cause of her sleeplessness: she had fallen in love with a dancer name Pylades.

In Rome, Galen's fame grew to such an extent that citizens throughout the provinces were ready to accept his medical advice by mail. (Given the size of the Roman Empire his prescriptions must have arrived long after nature had cured or killed the patient.) He remained in Rome for four years, writing, teaching, and heaping scorn on his rivals, until, fearful that those rivals were about to assassinate him, he left in a hurry. The presence of a plague in the city may have spurred his retreat, for Galen was well aware that pestilence had no sense of discrimination or respect, even for such a great man as himself. He returned home to Pergamum.

A year later Galen was summoned back to Rome by the Emperor, Marcus Aurelius. One of his patients during this period was the Emperor's rude and brutish son, Commodus, who rivalled even the Claudians for beastliness. "Immersed in blood and luxury" (Gibbon), Commodus fancied himself as a premier performer in the Roman amphitheatre. Attired in helmet, sword, and buckler, he despatched a total of 735 opponents — after ensuring his own safety by arming those opponents with inferior weapons. His thirst for blood was matched by his appetite for sex. He had a brothel of three hundred beautiful women and three hundred comely boys, and had his way with quite a number of them — in quite a number of ways — every evening. He was finally poisoned by one of the ladies, and, to make sure he stayed dead, was throttled for good measure by one of his wrestlers.

Among Galen's clientele were many public men who had seen a considerable number of their friends and relatives murdered by the tyrant, so it is safe to assume that Galen learned not to brag that he had once saved Commodus' life.

Galen was a tireless historian of ancient medicine as well as being a physician of genius. He gave valid descriptions of a number of maladies. One of his more important observations was that consumption was contagious. He also invented cold cream. He made excellent contributions to anatomy, and the names he gave to certain muscles are still in use. He proved that the arteries contain blood, though for four hundred years the

Alexandrian school had taught that they were filled with air. He was the first to explain the process of respiration, and he made noteworthy contributions to neurology, describing the spinal cord and determining that it was an offshoot of the brain, the central organ of the nervous system. His practical work was of great value, and his awe at the perfection of the interacting parts of the body was to win him the praise of the Christians. "In writing these books," Galen said in one of his anatomical tomes, "I compose a true and real hymn to that awful Being who made us all."

He made mistakes, over two hundred of them in one anatomy textbook alone. He claimed that woman had two uterine cavities, one for the male fetus and the other for the female. He saw passages in the body where none existed, and failed to see many a bone that did. His greatest error, though, was in his dogmatic theorizing. "Hippocrates left medicine free, but Galen fettered it with hypotheses." He explained everything physical, philosophical, and metaphysical, and had no doubt that his work in co-ordinating all the medical knowledge of the ancients he was recording the whole truth and nothing but the truth.

When he died in 200 A.D. the creative age of Greek science died with him. The experimenters were suppressed. Magic was restored to medicine, and a fog of dogma was released that was not to lift until the revival of learning that the invention of printing helped to inspire.

Until the Renaissance, Galen's precepts were followed uncritically, so that where he had made mistakes, the mistakes were perpetuated. The situation was further complicated by the fact that his doctrines had become misshapen after undergoing Arabic, Syrian, and Hebrew translations and retranslations. At the University of Paris, the headquarters of the reactionary medical Establishment in the Middle Ages, there was no attempt to check Galen's assertions by experimentation. There was little significant practice—surgery and bedside examination were actually forbidden at the university in the thirteenth century. If a dispute arose among the scholars and dialectitions as to whether the semen of a negro was white or black, it would not occur to them to see for themselves; they would repair to an ancient source, such as Hippocrates, to see what he had to say about it. (He said it was black.)

Almost any definition of the Renaissance—the revival of learning in the fifteenth century; the combination of forces that released intelligent man from the prison of scholasticism and feudalism of the middle ages; the new, intense interest in humanity and its literature, art, and science—is dark with abstractions. The illumination is in the flaring lives of individuals, like François Rabelais, a graduate (1530) of the faculty of medicine at Montpellier. He began by publishing the usual traditional works of medical vulgarization of Galen and Hippocrates, but ended up writing *Gargantua and Pantagruel,* which expressed the reality behind the Renaissance. The world, he said, was to be enjoyed with full, rich exuberance, instincts were to be followed, not suppressed, the body was for joy, and the mind for the fullest consummation of intellectual curiosity and study.

The birth of his roisterous character Gargantua summarized the spirit of the age. "As a result of Gragamelle's discomfort, the cotyledons of the placenta of her matrix were enlarged. The child, leaping through the breech and entering the hollow vein, ascended through her diaphragm to a point above her shoulders. Here the vein divides into two; the child accordingly worked his way in a sinistral direction, to issue, finally, through the left ear.

"No sooner born, he did not, like other babes, cry: 'Whaay! Whaay!'; but in a full, loud voice bawled: 'Drink, drink, drink!' as though inviting the company to fall to. What is more, he shouted so lustily that he was heard throughout the regions of Beuxe (pronounced 'booze') and Bibarois (which in sound evokes bibblers and is how the Gascons pronounce 'Vivarais')." Rabelais does admit, though, that we might find this strange nativity a shade unbelievable, because "there is no evidence. And I reply in turn that for this very reason you should believe with perfect faith. For the gentlemen of the Sorbonne say that faith is the argument of non-evident truth."

Which of course was the kind of thinking that the men of the Renaissance were revolting against.

A major symbol of the new individualism was Paracelsus, whose life was one long uproar of aggression and controversy. Born near Zurich in 1493, he began to study medicine under his father, who was learned in all the usual occult sciences, such as astrology and alchemy. His father was affronted when Paracelsus began to bully physicians into abandoning alchemy for chemical pharmacology and therapeutics, of which he was the founder.

Coarse, quarrelsome and vulgar, Paracelsus' humour was of the kind that tended to progress, in George Moore's words, "from the obscene into the incomprehensible." His appearance, particularly his face, angry-eyed and contemptuous of mouth, did not endear him to his colleagues. With his patients, though, he was humane and deeply concerned. Travelling widely throughout Germany, often in the company of gypsies, midwives, executioners, and other riff-raff, his record of cures was varied and exceptional. He restored a soldier shot in the chest by an arrow, a girl who had eaten stones and chalk, an epileptic, a victim of a snake bite, a syphilitic, an impotent, and hosts of people suffering from every conceivable type of disease. His fame brought him an invitation to teach at the university at Basel, where he amazed the students and faculty by instructing them, not in highflown Latin but in vigorous common German, hitherto a language considered fit only for ordering harlots to haul up their skirts.

Worse was to follow. His footloose practice had convinced him that much of the theoretical science he had been taught was garbage. In the lecture hall he had at his elbow some of the best medical works of antiquity. He proceeded to stoke up a brazier, and dump the sacred books into it, shouting that his shoebuckles had more sense than Galen.

Some of his own writings were also rubbish, adulterated as they were with much of the occultism he despised, and with all kinds of obscurities and mystic dross. But gleaming through them were many remarkable insights and reflections of original thought. He had valuable comments to make on open wounds and the value of mineral baths, on syphilis and cretinism, and he was one of the first to write on occupational diseases.

He died as violently as he had lived, in a tavern brawl, his swagger and courage undimmed, but with his physique flayed by self-indulgence in the low company he preferred, and a mind maddened with frustration over his inability to fully understand the human body.

Though not a doctor, Leonardo da Vinci was another great contributor to the Renaissance, through his anatomical sketches, which, astonishingly, were made with the actual dissected subjects as a model.

Described by William Hunter as, "the greatest anatomist of his epoch," da Vinci epitomized the changing attitudes of the time. At first he believed as intensely in Galen as everybody else; but the more he advanced in an understanding of anatomy and physiology, the further he resisted the medievalist inertia. "They scorn me who am a discover," he wrote, "but how much more do they deserve censure who have never found out anything, but only recite and blazon forth other people's works. Those who study only old authors and not the works of Nature are stepsons, not sons of Nature."

Leonardo was among the first to draw the human skeleton as it really is. His studies in a Roman hospital (until the Pope ordered him out of the hospital as a heretical and cynical dismemberer), resulted in masterly drawings on the dynamics and inner workings of the body. They were a revelation even to the professional anatomists, including Mundinus, one of the doctors of the time who had actually dissected a body or two.

The anatomy taught in the medical schools was still influenced by Galen. A picture of Mundinus, published when Leonardo was forty-one, sums up the instruction methods of the day. It shows Mundinus, seated in an imposing chair, teaching anatomy from a Galenical textbook which reposes in his lap. The actual demonstrating is being done by an assistant, who is shown to be pawing somewhat squeamishly at the viscera of the subject on the morgue table, using his bare hands—or possibly her bare hands—Mundinus' assistant may have been a girl named Alessandra Gilliani.

Meanwhile, the medical students looked on passively, without trying their own hands at dissection. As Victor Robinson puts it, "The advantage of this method is that it saved the student's fingers from contact with cadaveric material, and the disadvantage is that the student did not learn any anatomy."

It was scenes such as this that caused the great Vesalius (1514-64) to snarl with impatience. On one occasion he became so annoyed at the ineptitude of the demonstrator that, seizing the knife, he performed the dissection himself.

Though there is some controversy as to the real merits of Vesalius, he is certainly the most commanding figure in European medicine between Galen and Harvey, the discoverer of the circulation of the blood. Vesalius was said to have dethroned Galen and turned anatomy into a working science, making dissection very nearly respectable.

Vesalius' career has been described as one of the most romantic in medical history. He was born in 1514 in Flanders, five years before Leonardo da Vinci died. At first, like so many other great medical men of the time, Vesalius was an entirely conventional follower of Galen. He could hardly have been anything else, for he was taught at the University of Paris, the principal stronghold of Galenism. What little dissection was done there was mostly performed on animals. He received his degree in Padua and began lecturing there at the age of twenty-three. His enthusiasm for dissection was quickly transmitted to his students. Vesalius was no passive pedant, lording it on a throne with textbook in one hand and, in the other, a wand for pointing out the various features, while somebody else did the dirty work. He did his own cutting, sawing, and teasing, and his audience rapidly increased, marveling at his skill. The most perceptive among them noted with wonderment that the name of Galen was mentioned with less and less frequency, and more and more disrespect.

Convinced that he was now competent to write a book on anatomy, Vesalius had first to ensure that it would be properly illustrated. He set about luring Titian's favorite artist, John Stephen, into the mortuary, to make the drawings. Vesalius had considerable difficulty in persuading Stephen, for mortuaries were not considered fit places for artists, who were used to drawing and painting from life. Preservative fluids were not used and viscera decayed rapidly. While supervising the dissection of one female body, even Mundinus could tolerate the smell only for the time it took to deliver four lectures. Nevertheless the artist was prevailed upon to undergo the ordeal, and in due course the wood blocks cut from Stephen's designs went to the printer in Basel. There Vesalius spent six months supervising both the printing of the blocks and his monumental text.

Printing, then only a hundred years old, was still a laborious process. The most remarkable of the illustrations are the ones showing the muscles, layer by layer, the standing figures being presented against an attractive landscape, perhaps in the hope that this would help to soften the contemporary prejudice against dissection.

In 1543, this work that was to overthrow Galen was published. Though Vesalius had been lecturing for five years with decreasing reference to Galen's precepts, nonetheless the work caused a sensation. Like many pioneer medical works, it also produced an uproar of disbelief, derision, and abuse. Sylvius, the best of his teachers, turned on him with bitter fury. Sylvius refused to believe that the great Galen could be wrong in even a single detail. Galen, for instance, had laid down that an intermaxillary bone existed. Vesalius could not find it, and said so. When he challenged Sylvius to find it and point it out, Sylvius blustered, "Man had this bone when Galen lived. If he has it no longer, it is because sensuality and luxury have deprived him of it." Presumably nobody dared to ask Sylvius how the bone had managed to survive all that Roman sensuality and luxury long enough for Galen to have discovered it in the first place.

The authorities, too, joined in the condemnation of Vesalius. He was subjected to considerable persecution. Vesalius, shown in a contemporary portrait as a man with a somewhat arrogant set to the lips and a gaze not particularly tolerant, was so enraged that he destroyed his manuscripts and left Padua forever.

The treatise that had caused the sensation, *The Fabric of the Human Body (de Fabrica Humani Corporis)* reconstructed the knowledge of man. As summarized by Victor Robinson: "Galen believed there was no marrow in the bones of the hand; he believed that during parturition there is a separation of the bones of the symphysis; he believed that the inferior maxilla consists of two pieces; he believed that the ascending vena cava arose from the liver; Vesalius proved that in each instance Galen was incorrect. Vesalius showed that Galen was wrong when he assumed the existence of a general muscle of the skin, an imputrescible bone of the heart, the ox intermaxillare in adults, a decided curvature to the bones of the thigh and the upper arm. Before Vesalius finished with the Prince of Physicians, he demonstrated and corrected over two hundred Galenian errors.... Pre-Vesalian anatomy is antiquated anatomy; Vesalian anatomy is modern anatomy."

In history, no account should be accepted as being wholly reliable. History's raw material, the facts, or what are thought to be the facts, are perceived through the colour-filter of the historian's eye. In the story of Vesalius, though some writers view him with admiration, others do so with scorn. One source characterized Vesalius as being energetic, ambitious but ignorant. "To these he added the further useful and stimulating qualities of a consuming jealousy of other men and their knowledges, an unflagging exhibitionism, a shameless boastfulness, a torrential and incomprehensible vocabulary, and a most insensitive attitude towards the truth." The modern researcher, W. M. Ivins, Jr., goes on to say that many among Vesalius' contemporaries made contributions to knowledge that were no whit inferior to those credited to Vesalius, but rather that the *Fabrica* "was a normal step in an evolution that had been under way for many years...."

Certainly Vesalius' life after he left Padua was hardly as rich in accomplishment as the portrayal of his character by loyal Vesalians would lead one to expect. He became a physician to the Spanish court, and "laboured faithfully on the gouty toe of Charles V." He developed a skill in foppish manners and empty chatter. Though dissection was not permitted in Spain, it seems doubtful that he cared whether it was or not, though at one point he did complain that he could not get his hands on so much as a dried skull.

Perhaps it was the success of one of his pupils, Fallopius, that finally forced Vesalius to face up to his wasted years of obsequious mummery at the court of the Emperor. When he received a copy of Fallopius' *Observations on Anatomy* in 1561, Vesalius read of discoveries about which he knew nothing. Fallopius, who gave his name to the oviducts (Fallopian tubes), made things even worse by correcting errors that Vesalius had made. Fallopius, a generous man whose praise of Vesalius was unstinting, received a vicious response from his master. In his last book Vesalius attacked Fallopius—on the grounds that his anatomical observations were not according to the teaching of Galen.

There is no evidence that Vesalius made any attempt to check Fallopius' discoveries by returning to the dissecting table.

His end was no more dignified than his years at court. He set out on a pilgrimage to Jerusalem, possibly in order to get away from the Imperial hothouse, but just as possibly because of the terrible penalty he paid for denying the profession that had given him such fame. One day in Spain, he was asked to perform an autopsy on a nobleman, whom he had pronounced dead; but when he opened the chest he found that the heart was still beating. The pilgrimage to Jersualem may have been a penance, or an escape from the Inquisition. He died in 1564, alone and friendless, on the island of Zante.

William M. Ivins, Jr. ascribes much of Vesalius' fame to the handsome appearance of the *Fabrica,* and speculates that had it been a small book, badly printed and illustrated in humdrum fashion, it would now have earned a heroic reputation for its author. This conjecture, however, is put in doubt by the appearance, eighty-five years after the publication of the *Fabrica*, of a work that was indeed small, meanly printed, and inadequately illustrated, but which marked the most momentous event in medical history. It was William Harvey's *Anatomical Exercise on the Motion of the Heart and Blood in Animals*.

Harvey had also attended the University at Padua, and had studied under Fabricius, a pupil of Fallopius. He returned to England in 1602, the year that *Hamlet* was published. Though he announced his discovery as early as 1616, he held on to his proof for another dozen years before finally handing it over to a Frankfurt printer. He did so with some trepidation, for he was well aware that Galen, whom he was contradicting, was still worshipped. Harvey knew that his demonstrations as to how the blood circulated in the human body were likely to earn him rage and outrage. "Galen's false concept about the pores in the ventricular septum diverted all speculation into the wrong channel for fourteen centuries," wrote Fielding Garrison. "In the drawings which Vesalius had made, indicating the close proximity of the terminal twigs of arteries and veins, the truth about the circulation was literally staring in the face of any observer who had eyes to see or wit to discover it. Yet anatomists continued to see everything in the light of Galenical prepossessions.... But Harvey, who knew the whole history and literature on the subject, first made a careful review of existing theories, showing their inadequacy, and then proceeded, by vivisection, ligation, and perfusion, to an inductive proof that the heart acts as a muscular force-pump in propelling the blood along, and that the blood's motion is continual, continuous, and in a cycle or circle."

In his 1628 work, Harvey gives some idea of the problems that faced him. "When I first gave my mind to vivisections, as a means of discovering the motions and uses of the heart, and sought to discover these from actual inspection, and not from the writings of others," he wrote, "I found the task so truly arduous, so full of difficulties, that I was almost tempted to think, with Frascatorius, that the motion of the heart was only to be comprehended by God. For I could neither rightly perceive at first when the systole and when the diastole took place, nor when and where dilation and contraction occurred, by reason of the rapidity of the motion, which in many animals is accomplished in the twinkling of an eye, coming and going like a flash of lightning; so that the systole presented itself to me now from this point, now from that; the diastole the same; and then everything was reversed, the motions occurring, as it seemed, variously and confusedly together."

For year after year, he had dissected or vivisected over eighty species of animal, accumulating facts that could be demonstrated, instead of theories based on beautiful imagination; and all the facts pointed in one direction. No matter what others said, the only possible way that the blood could flow was in a circuit, and *not* in an ebb and flow manner. It went from heart to arteries, from arteries to veins, veins to heart, heart to lungs, lungs to heart, and heart to arteries, and so on, and on, and on. A staggering discovery.

As a person, Harvey was so preoccupied with his work that he appears to have been totally indifferent to the colourful and riotous times in which he lived: to the vulgar, brawling first performances of Shakespeare's greatest plays, John Bull's music, or the intrigues of his friend Francis Bacon. He was not even interested in Cromwell's Civil War. There is no mention of his wife in his writings, except in connection with her pet parrot — and then only because he dissected the parrot. When his lodgings in Whitehall were broken into and all his furniture, museum specimens, and much of his paperwork, including his writings on insects, were stolen, the most he could manage was to "give vent to a sigh." When he visited a witch, he was more interested in her toad than in her supernatural abilities. (He also dissected the toad, to prove that it had no magical powers, and "in no way differed from other toades.")

Harvey's manner was so distant that it took even that ebullient diarist, John Aubrey, half a lifetime to summon up the courage to approach him. Harvey was then seventy-three. Aubrey thought he might have mellowed by then. Were it not for Aubrey's joyous gossip, we would have had to rely for an idea of Harvey's appearance on the impatient portraits of him. According to Aubrey, "He was not tall; but of the lowest stature, round faced, olivaster complexion; little eye, round, very black, full of spirit; his hair was black as a raven, but quite white 20 years before he died." And: "He was, as all the rest of the brothers, very choleric; and in his young days wore a dagger…this Dr. would be apt to draw out his dagger upon every slight occasion." Aubrey also wrote that, "For 20 years before he died he took no manner of care about his worldly concerns, but his brother Eliab, who was a very wise and prudent manager, ordered all not only faithfully, but better than he could have done himself."

This, then, was the rough state of medical knowledge as it was brought to Acadia and Quebec by the European explorers: contained in a script four thousand years long, crudely expressed, scientifically primitive, but striving for the truth that was beginning to be revealed through the experimental methods of Harvey.

It was while Harvey was just beginning to suspect that the heart might be a pump in a sanguinary circuit, that Champlain was founding the first permanent colony in the land that would be Canada.

4

Botchers,
Bunglers,
and a Genius or Two

Among the first Indians that Jacques Cartier met at Quebec in 1535 were three medicine men who became thoroughly agitated when they learned that he proposed to sail further up the St. Lawrence toward Hochelaga-Montreal. The medicine men, wrapped in the skins of black and white dogs, "their faces besmeared as black as any coals, with horns on their heads more than a yard long," danced and wailed and frothed forth warnings that the spirits would surely strike the white men dead if they ventured any farther.

With the lamentations and incantations of the medicine men fading into the oppressive silence of the seemingly endless forests, Cartier sailed onward up the narrowing river, watchful for hostile signals. His uneasiness was quickly dispelled by the warmth of the reception he received from the Indians he found camped below Mount Royal. Their chief, Agouhanna, welcomed Cartier personally, though he had to be brought forward on a litter, for his arms and legs were paralyzed. Impressed by the white chief's appearance—Cartier, a stocky man in his early forties, with a broad brow and direct, fearless eyes, had the aura of power and self-confidence of a born leader—Agouhanna asked Cartier to treat him. Responding with a confidence he probably did not feel, Cartier, the continent's first white physiotherapist, massaged the chief's limbs. The chief paid handsomely for the treatment in real estate. Appropriately enough, part of his gift of land is now the site of McGill University and its famed medical school.

On his return to the camp at Cap Rouge, Cartier was alarmed to find that scurvy, the ugliest name ever invented for a disease, had broken out.

Scurvy was caused by a shortage of vitamin C. The body cannot store that vitamin in quantity; consequently a low vitamin-C diet soon brings on a deficiency that can cause hideous effects. At the time there was no understanding of vitamins and their significance. But at least Cartier made an effort. He ordered an autopsy on one young victim among his crew in the hope that the morbid changes noted would provide information as to the nature of the disease and inspire his medical staff to work out a cure.

A barber-surgeon, or possibly an apothecary, performed the autopsy, with Cartier observing. "They found the heart to be all white and withered, surrounded by more than a pitcher of water as large as a spleen. The liver was fine but the lungs were black and mortified.... They made an incision in his thigh which was quite black on the outside but inside the flesh was found to be normal enough."

The sight of the dreadful lesions, however, failed to inspire the medicine men with anything other than apprehension that their own insides might soon look like that. Unless, of course, the Indians killed them first. So Cartier was forced to fall back on the white man's magic of prayer and psalm-singing. He placed an image of the Virgin Mary in a tree near the fort and ordered his men to attend a mass on that site. His men continued to die, of scurvy at the rate of more than one a week.

One bitterly cold winter's day while he was out walking, Cartier caught sight of an Indian named Damagaya who, only two weeks previously, had been suffering so badly from scurvy that his knees were swollen "as big as the body of a two-year-old child." Cartier stopped and stared. Damagaya not only appeared to be cured but to be in unusually good health. He was striding purposely over the ice on the river, taunting the intense cold in a thin sealskin coat and leggings.

When Cartier questioned him, the Indian replied that he had cured himself by drinking an old Indian remedy and then using the dregs as a poultice for the inflammation and swelling of his limbs.

Cartier was seriously alarmed by his casualty list. This was his first winter in Canada. He had started out from France with 112 men in three ships. Now, eight months later, he had barely enough men left to crew two of the vessels. His force was so depleted that he was in danger of being overwhelmed by the natives who were now beginning to realize that the white visitors were not merely tourists but might one day attempt to settle permanently in their territory. The hostility of the Indians was such that Cartier already felt compelled to bury his scurvy victims under the snow in the dead of night so that the Indians would not realize how grave the situation was.

A few months before, Cartier would probably have dismissed the remedy as just another example of aboriginal hocus-pocus. Now he was desperate enough to try anything. Learning that the potion had been brewed from the twigs and bark of a tree called "Annedda"—white spruce or hemlock—he tried it out on his own men. Within weeks the scourge had been eliminated from both the ships and his shore establishment.

It must now have occurred to Cartier that Indian medicine was not entirely a matter of conjuring tricks and frantic incantations. There was more to their culture than he had suspected. The odorous oils and fats with which they smeared their bodies certainly seemed to help them withstand the heat, the cold, and the mosquitos. And was it possible that the long Indian hair was befouled with other greasy concoctions because it helped to shed the rain, or perhaps even to help them lubricate their way more smoothly through the tangled forest while hunting game? Many Indian practices made quite a lot of sense—their resuscitation methods, for instance. Spending much of their time on the water, in frail canoes, near-drowning was a not uncommon occurrence. To revive a victim the Indians suspended him from a tree. Next, an animal gut was filled with tobacco smoke, which was then blown into the patient's lungs. If the rescuers were not too late, his violent coughing helped to bring up the water, and restore normal breathing.

The Indian sweat bath was not to be despised, either. To treat a fever, the patient sat in an enclosed space while his friends threw water over hot stones to produce a steam. The steam caused copious sweating. The bather then jumped into the river to cool off.

Childbirth was equally hygienic. The Indian woman delivered the baby while squatting on her knees or on hands and knees, and was revived afterwards with a decoction made of leaves of yellow ash. The baby was washed and given fish oil or animal tallow, and from then on, received mother's milk. There was room for improvement, though, in the way the child was carried on the squaw's back, with the feet dangling and set close together. That position tended to dislocate the baby's hips.

In many respects, Indian medicine was as effective as the white system, but it was to break down after prolonged contact with the white men and his unfamiliar afflictions. The Indians were used to medical problems associated with a hard and dangerous outdoor life, and had little resistance to the new imports: measles, typhoid, typhus, diphtheria, and yellow fever. (Some historians claim that the Europeans also introduced venereal disease to the Indians, but apparently there is some doubt about this. Fallopius, among others, maintained that syphilis was imported by the Spaniards from America. Certainly an epidemic of the disease, which had not been clearly defined in Europe until then, broke out in Italy and France not long after the return of Christopher Columbus' expedition.)

An example of how the Indian system of medicine broke down was their response to smallpox, the most dreadful of the scourges. The Indians applied the sweat bath method in an attempt to overcome it. Unfortunately, sweating a smallpox victim and then shocking him with icy water was just about the worst treatment possible. It merely hastened the patient's demise.

Smallpox, introduced and reintroduced by shiploads of immigrants, caused as much anguish among the white settlers, and were to keep the doctors and nurses desperately busy for over two centuries. Bonnerme, Quebec's first surgeon, lasted only one year before being carried off by the disease. Casualties among the nursing sisters were particularly heavy. It was fortunate for the colonists that they had the advantage of the French tradition in nursing rather the English. In the very year that Jacques Cartier sailed for Canada, Henry VIII, in defying Rome, was suppressing the Catholic sisterhoods that had served the London hospitals so devotedly. As a result, English nursing fell into a dismal state of neglect and incompetence and was not to recover for three centuries, until Florence Nightingale illuminated the scene. But French nursing maintained its traditions, and the colonists of New France benefited from the intense missionary zeal that the nursing sisters brought to Canada and to its first hospital, the Hôtel-Dieu.

The first physician at the Hôtel-Dieu (four rooms, two closets, beds made out of tree branches) was Robert Giffard, who came to Quebec in 1627 as a barber-surgeon. Maude Abbott explained in her *History of Medicine in Quebec* that, "The curious custom then in vogue of combining the two offices of barber and surgeon in one person was probably due to the practically universal employment of *bleeding* as a panacea for almost every ill, and that the performance of this operation was thought to require no other knowledge than how to sharpen a knife and the proper location for the incision into one of the great veins." (The barber pole was a symbol of the barber-surgeon of those days, the red stripe representing the bloody wound and the white stripe the bandage enwrapping it.)

There is not much evidence as to Giffard's skill as a doctor, though he is mentioned frequently in church records as delivering Indian infants and baptizing children. However, there is plenty of evidence of his enthusiasm for the pioneer life. His was a spirit undaunted by danger. While returning from a trip home, he was captured by the English in the Gulf of St. Lawrence, but was put ashore at St. Pierre. The Basques living there, having no use for him either, promised to kill him within the hour if he did not leave immediately. Fortunately they made this possible by providing him with a small boat and a few biscuits. A couple of days later, after some hard rowing, he was picked up by a French ship and found himself back where he had started, in France.

Giffard seems to have contributed more to the colonizing of the new land than to medicine. What with the threat of famine, not to mention the murderous Iroquois, he probably had his priorities right. It was not much good curing people of typhus if there was nothing for them to eat afterwards. Nor did he wish to suffer the fate of such colleagues as René Goupil, a young man of singular beauty, who was tortured for six weeks by the Iroquois before being finally, mercifully, despatched with a tomahawk. So as well as tilling the soil, sowing corn, and transplanting vines, Robert Giffard ensured the survival of himself and his people by putting up secure quarters, a manor-house at Beauport. Within three years of bringing his family over from France, his success as a farmer enabled him to support twenty people on his produce, a more important contribution to the colony than his surgical skills.

Even so, ten years later the population of New France still numbered only two or three hundred persons. It was in the second half of the seventeenth century that tides of immigrants began to sweep onto the Royal shores. Not a few of them were barber-surgeons, apothecaries, midwives, quacks, and even a few qualified physicians—among whom was the first major Canadian contributor to medical and allied sciences, Michel Sarrazin.

From the moment he stepped ashore in New France, Sarrazin was so swamped with work that though he had every intention of marrying, he was fifty years old before he had an opportunity to do so. He even arrived with a boatload of patients, for his ship imported not only colonists but an epidemic. Sarrazin's work among the sufferers rapidly earned him an appointment as surgeon-major to the French troops in Canada. This in turn provided him with some much-needed experience in surgical work, such as removing Indian arrow heads and probing the wounds of officers who had duelled not wisely but too well.

He must also have assisted in caring for the wounded during the Siege of Quebec in 1690. Under Frontenac, the governor, the French had been making damaging attacks on the New England colonists. In revenge the colonists riposted with Sir William Phips. Phips, an early example of the American dream, having started out as a penniless Maine fisherman and worked his way up to early fame and fortune, was given command of a fleet of thirty-five ships, with orders to seize Quebec. For a few days he caused some apprehension among the defenders. At the Hôtel-Dieu, the nursing sisters were ordered to abandon the hospital, though Frontenac later countermanded the order.

The sisters willingly remained, though Phips lobbed a total of thirty-six cannon balls into the hospital. But the ladies had gone through far worse experiences than a mere bombardment, which ended soon enough anyway when Phips lost heart, abandoned the siege, and sailed for home, morosely practicing carpentry.

Three years later, Sarrazin became official physician to the Hôtel-Dieu, where his skill and efficiency earned him the approval of the sisters, who had hitherto not been too impressed with the quality of the doctors they had worked with.

Sarrazin did not greatly admire his own competence, though. Frustrated by a lack of basic medical knowledge, he resigned his official posts and went back to France to study at Rheims. After six or seven years of practice in Canada he had no difficulty in obtaining his M.D. On his return from Rheims, once again he found himself in the midst of a severe epidemic of typhus—a disease encouraged by cold, damp, poor food, and worse sanitation. A similar epidemic a dozen years previously had killed more than eight hundred colonists and immigrants. This time, nearly all the victims who packed the wards and corridors of the Hôtel-Dieu recovered. This extraordinary success was credited to Sarrazin's skill and dedication.

There are no details as to how he accomplished this, but we can guess. In France, Sarrazin must have been electrified by the changes in medical thought inspired by Harvey, Thomas Sydenham, and others. Sydenham was one of the new clinicians, a clinician being one involved in the direct observation of the patient. A new clinician really looked at the patient, clearly and objectively, instead of appearing at the bedside arm in arm with preconceived ideas. Sarrazin, given his character and professionalism, must have absorbed the new clinical ideas and applied them to his typhus patients, and, his mind enriched by new principles in physiology and pathology, applied them effectively.

After his triumph over the epidemic, Sarrazin became the most famous man in the colony, and was besieged by patients and colleagues alike, for treatment and consultations. Within months he had a practice extending from Three Rivers to Montreal.

Sarrazin was apparently just as successful in general medicine. In dealing with pleurisy, for instance, he combined the Indian sweat bath method with blood letting, with remarkably good results. His work in botany and zoology was said to be outstanding. His dissection of the beaver provided the original anatomical knowledge of this animal. He tried to do the same for the skunk, but though accustomed to the miasma of the charnel-house, the odour of the skunk was too much for him.

Sarrazin's botanical work was outstanding. He catalogued two hundred native plants and detailed their pharmaceutical properties, and how the Indians used them to sweat their patients, or to vomit or purge them of impurity. He also received the credit for the industrialization of maple sugar. Maude Abbott noted that as a member of the *Conseil Supérieur*, Sarrazin was asked to look into the question of harvesting and sowing grain. She went on to quote an eighteenth-century Swedish botanist: "Dr. Sarrazin had procured in Sweden a small quantity of winter wheat and barley. This was sown by him in autumn, passed the winter without damage, and produced fine wheat the following summer, with grains a little smaller than the wheat of Canada, but this winter grain gave a larger amount of fine flour than the summer wheat. I have never been able to understand why this experiment was not continued.'" Maude Abbott added that "In view of the modern transformation in the harvest acreage of Canada through the introduction of wheat adapted to a short summer, this practical application at that date of Sarrazin's scientific intelligence is truly astounding."

At fifty, Sarrazin married a young lady of rank, who owned considerable property in the Gaspé area. It was a union which simultaneously raised him still higher in influence and prestige, and diverted him onto the beaten path to ruin. He had arrived in the country almost penniless, and had risen to become King's physician and a major property owner, but his attempt to exploit the Gaspé property for its valuable slate ultimately wiped him out. He was almost poverty-stricken by the time he died in 1734, after being infected by one of his patients in the Hôtel-Dieu. According to a contemporary source, his "unparalleled devotion for every class of patient rendered him able to perform with joy and grace all that lay in his power for the relief of the sick under his care."

Sarrazin had the further distinction of being fully qualified for the job. A few other doctors were licenced to practice, such as Tim Sullivan (known to the French as Timothée Sylvain) who passed an examination in front of Sarrazin before being allowed to practice in Montreal; but not only were most practitioners earning a living without official permission, they had little or no grounding in the art. Some of them could not even read or write.

The Mother Superior of the Hôtel-Dieu thus had some difficulty in replacing Sarrazin. She complained that the average surgeon could hardly do more than apply dressings. Often the parish priests knew more than the country practitioners. One of them, Father Boispineau, became so knowledgeable that even Sarrazin consulted him. But generally, even many years after Sarrazin's death, the Quebec countryside was infested with ambitious bunglers and botchers. Which was hardly surprising, as there was no formal medical teaching in the country, and no real attempt to enforce professional standards. The authorities were strict enough though, with practitioners who made mistakes in other fields, such as the local currency. While the death of a patient through a doctor's incompetence might earn barely a shrug from the authorities, the doctor as forger was another matter. He could be condemned to death for such a crime. A general pratitioner, Jean Lacoste, who counterfeited a five *livre* bill, worth about a dollar, escaped the ultimate penalty, but "was condemned to be conducted naked through the town of Ville Marie, lashed at its four corners, branded on the face and then despatched by the first ship sailing for France to serve there as a galley slave for life."

While conditions in New France were not exactly those of sybaritic ease, outside the boundaries they were growing dangerous. Since the beginning of the century, relations between the French and English in North America had been steadily deteriorating. Sir William Phips' attack on Quebec had been only one episode in a series of skirmishes, ambushes, massacres, and outright battles between the nations. In June 1759 the decisive confrontation began when James Wolfe arrived off the French bastion with his fleet and a force of 8,500 men.

Wolfe was such a distinctly odd person that even before he set out for Quebec Prime Minister Pitt had begun to wonder if he had backed the right man, especially after he had entertained Wolfe at dinner. During the meal the youthful general, who looked like a red-haired rat, stood up and marched round the table, waving his sword and uttering extravagant boasts and generally exercising his legs, his extreme vanity, and his egomania. Well aware that the decision at Quebec was likely to be most momentous, Pitt was appalled. "Good God," he said to another guest, Lord Temple. "That I should have entrusted the fate of the country and of the Administration to such hands."

He must have been even more anxious when September arrived and the enemy citadel had hardly been dented. Wolfe had achieved a few hits on the Hôtel-Dieu, but instead of fuming outside the hospital he ought to have been inside it. Never very strong, and suffering from lifelong rheumatism and occasional attacks of scurvy, after three months of bankrupt tactics he had become deathly sick. The medicines he was dosing himself with did not help. One of his potions was composed of the ingredients of soap, which did nothing to clean up his diseased kidneys and bladder. On August 19 he was so ill he could not rise from his bed, but he would not give in. He insisted that his surgeon bleed and drug him to his feet.

Though a redoubtable general and recklessly brave, it was luck, perhaps, that enabled Wolfe to surmount the cliffs along the St. Lawrence that had stultified so many attacks in the past. Or perhaps treachery. Certain high officials in Quebec, including François Bigot, may have deliberately weakened the defences at a critical point two kilometres above the citadel, in the hope that an English take-over would cover up their corruption. Bigot's exploitations for the sake of a fast *livre* had extended even to medicine. Nine years previously he had passed a bill making it compulsory for those who wished to practice medicine to undergo an examination before the King's physician — then he extorted bribes in return for the Letters Patent.

In any event, Wolfe seized the opportunity, and by the time Montcalm, the French commander, who had commandeered Dr. Robert Giffard's manor-house at Beauport as his headquarters, arrived on the Plains of Abraham in front of Quebec, the British thin red lines were already ruled across the bright green grass, ready for the kind of set-piece battle that they usually won by sheer brainless fortitude. Wolfe, in the forefront of the battle that followed, was mortally wounded, as was a defeated Montcalm. Thus the operation was successful, but the generals died, and the Bourbon flag was lowered for the last time from its mast in the citadel, signaling the beginning of the end of French rule on the North American continent.

5

"Fleglottomy" and Other Emergencies

THE EARLIEST INHABITANTS of English Canada, huddled in settlements mashed between endless forests and seemingly sourceless rivers, or lakes like inland seas, depended for medical support on British army or navy surgeons. One of the first of the army surgeons was an unlucky man by the name of James Connor, who had served under the equally unfortunate Gentleman Johnny Burgoyne. Burgoyne was the charming general who brilliantly defeated the American revolutionaries on paper, and couldn't understand it when they won the actual battle, at Saratoga. The swine had failed to dispose themselves in accordance with Burgoyne's battle plans.

After his demobilization, Dr. Connor suffered a long illness that reduced his family to poverty, and ultimately led to his arrest as a debtor. He made a desperate appeal to the authorities in Quebec to be forgiven his dastardly crime of ill luck. The appeal was successful, and he managed to establish a new practice in the Kingston area. There he continued not to prosper, though his knife work was competent enough. He is said to have carried out the first civilian operation in the province, successfully excising a settler's neck tumour.

Just as he had great difficulty in overcoming his own misfortunes, his intercession on behalf of others was equally unlucky. In 1788 he appeared at a trial held at Finkle's Tavern in Ernesttown, to speak up for a settler who had been accused of stealing a watch. The accused maintained that he had bought the watch off a pedlar, but as the pedlar could not be found, Dr. Connor's appeal for mercy was ignored. He was hissed down, and the accused was strung up. Subsequently the pedlar reappeared, and corroborated the man's story.

Thus Canada's first hanging also turned out to be its first major miscarriage of justice.

Just as the American Revolution helped to unite Quebec by supplying its French and English citizens with a common enemy, it also helped to populate Upper Canada. The rush of United Empire Loyalists fleeing from democracy brought not only a large number of badly needed colonists to this frontier but a proportional number of private practitioners, some of them quite competent. Further, as living conditions improved, a few physicians from the mother country ventured to risk the frontier life.

The quality of some of these medical men can be judged from the pen portraits of William Canniff in his *The Medical Profession in Upper Canada, 1793-1850.* Among them were Dr. Pitkin Gross, a genial, kind-hearted man and a bold surgeon, who must have left the United States in something of a hurry, for he settled in Brighton, on Lake Ontario, with but one instrument, a lancet.

Gradually Dr. Gross built up a tool-chest of home-made instruments. "On one occasion a lumberman...met with an accident and gangrene resulted within the abdomen, Dr. Gross made an incision and removed a portion of the omentum, washed out the cavity and the patient got well. Finally the patient ran away to escape paying his bill. On another occasion he had been called some distance to see a patient, and while absent a messenger over took him to secure his services to see a man still further away, who had met with an accident. Dr. Gross proceeded on his way with as much speed as the path through the woods and a jaded horse would allow. Having reached the log-house of his patient, he found the nature of the injury to the man was such that, to save his life, amputation of the thigh was immediately necessary. He had positively nothing with him either to amputate, to arrest the haemorrhage, or unite the flaps. But his skill, courage and ingenuity were equal to the occasion, and the man's life was saved. He obtained a portion of a scythe or sickle, to which, by means of a thumbscrew—however he got it—manufactured a tourniquet, and made a hook to take up the arteries; finally with a darning needle and linen thread he prepared to stitch the flaps. Having completed his arrangements—which took twenty-four hours—he, with scarcely any assistance, accomplished the operation. The instruments made to meet a pressing emergency, were afterwards repeatedly employed to perform surgical operations."

Two decades later GPs were still improvising. While on a fishing expedition up the Ottawa River, Dr. James Richardson met a French-speaking Canadian who was in agonies through retention of urine.

Naturally the doctor had no surgical instruments on him, but after searching around for something that could be used as a catheter for drawing off the urine, he found a goose's wing which was being used for dusting. Richardson cut the quills of the wing into sections and joined them together with shoemaker's wax, and with this home-made catheter relieved the French-Canadian's ballooning bladder. Dr. Richardson was so proud of the instrument that he kept it as a memento.

Patients in those days appear to have been a constipated lot. At least one physician found it necessary to carry in his bag an ivory tube with a bladder attached to it, which he used to administer enemas. But, "On one occasion he had left it at home, and it was too far to go back for it; but an old woman who was present went out to the bush and procured a piece of elder, trimmed it up, and attached a bladder, which worked very satisfactorily. Shortly after, he was similarly placed—his ivory tube was left at home." Remembering the old woman's substitute, he obtained a piece of elder, trimmed it, affixed a bladder to it, and attempted to inject the appropriate solution, but found that he could not empty the bladder. On withdrawing the elder from the rectum, he found he had neglected to take the pith out of the piece of elder.

The United Empire Loyalists had hardly settled down in their new country before they were called upon to defend it. In 1812, the United States, announcing that it was their manifest destiny to own all the real estate in North America, invaded Canada once again. At Detroit, General Hull made the first move. "Raise not your hands against your Brethren," he told the Canadians. "The arrival of an Army of Friends must be hailed by you with a Cordial Welcome." His army then proceeded to plunder every barn, store, and home distillery in sight. Luckily, Hull was a particularly inert general and was tricked into surrendering by his opposite number, General Isaac Brock, who later had his brains blown out by a bullet through the heart, thus becoming Canada's first national hero.

By 1813 the war had reached Toronto (renamed York, later renamed Toronto), a bustling metropolis of 900. The Americans landed a strong force at Sunnyside Beach and after brushing aside the opposition, rambled into the garrison headquarters. Shortly afterwards the powder magazine blew up. William Baldwin, a doctor turned lawyer, was helping out by dressing a soldier's wounds when the explosion occurred. "He was conscious of a strange sensation—it was too great to be called a sound— and he found a shower of stones falling all around him, but he was quite unhurt." The American troops in the garrison at the time were not as lucky. Fifty-two of them were killed.

Some time previously, Dr. Baldwin entered upon the study of law, as apparently, medicine had not kept him sufficiently occupied. Still, he was always willing to provide medical relief when called upon, even when the calls clashed with his legal responsibilities; like the time he was arguing a case before a judge when he was summoned "to attend the advent of a little stranger into the world." The judge obligingly adjourned the case, and when the doctor returned, expressed the hope that all had gone well with the patient. "I have much pleasure in informing Your Lordship," Baldwin announced rotundly, "that a man-child has been born into the world during my absence, and that both he and his mother are doing well."

In the 1812 war, just as generals were expected to lead their men rather than to exhort them from comfortable quarters well behind the enemy lines, surgeons were also expected to be on the spot when the balls flew and the smoke swirled; though naturally, after the emergency was over, the doctors were as likely to be as shabbily treated as any other veteran. A colleague of Baldwin's in the war, Dr. Nathaniel Bell, a six-foot United Empire Loyalist, had the misfortune to be captured by the Americans, and while escaping was shot in the leg. He was still fighting for his rights to a disability pension a quarter century later.

One particularly individualist medico who took part in the war was John Lafferty, whose large, portly presence, a head of bushy gray hair, loud, sonorous voice and forcible language made him a conspicuous figure in society. "He swore profligately, but this did not deter him from taking the place of the local clergyman whenever he had the chance. Once, while reading the service, he happened to glance out the window and saw that a flock of sheep had escaped into a nearby pasture. With hardly a pause in his sacred function he leaned out the window and bellowed at his son to 'take the d—— sheep back again.'"

The sheep were probably his, for Lafferty carried on farming as well as medicine. He was particularly fond of horses, and during the war, "when he was amputating a soldier's leg he suspended the operation to have a look at a fine horse going by." He became a member of the legislature, where he kept boring his colleagues in that already sluggish chamber with the same anecdote, repeated ad nauseam. However, he spared them his favorite song "Twelve Bottles More," which was also the only one he knew.

The contents of his house were as interesting as their owner. They included, as well as a mammoth's tooth and stuffed owls, pigs, and rattlesnakes, "A wild goose tamed; this animal was very polite, indeed, and bowed to those who fed it, with dignity." There were also a number of human bones scattered around, and military sashes, daggers, cats and dogs, mortars and pestles, Lucan's *Pharsalia* (1636), an "electrifying machine," and of course the inevitable doctor's phials, bottles, and jars filled with fluids, unguents, and powders.

There was no stethoscope to be seen, though. Lafferty did not approve of that newfangled instrument, which was just coming into use in Canada in 1832.

Dr. Ashern Augustus Chamberlain was perhaps the most typical practitioner of the time, and Canniff's account gives us an equally typical picture of contemporary living conditions. Born in Vermont, Chamberlain came to Upper Canada in 1815 with his mother and stepfather, Timothy Smith. The family "pitched their tent in what was at that time a comparative wilderness, about four miles from Rideau Lake in the township of Bastard, on the bank of a small stream. They built a log shanty, covering the roof with wooden troughs made by scooping out basswood trees, cut of sufficient length and split in halves. After a little time Mr. Smith built a rude grist-mill on this stream and named the place 'Smith's Mills.'" He died in 1830, passing on to young Chamberlain the responsibility of bringing up a large brood of younger brothers and sisters. "In order to meet the necessities of the family and to pay his board while attending school in the winter, he was obliged to leave home and seek employment during the summer months. His education was procured at Potsdam, N.Y., to which place he would travel each fall on foot to the St. Lawrence at Brockville, and cross the river in a canoe, and then on to Potsdam. Returning in May, he would look after the family and prepare the means for the next winter's schooling. In this way he obtained sufficient education to enable him to lay the foundation for his subsequent professional studies. During this time settlers had gradually found their way into the back townships. The bridle-paths marked by blazed trees gradually became enlarged to public highways. Small clearings dotted the woods at intervals of half a mile or more, and that kind of prosperity which after a time rewards the early settler for his suffering and deprivation, began to be realized by the inhabitants of that section. Soon the necessity for medical assistance became so great, and the number of medical men so few, young Chamberlain decided to prepare himself for that profession, and he bent all his energies in that direction. The other children had now become sufficiently large to look after the farm and mill. He arranged matters for their comfort during the approaching winter, and left home for Fairfield Medical College, N.Y., where he attended the lectures and completed his medical course."

Quite a number of Canadian doctors attended Fairfield College, which was one of the few in the United States where a thorough medical training could be obtained. A fellow graduate of Fairfield College, John Crombie, also exemplified the spirit of self-sacrifice that imbued a high proportion of pioneer doctors. "Many a time," writes Dr. Canniff of John Crombie, "has the familiar form of the 'Old Doctor' been seen on horseback, with a basket of provisions on his arms and saddle bags behind him, wending his way through the woods to the relief of some poor family in distress by sickness and poverty where, instead of claiming a fee, he left them the wherewith, not only to relieve their suffering, but to supply the want of necessities of life."

Not that all doctors were indifferent to the confused currency of pennies, cents, dollars, pounds, scrip, and credits. While Crombie was performing as a good samaritan in one part of the province, there was a Dr. Muttlebury who was dying of cholera in another. A colleague was called in from York who after examining the patient, bluntly informed the sons that their father would soon be dead. "There is no hope," he said, "and now where am I to obtain my fee? I must be paid immediately."

Nor were some doctors prepared to put up with the savage conditions. Dr. Howison, practicing in the Niagara Peninsula, quickly gave up the frontier life and went home to England where he wrote a spiteful description of the early settlers, saying that "the country was unfit for a professional man of good education, who expected to make an income...."

It was certainly true that a country doctor could not expect much in the way of financial rewards. "If the Doctor got a bag of oats, a small quantity of flour, a few pounds of bacon, part of a quarter of beef, or even a bunch of shingles, he did not repine. Fees were very low and money very rarely seen. Long rides through the bush, only a road cut through where sawlogs were drawn to the mills, made the Doctor's life one of toil, as well as tedious, arduous and irksome in the extreme." On one occasion, a highly qualified surgeon by the name of de la Hooke received a pair of live ducks in part payment. "I put them in my buggy," Dr. de la Hooke recounted, "and on my way home met a gentleman. While we were conversing, the ducks began to quack , and he remarked that this was a novel way of advertising, and he had no doubt it would prove a very successful one. I felt very much chagrined...."

The doctor had reason to be chagrined, for before and after the 1812 war, a good many quacks or ill-trained physicians came waddling across the border. "Sometimes they had a degree of medical education which had been acquired in the U.S. medical schools; sometimes they knew a little about the use of drugs; but too frequently they only knew how to deceive the people by arrant quackery." Granite-faced Bishop Strachan, who was chief mouthpiece of the Family Compact (the Upper Canada Establishment of churchmen, bankers, law and Crown representatives, and other privileged persons) felt very indignant about the situation. These self-made physicians, he wrote, "cure all diseases with two specifics, opium and mercury. Is a patient in great pain, he must swallow a large pill of opium. Is a practitioner in doubt about his disease, a dose of calomel is the remedy. I was lately visiting a young woman ill of a fever. The Doctor came in, felt her pulse with much gravity, pronounced her near a crisis. 'She must take this dose,' said the gentleman, pouring out as much calomel on a piece of paper as would have killed two plough-men....On another occasion I found, on going to see a man ill of a bilious complaint, that the doctor had ordered three large blocks of wood heated in boiling water, one for his feet and one for each of his sides. The poor man was sweating himself to death. I commanded the blocks to be removed, ventilated the room, sprinkled the room with vinegar, washed his head and hands with it, and he began to breathe—another hour would have killed him, for you could hardly discern life in him when I entered."

Actually these and similarly irascible anecdotes from the same source suggest that the bishop was rather more concerned to show how clever he was than to expose a parlous state of affairs. Still, the situation was dangerous enough—a countryside swarming with bunglers. Many of them were well aware of their own deficiencies. As a Reverend gentleman of the period observed, "American physicians do not commonly place themselves in any situation in which competition with Europeans is hazarded."

Almost as bad as the outright imposters, according to an article in the *Western Mercury*, were the "licenced quacks" who deceived the public into thinking they were entitled to practice physic, surgery, and midwifery, when they were licenced to practice only one of these branches. Nevertheless, a fair number of these objects of righteous indignation managed to learn something of medicine by actually practicing it. Among these were Dr. Alex Burnside, an imposing, portly New Englander, who always wore a large gold seal. He was characterized as being an ignorant man but a fine money maker, "whose benefactions are now doing good to thousands, but whose name will ever be remembered as the promoter and encourager of church music, both vocal and instrumental." Another American, Elnathan Hubbell, who settled in Brockville, also managed to learn on the job. "Dr. Hubbell was remarkable for his large size, and a face marked by numerous nodules of the skin. It was stated that his education, both general and medical, was of doubtful extent." But he was highly successful. He built up a large practice, "especially in midwifery, though there were some who doubted his skill."

Hubbell, yet another doctor who had had a rough time during the 1812 war—he was captured by an American party, though later released on parole—was one of a host of medicos who compensated for a lack of basic training by a presence and a manner that suggested he knew what he was doing—qualities that have fooled many a patient into getting well. He had another redeeming feature. "He was very fond of hot cakes." Apparently a taste for hot cakes was regarded as an endearing characteristic of United Empire Loyalists.

Otherwise there were too many incompetents in the profession who had not even the decency to cultivate a bedside manner. A series of letters published in the Kingston *Gazette* in 1812 described some of these unworthies. One complaint about American doctors was that they did not use opium or calomel, but charms. One such fraud had treated a tumour by stroking it and delivering incantations to drive away "the devil's swelling." Another letter told of a practitioner who was in fact a shoemaker, and who, on being called in to see a case of dropsy described it as pleurisy, and declared that "fleglottomy" was needed to reduce the patient to his normal size. However, on being exposed by the writer of the letter, the humbugger hastily departed, speeded on his way, perhaps, with the reminder that the shoemaker should stick to his last.

A fortissimo chorus of similar complaints led to legislation, enacted at the end of the war, to regulate the profession and licence practitioners in "physic" and surgery. Unfortunately it was drawn up too hastily and the irregular regulations had to be repealed. They were replaced by an act establishing a medical board.

One of the first persons to be examined by the board was an English doctor who had come to Canada with his six children on the rather surprising grounds that the climate might be good on his ailing constitution. His constitution had been nearly ruined even before he experienced the climate. He had loaded his luggage on board ship in England but was delayed, and the ship sailed without him or his family. The delay saved his life, for the ship was never heard of again.

As the doctor's credentials had been packed with his luggage, he had to appear before the medical board in Toronto without proof of his qualifications. However, he was allowed to practice, after showing himself a worthy enough heir to the two centuries of medical progress that had followed Harvey's discovery of the circulation of the blood.

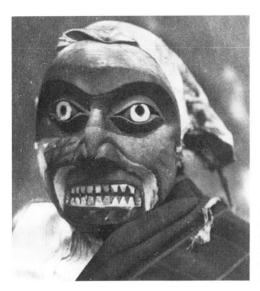

LEFT: Spirit of the medicine man. (Public Archives Canada/C30917) BELOW: Medicine man—nobility and hysteria. (PAC/PA9318)

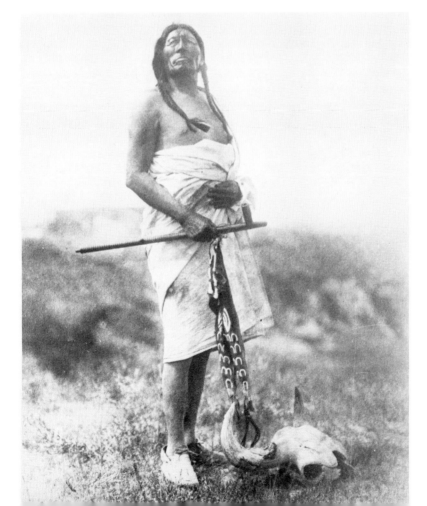

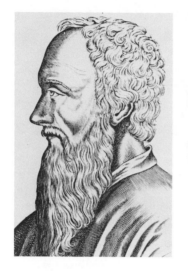
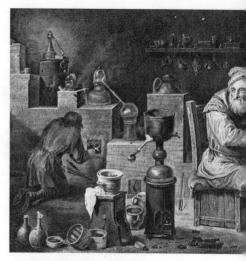
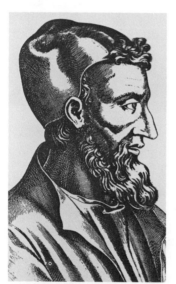
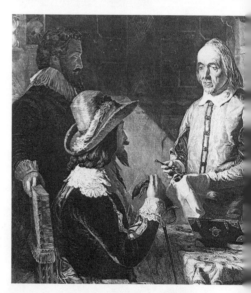

TOP LEFT: Hippocrates. (Museum, Academy of Medicine, Toronto) LOWER LEFT: Galen. (Museum, A of M) TOP CENTRE: The alchemist—whose aim was to find the earth-born substance that was thought to generate valuable metals. (Museum, A of M) LOWER CENTRE: Harvey demonstrating to Charles 1 his theory of the circulation of the blood. (Museum, A of M) RIGHT: The frontispiece of *de Fabrica Humani Corporis* showing Vesalius demonstrating at Padua (Museum, A of M)

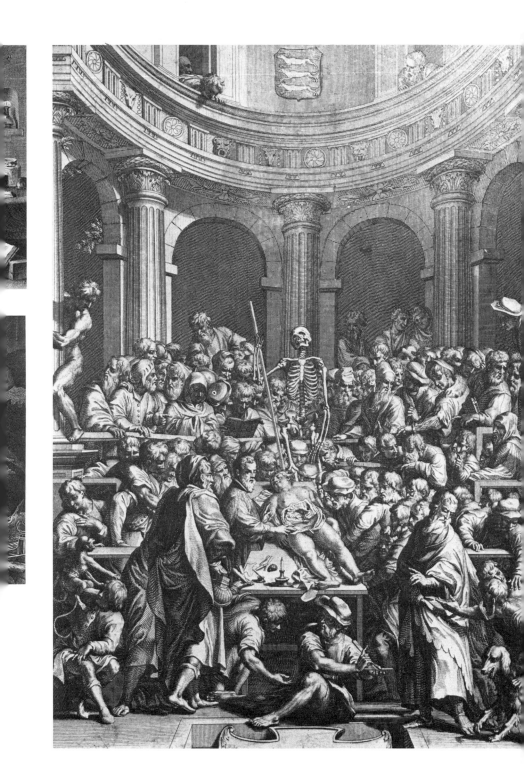

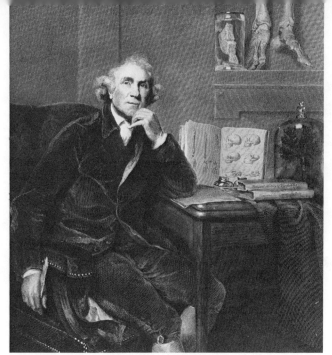

Joshua Reynolds' portrait of John Hunter. (Museum, A of M)
Edward Jenner giving his first vaccination. (Museum, A of M)

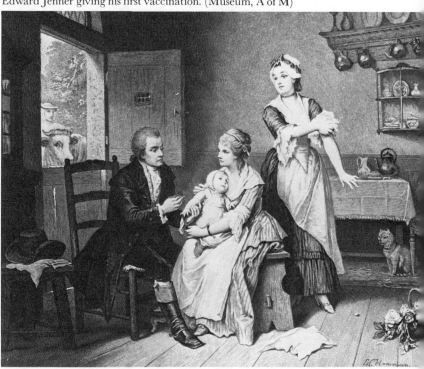

6

Perspective:
From Circulation to Vaccination

I N THE TWO centuries between the founding of the first permanent colony in Canada and the second threat to its independence from American republican rowdyism, medicine had advanced first in a rush, then at a saunter.

Medical progress was one of the glories of the seventeenth century in Europe, even though there were few contributions from two of its most scientifically oriented countries: Germany, torn apart by the Thirty Years War, and France, paralyzed by its Paris Faculty, which allowed doctors to graduate only after they had proved that they had no practical experience. The finest scientific achievements came from England, Holland, and Italy.

Italy's brightest star was Malpighi, who was born in the year that Harvey's work on the circulation of the blood was published. He was the founder of histology, the branch of science concerned with the structure of plant and animal tissues as seen through the microscope. He also made valuable contributions to embryology and physiology, through his work on the structure of the liver, spleen, and kidneys. He described the red blood-corpuscles — "fat globules looking like a rosary of red coral." And he demonstrated the true nature of the lungs after he had discovered the capillaries. (Harvey had predicted that the capillaries must exist, but lacking a microscope, had not been able to prove it.) With this superb achievement, Malpighi established the anatomical foundation for the true understanding of how we breathe.

In internal medicine, the peculiar character of Englishman Thomas Sydenham dominated the latter half of the century. A Puritan captain in

the Civil War, he ignored the medical theorizing and scientific experimentation of the time (mostly because he knew nothing about its greatest
representatives, Vesalius, Harvey, or Malpighi). Sydenham skipped
modern science and went back to his beloved Hippocrates. Even so, his
accounts of epidemics and their periodic recurrence were still being
studied two hundred years later. His treatise on gout is considered his
masterwork, but he also produced first-rate accounts of measles, hysteria,
and the widespread malarial fevers of the time. As we surmised, his
Canadian contemporary, Sarrazin, was one who appeared to have
benefited from Sydenham's clinical study of epidemics.

The many scientific advances of the century were an expression of
individual drives. It was the painstaking labour of the lonely experimenter
and observer, and his personal flashes of inspiration that enriched science
and stimulated spiritual and intellectual freedom. The seventeenth century danced to the rhythm of Shakespeare and Milton, Bach and Purcell,
Rembrandt, Velasquez, Newton and Spinoza. By contrast the eighteenth
was leaden-footed, plodding at the pace of a Linnaeus, who classified
things.

It was essentially an age of theorists and system-makers. "Linnaeus
established the vogue of classification in medicine as well as his own
science (botany) and seems to have set the pace everywhere. In this
respect, eighteenth-century medicine is as dull and sober-sided as the
Arabic period."

Still, the century had its great men. There was von Haller, the master
physiologist, who wrote Latin verses at ten, was correcting his medical
instructors at the age of sixteen, and by old age had written 13,000
scientific papers. There was Auenbrugger, who formed a way to determine the internal condition of the human thorax by tapping the chest
and listening to the resonance of the sound produced. (This, percussion, is
one of the four features of physical diagnosis: inspection, palpation,
percussion, and ausculation.) And, in Italy, where Versalius had described
the normal body, Morgagni described the diseased body, thus establishing
the science of pathology.

There were also advances in pharmacology, though in many ways the
science of drugs was not much better than it had been in the days of the
ancient Egyptians. While Harvey was studying the valves in the veins,
the London Pharmacopeia was still touting the therapeutic virtue of goat
urine, woodlice, the intestines of wolves, and the ground-up skull of a
criminal who had been hanged by moonlight. A century later, while
Dominique Anel was treating traumatic aneurysm (a weak spot in the
wall of an artery) by ligation of the brachial artery, a French catalogue of
drugs was extolling the products of men and women, their excretions and
excrements, as aids to good health. Burning hair was good for counteract-

ing the vapours, according to the catalogue, and ear wax was beneficial against whitlows, while finger- and toenails made an excellent emetic.

Thus the ship of progress still tended to drag at the anchor of the past, with its superstitions, quackeries, and fanaticism, and its brutality (witch-hunting, debtors prisons, window taxes, public hangings). Not that the new science was incapable of creating its own diversions. Discoveries in electricity were current, so to speak, through the work of Volta and Priestley. Benjamin Franklin was writing on the treatment of nervous diseases by electricity, and through his experiments on muscles and nerves, Galvani was originating electrophysiology. But at the same time, exploiting scientific progress for fun and profit, were medical men like Mesmer, with his magnetic medicine.

Franz Mesmer, a Swiss, had studied medicine in Vienna. His graduating thesis was on the influence of the planets on man. In his experiments with the magnet, he convinced himself that both it and the human hand had properties that would enable him to detect disease and to heal various afflictions. He attempted to practice his "mesmerism" in Vienna, but the Viennese were not receptive to his therapeutic legerdemain. He was finally ordered by the Empress Maria Theresa to get out of town within twenty-four hours.

France was more tolerant. In Paris, the home of the physician as "sterile pedant and coxcomb, red-heeled, long-robed, big-wigged, square-bonneted, pompous and disdainful in manner," Mesmer was welcomed with praise and gold. His mesmerism was a great success. He established hypnotic *seances,* in which he would dress up in a lilac suit, and play the harmonica. Among his props were magnetic tubs, or *baquets,* containing various ingredients, including hydrogen sulphide. The magnetic tubs were provided with iron conductors, with a ring hanging from them. The patients were arranged around the tubs, holding hands, and were supposed to be mystically and magnetically influenced by the rings. And also by Mesmer, who groped selected individuals, and gazed deep into their eyes. Most of them were fashionable women, and the more famous they made Mesmer, the more susceptible they became.

Mesmer also employed assistant-magnetizers, handsome young men who each selected a woman and after staring at her intently for a while, in a silence broken only by distant incidental music, embraced her knees and rubbed her here and there, and gently massaged her breasts. Whether it was magnetism or not, the women certainly felt *something* surge through them. "The magnetizer generally keeps the patient's knees enclosed within his own," and consequently the knees and all the lower parts of the body are in close contact. The hand is applied to the hypochondriac region, and sometimes to that of the ovarium, so that the touch is exerted at once on many parts, and these the most sensitive parts of the body."

If the lady had a "crisis" (as they called it), Mesmer then took over. He would pick her up and carry her into his private chamber. What went on there was a private matter between the doctor and patient, but at least one contemporary gendarme was curious to know, suspecting that when a woman was magnetized, it might be all too easy to "outrage" her.

Still, the women did not appear to be outraged, for they kept coming back for more, until, after ten years or so, the spoilsports cracked down on the delicious treatment. Shortly afterwards the fashionable ladies had something else to think about, when the French Revolution came along.

Surgery, for another half-century after the death of William Harvey, was concerned mostly with war wounds and battlefield amputations. Ailments such as wryneck, cataract, and stone in the bladder, were left to the charlatans who wandered from place to place, offering their specious specialist skills. Dentistry was also in the hands of the itinerants. One eighteenth-century London dentist named Van Butchell, a short man with a long beard, rode a white pony up and down Rotten Row every morning, advertising his wares: "Real or Artificial Teeth from one to an entire set...also Gums, Sockets and Palate fitted, finished and fixed without drawing stumps or causing pain." To catch the jaded London eye he painted purple spots on his pony. But now the young surgeons in the hospitals ventured to compete with the itinerants. Their increasing success helped to put them on an equal footing with the hitherto much more highly regarded physicians. The most famous surgeon of the first half of the eighteenth century, William Cheselden, was soon able to perform a lithotomy (the operation to remove stones from the bladder) in as short a time as one minute, fifteen seconds. His knifework was so speedy that there was little bleeding and shock, so the patient had a much better chance of surviving.

Cheselden took pains to prove he was that fast. He usually had a small apprentice standing by with a large watch, to time him.

Cheselden's success lay in his application of up-to-date anatomical knowledge to surgical problems. Among those who benefited from the improved teaching of the subject were the Hunter brothers, who advanced the tradition still further. The elder brother, William Hunter, a graduate of the University of Edinburgh, came to London in 1740, where he established that city's first real medical school.

William was soon joined by his young brother, John, who was to become the century's biological titan. He certainly did not look the part of the great man. He had left school at the age of thirteen, and his naive and uncouth manner reflected this truncated education. The contrast between the brothers was further heightened by their appearance. William was strikingly handsome, with an aloof, solemn air perfectly suited to the hospital ward. John looked like a lout. He did not even have the decency to conceal his coarse, red hair under a fashionable wig.

To everybody's surprise, John took an immediate interest in his elder brother's anatomical research. He even offered to help him. Somewhat doubtfully, William took him into the mortuary, and after a brief introduction, handed John a human arm and asked him if he would like to try and dissect the muscles. John took the scalpel and with quite untypical care and application, laid back the layers of skin and fibrous tissue, and then the nerves, veins, and arteries, until the muscles were cleanly exposed. William was so impressed that he soon had John actively employed in the dissecting room.

John also turned out to be a splendid agent for the procuring of bodies from the sack-em-up men. This was a great help, for though it was professionally necessary for William to cultivate the body-snatchers, he much preferred the civilized pleasures of Covent Garden and Drury Lane. But John actually enjoyed mixing with the inmates of the brothels and grog shops that flanked those theatres.

Over the years John Hunter read before the Royal Society a large number of scientific papers and produced such influential works as the physiological, pathological, and surgical study *Blood, Inflammation, and Gunshot Wounds*. In his teaching he hammered home his belief, then a truly original one, that to know the effects of disease was not enough. It was more important to learn the cause. The structure of the body was important, he said, but function was even more important. In addition to his writing and teaching, he also studied birds, beasts, and fishes, and accumulated a magnificent museum of specimens and dissections. All subsequent museums of natural history have been modeled on it.

Among his many operations and experiments he performed the first high operation for aneurysm of the great artery that runs behind the knee. Until Hunter showed the way, surgeons usually either killed the patient by tackling the aneurysm without really knowing what they were doing, or evading the issue by amputating the leg.

He also experimented on himself, and it was one such experiment that ultimately caused his death. One of his most famous works was a *Treatise on the Venereal Diseases*. The project began when he innoculated himself with gonorrheal pus. Unfortunately he was not aware that the donor also had syphilis. This distorted his findings on the controversy as to whether syphilis and gonnorhea were different diseases or manifestations of the same disease. In order to study what he thought was the progress of gonorrhea he kept halting the treatment to see what happened, with the result that the syphilitic spirochetes established themselves in his system, and killed him a quarter century later.

John Hunter's principal achievement was in the enhancement of surgery. Through his work and his impact on his students, surgery ceased to be regarded as a mere technique in treatment, and took its place as a branch of scientific medicine, firmly based on physiology and pathology.

Incidentally he may have had Canadian connections. According to Canniff, Upper Canada's second governor was Peter Hunter, "who came to Canada in 1799. He was a brother of the great Dr. Hunter," presumably meaning John Hunter. If so, James must have been one of the Hunter family's first four surviving children to be born in East Kilbride.

Among Hunter's many gifted pupils was Edward Jenner. He was a stocky young man with a deep, rich voice, very nattily attired. A gentleman but no "macaroni," as they would say at the time. He was the first student to be taken on by Hunter. Hunter was acutely disappointed when Jenner turned down an offer to become his assistant. Instead, Jenner returned to Berkeley, Gloucestershire, to practice medicine, study cuckoos, and ponder on the dreadful disease of smallpox.

Smallpox was the world's most effective form of population control. It had killed and was still killing by the million, and where it left survivors, they were likely to be maimed or crippled for life, or to be so disfigured with pock-marks that their faces hardly looked human.

As virulent in the eighteenth century as in one thousand B.C., it had led to countless tragedies. If a baby caught the disease, which was not unlikely, the mother was faced with an agonizing dilemma. If she continued to wean it she would likely perish herself. If she did not, the child would die. Often she could not bring herself to abandon the child, so that both of them perished, or were marked for life.

As a youth, Jenner had overheard a milkmaid remark that she could not catch smallpox as she had once had the cowpox. Jenner was a countryman, and knew that old wives' tales were not always rubbish. The remark simmered in his mind for years before he started to amble along the line or enquiry suggested by her remark.

His was a leisurely age. Gentleman might take all morning to dress, and then dawdle for another two hours over dinner. Even so, Jenner's pace was remarkably measured. He began a systematic study of cowpox in 1778, and slowly built up an understanding of the disease, which until then had not been described. He came to the conclusion that cowpox was a different form of smallpox, and that it came in a spurious form as well as a genuine form. After four years he satisfied himself that he could distinguish between them.

By then he was married, and a child was on the way. Sharing the terror or resignation with which parents throughout the world, from plutocrat to pauper, regarded the almost inevitable onslaught of smallpox, he decided to innoculate the child with cowpox. He awaited the birth with his ivory lancet at the ready.

This decisive experiment depended of course on the availability of the cowpox virus. Unfortunately when his son was born there was no convenient outbreak, and none was to appear for eighteen months.

Worse, by 1791, he had learned that it was still possible for a person who had contracted cowpox to catch smallpox afterward. It was "a painful check to my fond and aspiring hopes," Jenner wrote, "but I resumed my labour with redoubled ardour." It took him another three years to understand why, at the end of which period, "I was struck by the idea that it might be practicable to propagate the disease by innoculation... first from the cow; and finally from one human being to another. I anxiously waited for some time for an opportunity of putting this theory to the test. At length the period arrived."

It was 1796 when Jenner took matter from the hand of a dairymaid who had become infected with cowpox, and conveyed it to the arm of a boy of eight, James Phipps. A year later James was subjected to a quantity of smallpox matter that would normally have killed him. The boy was unaffected. He had been vaccinated (from the Latin *vaccinus*— of or from cows).

Another year passed before Jenner was able to build up sufficent proof to convince the world of the advantages of cowpox innoculation. By June 1798, he had twenty-three case histories completed, which were embodied in his *An Enquiry into Cause and Effects of the Variolae Vaccinae*. It cost seven shillings and sixpence, and it was typical of a rigid and jealous age that some of his most eminent colleagues declared that it was not worth tuppence.

Though Jenner's vaccination method was introduced to Canada within four years by a Dr. Bond of Yarmouth, Nova Scotia, smallpox continued to ravage the country for more than a century. One of the worst epidemics of the disease occurred in Montreal in 1885. It touched off riots among citizens opposed to compulsory vaccination. Even after many people had died, the mob continued to oppose vaccination along with the sanitary measures designed to prevent smallpox from flourishing. It was not until the casualty list reached the thousands that the people began to comprehend the value of Jenner's discovery.

The issue was clouded to a certain extent by the fact that cowpox vaccination was not invariably effective, and because there was a longer-established method of fighting smallpox: the innoculation of a healthy person with a small quantity of smallpox matter, so that a mild attack could build up the body defences against a severe attack. Sometimes it worked. Often it killed, and there was always the danger that the practice might start an entirely gratuitous epidemic. "The Elysian Fields are filled with innoculated smallpox victims," as one nineteenth-century letter-writer put it. The practice was abolished in Canada by Act of Parliament in 1853, though thirty-nine years later during an epidemic in British Columbia, that province's best-known doctor was advocating the use of humanized lymph rather than waiting for a batch of bovine lymph to arrive from Eastern Canada. "Wait until tomorrow?" he asked. "Bah! Procrastination in an emergency is not the motto of J. S. Helmcken."

To understand the resistance to vaccination from the perspective of an age that is accustomed to fast action in everything from aspirin to armed aggression, we need mentally to impersonate a nineteenth-century citizen and decelerate to his more ponderous pace, wonder at his not overly-developed social conscience, and sympathize with his difficulty in absorbing new ideas. Rudimentary communication was the causality. The authorities did not care enough, and so the public did not understand. This accounts for the situation in which Jenner's discovery, which should have slammed the door on humanity's worst scourge, had not been universally adopted three-quarters of a century later in a more medically sophisticated Europe. In the Franco-Prussian War of 1870, the vaccinated German army lost 297 men to smallpox. The unvaccinated French army lost 20,000.

Incidentally, the story of smallpox ended only recently, when the World Health Organization reported that the disease had finally been eradicated from the earth, in 1979.

7

Pork, Pickles, and Pock-Marks

THE TRAGEDY OF the Canadian Indian was that his culture was too strong to blend satisfyingly with white civilization, but not strong enough to avoid being corrupted by it. The story of the Six Nations Indians near Brantford, as researched by Sally Weaver in her *Medicine and Politics Among the Grand River Iroquois,* illustrates the native frustration, and serves to bring Indian medical history up-to-date.

In 1838, the Lieutenant-Governor of Upper Canada took a trip along the Grand River and was disturbed enough by the sufferings of the Indian families to recommend that a physician be appointed to attend them. This was done, but half a century later the Indians had still not unreservedly accepted the new medicine. "Western medicine was turned to largely as a last resort when traditional [Indian] methods were perceived to be unsuccessful, or in extreme cases such as the threat of a smallpox epidemic.... These were the methods that had served the people in the past...." The resistance still existed in the 1890s. A white physician reported that, "Among the Pagans, it is quite common to find a patient's bed surrounded by curtains to keep him or her from being defiled by contact with the outer world. The sick person may be kept for days in this seclusion and fed on white chickens and white beans, this diet being symbolical of purity. The Indian medicine women.... administer some medicine, usually herbs or roots, in the efficacy of which they themselves have no faith, but put all their trust in superstitious ceremonies, and invocations to the Great Spirit. A physician is only called after this method of treatment has proved to be of no avail, or after some intelligent advisor has succeeded in getting the patient's consent to have the doctor.

47

This condition of affairs is, however, fast improving, and I am of the opinion it will not be many years before the Pagans will all recognize the efficacy of modern medical treatment."

Only at the beginning of the twentieth century was it finally recognized that compulsion in preventive medicine is essential for the common good. "During the spring and early summer of 1901," Sally Weaver recorded, "an epidemic of smallpox broke out on the reserve, causing the health officials in the adjacent townships considerable apprehension. Fear of smallpox spreading into adjacent areas led them to pressure both the Indian Agent and the Medical Officer to quarantine the entire reserve."

The Indian Council on the Six Nations Reserve acted promptly enough. "Guards were employed and placed at strategic locations around the six quarantined blocks....to ensure that no one violated the quarantine. In addition, the local Six Nations constable patrolled the roads by horse and buggy to give even further assurance against violations. Food supplies and other necessities were brought to the families in the quarantined areas and left at the road to be picked up by someone in the household. A house near Number 6 school was 'turned into a pest house' for the sick, and additional tents were brought in and set up in the other blocks for the same purpose....Dr. E. Secord was brought to the reserve from Montreal for a period of four months to take charge of the quarantined areas."

The council had agreed to support the measures, but a month later the chiefs changed their minds. Concerned with the high cost of the quarantine, they convinced themselves that the epidemic was not of smallpox but of chicken pox. They proved this to their own satisfaction by feeding the patients pork and pickles. When the patients lived, the chief felt vindicated. If the patients had been suffering from smallpox this diet would have killed them. Therefore, it was not smallpox at all.

When the white doctor insisted on maintaining the quarantine, the chiefs voted $100 to bring in a more competent medical officer. To their chagrin, the new officer verified that it was smallpox all right, and that the disease was rampant.

The epidemic ended in September of 1901, but returned the following year. Fortunately there were no fatalities, and only a few were left permanently scarred. "For the remainder of this period, however, the threat of smallpox was continuous....Immunization was repeatedly urged by the Indian Department, but although many had been and were vaccinated during this time, there was no systematic infant or child immunization program, isolated cases of smallpox appeared through this period, and it became more frequent in 1920 and 1921."

Sally Weaver gave an example of the quarantine experience. "One informant recalls a quarantine being imposed on her family when her father suffered from the disease. The Council hired two men to enforce the quarantine for a six weeks' period; one was a 'day guard' and one a 'night guard.' These men were ideally to remain outside the house at all times, but 'one came in every afternoon for a cup of tea.' They performed the necessary 'chores,' chopped wood, milked and fed the cows, and ran errands. At the beginning of their isolation, all the food in the house had been 'sealed up' by the doctor, so the informant said, because of 'germs in it,' and they were given new supplies at regular intervals. Her father was confined to bed for about three weeks; after he was feeling 'good' he was allowed up and one day 'ran away,' taking a walk up along a creek bed out behind their property beyond quarantined limits. The guard, she said, did not inform on her father because his pay would be 'docked' by the Council."

The medical history of the Grand River Indians is the story of a clash of cultures. White physicians were first appointed to the reserve in the mid-nineteenth century, but though the Indians came to rely more and more on Western medicine, a resentment toward it floated just under the surface. In his heart the Indian believed that his own medicine had served him well in the past, and deep down he did not really believe that the imported methods were superior. The depth of his resistance to white culture has rarely been properly appreciated, and just as rarely sympathized with. Too often the Indian behaviour, a manifestation of this resistance, merely appeared to be obtuse.

The clash of cultures was dramatized in the relationship between the white doctors and their Department of Indian Affairs on the one hand, and the Indian chiefs and their people on the other. The chiefs ultimately discharged Dr. Secord because he refused to live on the reserve. The next medical superintendant of the Six Nations, Holmes, was also fired. There had to be sympathy between the patient and the doctor, said the chiefs, but none existed. Moreover, "The Council is of the opinion that, as Doctor Holmes is paid out of the funds of the Six Nations, he should at least have been courteous enough to the Six Nations Council to have attended the meeting when summoned instead of writing an insulting letter to it in which he refused to come."

Dr. Holmes had also blotted his copybook by taking leaves of absence. "Since last Spring he was away to Military School about two weeks, Camp at Niagara two weeks, attending Courts at Toronto for days at the time, attending races, and frequently away to Muskoka shooting deer."

The situation was not improved by a growing antipathy to the federal government. The Department of Indian Affairs appointed another doctor in Holmes' place without properly consulting the chiefs. A year later the chiefs fired this doctor as well. Of course, the strained relationship was not all the fault of the doctor. The physicians often felt that they were being called upon unnecessarily. It was not unknown for the patient to be out when the doctor drove up in his buggy. Sometimes the Indians would not submit to the long course of treatment necessary, for example, with syphilis. It seemed to the Indians that the treatment was worse than the disease. If they did not understand the treatment, or disliked the procedure, as often as not they would abandon it, and attempts at compulsion only led to further resentment.

Another example was the treatment for typhoid fever. At the time part of the treatment was to deprive the patient of food, but, "As one Indian phrased it, 'They used to starve you to death, you were nothing but skin and bone when they finished with you.'"

The strained relationship was, in a way, worsened by the fact that the Grand River Indians had at one time been attended by a physician whom they considered to be an unusually flexible, sympathetic, and self-sacrificing person. His name was Walter Davis. "When Dr. Davis was an infant, it is said, his white parents abandoned him on the doorstep of an Indian home on the reserve, and an Indian couple raised him. He went to public school on the reserve and as a teenager walked several miles to attend high school in one of the nearby towns. After graduating from the University of Toronto medical school, he began practising medicine on the reserve in 1914....In spite of his being white, 'he was different....People didn't consider him a white man. He was one of us.'

"As a physician, he is best remembered in the 'horse and buggy days' when 'he would always come when you called at any time of day or night. You could always depend on him.' It is said that he knew the people who made unnecessary demands on his time and energy, but it is seldom stated that he refused to make future calls in these cases....

"Despite the minor limitations of his medical knowledge and skill, one seldom hears unfavourable comments about this physician because it was felt 'he tried, he tried his very best.'

"Dr. Davis's popularity on the reserve arose from many factors, among which was a certain understanding of medical beliefs and practices of the [Indian] people... 'When his medicine didn't work, he'd tell us to use our own medicines.'"

Dr. Davis further endeared himself to the Indians by becoming deeply involved in the life of the community. He and his family supported the church and his children went to school with the Indian children. It was recognized that "he wasn't right up there in medicine," but his warm, personal interest in his patients more than made up for his deficiencies. He became the model from which all other doctors have been judged.

Sally Weaver concludes, however, that much of the discord was due to the antipathy between the chiefs and the Department of Indian Affairs. This was exacerbated during the 1950s by fresh government pressure to centralize the medical services on the reserves. The physician was now to base his activities round the hospital rather than through house calls. Thus personal relations were downgraded. Basically what the government was doing was treating the Indian as it did the whites. But the reaction by the Indians was one of "characteristic apprehension" that they were losing their valued status as Indians. A number of the Indians who had clung to traditional Indian healing methods could cope with the changes, but those who had come to depend on Western medicine were upset. They did not appreciate that the same adjustment was being demanded of North Americans in general.

However, the story of the Grand River Indians does not have an entirely unhappy ending. Today, Weaver concludes, "the Six Nations now hold a comparable position with whites regarding medical behavior demanded of them by the profession. In other words, they have had to change not only their expectations of the physician's role performance, but also their own role performance as patients."

8

Mercury and Venus

THE QUACKS HAD a field day when, two years after the signing of the peace treaty that ended French rule in Canada, an epidemic erupted in the St. Paul's Bay area, fifty miles downriver from Quebec City.

Both sides were blamed for the epidemic, the occupying Scotsmen for introducing it, and the *habitants* for propagating it by domestic habits which tended to prove that ignorance is filth. Over the next few years, the disease tardily identified as syphilis, became so widespread throughout the countryside as to bestir a normally pennypinching government into supplying free medicine, including mercurial drugs. The "Baie St. Paul Disease" yielded readily to treatment by mercury if it was administered properly and at the right time. But all too often it was not, and in the opinion of Dr. Charles Blake, then one of Montreal's most eminent practitioners, some of the medical countermeasures were even worse than the disease they were countering.

Blake was an American loyalist who had joined the British army as a surgeon during the War of Independence. At the end of the war he settled in Montreal and built up an enormous practice. Possibly as a guide as to how much he should charge his patients, his statements of accounts included their occupations as well as their names: "William Smith the Gardener, Fynn the King's Carpenter, Simon the Cooper, Abraham the Jew a Tailor, Pickard the Butcher, Mr. Chewatt a Surveyor, Shiller the Bailiff, John Jones a Shoemaker and John Long a Publisher."

By the time he had been in practice for two years, Dr. Blake was able to afford a house on Notre Dame Street, another house on the river, and a farm "in the Quebec suburb." He also owned three black slaves, showing, as Maude Abbott points out, that slavery was in vogue in Montreal as well as in the United States in the late eighteenth century.

At the height of the St. Paul's Bay epidemic, Blake wrote a ferocious denunciation of the quacks and illiterates who were being allowed to thrive in the province. He described how he queried the account of one doctor who had administered no less than two ounces of pure mercury in a single dose. "On my remonstrating, he [the practitioner] strenuously insisted that he had actually done this, and as a sanction for his giving it said that a Canadian constitution would bear as much again as an English one. I have no occasion to tell you the man died.... I could give many other instances of murder being perpetrated by these imposters in the profession," Dr. Blake said, and went on to mention a childbirth case where a doctor, unable to deal with a baby whose head was caught in the pelvic opening, cut off its head and threw it into a bucket.

Several such cases of brute incompetence finally forced the authorities to clean up the medical profession, and in 1788 the British Parliament legislated that no one should practice physic and surgery in Quebec without a licence.

Naturally, with the state in charge of things, there were the inevitable abuses. The licences had to be obtained from government-appointed examiners, who showed themselves to be narrow-minded and prejudiced from the moment they tested the first applicant, Dr. Laterrière.

In his *Memoirs*, Laterrière, who had studied medicine in France and practiced it in Canada, described how, "I had lost my certificate of St. Come, and the documents of my apprenticeship in Paris, but I knew I had talent enough to pass an examination. I was the first to present myself before the medical bureau of examination at 8 o'clock in the morning in the presence of four practitioners and four councillors, and a very large assembly attracted by curiosity because there was a new institution in the country. The examination lasted until four in the afternoon. One question did not wait for another. However correct my answers were, my examiners, because of my failure to present my letters to them, did not wish to permit me to continue practising. It was necessary for me to go to another college to obtain other certificates. Their partiality, their hardness, their malice were so apparent that many of my friends, mere spectators, said to me, 'Go to Cambridge, near Boston, where in a short time, with the knowledge that you have obtained here, you would obtain what you now lack.' My examiners having seen that, and the reproaches that the public were making, rather through shame than friendship, said: 'Yes, if the candidate should go to Cambridge or elsewhere, we will give him a certificate favourable to the talents and knowledge which he has displayed.'"

Even after he obtained an M.B. at Cambridge, Dr. Laterrière had to submit to the ordeal again the following summer, even though there was a clause in the act to the effect that anyone with a medical degree was not subject to examination. There were no French-speaking Canadians on the examining body, and in fact none was appointed for a further forty years. According to J. E. Roy, the English examiners were often unjust to their French colleagues.

On the whole, though, the British treatment of the defeated French in Quebec, in contrast to their handling of the American Colonies, was quite extraordinarily tolerant. The French medical applicants had cause to complain professionally, but their language and customs were officially respected, and there was a minimum of interference with the French civil laws, and none whatsoever with the Roman Catholic Church.

The new administration in Quebec was, if anything, an improvement over the former regime (which would shortly get its come-uppance in the French Revolution). That the official tolerance was appreciated is shown by the response to the British offer after the signing of the peace treaty, to provide free transport for any colonist and his possessions who wished to return to the motherland. Hardly any of the colonists went home to Mother. Even Dr. Laterrière, despite his understandable annoyance, preferred to return to Quebec from Massachusetts, rather than go back to France, or remain in the American Republic, where the melting pot policy would have deprived him of his language.

The generally civilized treatment of the French (or at least of the ones who counted, the social elite and the clergy), paid off only a dozen years after the Conquest when the Americans invaded Canada during the War of Independence. The French colonists fought the invaders just as dedicatedly as did the English Canadians—or, to put it in terms closer to the human realities, they resisted the Americans with approximately equal apprehension, doubt, and pusillanimous self-interest.

In the nineteenth century, a French-speaking Canadian and an English Canadian in Montreal furnished two of the most amazing stories in Canadian medicine. The first concerned an illiterate voyageur who made a major contribution to the physiology of digestion—very unwillingly indeed; and the other concerned the longest-running solo performance in the world's medical theatre.

The first story began in Michilimackinac in Michigan. The scene was an American Fur Company store, packed with traders from both sides of the border: Indians and half-breeds, trappers, voyageurs, and company clerks. Suddenly there was an explosion. One of the shoppers had brought a loaded shotgun into the store. He had been jostled. The weapon fired, straight into the chest of a young fellow standing a few feet away. The young man was flung to the floor where he lay too shocked to make a sound. His shirt smouldered, then burst into flames.

A U.S. Army surgeon was called in from the fort. His name was William Beaumont, a Connecticut man whose knowledge of surgery had been gained as a medical apprentice. He added a great deal of surgical experience during the War of 1812, as a member of the American forces that had attacked Toronto. While the invaders were marching into Fort York, a powder magazine had exploded, killing and wounding many Americans. Beaumont tended to the victims for forty-eight hours without food or sleep. "My God!" he said later, "Who can think of the shocking scene when his fellow-creatures lie mashed and mangled in every part with a leg, an arm, a head, or a body ground in pieces, without having his very heart pained with the acutest sensibility and his blood chill in his veins. Then, who can behold it without agonizing sympathy!"

The victim of the shotgun accident at Michilimackinac was almost as shocking a sight. The young man's flesh was burned, the muscles torn, the ribs fractured, the stomach blasted open. There was a deep hole in the chest, below the left nipple. The wound was so deep that both the lungs and the stomach protruded. His chances of surviving were, to put it mildly, remote.

Yet he lived. Alexis St. Martin had spent his youth in the backwoods of French Canada and the West, and it had given him a toughness and vitality that saw him through the first critical weeks of his recovery. Miraculously the dreadful wound did not become infected, though when the shot entered his body it had carried into the wound pieces of clothing, wadding, and grains of gunpowder. All the same, it was a long time before Alexis was capable of earning a living.

Consequently he became a burden on the local treasury. As soon as he was more or less on his feet, the village elders demanded that he go home. As his home was two thousand miles away, it is unlikely that he would have survived the journey.

Dr. Beaumont came to his rescue, even though he was not at all well off, having a monthly salary of only forty dollars. He was so indignant at the callousness of the authorities that he offered to take Alexis into his own home. And for the next several years, "I nursed him, fed him, clothed him, lodged him and furnished him with every comfort," Dr. Beaumont related, "and dressed his wounds daily and for the most part twice a day."

Two years after the accident, Alexis was able to work, though there was still a gaping hole in his left chest. It was so large that Beaumont was able to see into the stomach. As related by Victor Robinson, "About three years after the accident, Beaumont realized that St. Martin's gastric fistula offered a unique opportunity for experiments in the physiology of digestion: 'I can pour in water with a funnel, or put in food with a spoon, and draw them out again with a syphon. I have frequently suspended flesh, raw and wasted, and other substances into the perforation to ascertain the length of time required to digest each; and at one time used a tent of raw beef, instead of lint, to stop the orifice, and found that in less than five hours it was completely digested off, as smooth and even as if it had been cut with a knife.' Beaumont began to make the most of his opportunities. He introduced all sorts of food into St. Martin's aperture, withdrew them, reintroduced them, and learned what the gastric juice did to each. He was the first who was able to collect, directly from the human stomach, gastric juice either pure or bright yellow bile."

Then Alexis took off, and it was four years before Dr. Beaumont caught up with him again. In the meantime the French Canadian had married, and was supporting two children on his wages as a voyageur for the Hudson's Bay Company. Beaumont managed to lure him back, and after a series of experiments, published in 1833 his *Experiments and Observations on the Gastric Juice and the Physiology of Digestion.*

By this time, though the doctor offered to support him and pay him a large sum of money, Alexis had had enough of being treated "as a stomach with a window." He vamoosed, this time for good, leaving behind a fuming Dr. Beaumont, who considered him an ungrateful savage. After all, had he not saved St. Martin's life?

On the other hand, Alexis had made Beaumont famous. He had submitted to 238 experiments, making Beaumont America's foremost physiologist; experiments that were not surpassed, according to Dr. Robinson, until Pavlov's researches into the digestive glands in 1897.

The story ended in Montreal half a century later, as related by Harvey Cushing in his biography of William Osler. Osler was then teaching at McGill University. One of his subjects was physiology, and he often mentioned St. Martin's stomach while discussing the processes of digestion. He learned that Alexis St. Martin, by now the father of twenty children, was living in Quebec, at St. Thomas, Joliette County. Osler, who was building up a splendid collection of pathological specimens, hoped to obtain the famous stomach. In 1880, when St. Martin lay dying, Osler laid his plans for an autopsy accordingly; but on the day of the voyageur's death, the local doctor sent Osler a telegram, warning him that the locals knew of his intentions, and that if he even attempted an autopsy, the locals would perform a crude equivalent on him, Osler. The warning was reinforced by the information that the grave was being guarded every night by French Canadians with rifles. So Alexis ended up by disappointing two doctors.

In the same year that Beaumont was serving with the American forces during the attack on Toronto, a Dr. James Barry was entering the medical service on the British side, as a hospital mate.

Dr. Barry's origins were mysterious. He would never admit the date of his birth, though it was later estimated as being somewhere between 1790 and 1795. It is still not known who brought him up after his parents died shortly after his birth; except that he appeared to have been placed in the care of a personage of considerable means. In those days an independent income was essential for an army officer, to enable him to keep up a fashionable front. James Barry's career was well financed; but who his patron was, nobody knew.

There were other mysterious influences on Dr. Barry's life. He rose through the army hierarchy like a Congreve rocket. The first promotion was understandable enough. Two years after joining up, six months after the Battle of Waterloo, he was made assistant surgeon. But after all, he was an Edinburgh M.D., and thus thoroughly qualified for the post. If anything, the promotion was overdue.

But from then on his rise, at a time when an army officer might remain at one level for fifteen or even twenty years, went at an accelerated pace that his qualities did not appear to warrant. His promotions we even harder to understand because he was often in trouble with his superiors over breaches of discipline. He was an extraordinarily difficult person, pretentious and almost pathologically sensitive to the slightest hint of disrespect. Unfortunately it was difficult for people meeting him for the first time to suppress their amusement or disdain, for the doctor was an even more absurd sight than General Wolfe had been. He was thin and undersized, but wore ridiculously large spurs and the longest, sharpest sword in the army. To match the sword he had a sharp voice, which he used on his subordinates in a rancorous way. He challenged to a duel at least two adversaries who had not been warned about the choleric medic. One of them paid for a verbal blunder with his life.

By the time Dr. Barry arrived in Montreal in 1857, he was inspector-general of the Canadian military hospitals. He was thought to have occupied a house at the corner of Durocher and Sherbrooke Street, and his physician was a Dr. Campbell who, though he got to know Barry quite well, could not have been overly perceptive.

The inspector-general soon became a familiar if not particularly popular figure around the hospitals, and in Montreal and Quebec military circles.

Even then, Barry's rise in the hierarchy did not falter. Within two years of his appointment in Montreal he became head of the entire army medical service, which confirmed in the minds of those who had never seen any intrinsic cause for Barry's success that his patron was very high up indeed. How else could he have got on so well when he had so often been guilty of breaches of discipline on account of his fiery temper and neurotic sensitivity? Of course, there was no doubt that he was a first-class medical officer, but since when had superior ability guaranteed success in the army? Was he perhaps the illegitimate son of a duke, perhaps even of the Prince Regent himself? And there was another strange thing about Barry, a contradiction that deepened the mystery of his background: although he had often shown bravery in the field, during his service he never received the military decorations that were his due. It was almost as if not one but two influences were at work on his behalf, and in conflict with each other.

It wasn't until James Barry's death in London in 1865 that one of the mysteries, at least, was cleared up, when a woman in the sickroom where he died became, so far as is known, only the second person in nearly half a century to see the unclad form of James Barry, and found it to be that of a woman. The finding was confirmed (as if confirmation were needed), by the autopsy that was ordered by an astounded War Office.

The only other direct witness, it seems, was the surgeon-general, Sir Thomas Longmore, who had attended Barry in Trinidad in 1844. She had been too sick to prevent a complete examination. Longmore had subsequently been sworn to secrecy.

The reason for the forty-six year impersonation has never been determined, though it was surmised that it may have originated in a love affair with the person who helped her to skip many of the rungs in the promotional ladder, a man of influence but of illogical standards, who could allow her to fool the entire army, but who could not bring himself to permit decorations for valour to be awarded to a woman.

Perhaps he was the father of her child. There were unsusbstantiated reports that the autopsy had revealed that she had once given birth to a child. It is just as possible that James Barry had a spirit that could not be satisfied in any other way except through a life of adventure in the army. Whatever the explanation, the experience must have caused an enormous strain on her personality. Maude Abbott speculates that, "some at least of her physical peculiarities were assumed in order to conceal her identity, and that the asperity which she showed to subordinates was a necessary part of the role she played."

She may have had to force herself, for forty-six years, to act tempestuously and temperamentally, for the opinion of those who knew her well suggested that her Wolfe-like qualities were not natural to her. That in reality she was quite an agreeable person.

9

The Tiger

IN LONDON, DR. WILLIAM Dunlop, "a carroty-haired, slovenly, coarse-looking Scotchman" (his description of himself), was one of the literary lions that prowled around such famous magazines of the day as *Blackwood's* and *Fraser's*.

Though not a writer of the stature of his contemporaries Coleridge, Southey, Hazlitt, and Walter Scott, Dr. Dunlop was a gifted essayist and much admired for his storytelling ability and personality. The great Thomas Carlyle, who had married William's cousin, Jane Welch, came to share the general admiration once he had gotten over the shock of his first meeting with the Canadian backwoodsman. "The door opened," as the scene is described in the *Dunlop Papers* "and there was ushered in an enormous giant of a man with long red hair; so strange and immense did he look at first sight, and like an Ogre, that Carlyle felt timorous, expecting he would proceed to devour some of the party; while his wife made one spring on this tremendous apparition and caught him round the neck and embraced him. For a few seconds Carlyle thought he had married a woman who was wrong in the head."

In London, Dunlop had also been the editor of a Tory newspaper, and had prepared for the British market an American work, *The Elements of Medical Jurisprudence*. Yet "Tiger" Dunlop was to feel truly at home only in the crude, far-from-literary Canadian backwoods, where his riproaring way of life, and his learning, his wild humour, and love of unpretentious people, were to make him a legendary figure.

Within months of his return to Upper Canada in 1826 as an employee of the Canada Company, he was using his rackety, dramatic personality to dominate every sort of company from tavern brawlers to the sluggish toffs of the colonial aristocracy. He could create drama out of disrobing. Once, after a day in the sodden forest, upon joining a woodland party of Canada Company officials, he flung off his clothes and danced naked around the camp fire, singing violently. He was regarded with deep appreciation by the Indians, and with even deeper effrontery by his boss, the distinguished but utterly circumspect novelist, John Galt.

Dr. Dunlop made a production number even out of snuff-taking. He would toss handfuls of the stuff into the air, and, catching some of it on his upturned face, would snort up as much as possible, before the remainder rained onto his coarse canvas trousers and half-Wellingtons.

When the company sent an unpleasant little Cockney named Smith to investigate Dunlop's affairs as "Warden of the Forest," the good doctor led him into the woods, programming him all the way with frightful tales of man-eating wolves. That night, Dunlop slipped into the darkness and proceeded to howl from every point of the compass. Smith was so agitated that he flung himself upon his horse and fled in almost as many directions, until he was swiped out of the saddle by an overhanging branch. Smith never again attempted to supervise "the Tiger," enabling Dunlop to go on enjoying the free life of a Canadian settler, "which is lacking in a more civilized country."

Such sentiments, expressed in his best-known work, *Statistical Sketches of Upper Canada* (containing hardly any statistics), did much to attract settlers to Canada, especially to the area he was particularly interested in, the Huron Tract, which was roughly between Stratford and Lake Huron. He built his own house near Goderich, and nobody was allowed to pass the front door without being dragged in for a meal, or a gallon of whisky, or both.

By then he had brought his brother Robin to Canada, and the two of them were faced with a delicate problem. They had a housekeeper, Louisa McColl, staying with them. Though Louisa, who was as affectionate as she was sharp-tongued, was forty years old, the neighbours felt that it was not right for a single lady to share a house with two eligible bachelors, and the brothers were continually being nudged with hints to this effect. Neither was keen on marrying, but they recognized that Louisa had brought splendid domestic order to their wild paradise, and they were reluctant to see her swept out by the broom of propriety. They agreed that one of them would have to wed her. But which? They decided to toss for her, the loser to get the merciful beldame. He turned out to be Robin.

It was in the same house that Dr. Dunlop made his famous will, in which, "being in sound health of body, and my mind just as usual (which my friends who flatter me say is no great shakes at the best of time)," he left his property to his sisters Helen and Elizabeth, "the former because she is married to a minister who (God help him) she henpecks. The latter because she is married to nobody, nor is she like to be, for she is an old maid, and not market rife.

"I leave my silver tankard to the eldest son of old John, as the representative of the family. I would have left it to old John himself, but he would melt it down to make temperance medals, and that would be sacrilege—however, I leave my big horn snuff-box to him: he can only make temperance horn spoons of that.

"I leave my sister Jenny my Bible,... and when she knows as much of the spirit of it as she does of the letter, she will be another guise Christian than she is....

"I leave Parson Chevasse (Magg's husband) the snuff box I got from the Sarnia Militia, as small token of my gratitude for the service he has done the family in taking a sister that no man of taste would have taken.

"I leave John Caddle a silver teapot, to the end that he may drink tea therefrom to comfort him under the affliction of a slatternly wife."

And so forth. Louisa was naturally mentioned in his will as well, but without comment, because as W. H. Graham says in his biography of Dunlop, "the reference to Louisa in the original draft of the will was so outrageous she flew into one of her famous rages and pursued the Tiger about the kitchen, beating and scolding him until he then and there revised it to its present simple form, showing 'more respect for her reverence.'" When the other heirs read or heard of the will, no doubt they must have wished that they had been on the scene as well, to effect similar emendations.

Dunlop's medical career began at Glasgow University when he was fourteen. He completed it in London to enable him to pass the army medical exams and qualify as an assistant surgeon. He had anticipated a trip to Spain to fight Napoleon. Instead, he found himself in a country that entranced him from his first glimpse of its loon-lonely rivers and the fan-tracery of its cathedral-high forests.

In 1813, the Canadian-American war was at its height, or depth—the incompetence on the one side nicely balancing the ineptitude on the other. Shortly after Dr. Dunlop's arrival in Montreal, the first real threat to the city developed with the American crossing of the St. Lawrence, eighty miles up river. It could be justifiably said about most of the British Army leaders that they had every soldierly quality except skill, knowledge, imagination, dash, intelligence, and prudence; but on this occasion they acquitted themselves splendidly at the Battle of Chrysler's Farm, and the American invasion was repulsed. Dunlop was despatched from Montreal to look after the men who had been wounded during the battle. For the first time he was called upon to put his surgical training into practice, and he was charactistically candid about the results. "My patients gradually began to diminish," he wrote. "Some died, and these I buried—some recovered by the remedies employed, or spite of them."

Dunlop may have fallen instantly in love with the silent beauty of the Canadian forests, but he was always careful not to let the same emotion get out of hand in his relations with women, or "the fair," as he called them. He was determined to remain a bachelor all his life. Not that he was above amorous dalliance. While attending to the Chrysler's Farm wounded, he boarded in the same house as a Pennsylvania Dutch lass, whom he courted with a boisterousness that somehow suggested that he was not really to be taken too seriously as a lover. His kisses were hearty rather than insinuating. In fact his friends compared the sound of these osculatory assaults to "the slap of a wet brogue against a barn door."

Dunlop's first Canadian winter was otherwise uneventful, but he was vastly enjoying the frontier life, especially as he could drink all he liked and nobody seemed too worried about his disheveled appearance. When he first arrived in Montreal he was quite reasonably caparisoned in a red coat, white trousers, and cocked hat. Unfortunately he was still a growing lad, and his giant fists were pushing further and further out of his scarlet sleeves, while his red hair continued to flourish six feet three inches above his gaitered pedal extremities.

This was the sight that greeted his next hostess, Peggy Bruce, when he took up quarters in a log hotel in Cornwall in the spring of 1814. "Peggy," he wrote, "was the daughter of a respectable Irish farmer, and had made runaway match with a handsome young Scotch sergeant. She had accompanied her husband through the various campaigns of the revolutionary war, and at the peace, his regiment being disbanded, they set up a small public house, which, when I knew her as a widow, she still kept....

"Bred in the army, she still retained her old military predilection, and a scarlet coat was the best recommendation to her good offices. Civilians of whatever rank she deemed an inferior class of the human race, and it would have been a hard task to have convinced her that the Lord Chancellor was equal in dignity or station to a Captain of Dragoons."

Already sharply individual himself at the age of twenty-three, Dunlop recognized a character when he met one. Peggy was a properly vigorous product of the frontier life. She was quite likely to take a broom to any guest she did not like, but there was nothing she wouldn't do for the ones she did, as Dunlop somewhat ruefully discovered. "It was my luck," he said, "to be a prodigious favorite with the old lady; but even favor with the ladies has its drawbacks and inconveniences, and one of these with me was being dragged to the bedside of every man, woman and child who was taken ill in or about the village. At first I remonstrated against my being appointed physician—extraordinary to the whole parish, with which I was in no way connected; but Peggy found an argument which, as it seemed perfectly satisfactory to herself, had to content me. 'What the d—l does the king pay you for, if you are not to attend to his subjects when they require your assistance?'

"I once, and only once, outwitted her. She woke me out of a sound sleep a little after midnight, to go and see one of her patients. Having undergone great fatigue the day before, I felt very unwilling to get up. At first I meditated a flat refusal, but I could see with half a glance, that she anticipated my objections, for I saw her eye fix itself on a large ewer of water in the basin stand, and I knew her too well for a moment to suppose that she would hesitate to call in the aid of the pure element to enforce her arguments. So I feigned compliance, but pleaded the impossibility of my getting up, while there was a lady in the room. This appeared only reasonable, so she lit my candle and withdrew to the kitchen fire, while I was at my toilet. Her back was no sooner turned, than I rose, double-locked and bolted the door, and retired again to rest, leaving her to storm in the passage, and ultimately to knock up one of the village doctors, whose skill she was well persuaded was immeasurably inferior to any Army medical man."

But over the next few days Dunlop had such a rough time of it from her broom and tongue, that he was finally forced to promise not to do it again. To make sure that he did not, on the next occasion Peggy remained in his bedroom, watching him like a hawk while he stumbled, mumbling, into his underwear.

Even then his tribulations were not over with. Peggy had decided medical opinions of her own, and insisted that he consult her before treating the patient, "which, like many other medical consultations," Dunlop observed, "generally ended in a difference of opinion."

Peggy's method was to feed the patient with as much food as could be stuffed into him, by bullying and cajolery. A herb bath with herbs infused in it was her favourite remedy, while, "Her concluding act at the breaking up of the consultation was generally to dive into the recesses of a pair of pockets of the size and shape of saddle bags, from which, among other miscellaneous contents, would she fish up a couple of bottles of wine which she deemed might be useful to the patient." Finally when the patient had been rendered suitably turgid, the consultants would retire to the log hotel to congratulate each other and reward themselves with hot brandy and water.

In the summer of 1814, Dunlop was despatched to Butler's Barracks at Queenston to take care of the wounded, following the Battle of Lundy's Lane. Though it must have been obvious that most of the fighting would take place on the Niagara Peninsula, most of the army medical support service had been held back at Quebec. Dunlop found himself having to care for scores of badly wounded men without medical equipment, except for what he carried with him, and assisted only by a sergeant. He obtained what he could from the local people in the way of beds and bandages, and worked for two days and nights in the hot, miasmic barracks, hurrying from patient to patient, from straw mattress to tiered bunk, probing for musket balls, tweezering cloth shreds from ragged wounds, and doing amputations, some of which would have been unnecessary if he had had more time and more help. On the morning of the third day he was so exhausted that he keeled over and slept, with one arm around a bedpost. As it was impossible to wake him, he was allowed to snore ebulliently for a few hours.

From Queenston, Dunlop was sent to Chippawa, near Niagara Falls. "My duty here," he informs us, "was to keep a kind of medical boarding house. The sick and wounded from the Army were forwarded to me in spring waggons, and I took care of them during the night, and in the morning I forwarded them on to Niagara by the same conveyance, so that my duty commenced about sun-set, and terminated at sun-rise."

The duty also made him restless. Dunlop had an appetite for adventure proportional to his enormous frame. He delighted in the independent frontier life, and in eloquent, roistering company. He was not likely to find this in a hospital. Accordingly he offered to change places with another surgeon, who was attached to an infantry unit that was preparing to attack Fort Erie, then in American hands.

Dunlop could not help noting the eagerness with which his opposite number agreed to the exchange of postings; but the other's evident relief failed to warn him. He duly reported to his new commanding officer, and looked forward excitedly to the coming night assault on the fort. The experience changed the direction of his life. "I had not proceeded many yards," he wrote of the attack, "when I stumbled over a body, and on feeling, for I could not see, I discovered he was wounded in the arm and the blood flowing copiously. He had fainted and fallen in attempting to get to the rear. I flexed a field tourniquet on his arm, and throwing him over my shoulder like a sack, carried him to a ravine in rear, and delivered him to the care of a Naval Surgeon I met with there."

Instead of remaining at the dressing station, Dunlop rejoined the infantry, and had just reached the fort when the powder magazine went up. "At first I thought it was a shell had burst close to me, for the noise was not greater if so great as that of a large shell; but the tremendous glare of light and falling of beams and rubbish soon demonstrated that it was something more serious...those not killed by the shock fell on the fixed bayonets of their comrades in the ditch, and thus, after we were in possession of the place, in one instant the greater part of our force was annihilated."

Braving a metallic blizzard of grape, canister, and shot, Dr. Dunlop did what he could for some of the wounded, and carried others to safety; but the activity, though satisfying the man of action, did nothing for the medical man. It is likely that the experience had a much greater impact on him than he was prepared to admit in his memoirs. One of the casualties of the battle was his interest in medicine.

Admittedly he returned to the profession a few years later, to deliver a course of lectures on forensic medicine in Edinburgh, to the delight of the students, who found his methods unforgettable, the lectures being a heady mixture of fun and learning, law and science, "blended with rough jokes and anecdotes not always of the most prudish nature." But the lectures were inspired not by a devotion to medical science but by pressing economic reasons. He needed the money.

Still, he deserves a place in the story of Canadian medicine, for it was as a surgeon that he experienced that love at first sight for the Canadian scene that was to lead to a worthwhile contribution to its cultural and economic development. If he lost interest in opening up patients, there were compensations. He helped to open up the country instead.

A surprising number of early medical men abandoned the profession. Some, like the previously mentioned Dr. Baldwin, did so on the grounds that there was not enough work for them in medicine, but most of them took on what they considered to be more important work in government. Whereas Brtish doctors tend to become authors, Canadian doctors tend to become politicians. Given the state of affairs in Upper and Lower Canada, politics often *was* more important. The fortunes of Lower Canada were determined by a clique of French seigneurs and Scottish businessmen who were not sufficiently sensitive to the interests of the rest of the population, while Upper Canada was governed by an impervious establishment of churchmen, legal types, and various privileged toadies huddled around the lieutenant-governor, most of them with far too large a share of the available land, votes, money, and legislative power.

By the 1830s, the demand for political change had become raucous. The Reformers compared the second-rate oligarchy with the thriving Republic to the south, and found it wanting. Instead of an Andrew Jackson they had a spokesman for privilege, Bishop Strachan, and a lieutenant-governor, Francis Bond Head who, it was rumoured, had been appointed in error. The appointment was supposed to have gone to a brilliant fellow named Edmund Head, but the colonial secretary had made a mistake and sent his message to Francis, thus giving the wrong Head his head.

Dr. Charles Duncombe was one Reformer who objected strenuously to the result. By 1836 he was so unhappy about the appointment that he traveled to London to present a petition to the Imperial Parliament, urging the recall of Bond Head. He presented sufficient proof of the lieutenant-governor's unsuitability for the position to make a considerable impression on the government, but the colony sputtered into armed revolt before they could do anything about it—unfortunately for Duncombe, who was implicated in that 1837 rebellion.

Duncombe was another doctor to abandon medicine for politics. A benign, round-faced native of the United States who had settled in Burford a few years after the War of 1812, Duncombe was one of the first to be passed by the medical board that had been set up in 1818 to regulate the profession. He was sufficiently well thought of to be appointed subsequently to the board himself. For a while he continued in private practice in the Brantford area, where his skill in physic and surgery and his sympathetic manner made him a rich man, though as Canniff quickly points out he was no money-grubber, but "would ride mile after mile, through swamp and forest, to visit patients too poor to give a fee."

In 1834, "his popularity caused him to be sought out as a fitting person for parliamentary honours." Actually, according to Edwin Seaborn in his *March of Medicine in Western Ontario,* Duncombe had made an attempt to climb into Parliament ten years previously, using Colonel Thomas Talbot as a stepladder. Talbot was the famous backwoods baron who governed a vast realm along the shore of Lake Erie, issuing curt, unquestionable orders to his tenants from a log manor-house named Castle Malahide. To achieve election, Duncombe needed the local support that Colonel Talbot could easily supply, merely by ordering his settlers to supply it. (In those days the elector did not cast his ballot in secret. He was required to call out his preference for a candidate in public at the hustings, so there was no way for the settlers to double-cross the old man.) There was just one snag. Duncombe had mild Reform sympathies, while the feudal chief was loyal to the Family Compact. Which was hardly surprising, as it was the Family that had made it possible for him to acquire somewhat more than his fair share of crown land—650,000 acres, instead of the usual fifty.

To overcome the difficulty, Duncombe and an equally radical friend of his, Dr. John Rolph, devised a little plot. First they got into the colonel's good books by organizing a lavish and festive picnic to celebrate Talbot's accomplishment in attracting immigrants to the Lake Erie region and forcing them to build roads, mills, and bridges. The picnic, attended by settlers from a hundreds miles around, was a great success, and pleased the colonel immensely. While he was in one of his rare benign moods, Rolph then proposed that Talbot should further immortalize his name by supporting a medical clinic for the poor, to be called The Talbot Dispensatory. And while he was at it, why not subsidize a few improving lectures to the public, for a fee of say, a bushel of produce? Before Talbot knew what was happening, the dispensatory had become a medical school with staff members and twelve students. Duncombe lectured on the theory and practice of medicine, and Rolph on anatomy and physiology.

But, as Seaborn puts it, "The colonel by now had smelt a rat. The scheme had been to secure the political support of the colonel for the election of Dr. Duncombe to Parliament and in support of the Reformers." And when that d——d Reformist journal, *The Colonial Advocate*, started to publicize the two doctors, Talbot's suspicions were confirmed. He withdrew his support, and Duncombe failed in this first election bid—though his friend Rolph succeeded in reaching the Legislative Assembly later that year.

Ten years passed before Dr. Duncombe reached the legislature, where he quickly made his mark. Though a reformer, he was not then an extremist like that fellow William Lyon Mackenzie, the mayor of Toronto. Duncombe thus avoided the fate of several others of his ilk, who, though properly elected, were repeatedly denied a seat in the House. He was certainly considered fit enough to be appointed, in 1836, along with two other doctors, to an important commission which was charged with evaluating American educational methods.

Unfortunately from the point of view of the governing clique, the research trip to the United States also reinforced Charles Duncombe's impression that the colonial system he was representing was sadly deficient, compared with the American system; and to notice that while President Jackson was handing over more and more power to the people, the Family Compact was just as enthusiastically withdrawing it. He returned from the United States convinced more than ever that he was serving a second rate oligarchy. The Goderich pier was a good example of the way the clique ran the province. Little work had been done on it—until the lieutenant-governor was scheduled to pay a visit. Whereupon the contractors, the Canada Company, hastily allocated additional men to the project, so that when the governor arrived there was a scene of most impressive activity, the air vibrant with barked orders and the thud of pile drivers and the chip-chip of busy adzes. The governor was then taken to the Colbourne Bridge, which, after a delay of about a dozen years, was now supposed to be in the process of construction. The lieutenant-governor's retinue however, took him the long way round. This was to enable the contractors to transfer the same workman from the pier to the bridge. Luckily the lieutenant-governor failed to recognize any of the men. He was really impressed by all the activity, which, of course, resumed its former sluggish pace as soon as he had departed.

The governing clique was often tyrannical as well as self-seeking. One of its victims was the reformer Robert Gourlay. He had been ordered to leave the country after uttering several fiery, anti-government speeches and newspaper articles. When he refused to exile himself, he was jailed and kept in solitary confinement throughout the winter in an unheated cell, with little ventilation and no light whatsoever. When he was finally brought into court the following August he was a wreck of a man.

Dr. Duncombe's work on the education commission was highly praised, but his journey to London the same year, to complain about Sir Francis Bond Head and the Family Compact, was not viewed with nearly so much approval. It was indignantly pointed out in the legislature that he had no right to claim that he had been speaking for all Canadians in demanding constitutional reform. But the medical profession sticks together, even in politics. Several other doctors supported him, including Dr. Baldwin, who not only endorsed Duncombe's demands for reform but his violent attack on Bond Head.

Thus the doctor-reformers, with a few notable exceptions, such as Tiger Dunlop who thoroughly enjoyed the *status quo,* had considerable support from their colleagues. Most of them, however, stopped short of treason. Duncombe did not. He became the leader of the rebels in the western part of the province. When the rebellion broke out in 1837 he attempted to raise an armed insurrection in support of William Lyon Mackenzie.

The result was as farcical as Mackenzie's effort in Toronto, and Duncombe was forced to flee. For a month he lay concealed at the house of his sister, Mrs. Shennick, a few miles from London, until a friend, Tilden, persuaded him to make a dash for the border. But he could hardly travel as himself, for by then a reward of £500 had been offered for his apprehension as a traitor. All over the district the Indians of the Grand River Reserve were on the lookout for his scalp and the blood-money it would bring. Duncombe decided to disguise himself as a farmer's wife. His smooth, round face made the impersonation plausible enough—though Mrs. Shennick thought that his aggressive stride perhaps needed a little work.

Next morning, accompanied by Tilden, Mrs. Shennick and her nine-year-old daughter, the medical female impersonator set off in a box-sleigh. Tilden drove, while Duncombe and his sister sat side by side, gossiping nervously, and Mrs. Shennick's little girl repeatedly addressed him, as she had been instructed to do so, as "Auntie." "All day they drove through the countryside without molestation. At night they stopped at a country hotel where, there not being sufficient accommodation, Charles Tilden had to sleep with one of the hotel-keeper's boys, while the three 'womenkind' had a room to themselves. Unable to sleep from the excitement of his position, Dr. Duncombe sat up all night. At early dawn they drove away breakfastless, and arrived, after a journey of several hours, at the crossing place, which was at a village opposite what is now

Marine City, Michigan. They drove into the yard of a tavern where were the soldiers of a party in command of a sergeant, posted there to watch the crossing place, and, if possible, arrest the 'rebel' chief. Very calmly Tilden watered his horses, and then addressed the sergeant in command as 'Captain,' asked if the ice was safe, and if he would kindly send one of his men to guide them to the right track. The sergeant asked whence he came. Tilden replied, truly enough, that he came from London, and was going with his aunt and mother, to visit some friends, whose names he mentioned, on the opposite coast of Michigan. The sergeant ordered one of his men to accompany them across the ice. When they had got half way across the river, the young soldier said that they could easily find their way for the rest of the track, and was about to leave them. Dr. Duncombe handed Charles Tilden fifty cents for the soldier, and while the latter was thanking them, felt very much inclined to send Dr. Duncombe's compliments to the sergeant who had furnished them with a guide, but refrained, lest he should spoil the chance of some other unfortunate, who might try the same stratagem for evading the blood-hounds of the Family Compact government."

A few minutes later Dr. Duncombe was on free soil, though he had one more small ordeal to undergo. When the Americans realized that there was a man under the skirts and bonnet, they insisted on his standing up in the village square and making a speech in his woman's dress. No doubt Duncombe felt that this was a small price to pay for having escaped almost certain death at the hands of the vengeful authorities.

Duncombe's friend John Rolph was implicated in the rebellion as well, and was also forced to flee. On his way to safety across the Niagara River he was captured by the loyalists, and was only saved by the intercession of some former students of his. They argued with Rolph's captors that a great man like Dr. Rolph could not possibly have been involved in the uprising.

Rolph's persuasive appearance aided and abetted their arguments. "He had a noble and handsome countenance," according to Dent, in the *Story of the Upper Canadian Rebellion,* "a voice of silvery sweetness and great power of modulation...a pair of deep, clear blue eyes, surmounted by rather heavy eyebrows, glanced out from beneath his smooth and expansive forehead. He had light brown hair, a well-moulded chin, a firmly set nose, and a somewhat large and flexible mouth, capable of imparting to the countenance great variety of expression."

Convinced that someone as noble and handsome as Rolph could not have been involved in such a sordid affair, the soldiers let him go, and he was able to make his escape across the Niagara River. Had it not been for the students, the loyalists would have found themselves the captors of the second most important figure in the reform movement. It is quite possible that Dr. Rolph would have become chief of the provisional government that was to be declared as soon as the rebels had seized the loyalist arms in the City Hall and imprisoned its chief officials.

Dr. Rolph tended to create turmoil wherever he went. "Throughout the turbulent history of Upper Canada whenever there was a controversy John Rolph was in its midst, and if there was no controversy, John Rolph succeeded in creating one." His very first appearance on the continent created alarm and confusion. While on his way from England to Canada via New York, the American authorities took one look at the nineteen-year-old, and promptly accused him of being a spy. Presumably John had not yet developed that nobility of countenance. After serving as paymaster for the London district during the 1812 war, he returned to England where he studied not only medicine but law, and qualified in both. Returning to Canada, he practiced these professions simultaneously until 1828, when he stormed out of the courtroom forever, following an adverse verdict from a Mr. Justice Sherwood.

Though a competent physician, Rolph's talents and ambition inclined him toward teaching rather than practice. His association with Duncombe at the school in the Talbot settlement was his first experience of teaching, and the ambition to establish a school of his own sustained him throughout his subsequent political career and exile. After an amnesty for the rebels was declared, he returned to Canada, and founded the second of Toronto's confusing complex of medical schools. It was located in his house on Lot Street (Queen Street). The accommodation was shared by his horse and a cow.

It had become increasingly obvious over the years that Upper Canada badly needed a medical school, if only to counteract "the evil and danger of the young men of Upper Canada going to the U.S. for a medical education" (where the young men might be infected with democratic ideals). The only tuition available in the province was through the apprenticeship system, where a pupil would be taken on by a general practitioner and trained on the job. Initially, much of the apprentice's work was of a humble nature: fetching and hauling, looking after the horse, digging his master out of the snowdrifts, or putting him to bed after a tavern carousal. Gradually the apprentice would progress to dressing wounds, pulling teeth, and bleeding the feverish, familiarizing himself with the materia medica and learning to make up unguents and ointments, tinctures and plasters, and to pound raw roots and bark.

When he had completed the contract with his preceptor, there was then nothing to stop him from going into practice for himself. Even after the establishment of the medical board, many pupils simply ignored its examinations and set up shop regardless, to practice the art of looking as if they knew what was wrong, and to render accounts such as the one that was sent to the widow Gould, which read, "To Dr., For Medsin and attendants whene he was chokd with a large pease of Butter no of meat, £3."

Such an apprenticeship system was hardly likely to produce doctors who were up to European standards; hence an increasingly urgent need for medical schools. The first true medical school was the Montreal Medical Institution, later absorbed by the Medical Faculty of McGill University. Upper Canada's first medical department was established in King's College, Toronto, whose president was that pillar of the undeserving rich, Bishop Strachan—still laying down the law in the 1840s, despite the increasingly effective reform agitation. His school taught theology as well as the normal medical subjects.

For once, however, Strachan did not have it all his own way, and by 1850 he was storming across the Atlantic to complain to the Imperial Government that the new University of Toronto had ruined his King's College, "whose Royal Charter it has repealed, under the pretence of amending it, and whose endowment of eleven thousand per annum it has seized and appropriated to itself." His contacts in London smiled, sympathized warmly, and did nothing about it whatsoever.

John Rolph's school further infuriated the bishop. It was competing all too effectively for the few available students. With his redoubtable intellectual powers, a style of eloquence at once ornate and almost abnormally logical, and a majestic presence, Rolph was proving to be a truly inspiring instructor in the science of medicine.

Strachan, though, had one useful weapon. He controlled the medical board. Rolph's students found it increasingly difficult to get past the board, while the students of Strachan's King's College, who were certainly no more knowledgeable in chemistry, mathematics, materia medica, anatomy, physiology, obstetrics, practical anatomy, and surgery, were sailing through the exams.

The struggle for power between the various rival medical schools (which changed their names and allegiances so often it was hard to tell which was which) continued for some years. Rolph was by no means innocent of scheming and skulduggery himself. Halfway through the century he had talked his way back into politics. Three years later he was using his influence in the government to clobber his enemies. At one point he suppressed the medical faculty of the University of Toronto.

He finally had his come-uppance in 1870, when his school forcibly became the medical department of Victoria University. It's new dean: none other than our Dr. Canniff.

In his book, Canniff deals tactfully with the upheaval that finally ended Rolph's often pernicious influence. He describes at length the opening ceremonies of the Victoria University Medical Department, and ends up by quoting himself. Responding to a toast by the late venerable dean, the Hon. Dr. Rolph, he writes, "He [Dr. Canniff] referred to the many excellencies of the veteran teacher of medicine, [Dr. Rolph], whose ability to teach he had never seen equalled in the new or old world. He concluded by expressing not alone his personal regret...that the hope always entertained by them that Dr. Rolph should continue to hold, as long as he lived, his position of Dean, had been unfortunately destroyed."

The truth behind this kindly obscurity was that the staff had become so fed up with Rolph that they all resigned, forcing him into retirement.

Though a high proportion of Upper Canada practitioners were political radicals, not all of them despised the establishment. The one who set the best example that evolution achieves more in the end than revolution, was an old regimental surgeon, Christopher Widmer.

Medical men enjoy labels just as much as art critics, and Widmer's tag was the Father of Surgery in Upper Canada; though in fact there is little specific evidence of his skill, except through the assertions of his contemporaries. One of them was Francis Mewburn who knew Widmer when he was on the staff of the York Hospital (later the Toronto General). He described Widmer as stalking the wards in riding breeches, top boots and riding crop. (He probably operated in this costume as well.) Mewburn added that Widmer "was notorious for two things, his awful swearing and his good surgery. His theological views at that age were looked upon with horror. But he was an amazing favourite with the ladies, and also, I believe, with old Dr. Strachan. That only proves that old ladies and parsons rather prefer their doctor to have a certain quantity of the devil in him; and old Widmer had it fully developed. However, he was kind and attentive to the sick poor, never neglecting them; and no doubt this covered a multitude of sins. I saw him amputate a thigh for a gunshot wound of the knee. There was secondary haemorrhage and the man died."

But then, of course, those were the days of, "In surgery, no chloroform; and no words can express the unspeakable horror of some of our cases; no pulley and weights for broken thighs; no regular wound drainage; no opening into joints; no hot water to stumps; but there was good surgery even then." And Widmer was as highly qualified as any surgeon on the continent, with a fellowship in the Royal College of Surgeons.

There are more specific accounts of the work of another F.R.C.S., William Rawlins Beaumont, who arrived in Toronto four years after the rebellion, and who might just as easily be categorized as the Father of Surgical Instruments in Upper Canada. He invented instruments for tying polyps, a pair of sliding iris-forceps, a speculum, and a probe-pointed lithotomy knife. The most interesting to a layman was an instrument for passing sutures (the material used to sew parts of the living body) in deep-seated parts, as, for instance, in his operation for cleft palate. Beaumont first demonstrated it in 1838. It was reputed by Tiemann, the surgical instrument-maker of New York, to have been the origin of the machine which Isaac Singer patented thirteen years later.

Beaumont's instrument was described in an 1866 issue of the *Lancet*, showing that it could be used to sew a continuous chain of stitches. So Beaumont was probably right when he claimed that he had invented the principle of the Singer Sewing Machine.

10

Maritime Lancets

"A GREEABLE TO YOUR request, I examined the black man's skull," Dr. Moore reported at a 1784 trial in New Brunswick. "I am perfectly satisfied he was murdered."

The accused was a Nancy Mosley, who had attacked the victim with a "fork" — presumably a pitchfork. Dr. Moore had already shown the jury the damage it had done, for the jury were all spectators at the post-mortem. As it turned out, Nancy was found guilty of manslaughter, and her punishment was lenient. She was ordered to be branded on the thumb with the letter M, and was then set free.

Nothing else is known about Nancy Mosley, but the doctor, Sam Moore, was one of the fair number of American Loyalists who settled in New Brunswick, Nova Scotia and Prince Edward Island, to escape the sordid Republican experiment going on in the south. As the years passed, men of ambition, like Dr. Moore, must occasionally have wondered if they had made the right decision. The United States might be uncouth, intolerant and egalitarian, but, by george, it got things done. In 1817, while Andrew Jackson was acquiring large chunks of real estate for his compatriots by annexing Florida, the inhabitants of many a Canadian Maritime settlement were abandoning even what little land they owned. The settlers were demobilized soldiers who were not ready for the self-reliant life of the pioneer farmer. Admittedly, tilling the Maritime soil was exceptionally hard work. Too often the spade struck rock only inches below the splendid scenery. Still, there was always logging and the fishery to supplement a meager income. Nevertheless, too many of the former redcoats drifted to the comparatively easy life of the tavern-anddoxy-riddled towns, to search for an employer who would behave like an officer and tell them what to do.

The Atlantic provinces were not only largely populated by ex-soldiers but governed by them. The lieutenant-governors were likely to be former generals in Wellington's army. Naturally they had a fashionably low opinion of democracy. All the same they had nothing much to put in its place, except a transplanted privilege that was as out of place on the seaboard frontier as a string quartet at a barn-raising bee.

Maritime medical men, though, were energetic enough, judging by contemporary accounts of their lives and their achievements. One of them discovered a substance that was to light a continent, a by-product that today enables a native of Halifax to reach Vancouver faster than it took the pioneer physician to reach his patient fifty miles away.

The discoverer was stern, sidewhiskered Abraham Gesner, who set up in practice in Parrsboro in 1824, after an adventurous life that had already seen him twice shipwrecked in the British West Indies. The son of a loyalist colonel from New York, Gesner was born in Kentville in the Annapolis Valley. He had just returned from five years study at Guy's and St. Bartholomew's hospitals in London when he bought the house in Parrsboro.

If he was not as dedicated a physician as some of his confrères, it was only because of his passion for the glorious Nova Scotia landscape, and the secrets of its geological formations. He spent much of his time on field studies. A dozen years after establishing his practice, he published an account of the geology and minerology of the province that became a standard reference work. By then his reputation in this field was sufficiently high for the Prince Edward Island and New Brunswick authorities to invite him to conduct a geological survey of their provinces as well.

It was at Charlottetown that he first demonstrated his method of producing a liquid from coal that would burn in a lamp. In 1852 his experiments were sufficiently advanced for him to patent the substance, kerosene.

His progress then took an all-too-familiar when, unable to get financial backing for the production of kerosene in his own country, he moved to New York, where he surrendered his patents to the North American Gas Light Company, in return for a job as a consultant chemist. He returned to Nova Scotia about ten years later to teach natural history at Dalhousie University.

Many a Maritime doctor turned to other occupations, partly because the simple medicine of the time was not enough of a challenge for the superabundant mental energies so often produced by the Scottish Calvinist tradition; and perhaps to some extent because the life of a nineteenth-century Maritime physician was hard and materially unrewarding.

John Clarence Webster of Shediac, for instance, established a second career as a historian. A fellow New Brunswick man, Murray MacLaren, entered politics, and became a government minister. And Sir Andrew MacPhail turned to authorship.

MacPhail, born in rural Prince Edward Island in 1864, had a considerable impact on the intellectual life of English Canada prior to the First World War, through his work as a pathologist and as professor of the history of medicine at McGill, and through his creative and critical writings. (Author's note: my grandfather, the Reverend Mr. Murdoch Lamont, went to school with MacPhail in P.E.I., and MacPhail mentions him in his autobiographical work, *The Master's Wife*, as delivering a sermon in a Gaelic that some purists among the congregation found fault with, though MacPhail confides that he could detect no difference between the "pure" Gaelic and the minister's version.)

In the same work, MacPhail described his ability to make money by his pen even before he had graduated from McGill Medical School. "The danger of reading is that it engenders the desire to write," he wrote, "even if one has nothing to say." He earned enough as a graduate to pay his tuition expenses, and to save twelve hundred dollars besides. Part of this considerable sum was the proceeds from a competition organized by a newspaper, in which competitors were asked to submit essays for and against vivisection (experimentation, sometimes distressful, on living animals). MacPhail won first prize with his essay in favour of the practice. When nobody else argued effectively enough against vivisection, he entered a second essay condemning it — and won that first prize, as well. MacPhail had, as he wrote, "that fatal capacity to see the paradox of things, that is, both sides of the subject at the same time."

Another Maritime physician who turned to other fields of endeavour was Sir Charles Tupper of Amherst. He returned to general practice whenever he was defeated in his bids for political office, which was fairly frequently, but his heart was really in politics, which ultimately brought him the position of Conservative prime minister, in 1892.

Many of the Maritime provinces' early doctors were quite highly qualified, being members or licentiates of the Royal Colleges of Edinburgh, London, or Dublin. They exerted, in the words of one of them, Daniel Parker, "an elevating and salutary influence on the communities where they lived and laboured."

The inevitable quacks were almost as influential, in their own way. "These men were generally illiterate," Dr. Parker recalled, "but shrewd and insinuating, and would sometimes exert no small amount of influence on the simple-minded settlers, prejudicing seriously the interests of the qualified men and in many instances largely reducing the already meagre incomes of the latter.

"In those districts where the schoolmaster had not been abroad...the illiterate people were often led to believe that the educated man was the quack, while *he* had been born a doctor, and had received his knowledge of the healing art by intuition."

Dr. Parker went on to describe one such interloper "who had obtained a diploma from a western United States manufactory, whose portals had never been darkened by his presence; but on remitting $100 or $150, with a commendatory letter signed by several of his neighbours, received from the authorities of the so-called medical school the document he asked for—a diploma."

Parker cited an example of this man's diagnostic ability. The American doctor claimed that a certain child was suffering from a severe rupture. To treat it, the quack applied a truss with a strong steel spring, causing the child considerable pain. When Daniel Parker examined the boy, he concluded that the problem was not a rupture but a retained testis.

Such cases gradually convinced the public that a regularly qualified practitioner might just possibly be preferable to a doctor who had learned the art by "intuition."

Another kind of amateur practitioner made a rather more favourable impression. This was the Presbyterian minister, who had learned something of therapeutics during his college course in Scotland. Owing to the scarcity of doctors in remote areas, the ministers often substituted for them, and enthusiastically dished out Epsom salts, sulphur, molasses, and moral homilies. Dr. C. Lamont MacMillan recounted that in Cape Breton Island, all homes in the countryside had a spare bedroom ready for the Presbyterian minister on his monthly call. "It was the custom in winter to send the maid to that bed early in the evening to warm the bed," MacMillan said, quoting a predecessor. "When bedtime came, the hostess would awaken the maid and send her to her own room. In those times the Scottish clergy were not against a little good Scotch whisky on a cold winter night just before bed. On one occasion the wee drop must have been repeated, because the hostess forgot to wake the maid. The minister was given his candle, and he started for the spare bedroom. When he opened the door and saw the beautiful girl in bed, he raised his candle a little higher to make sure and said, 'Oh Lord, the companionship was good, the prayers were good, the whisky was good but this is certainly the height of highland hospitality!'"

Even as late as 1838, the system of medical apprenticeship still obtained in the Maritimes. Daniel Parker was one who commenced his career in this fashion. One of Nova Scotia's most prominent doctors, who did a great deal to improve the province's medical services, Parker was apprenticed that year to Dr. Almon of Halifax, to learn according to the indenture, "the science profession and practise of a physician, and the art and mystery of a surgeon, and the trade and business of an apoethecary and druggist…until the full end and term of four years thence ensuing….

"During all the term aforesaid," the contract continued, "the said Daniel McNeill Parker his said master faithfully shall serve after the manner of such an apprentice, his secrets conceal, his lawful and reasonable commands, everywhere, readily perform and obey, that his said master's goods or estate of any kind he shall not waste, embezzle, purloin or lend unto others and will not suffer to be wasted, embezzled, purloined or lent unto others without giving notice thereof to his said master. That he shall not frequent taverns or ale-houses or play at any unlawful games or contract matrimony."

Parker also had to pay Dr. Almon a hundred pounds.

At the conclusion of his term of indenture, Daniel Parker completed his studies at Edinburgh University. Home again, he expressed apprehension at the prospect of being sent out into the world to practice what had been preached to him. In that moment of fear and self-doubt, Parker confided to himself that after all those years of slogging and clinical analysis he felt he knew almost nothing. He longed to scuttle back to the comfort and safety of the morgue, ward, and lecture hall.

However, the necessity of earning a living had overcome his fears by the time he entered Halifax's apology for a hospital. This was the Poor's Asylum at the corner of Queen Street and Spring Garden Road.

"It was at this Poor House, under the direction of Dr. Almon, that I began 'to learn the rudiments,' drew first blood, and ere long became the Phlebotomist of the house. Those were the days," Parker said, "when the lancet (now an almost forgotten surgical instrument) was in constant use."

By Daniel Parker's time, the lancet, or its distant ancestors (flints, sharp roots, hardwood splinters) had been tapping into human veins for thousands of years. The ship of medicine had sailed across oceans of leeched, let, and cupped blood. Even to prehistoric man there seemed to be a wealth of signs to indicate that losing blood was good for you. For example, the beneficial effect of sucking blood from a snake bite wound. Garrison also remarks that, "the natural and periodic process of menstruation, suggested, no doubt, the advantages of blood-letting, which was to become a sort of therapeutic sheet-anchor through the ages."

One seventeenth-century medic, Guy Palin, kept score of his sanguinary endeavours. "He bled his wife twelve times for a fluxion of the chest, his son twenty times for a continued fever, himself seven times for a cold in the head, while his friends, M. Mantel and M. Consuiat, were bled thirty-six and sixty-four times in a fever and a rheumatism respectively." Two hundred years later, Dr. Francis Mewburn of Toronto was still tapping his patients by the bucketful, and, in retrospect remarking, "what recklessness there was at that time about bleeding."

In the Nova Scotia of Parker's day, the bloodletter was often an otherwise untrained man, "with his little sharp-pointed knife, which he carried in his vest pocket but sterilized in boiling water before using. He was always ready to draw his victim's blood, and to continue drawing it until the said victim fainted, or until the operator was satisfied that the so-called 'Inflammation' was removed. These men sometimes travelled great distances in pursuit of their voluntary calling: no matter what hour, whether day or night.... the call for extracting blood was responded to with the greatest alacrity."

Still, "they occasionally accomplished much good, and... the early opening of a vein by the *bloodletter* saved many a case of an inflammatory nature from advancing beyond the congestive stage," wrote Dr. Parker. Nowadays, bloodletting is occasionally employed in cases where blood cells are too abundant, or in conjestive heart failure where blood pressure needs to be reduced. The main objection to it as practiced in the past was not that it did much harm to the patient but that it was done to excess and for the wrong reasons. The medieval doctors and their successors believed that it eliminated the cause of disease—an imbalance in the "morbid humours," blood, yellow bile, black bile, and phlegm.

In 1845, the Poor's Asylum in Halifax, where Daniel Parker was chief bloodletter, and a dispensary, were the only medical institutions in the province. The asylum, Daniel thought, was a miserable place. As for Dispensary No. 1, it was no more than a dank room in a tiny, mildewed house. When it was destroyed by fire, he considered that, "the loss to the community was unimportant."

Parker was utterly frustrated by a lack of the facilities that he had gotten used to in Edinburgh. He could add almost nothing to his pathological knowledge, for post-mortem examinations were rare. The public was too hostile to the idea. He could do no histological work—the microscope was not in practical use. Even stethoscopes were rare—only the younger, up-to-date men had them. Perhaps most of all, he regretted the lack of periodicals and reference works. He had to make do with tired standbys, like Cooper's surgical dictionary, the published lectures of Astley Copper, *Bell on Wounds*, and *Lawrence on Hernia*.

In his later years, Parker did much to overcome these deficiencies, and was the main driving force behind the establishment of city and provincial hospitals. He also helped to found the Nova Scotia, Maritime, and Canadian Medical Associations. In the meantime, as a general practitioner, he did what he could, using his training and his memory, and sent his most difficult cases to American hospitals. In Halifax there were no surgical specialists to whom they could be referred. When he performed an operation himself, it was usually in primitive conditions, often in the middle of the night with only a tallow dip or candle for illumination, and with the unanesthetized patient strapped down, or held down by beefy neighbours. In one case the patient broke free, and Parker had to finish the operation on the floor.

The mode of transport was by horse. Dr. Parker kept three of them in a stable on Argyle Street, using them a day each in turn. During one ferociously cold night on a trip to Windsor, Dr. Parker was so worn out by nightly summonses from the bedside night bell, that he fell asleep and drooped over the horse's neck. He was held in place only by his saddle-bags. But, "many long and lonely rides by day and night had established a perfect understanding of each other and a mutual affection, and the horse, sensing his master's insensibility, moved carefully into shelter under a spruce tree, and remained there until daylight."

Occasionally he traveled in a light carriage, and if the journey was a long one, would transfer to post horses en route. One day, on his way to perform an emergency operation, he found that the only available horse at one coach house had recently attacked and injured its rider. For this reason, the innkeeper at first refused to hire it out, but Parker insisted on taking it. While traveling along a lonely stretch of road, the stallion started to thrash about in the harness, threatening to upset the carriage. Parker got out and tried to take it by the head, but the beast struck at him with its hooves. Parker was not noted for an phlegmatic temperament. In a fury, he darted in, and grabbed the reins close to the curb bit. At this, the choleric nag lost its temper completely, and reared again and again, swinging the doctor high into the air, then dashed him back to the road again, flailed at him with its hooves, and attempted to sink its yellow teeth into the doctor's hide.

Parker held on, by now aware that to let go could mean far worse injury than the animal's forelegs were already inflicting on him, until a wagonload of farmhands appeared and helped to bring the brute under control. Bruised, dizzy, and by now in a ferocious temper of his own, Parker lashed the stallion onward to the next post at full speed, until exhaustion finally took the stuffing out of it.

Another doctor, practicing in Cape Breton Island, described an incident where he had to roll his fallen horse part of the way, to get to a patient at North River Bridge. When the doctor reached South Gut in his horse and sleigh, there was a blizzard raging, and even the mail driver, Murdoch Dan, had given up. When the doctor and his driver, Jimmy MacIver, announced that they intended to press on, Murdoch reluctantly agreed to accompany them with his sleigh.

The trio floundered on through the storm. Two miles short of their destination they got stuck in a snowbank, whereupon the doctor's horse strained so hard that it broke the harness three times. Three times they had to take the horse out of the sleigh so that Jimmy could patch the harness. "Jimmy always carried an auger, leather straps, brads and a hammer with him, and he could patch up any harness that broke on a trip," the doctor said. "But we still couldn't get through the snowbank."

Then the horse fell, and this time was unable to rise. The trio were forced to seize the horse and roll it sideways over to the ditch, then across the ditch and up into the field where the snow was not so deep. There the horse finally managed to get its hooves onto solid ground, and struggled up.

On another occasion, the same doctor was on his way home after treating a girl who was suffering from pulmonary tuberculosis. He was driving "one of those dancing, prancing creatures, a beautiful horse, spirited and easy to drive, elegant to look at when in a sleigh." Crossing the ice at North River the horse went through it, followed by the driver, Red Roddie. While trying to rescue him, the doctor went into the water as well. Next, trying to get out, Roddie hauled the sleigh into the ruin, sending the doctor's bags to the bottom.

By the time help arrived, the two men had managed to clamber out but the horse had reared over backward and drowned. The rescuers found the doctor, still in his soaked sheepskin coat, attired in the brown paper that he had stuffed inside the front of the coat to keep warm. The doctor was just standing there, looking at the big hole in the ice and shivering. It was a long time before he would speak.

This was the late thirties. The late *nineteen* thirties.

The doctor, C. Lamont MacMillan, remembered that "In winter and spring my practise differed in no way from the days when the first pioneer doctors worked in the area." Accordingly his tale is one of hardship and of triumph over the geographic and climatic conditions that until recent times made the life of the Canadian country doctor unique in medical experience.

Dr. MacMillan first arrived in Baddeck in 1928, after graduating from Dalhousie University, Halifax. Gruff, abrupt, absent-minded, and possessed of a sixth sense as well as a "terrific bedside manner," he must have been as thoroughly admired by his hardworking, humorous Cape Breton patients as he was loved by them. He was dedicated to the point of selflessness.

One evening, he received a call from a lumber camp at Upper Baddeck River, where a man had chopped himself with an axe, and was bleeding badly. He set off in his sleigh, in a storm so severe that he could hardly breathe when facing into the wind. Inevitably he was held up on the way, this time by a fallen tree. There was no way around it through the woods. He considered unharnessing his mare, Gypsy Queen, and jumping it over the tree, but decided against it because he had two bags to carry, and no saddle. He had to lift the horse across in four stages, in turn picking up the hooves and lifting them up and over the tree trunk.

So there he was, with the mare on one side of the tree and the sleigh on the other. Not daring to lift the sleigh from the front in case the horse moved and pinned him against the trunk, he went behind the sleigh, "burrowed a deep hole through the snow, down to the ground, and then burrowed a hole up underneath the sleigh until I could crawl up to the front of the sleigh. Taking the sleigh on my shoulders, I raised it up enough so that I was half standing. I said, 'Get up.' The mare took one or two steps ahead and the sleigh was over the tree."

That was the easy part. After getting bogged down several times over the next mile, the mare got stuck in a snowbank and seemed unable to move. In trying to extricate it, MacMillan grew so exhausted that he had to give up temporarily. He picked up his bags and took shelter behind an abandoned community hall. "I was standing there, half bent over, panting for breath when something hit me in the back and hard enough to drive me headfirst into the snow. I couldn't imagine what it was. I lay there for a few minutes without daring to look around. I finally found the courage to turn around to see what hit me, and there was Gypsy Queen. When she had seen me go behind the building, she'd put an extra effort into getting out and followed me to shelter."

Unfortunately she had also overturned the sleigh, burying his buffalo robes, lantern, shovel, and the rest of his equipment. They were not recovered until the following May.

When MacMillan finally reached the lumber camp at midnight after digging out the horse once more, he found that his patient hadn't needed him after all. The axe laceration would have healed without stitches.

Like most country doctors, C. Lamont MacMillan was a man who could improvise. While at North River one day in 1946 he received a call to visit Red Jim MacNeil at Jamesville who had a piece of meat stuck in his gullet. Realizing that he would need an instrument called a bougie, but not having one with him, MacMillan called in at a garage on the way, and got the mechanic there to make him a makeshift instrument. With this in his wee black bag he continued on to the patient's home. Jim was having great difficulty in swallowing. After studying him for a few minutes, MacMillan urged him onto the kitchen table, then bent his head well backward, and told him to swallow. Just as he did so, MacMillan introduced the makeshift—a speedometer cable that the garage man had polished smooth on an emery wheel—and Red Jim obtained instant relief.

Frequently the weather was such that it was difficult to leave the scene of the emergency as it was to reach it in the first place. MacMillan was once called out, during a January thaw, to a house in Plaster, six miles from Baddeck. When he got there he found that the patient, Johnie, had a ruptured appendix. The problem was that the nearest hospital was at North Sydney, thirty-five miles distant.

With the patient and two helpers, Dr. MacMillan set out in his car for Ross Ferry, five miles away, intending to cross the Boulardarie. At first the captain of the ferry refused to cross in rough waters, but was persuaded to try. The doctor's helper, Roddie, who was driving the car (the doctor was not noted for his driving ability), studied the waves for several minutes, while the ferry pitched and tossed in the rough seas. His intention was to race the car over the edge of the wharf during the split-second that the ferry was exactly level with it.

He managed this exceedingly risky procedure, but just as the car drove off on the far side of the bay, the engine conked out, and they spent an hour in a rain storm drying out the distributor.

They continued on. "By this time, whenever we had to get out to shovel we were wading in snowbanks and slush up to our waists. There was a long snowbank at Big Bras d'Or through which we tried to push the car. We'd back up and then ram it ahead again and again. For a while we made progress, but then we seemed to come to an end of forward motion. I said to Roddie, 'Let me try.' I backed up about a half mile and got the car going. I hit that snowbank and drove in, I suppose, a hundred yards. Then the shaft broke. So there we were—in a crippled car, in a pouring rainstorm, with a man with a ruptured appendix in the back seat."

The other men went for help, and ultimately the patient was back in the old mode of conveyance, a horse and sleigh. At the other end of the snowbank they changed to another car, and finally arrived at the hospital after twelve hours on the road.

The patient recovered, and was home again in a few days.

It was conditions such as these that, right up to the 1950s, made the life of the Canadian country doctor one of spine-torturing effort. Small wonder that doctors such as C. Lamont MacMillan grew slightly ruthless where their own well-being, and therefore that of their patients, was concerned. His assistant in Baddeck, Phyllis Lyttle, a public health nurse, once reminded Dr. MacMillan that, "Regardless of whether there was a bed or not, you always managed to get a little sleep. If there wasn't a bed readily available, you would talk the expectant mother into getting up and taking a little walk. 'It'll be better for you,' you would say. And then as soon as she was out of bed you were in it."

Frequently the conditions were even worse for Phyllis. She had to keep the same hours as the doctor, but without the benefit of an occasional nap. "I remember an instance in 1941," MacMillan wrote, "when the nurse assisted me in three maternity cases, one after the other, without any chance for rest, although I got some sleep on each of the cases. These three cases kept me busy from some time during the day of June 19 until six o'clock in the morning of June 21."

The conditions also led to all sorts of trials and tribulations for the nurse. During one long confinement case that Miss Lyttle and Dr.

MacMillan attended, she was up all night while the doctor slept. In the morning at ten o'clock she disappeared and the patient was in heavy labour before she returned. MacMillan wondered where she had been.

With some embarrassment she confided in him that by mid-morning she desperately needed to use the toilet. She went out and followed the path over toward the outhouse in the woods, but after slogging part of the way through the knee-deep snow she was too tired to go on. Besides, she was out of sight of the house and there was nobody else around for miles. She decided that there was no need to go as far at the outhouse toilet. So she went a little way into the woods and tramped down a place in the snow. "Just then she happened to see two barrel staves there and she thought, 'That's a great place to put my feet.' The instant she got both her feet on the barrel staves, they began to slide, and she found herself, shooting down the slopes and through the trees, and over the brow of the hill and down." She lost the "skis" but kept on sliding wildly down the hill, and ended up in the shrubbery.

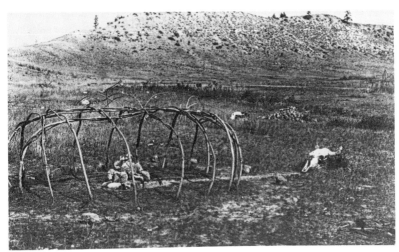

Sweat lodge frame: Cartier was impressed. (Public Archives Canada/C30233)

The famous Hôtel-Dieu. (PAC/PA65407)

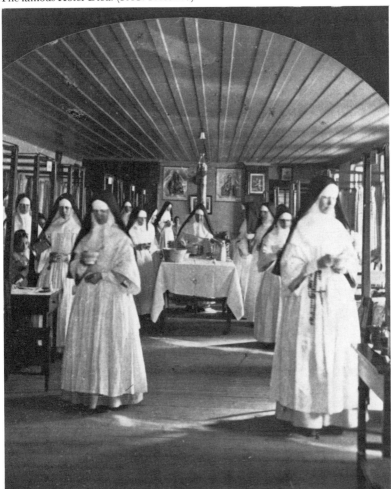

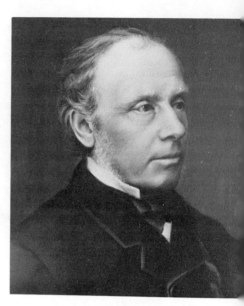

UPPER LEFT: William R. Beaumont of Toronto, who invented many ingenious surgical instruments. (Museum, Academy of Medicine, Toronto) LOWER LEFT: Upper Canada—the student examined. *Left to right,* Christopher Widmer, James Bovell, John King, George Herrick, Joseph Workman, and the candidate, John Gamble. (Museum, A of M) FAR RIGHT: Three impressions by English artist James Gillray of the state of medicine in 1804. "Breathing a Vein" (*top left*); "Gentle Emetic" (*top right*); "Brisk Cathartic" (*lower right*). (Museum, A of M)

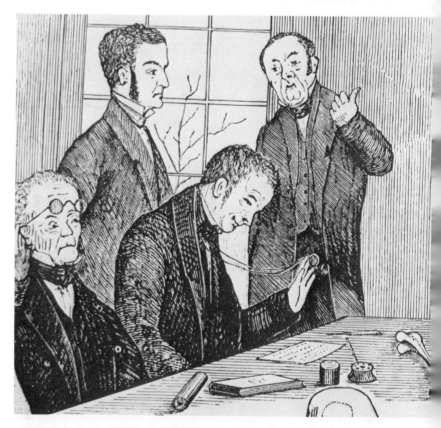

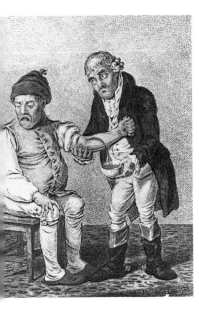

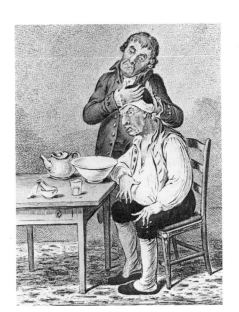

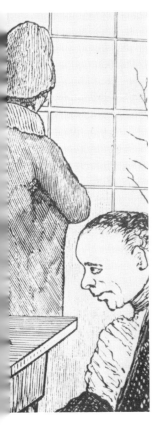

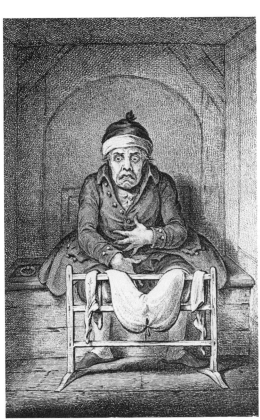

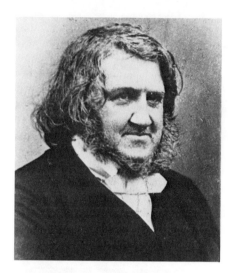

LEFT: Sir James Young Simpson, the discoverer of chloroform. (Museum, A of M) BELOW: Chloroform apparatus. (Museum, A of M)

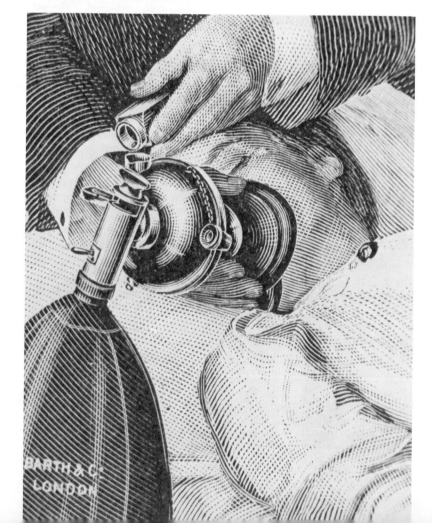

11

The Forty-Below Execution

THE START OF Dr. John Richardson's career as one of Canada's greatest explorers would not appear to have been particularly auspicious. During the first of the explorations that established his reputation as the founder of arctic biology, this graceful naval surgeon, naturalist, and man of letters, personally executed his Indian guide.

He was born in 1787 in the border town of Dumfries, the son of Gabriel Richardson, a brewer, who was on friendly terms with Robert Burns. Burns often visited the Richardson home on a Sunday evening to indulge in the old Scottish custom of memorizing psalms. On one occasion when the talk turned earthy—Burns and his host discussing the transitory nature of human existence—Burns took out a diamond-pointed pen, which he used for inscribing poetry on whatever glass surface happened to be handy. In this case it was a whisky tumbler, and Burns proceeded to write an epitaph on it, in verse.

John Richardson was the same age as the poet's son, and attended the same school. On the first day, the boys were escorted to school by their respective fathers. As they plodded along the road, Burns, in the eighteenth-century fashion of earnest philosophizing, speculated as to which of the boys was likely to become the greater man. His conclusion— for eighteenth-century philosophy required a firm conclusion, usually a complacently obvious one—is not recorded, but ten years later when John was a qualified surgeon on board H.M.S. *Blossom*, he must have felt entirely eliminated from the competition when he was accused of being privy to mutiny. The chances of his being destined even for mediocrity seemed slender, for the penalty for mutiny in the Royal Navy was death.

Blossom was Richardson's third appointment since receiving his licentiate from the Royal College of Surgeons of Edinburgh, and it was the most dangerous so far, not so much through the threat of enemy action as through the aberations of the captain. Captain Probyn was that not uncommon phenomenon in the Royal Navy of the Napoleonic era, a tyrant unbalanced by his own godlike power. Probyn was pathologically suspicious of his officers, a situation exacerbated by the machinations of a sycophantic purser, who spied on the officers and further inflamed the captain's paranoia with tattle-tales.

The captain became convinced that Dr. Richardson and the first and second officers were conspiring to take over the ship. Probyn was unable to place Richardson under close arrest, for he could not do without the services of the ship's surgeon, but he confined the other two officers throughout the voyage—for six months—under such vindictive restrictions that their health broke down.

At the court-martial in England, all three of the accused were exonerated. The behaviour of the captain had startled the court; that of the purser had made them deeply suspicious. It was Dr. Richardson who ended the purser's scheming ways. Despite his youth, Richardson must already have developed a force of personality, for he confounded the purser at the court-martial, by standing there and looking at him in silence. The purser was so affected that he "became confused, sick and fainted," as John later described the scene to his father. "After that he could not say another word, and was obliged to be taken out of court. The poor captain, who is nearly deranged, will long have cause to repent his having listened to the purser's tales."

In fact, Probyn was subsequently court-martialed himself, and dismissed from his command.

It was not the last time that the short, untidy surgeon with the broad cheekbones, wide mouth and gray eyes, and the mass of brown hair surging back from a high, sloping forehead, was to bring the carronade of his moral indignation to bear against a dangerous adversary.

In 1814 Richardson paid his first visit to Canada, when he was posted to a Royal Marine battalion at St. Jean on the Richelieu River, between Lake Champlain and the St. Lawrence. He made his way inland via Montreal at the same time that another Scots surgeon, Tiger Dunlop, was on his way to the fighting on the Niagara frontier. Richardson was as enthralled by the scenery as Dunlop. He was especially impressed by the distinctive French-Canadian churches, arising like silver halberds from the dark green woods. He thought they had a particularly fine appearance by moonlight.

From then on, though, he had little time to admire the tin spires, for he was involved in several forays into the United States. During the first two years of the War of 1812, a shortage of troops had forced the British to improvise in their tactics against the greatly superior American forces. Fortunately this uncomfortable strain on the British imagination was relieved in 1814, when twelve thousand of Wellington's finest fighting men arrived on the scene. With a handsome superiority, the British could, now, in the absence of a Wellington, squander their human resources, and overwhelm themselves with their own numbers.

It was the worst possible situation for a British general to find himself in, and the commander-in-chief, Sir George Prevost, was the worst available. Richardson was witness to the result of Sir George's attack from Montreal towards Lake Champlain. Prevost's progress was so sluggish, his tactics so cretinous, and his leadership so inept, that the Americans thought it was a trick to lull them into a state of shock and confusion. But the incompetence was entirely genuine. The attack was so bungled that in a rage, large numbers of Wellingtonian veterans stumped off into the sodden landscape to join the enemy.

Richardson was no more impressed by the overall strategy of the war, particularly that part of it that saw value in the burning of Washington, a reprisal for the attack on York. Luckily he had enough work to do to take his mind off the revenges and revanches of the conflict. In the winter of 1814, the prevalance of frostbite among the troops provided him with a great deal of experience in amputations. His references to frostbite, and "from seventy to eighty men ill at a time with chillblains" are among his few references to his actual work as a surgeon in North America.

It was his experience in caring for troops in a severe climate, and his high qualifications—he was an Edinburgh M.D., as well as an L.R.C.S. —that brought him an invitation to join Franklin's first expedition to the Canadian Arctic in 1819.

The purposes of the expedition were to determine the latitudes and longitudes of the Arctic coastline, to take scientific measurements, and to continue the search for the Northwest Passage. Part of the expedition was to journey by land, and another group, led by Lieutenant Parry, by sea. The expedition as a whole was under the command of Lieutenant John Franklin, R.N., a cheerfully religious friend of Richardson's, who had also served in North America in the War of 1812. Franklin's party would travel overland, via York Factory, and Fort Cumberland on the Saskatchewan River. Its members, besides Franklin and Dr. Richardson, included two other officers, George Back and Midshipman Robert Hood, and a staunch, loyal and hardworking seaman, John Hepburn. Additional help would be hired en route.

While Franklin went ahead with the advance party, Richardson spent the winter at Fort Cumberland. His most intense impression of this part of the country was the silence, a silence so deep that the sudden cry of an animal or trill of a bird had the shocking impact of an alarm bell. The loneliness of the land was another near-trauma. In a letter to his wife he said that, "When in my walks I have accidentally met one of my companions in this dreary solitude, his figure, emerging from the shade, has conveyed, with irresistible force, to my mind, the idea of a being rising from the grave. I have often admired the pictures our great poets have drawn of absolute solitude, but never felt their full force til now.... How dreadful if without faith in God."

Eight hundred miles ahead, at Fort Chipewyan, Franklin was fretting over other problems. He had anticipated friendly co-operation from the Hudson's Bay Company and the North West Company, but soon found that these commercial rivals were decidedly hostile to each other—though they were due to merge the following year—and totally indifferent to him. Franklin had much difficulty in obtaining supplies, transport, and local help. "The situation was not improved," according to Richardson's biographer, Robert E. Johnson, "by the discovery that a large amount of the provisions brought by Richardson had been eaten along the way by the French-Canadians."

The supply shortage was still a problem when Richardson joined Franklin's advance guard in July 1820. Nevertheless they pushed onward, up the Yellowknife River. On reaching Winter Lake, they prepared for another winter by building Fort Enterprise. It comprised a main building, a kitchen, a storehouse, and another dwelling for their party of French-Indian voyageurs, interpreters, and Copper Indians. The buildings were of logs plastered with clay, and the windows were fashioned from reindeer skin.

It was July 1821 before they obtained their first awed view of the Polar Sea. They had barely commenced their exploration of the coast eastward when their supernumerary Indians of the Copper tribe decided that they had ventured far enough into unknown territory, and took off. In Richardson's indignantly expressed opinion, they were deserters. The Indians, though, were far more aware of the dangers of a coastal journey than was Richardson.

For a while, the exploration went fairly well. In four weeks, Franklin and Dr. Richardson managed to survey 550 geographical miles of coast from the Coppermine River eastward, measuring terrestrial magnetism, recording temperatures, erecting cairns as guide-markers for ships, and ascertaining latitudes and longitudes of headlands and inlets along a coast that had never before been seen by white men. But low rations and foul weather finally forced the party of twenty Britons, French-Canadians, Indian and Eskimo interpreters, and the one cheerful and respectful Iroquois Indian, Michel, to turn back overland across the barrens.

On the way back, in gale winds and snow flurries, increasingly short of food and with no fuel except wet moss, Franklin made a grave mistake in navigation which cost them precious days, and took them close to the full fury of winter. "Now symptoms of distress became frequent," writes Johnson, "as cold, hunger and exhaustion weakened them. Loads were lightened by abandoning everything inessential including books and, inadvertently, the fishing gear. Richardson kept a bag of rocks and minerals he had collected on the shores of the Polar Sea, but a week later he did not feel strong enough to carry them any further. The going was hard. Feet in moccasins were cut to pieces by the rocky ground. Occasionally they found berries, partridge, rarely a deer, once a muskox. They could not fish. Their diet was mainly the lichen *tripe de roche* and 'swamp tea.' Diarrhea further weakened them, especially Hood and Vaillant. Oedema of the legs ('famine oedema') appeared. The party began to straggle. Franklin fainted once from exhaustion. He had to drop back at his own pace and Richardson took the lead, while Back and the hunters scouted ahead for game."

When they reached the Coppermine River it took them a week to cross it. Richardson attempted to swim across with a line round his waist, and almost made it before sinking in the icy waters. He was pulled out more dead than alive, and when the others removed his soaking clothes, "His emaciation astonished and grieved his companions, and it was the next summer before he recovered complete feeling in his left side. In the end a small canoe was made from willows and canvas and one by one they were carried across."

Desperately worried about the safety of his men, Franklin ordered George Back to forge ahead in company with the strongest of the French-Canadians, instructing him to pick up and return with the provisions that should by now have been delivered to Fort Enterprise. Franklin's party struggled on, but after two of the voyageurs had been lost, and when Robert Hood, the young midshipman, could no longer walk, a further split-up was decided upon. Dr. Richardson and the seaman, Hepburn, offered to stay behind with Robert Hood and look after him. The idea was that Franklin would continue on to Fort Enterprise and then return to the rescue with provisions from the fort.

Franklin agreed and said goodbye as Hepburn and the doctor pitched a tent and prepared for what they knew would be a long wait. Shortly afterward however, the Indian, Michel, appeared at Richardson's camp bearing a note from Franklin to the effect that he, Michel, and one of the French-Canadians, Jean Baptiste Belanger, were being sent back to join the doctor as they were no longer able to keep up.

But Michel, whose behaviour had greatly deteriorated over the past few weeks from a cheerful and helpful attitude to one of sullen resentment, arrived without his companion. When Dr. Richardson asked where

Belanger was, Michel said that the French-Canadian was missing. In the violent snowstorm of the past two days, he must now be presumed dead.

There then followed at Richardson's camp that October, a scene of hatred and violence that would live vividly in the memories of the two survivors. Only John Richardson and the sailor, John Hepburn, lived to tell the story when, giving up all hopes of being rescued, they struggled on and finally reached the comfort of Fort Enterprise on October 29, 1821; or what they hoped was comfort.

There they received a further shock. Franklin had managed to reach Fort Enterprise several weeks previously, but found what George Back had already discovered, that the North West Company had failed to ensure, as had been arranged, that provisions would be waiting there to see the expedition through the winter.

Dr. Richardson understood now why Franklin had failed to return to the rescue of his closet friend. When he saw the state that Franklin's party was in, he was appalled. It hardly seemed possible, but their condition was even worse than that of Richardson and Hepburn. Two of Franklin's French-Canadians had died of starvation within two days of their arrival at Fort Enterprise. Another two had succumbed to what Richardson had now come to recognize as the classic progress of malnutrition and cold stress—from emaciation and famine oedema to asthenia, decubitus ulcer, dementia, and finally, cardiovascular collapse.

"No words," Richardson wrote, "can convey an idea of the filth and wretchedness that met our eyes on looking around. Our own misery had stolen upon us by degrees, and we were accustomed to the contemplation of each other's emaciated figures, but the ghastly countenances, dilated eyeballs, and sepulchral voices of Captain Franklin and those with him were more than we at first could bear." Fortunately, Richardson had enough strength to take over at Fort Enterprise. He made John Franklin and the surviving voyageurs and interpreters as clean, dry, and comfortable as he could, and attempted to distract them from their sufferings by organizing religious services. For nourishment he went out every day to search for lichens. Fortunately there was no shortage of fuel for warmth and for drying clothes and blankets. It was only three months since they had put up the outbuildings of Fort Enterprise, for which the voyageurs had shaped tables and chairs with their knives and hatchets. Now this furniture was broken up for firewood.

Gradually, order and comfort were restored, and hope revived. As it turned out, the hope was justified, for nine days after Richardson reached Fort Enterprise, so did the Copper Indians, who, having been alerted by George Back, arrived with two sledges loaded with venison, fat, and tongue. Only then did Dr. Richardson tell Franklin exactly what had happened after Michel the Iroquois had turned up at the tent, five weeks previously.

When Michel arrived with the note from Franklin, Richardson, Robert Hood the midshipman, and John Hepburn were disturbed to hear that Michel's companion, Jean Baptiste Belanger, had become lost on the way in a snowstorm. However, their regret—and a vague uneasiness—were soon outweighed when they saw what Michel brought with him: food. And no ordinary food such as frozen scraps left by wolves and ravens, but delicacies associated with supper in a London club—meat said to be hare and partridge, killed just that morning, fresh and succulent and only slightly frozen.

The three white men were deeply religious. During the two days before Michel arrived, they had spent their time huddled in the stormbound tent, reading to each other from the few religious books they still had the strength to carry with them. Now they saw Michel as an instrument of God in the cause of their deliverance. George Hood was so grateful that he offered to share his buffalo robe with Michel. Richardson gave him one of the two shirts he wore. The sailor, John Hepburn, who did not entirely trust Michel, hoped fervently to find it in himself to love the man. After all, he had saved their lives, temporarily, at least.

But the story which began with such warmth of feeling and reverence, with morning and evening services, and with calm and cheerful conversation, "dwelling with hope on our future prospects," changed from love and gratitude toward the Iroquois guide, to a growing uncertainty about his attitude; and from uncertainty to mistrust; and finally from mistrust to dread. Robert E. Johnson's account, in its directness and simplicity, cannot be improved upon. The note that Franklin had sent back with Michel, he writes, "had recommended a change of camp to a stand of pines a mile further on, and in this laborious move, taking many journeys back and forth, Michel gave minimal help. He absented himself for long intervals and reappeared with specious excuses. He talked more and more of rejoining Franklin's party if only he knew the way. He grew increasingly idle and sullen until Richardson considered sending Hepburn with him, although by this time the non-arrival of Indian help made them fear for Franklin's survival.

"Michel's whole character had changed. Up to this period his conduct had been good and, as Richardson said, respectful to the officers, who indeed had earlier decided to reward him when they reached safety. Now he seemed to show by his tone and bearing that he held the three men in his power. Richardson believed it was the lack of Christianity that let Michel go to pieces under stress.

"They were all affected by the hopelessness of their situation. Hood was so weak he could hardly sit up and said the wind seemed to blow through him. Richardson and Hepburn could not manage between them to carry a log of wood to the fire. Richardson said, 'With the decay of our strength our minds decayed, and we were no longer able to bear the contemplation of the horrors that surrounded us.... Yet we were calm and resigned to our fate, not a murmur escaped us, and we were punctual and fervent in our addresses to the Supreme Being.'

"Hood, however, did point out that Michel would be cruel to leave them without making an effort to provide them with firewood and food. At this Michel was very angry, saying, 'It is no use hunting, there are no animals; you had better kill and eat me.'

"On Sunday, 20 October, after morning service, while Richardson was gathering *tripe de roche*, and Hepburn was cutting down a tree for fuel, Hood was sitting outside by the fire and arguing with Michel. A gunshot rang out. Rushing back, the two men found Hood lying dead, shot in the back of the head. All evidence pointed to Michel, who, though not openly accused, kept repeating that it was an accident.

"With Hood dead, they were free to set out for Fort Enterprise. They placed his body among the willows behind the tent and read the funeral service with their evening prayers They were all on guard and did not sleep.

"They boiled and ate part of Hood's buffalo robe, and a few partridges which Michel killed, and taking the rest of the robe with them, they set out on 23 October. They were all armed, Michel with two pistols, an Indian bayonet, and a knife, in addition to his gun.

"The journey continued in suspicion against Michel. He threatened Hepburn, accusing him of carrying tales, and his arrogance towards Richards convinced them that he thought they were powerless against him. He seemed obsessed by the memory of wrongs inflicted by white men upon his race, including cannibalism. This and other references brought them the dreadful suspicion that he had killed and eaten Belanger on one of his mysterious absences, and perhaps Fontana and Perrault who had also wished to leave Franklin and return to Richardson's camp. They remembered meat that he had once brought in, part of a wolf killed by a deer, he had said, but now they supposed it was a man.

"They were certain that he meant to kill them as soon as he was sure of the way to Fort Enterprise. He was stronger than the two of them together and was heavily armed. When he dropped behind at one point, saying he would gather some *tripe de roche*, leaving them alone for the first time since Hood's death, they took counsel with each other and decided they must put an end to him. Hepburn offered to do it but Richardson said it was his responsiblity alone, and when Michel overtook them, he shot him through the head with a pistol."

Despite the ordeal of that first Franklin expedition, caused partly by its leader's poor planning, and by allowing an early winter to take him by surprise, Dr. Richardson was to venture twice more into the Arctic. In 1825 he again accompanied Franklin overland to the northern edge of

North America. By then they were fairly sure that a northwest passage was feasible, provided ships could get through the islands in the Canadian Arctic Ocean. To this end, Franklin and Dr. Richardson between them surveyed an astonishing eight hundred miles of coastline, whose violent contours had until then never been recorded. The expedition also added considerably to the knowledge of the Arctic, its physics, flora, fauna and zoology. Richardson's work, *Fauna Boreali-Americana*, in four volumes, written in collaboration with three other experts, "established Arctic biology as a branch of natural history, and was the first great work on regional zoology as we now know the subject" (Johnson). Richardson's contributions to the two expeditions established him as a leading Arctic explorer and as a scientist of the first rank.

Yet the search for the Northwest Passage, which had been going on for three hundred years, was still not complete. For a time the navy, finding it an expensive business, lost interest in the search. Then Thomas Simpson, nephew of Sir George Simpson, the governor of the Hudson's Bay Company, who had long urged the completion of Arctic exploration, carried out his uncle's ambitions so thoroughly that by 1845 only three hundred miles of coast lay unaccounted for. Whereupon "pressure rose to let the British Navy finish what it had so long undertaken, before some foreign government could steal the credit."

Which was when Sir John Franklin went back to the Arctic for the last time, and which in turn also inspired Dr. Richardson's last journey to the barrens, the tundra and the icy Polar Sea, to search for traces of that last, lost Franklin expedition.

As for the killing of Michel the Iroquois, it was not to stain Richardson's reputation and even years later people would still regard him with an awe that was not entirely due to his medical and naturalist accomplishments, his knighthood, and his scientific and literary writings. Though the act had been carried out with the cold precision of the executioner, it was apparently a case of self-defence. The fact that he believed Michel to be guilty of cannibalism must have added a Christian righteousness to the act of placing a pistol to the Iroquois' head without warning, and pulling the trigger. Cannibalism was an abomination. It was nearly as bad as incest. After all, even today, in the words of Flanders and Swann, there is no doubt about it that "Eating people is *wrong*."

12

Forceps and Fisticuffs

THE PRICE THAT the Indians demanded in return for the sexual favours of their daughters was modest enough: one pewter plate per girl per night. But when the girls were brought on board Captain Cook's ship, *Resolution,* the crew did not at first find them much of a bargain. Though the maidens were pretty enough, shy and well behaved—not like the noisy trollops the seamen had encountered in the South Seas—the West Coast Indian girls had daubed their hair and their bodies with substances that David Samwell, the ship's surgeon, thought revolting.

"However," he logged that day in 1778, "our young Gentlemen were not to be discouraged by such an obstacle as this which they found was to be removed with Soap and warm water, this they called the Ceremony of Purification and were themselves the Officiators at it."

According to Samwell the sailors soaped and washed and rinsed away at the light brown flesh in a spirit of pure piety. His next words, though, betray a certain conflict of interest, for he goes on to describe the young gentlemen as "taking as much pleasure in cleansing a naked young Woman from all Impurities in a Tub of Warm Water, as a young Confessor would absolve a beautiful Virgin who was about to sacrifice that Name to himself."

The naked girls, of course, were quite bewildered by the ablutionary devotion. In giving themselves a top coat of ochre, they believed they were making themselves more attractive. Still, they learned fast. The next day they came on board degreased and tolerably clean.

The white men were not nearly as adaptable to the foreign culture, particularly the medical customs. In British Columbia, the Indian medicine men, seeing illness as having supernatural causes, were still interceding with the spirits through trance-like dancing and wild incantations, the use of the soul-snatcher, and the magic tube for sucking out the evil influence; but the cold scorn or lukewarm skepticism of the Europeans would soon devalue the Indian faith.

Shamanism in the Pacific Northwest, which bore a remarkable resemblance to practices in Tibet that were very ancient indeed, was a magic that had no less common sense about it than much of the white magic that supplanted it. It was a common sense based on intelligent observation. The decoctions, oils, and ointments applied to the Indian patient were from genuine medicinal sources; the feverish were isolated and kept clean and dry; the newborn child was protected from contamination more effectively than many a European baby. Wounds were protected from infection by packing them with hot dry sand and binding them with leaf poultices. Fractures were set with soaked rawhide, which when it dried, also helped to immobilize the limb. But the white men perceived only the hocus-pocus, and many of them, wrapped in cultural intransigence, felt mainly scorn, impatience, or disgust, at the smelly coatings and barbaric ceremonies.

Their own contribution to the medical experience in British Columbia was not exactly salubrious. To the Pacific Northwest they brought a certain sophistication in medicine, but the Indians could be excused reservations of their own, for they also brought rats, cockroaches, and venereal disease; and smallpox, which devastated the Indian tribes.

As distinct from the ship's surgeons, who came and went according to their sailing orders, the first land-based medical men of British Columbia were the employees of the great fur companies. It was the policy of the companies to station medical men at their forts to maintain the health of their employees. Of course, the companies were not in business for altruistic reasons but to make money for their shareholders, so their surgeons were also expected to act as clerks. One such merchant-medico was William Fraser Tolmie who entered the service of the Hudson's Bay Company in 1832.

Dr. Tolmie was one of that breed of deadly serious, moral Scotsmen who have done so much to colonize various parts of the world and to set high standards of mental and physical discipline that the rest of the world has always found so hard to live up to. In his diary he increasingly reproached himself for indolence and other forms of backsliding, but the description of his activities suggests that the only time he was indolent was when he was asleep. From dawn to candle-lit night he toiled dedicatedly in the service of the company, trading and skinning, and whenever stationary, he made copious notes on botanical specimens and on the natural history of the region and its geography, languages, and dialects.

In case thousands of miles of travel by boat, horse, and on foot was not enough, he climbed mountains (Mount Tolmie in British Columbia is named after him). For light reading he read Walter Scott, and for inspiration, Cowper, Tennyson, and the Bible. Even fifty years after his arrival at Fort Vancouver on the Columbia River (in what is now the State of Washington), his seventh son, Simon Fraser Tolmie, could not remember a single instance when the old man was not active in self-improvement, or in the improvement of others.

Nevertheless, as his life as a trader and surgeon settled into routine, Dr. Tolmie reproached himself with increasing despondency for failing to cling to the pinnacle of the work ethic.

At first the sheer beauty of the country, with its unfamiliar flora, its glorious fiords and mountains, its seals and snakes, its mammals and molluscs, and the strangeness of the natives, kept him, as he saw it, morally up to snuff. He observed with awe and wrote without excitement. He packed anatomical specimens, and compressed botanical ones. He learned how to handle a rifle, a vital tool in a land "peopled by treacherous, bloodthirsty savages, with whom murder is familiar." At first, most of his shots went wide, but with typical perseverance he was soon able to place his balls in the same spot three times in succession from a distance of 100 yards—an amazing achievement. He learned how to cope with bears: if a wounded bear rushed at you the thing to do was to stand your ground and look him steadily in the eye. Whereupon the bear would rise on its hind legs, return the fixed gaze until it grew tired of the staring match, and then quietly take itself off. Or at least that was what a company servant told the new doctor. There is no record that he actually put the theory to the test.

He also learned how to handle a polecat. After shooting the first one he encountered, he carried it back to the fort, refusing to be put off by its diabolical smell. He was then supposed to skin it, but he never actually did so. He claimed that he did not have the opportunity. So he gave it to a colleague, Dr. Gairdner—whom he didn't particularly like.

He had no difficulty in holding his liquor, for there were very few occasions when he partook of a potation. "Passed the evening very agreeable," he commented at one point. "Sung several old Scotch ditties and the other gentlemen also tuned their pipes." The next entry rather smugly records that though he had been drinking "mountain dew" with the rest of them, he was the only person to awake in good trim, the others suffering the usual hangover. Eight years later he had become so abstemious that on a journey by canoe and on horseback all the way from the Pacific Ocean to the Atlantic (he was on his way home on leave) he refused to take a single drink of alcoholic liquor, much to the annoyance of his companion, who had "an adequate supply" of the stuff. Even

Tolmie's son was amazed at this temperance. "Surely," he said, "this must be a record for a Scotsman."

Above all, Tolmie learned to handle the natives with whom he traded, doing so with a sympathy that never degenerated into indulgence, especially if the weakness were likely to be detrimental to the company. When an Indian named Babyar wanted more than the regular price for his beaver skins and called in his cohorts to intimidate the company servant, Tolmie "stood firm, at same time endeavouring by soft words to pacify the savage." But when harsher methods were called for, Tolmie was ready with his fists and boots, even when the adversary was considerably taller than himself. As in the case of Charbonneau, a brawny, six-foot layabout, an employee of the company at Fort McLoughlin, up the coast from Vancouver Island. Tolmie discovered that Charbonneau, noted for his laziness and dishonesty, was using the back garden of Tolmie's house as a toilet, or as Tolmie put it, a temple of Cloacina. Feeling that he should make an example of Charbonneau, the doctor kicked the offending part of Charbonneau's body and followed it up by driving his fist into the man's face, "which drew claret." Charbonneau retaliated by scratching Tolmie's face, but another kick to the backside completed his punishment. Tolmie then informed his diary that "my pommelling him will show the others that I am not to be trifled with and with proudence and firmness I may for a long time find it unnecessary to resort to the same measures, which I cannot approve of, altho' the custom of the country &c render it almost necessary for a newcomer."

Later, at Fort Simpson, a further two hundred miles up the coast, Tolmie showed his spunk again, while preparing to sail from the fort to treat an employee who had sustained a compound fracture of the leg. "On Saturday morning rum had been sold to the Indians and some of them getting intoxicated were very turbulent and from noon till sunset when we embarked we were all under arms and in momentary expectation of having to fight our way on board or being butchered on the spot. They attempted frequently to beat down the slight barricade raised on the site of the bastions, but were deterred on seeing us ready with firearms to send a volley among the intruders. About a dozen or twenty Indians with muskets were posted on a hill immediately behind from whence they could fire with deadly effect into the Fort at any part. Outside the pickets they were numerous and armed with guns, boarding pikes and knives and endeavouring by their savage whoops and yells to intimidate us."

During a lull, Tolmie tried to finish the job of loading the boats on the beach. While one of his men was carrying a barrel full of miscellaneous articles, "several armed villains rushed out from amongst the bushes— and one more inebriated and thence more daring than the rest seized the barrel and with drawn dagger drove the man from his charge,...seeing the savage advancing with his knife aloft in a menacing attitude I stepped slowly to the gate and procured a cutlass from the doorkeeper." Thus armed, the surgeon-factor advanced on the malefactor, routed him, and temporarily subdued the other Indians as well. Ultimately, however, the fort had to be abandoned.

While his relationship with the Indians was reasonably good, he was wary of them because of their casual attitude to life. They were quite willing to pardon a murderer, provided he atoned for his crime with a hefty contribution of material goods to the bereaved family. As for Tolmie's attitude to his white colleagues, it appears to have been accommodating but reticent. Most noteworthy among these was Dr. John McLoughlin, the chief of the Hudson's Bay Company's fur trade along the Pacific coast. McLoughlin was a native-born Canadian. His grandfather had been with Wolfe at Quebec, where he commanded a Highland Regiment. After the battle he had settled at Rivière-du-Loup on the St. Lawrence, where John McLoughlin was born.

As with so many early Canadian doctors, McLoughlin studied medicine at Edinburgh, though most of his energy was to go into the administration of his furry empire, which stretched from Russian Alaska to Mexico. McLoughlin sat like a king in a banqueting hall at his base, Fort Vancouver. He allowed no skirted women to enter, but plenty of kilted pipers to entertain a stream of visitors from Canada, Britain, the United States, and the Sandwich Islands. Little Dr. Tolmie was quite impressed when he was first ushered into the presence. McLoughlin was another giant Canadian lancet wallah: six foot four, with a similarly lofty temper. When Sir George Simpson, the governor of the company, first met McLoughlin, he described him as "such a figure as I should not like to meet in a dark night." But Dr. Tolmie was a dutiful and respectful person, so he and McLoughlin got on quite well.

As far as one can tell from his cool, objective narrative, Tolmie seems to have gotten on tolerably well with nearly all his colleagues, even his first boss at Fort Nisqually. (Nisqually was Tolmie's first posting, following a training period at Fort Vancouver.) The boss was the chief trader, Mr. Heron. Heron was a stout, elderly native of Ulster with a grievance: he had been rousted out of a comfortable billet at Fort Colville far to the south, in Oregon territory. He didn't think much of Fort Nisqually at all. He thought even less of it when an earthquake occurred three days after his arrival.

However, he may have been slightly mollified when the local Indians credited the earthquake to him. "The Chief's medicine is strong," they said. "He has gone up the hill to shake the grounds." Mr. Heron must have been pleased to have had such godlike powers ascribed to him — unless, of course, the Indians were referring to his weight. Heron, unlike his namesake, was distinctly obese.

Heron appears to have been quite a character, as locquacious, boastful, and effusive as he was fast with his fists. On one occasion, Tolmie was having trouble with a native named Bourgeois, one of the men responsible for the market garden that was attached to the fort. Tolmie had been trying to encourage Bourgeois (whom he also referred to in his diary as Bourshow), with verbal exhortations to overcome his laziness and try harder. Heron's methods were more direct. When he saw the way Bourgeois was harrowing the potatoes, Heron got down from his horse and proceeded to harrow Bourgeois. He "pommelled the poor wretch heartily on the field and then chased him at a hard canter... to the house, where on his knees Bourshow begged pardon for past offense and made earnest promises of amendment."

Four days later, Heron was boasting to Tolmie about how much he had done to ameliorate the conditions of the poor Indians. "He says he has greatly civilized the Indians about Fort Colville so much, that in their disputes they refer to him as an umpire, the Seventh day is kept holy, and they travel any distance without even a knife as a weapon of defence."

Tolmie was impressed. In his own territory, he wrote, "the Indian never parts with his knife, clutched in his right hand, it is either concealed under his blanket or employed in scratching his chin or hands and legs and to go any length from home without a musket is never dream't of by those who possess the article."

Six weeks later, Heron suddenly appeared after a day's seclusion and lit into several men who were busy dusting and packing beaver skins. He cudgeled them, and cursed them as worthless rascals. His behaviour was so erratic that Tolmie began to suspect that Heron privately indulged to excess in ardent spirits. At first the twenty-one-year-old doctor found this hard to believe, because, during their conversations, Mr. Heron had never even mentioned the subject of wines or spirits. Tolmie's doubts increased when Heron started to overwhelm him "with the most fulsome flattery and professions of friendship."

Tolmie's response could not have been entirely satisfying to Mr. Heron. He replied that "many men's professions were hollow, but that I valued his, thinking them sincere—perhaps they are—most likely not."

During his tour of duty at Nisqually, Dr. Tolmie saved the life of a particularly valuable company servant. It was one of his few cases to be written up in detail. The servant was a forty-year-old Indian named Pierre Charles, the best deer hunter in the Rockies. He had struck his foot with an axe. When Tolmie examined the foot he "found a terrible wound extending from situation of astragalus in ancle joint, along skin half an inch of proximal extremity of great and second toes—Metatarsal bones being probably sliced. The point of penetration to the sole, where it left a gaping wound of more than an inch in extent." Tolmie looked after Pierre Charles through a series of crises lasting for weeks. He recorded every detail of the case, the first-known detailed report on a medical case written in the Pacific Northwest.

A year later while traveling by ship to Fort Simpson, Tolmie performed one of the earliest modern operations on the coast, though unlike his extensive notes in the axe case, he described it in a mere three or so lines: "On Monday removed a fatty tumour from the breast of one of the Vancouver's crew—it was the size of a large orange, but was unfortunately lost. Incision transverse—vessels secured by torsion—the man is doing well." When he first arrived he had been pleased to find "a very excellent supply of surgical instruments—an Amputating, two trephining, two eye instruments, a lithotomy and a cupping case, beside two midwifery forceps and a multitude of catheters, flexible and silver sounds bougies, probangs, tooth forceps and not yet put in order." So he was not short of implements to take care of the wounds that the pioneers and even the skilled native woodsman inflicted upon themselves in the course of their activities. He also made sure that his medicine chest was stocked, with such as "Jalap: 3 oz. Potass: Supect: 4 oz. Emplast Adhes: 1 yard Ungt Calam: 6 oz. acid: Citric. Suggested to G. [Dr. Gairdner] the propriety of ordering cupping glasses in making his requisition and requested him to demand for me two aneurism needles, one for the Carotid, the other of a size for the Radical."

Though his medical entries take up only a small proportion of his diary, his terse comments and his constant reading of medical literature support Dr. Robert E. McKechnie II's opinion that the wee Scot "was one of the new breed of surgeons, no longer content with being an artisan but a scholar in search of the knowledge that would inform the work of his hands." On a certain Sunday in May, after seeing an Indian patient with stricture and disease of the testes, he immediately ran to Abernethy on strictures. The next day, underlining his professionalism and concern for the patient, he was consulting Mackintosh on syphilis.

His own equipment was as up-to-date as his attitudes. He brought from Scotland what were probably the first stethoscopes seen in the Pacific Northwest. "Friday, November 8: Evg reading Mackintosh on Bronchitis, Hiria is affected with Chronic Bronchitis and I intend examining his chest with the stethoscope on Sunday. Have finished a sermon in Dwight on the Unity of God." That Tolmie's patients appreciated his efforts is indicated by reports that after he left Fort Nisqually in 1859, some of them followed him all the way to Victoria so as not be deprived of his services.

He made sure, however, that he was not followed by the relatives of any Indian who was likely to expire during treatment. In such an eventuality, the Indians were quite likely to come looking for him with a knife of their own. In the case of Kyeet, chief of a particularly intolerant tribe, Tolmie not knowing enough about Kyeet's illness, prescribed "Essence of ppt." The doctor reckoned that his luck would have to be exceedingly bad for the old man to die of peppermint. On another occasion when the sufferer seemed likely to journey at any moment to the Happy Hunting Grounds, Tolmie refused even to give him a placebo. This unprofessional inertia troubled the doctor. But of course, a pack of vengeful relatives would have troubled him even more.

As the months passed, Tolmie's own health started to decline, and it bothered him. "Sunday December 1: My fears have not been groundless — on getting out of bed this mg. I felt a sharp pain in the left inquinal region and on touching the spot perceived a tenderness and cannot doubt that it is occasioned by a small hernia." By the Tuesday he was unhappily reproaching himself for not anticipating the trouble and sending for a truss. By the following April he was complaining of a bruised forefinger. Later that month, toothache. "Had the actual cautery applied by means of a piece of iron wire — it diminished the pain in the tooth, but has irritated the different branches of the 7th pair and I have since suffered pain in the cheek, ear and temple of the same side."

Simultaneously his morale was declining. He felt increasingly troubled over his "indolence and ennuye," his procrastination, his "fagged" state. Suddenly we learn that his devotion to his work is not entirely wholehearted. "Now three years since I bid adieu to the shores of Britain, and my liking for the Hudson's Bay Service is by no means increasing."

Despite his self-sufficiency Tolmie was lonely. He had no friends. He had not gotten on well with the man he had come out with, Dr. Gairdner. McLoughlin was too high up in the company to be a confidant, and Heron was too old, and besides, he resembled Tolmie's father.

Even the precious communication with his family in Scotland was unsatisfying. The correspondence was his lifeline, but it was subject to the exotic vagaries of the mail service. "My letters," he moaned one day, "were too late for the *Ganymede* which contrary to all expectation sailed about the 20th of September." And, "On Wednesday I visited the *Bolivar* and found my packet of letters... lying on the beach at high water mark in tatters and all in a heap. Picked up the fragments and found part of all. The packet was in all likelihood given to one of the *Golivar's* crew by an Indian and he was rascal enough to open and destroy the letters." The doctor's subdued despair is quite audible: "Have all my writing to do over again." But even when the letters were delivered, the replies made him all the more aware of his isolation. "Received a short letter from my father and Alick, both well — it is too bad that they write such brief epistoles."

When Tolmie did meet a kindred soul at Fort McLoughlin, a fellow employee named Anderson, his new-found friend was all too soon posted to Vancouver. Their brief acquaintanceship, and their companionable activities—exploring, rifle-shooting, and long walks—only served to heighten his loneliness. "Thursday, January 9: went today to the lake where Anderson and self skated....Since his departure A. has daily occupied a share in the cogitations of my breast or to speak more sensibly I have been daily thinking about him. I have certainly taken a liking to him and wish we had been longer together to have known each other better, our communications can now only take place by letter...as he will probably have the first opportunity I will see on what footing he places himself—whether that of a friend or mere acquaintance—if he assumes that of the former I will not hesitate to respond in the same tone. I feel much the want of a friend to whom I might unbosom my joys and griefs."

This was one of the very few rents in the thick fabric of his quill-woven confidences where the intense loneliness of his life in the sopping forests showed through. To make matters worse, he was too much of a product of his catechist, emotion-suppressing upbringing to give way to mere sensual intercourse. He was certainly not indifferent to women, as his lingering description of the gorgeous Princess Charlotte shows. But to separate her from his longings he hurriedly throws up a palisade of objections, reminding himself of her passion for intoxication and extravagance. Besides, "she is now wedded to a petty portage Chief, who, jealous as Othello, bangs her frequently," he wrote, "with a paddle or the butt end of a musket." Yet he could have had the Princess if he had wanted her, just as, a few days later, he could have had a "paint besmeared beauty" who appeared outside the store, and made desperate efforts to interest the little white medicine man in a liaison. "But this is truly no temptation, and if never more strongly assailed I shall remain virtuous during my stay in this country without assuming any merit [for] self-control."

All the same, seeing so many women "in a state of nudity except having the corner of a blanket round loins," must have had a terribly tumescent effect. By the beginning of the following year his determination to avoid a sexual liaison was already qualified. "A wife is the only being to whom one could unreservedly pour out his soul, but one with whom could be enjoyed a sweet communion of mind is not to be met with in this country and it is only when I abandon the hope and wish of laying my bones in old Scotland that I will ever think of uniting myself in the most sacred of all ties with a female in this country. When a person has resolved to settle in the 'pays sauvage' say Red river or the proposed Wallamatte colony I think the sooner he takes a wife the better. Manson I am sure is much happier with his wife and two pretty children around him than were he a lone bachelor, and leading the sensual life, indulged in by most of the gentlemen, who live in single blessedness."

Later Dr. Tolmie compromised to a certain extent when he married the Scots-Indian daughter of a Hudson's Bay factor. But the struggle to crush his emotions and suppress the rebellion of a cultivated mind that was so deprived of contact with intellectual equals left painful scars. By the time he married, his face was cold, dour, and withdrawn. William Fraser Tolmie's misfortune was that he never had true cause to repent.

"Well here goes" was how John Sebastian Helmcken began his memoirs one May day, as if he had sat for fully half an hour at his desk, with virgin notebook at the ready and a blotter within easy reach, arranged just so, and his old pen with its coarse nib poised. After finally dashing down these words, he must have raced on in his doctor's scrawl to keep pace with the stream of his memories of his broken-down, heavy-drinking father who had worked in a London sugar refinery, and later unprofitably managed the White Swan pub, and his busy, florid mother, whose pots and pans looked like polished silver—a mother who insisted on being bled once a year and said it did her good, otherwise she was troubled with headaches and giddiness, and who said one day to John Sebastian, "Never mind, my son, you shall be a doctor if you like, even if I have to pawn my clothes to pay the cost."

In 1839, at the age of fifteen or so, John Helmcken, an undersized lad with an oversized head, was apprenticed to a kindly local practitioner, Dr. Graves, in the Whitechapel district of London. Under Graves, John learned to dispense tinctures, pills and powders, to cup, leech, and dress sores, and to steel himself against the awful poverty of the patients. In time, because his mother had saved every penny of his wage, he was able to enter the best of the London medical institutes, Guy's Hospital, to attend courses of lectures in anatomy, surgery, medicine, midwifery, chemistry, materia medica, dissections, anatomy demonstrations, botany, and medical jurisprudence. Now that his wage was cut off he had no pocket money, but as he boarded and lodged at home, his mother kept him going.

At the end of the session he won the silver medal in practical chemistry and another prize which he dismissed rather offhandedly in his memoirs as being "something in Materia Medica."

He continued: "The third session comes on and oh the work! Lectures at 8 o'clock in the morning—Midwifery—and three or four more during the day, dissecting or in the wards the rest of the time. By this time I was a clerk to Dr. Barlow—had to write down every case under his care—at the entrance fully—family history and all—examine the urine, microsopically and otherwise—we had the affix P.B. to our names—Piss Boilers. Making out these reports would keep me often until one or two o'clock in the morning. At the end of the session I received the prize of the Medical Society for the medical reports."

Helmcken described Dr. Barlow as being rather careless about dress. He appears to have been rather careless about post-mortems as well. With Helmcken in attendance he performed one on a lady who had died of peritonitis. Barlow did so in the victim's home, right there in her nicely carpeted living room, with results so ghastly that even Helmcken, hardened to the sights and sounds of a nineteenth-century hospital, was glad to get out of the house. During another post-mortem, Barlow wished to remove the heart, as he had a particular interest in that organ, but a guard had been placed on the cadaver to make sure he didn't get it. He enlisted John's aid. While Barlow distracted the guard, Helmcken quickly sliced it from the body and slipped it into his hip pocket. While he was crossing London Bridge on his way back to Guy's he was stopped by a pedestrian who said, "You must have broken a bottle in your pocket—for it is dripping behind."

"Barlow afterwards took me to a meeting of the Medical Society—and they asked me to give the details of a case—heart of course—but I could not say a word save that I was not accustomed to speaking. So Barlow did it. I say I was always timid and bashful before strangers—could not walk up to aisle of a church without bent head not looking to right or left."

Like many timid people, John Sebastian had a tendency to blurt. He endangered his chances by arguing once with his Latin examiner as to whether a certain word was an adjective or an adverb. On another occasion he had the temerity to dispute about a diagnosis with a qualified man, earning a severe reprimand in the process—not so much for differing with the doctor but for his bad manners in arguing the case at the bedside of the patient. This sort of thing simply wasn't done.

In his fourth and last session, Helmcken, loaded with honours and first prizes, became deeply involved in midwifery among the poor, who would send for the student when the time came. In turn, if the case was complicated, the student would send for the senior clerk, or the professor. (Helmcken's description of his obstetrical work among the miserable poor living around Guy's Hospital sounds exactly like [Dr.] Somerset Maugham's description three-quarters of a century later in his novel *Of Human Bondage.*)

Finally, the great examination. John Sebastian told nobody at home about it, in case he was "plucked," but he was forced to tell Dr. Graves, in order to borrow the ten-guinea registration fee. "Well the evening came," Helmcken scribbled in his memoirs. "I dressed respectably and I wended my way to the College and ushered into the room. At 8 o'clock a certain number were called—I was one and entered a large hall with several small tables. The first table I went to was presided over by two professors—the one gave me the anatomy of the hand—I had to dissect it, relating from memory all the parts I reached, beginning with the palmar surface first. I was nonplussed at the very beginning—the professor said, 'You have forgotten a muscle,'—I said nervously, 'I do not remember one'—he had his hand flat on the table. He said, 'Is there not a muscle here?' 'Oh yes, but that is only a skin muscle.' 'Well—that's all right—now go on' and so I did for five or ten minutes—and then the other professor went to some other anatomy. My quarter of an hour being up, I was transferred to another table—two professors likewise. One gave me hernia in general and then anatomy in particular, and some other matters. My quarter of an hour ended. I was transferred with my paper showing their opinion in hieroglyphics, to another table and so on through a couple or so more—and then the examination being over, sent into the 'funking room.' Where some of his fellow students were larking about, laughing and gossiping or leap-frogging over chairs, while others were silent and dejected, sure that they had failed. And as it turned out, the most confident and playful were the ones that were rejected."

John Sebastian passed. Some of his friends went off to celebrate over supper, and to organize a rowdy jaunt to the theatre, but Helmcken had no money, so he went home and showed his certificate to his mother. And she wept, and then John Sebastian's brothers and sisters flocked in and pounded him on the back, and called him a sly, deceitful fellow for having kept the examination secret, and then they shouted joyfully, "We might have known there was something up on account of you having dressed so carefully."

Exactly two years later, John Sebastian Helmcken, M.R.C.S., sailed into Esquimalt on Vancouver Island, having been taken on as a surgeon, and as private secretary to Governor Blanshard by the Hudson's Bay Company. His term was a period of five years at £100 per annum.

He was no longer the docile boy he had been, and quickly proved it. Soon after his arrival he was awakened from a sound sleep and informed that Governor Blanshard had at length arrived and wished to meet him. Helmcken admitted later that regardless of the hour, he should have gotten up at once to meet his boss, to "show off my best qualities if I had any." Instead he grumbled so peevishly at having to get out of bed, and was so tardy about doing so, that the governor finally sent word not to bother, as there would be plenty of opportunities for them to meet in the future. But the damage was done. Blanshard did not care for the new doctor after that.

Admittedly, even if Helmcken had hastened to present himself before the governor, it is not certain they would have taken to each other. Helmcken, short and slender, with a wide mouth and eyes deep and cool as a Pacific fiord set in a massive head (made all the more disproportionate by the huge hat he constantly wore), was a man who did not open up to strangers. His profound reserve often distanced him still further from potential friends and allies. Much later, when the historian H. H. Bancroft interviewed him on the early history of British Columbia, Helmcken was so unforthcoming that Bancroft was not able to do justice to Helmcken's part in that history; which in turn drew from Helmcken, offended by the result of his own taciturnity, the remark that "Bancroft tells lies."

Nor at first did Helmcken make a good impression on James Douglas, the chief factor at Fort Victoria; though later they got on tolerably well, especially after Helmcken married Douglas' eldest daughter, Cecilia.

Like Tolmie twenty years previously, Helmcken was to discover that coping with the condition of the country was almost as important as observing the condition of the patient. He had to learn how to keep a canoe on its heading, how to slash a way through the forest, and how to manage a horse. He had hardly ridden a horse before he came to Canada. Now he had to spend hours in a Spanish saddle, covering an enormous area from his base at Fort Victoria. But he soon grew accustomed to the life, and later boasted that he was the leading practitioner from the North Pole to San Francisco.

Not that there were all that many patients. The territory was still sparsely populated in the mid 1850s. Vancouver Island had a population of little more than four hundred. Governor Blanshard blamed the Hudson's Bay Company for this sluggish development. The accusation was more or less justified, though the company maintained that they were supposed to be in business to make money for their shareholders, not to do the work of the Colonial Office.

The discovery of gold in California had a lot to do with the stagnancy. The temptation to join the gold rush was too much for many colonists, and even the most loyal company people must have been tempted by rumours of nuggets the size of the human heart.

Helmcken met some of these amateur miners when they drifted into Victoria. He described them as "ragged—boots minus soles—unshaven, tattered, dirty and forlorn—miserable-looking beggars." However, his opinion of them improved enormously after they had outfitted themselves in new clothes. He found that many of them not only looked like gentlemen, but actually were—and even better, with their leathern bags choked with gold dust, *rich* gentlemen.

After a stint at Fort Rupert, Helmcken returned to Victoria in time for Christmas, 1850. There he got down to the serious business of courting Cecilia Douglas, undeterred by the pranks of her little sisters. The girls would gather, giggling, in the room directly above his, and pour water onto his bed through the cracks and holes in the ceiling. Obviously they were not afraid of the little man with the big head. "Cold, brave" Douglas, however, continued to regard the doctor with some misgivings until he had secured character references from John Sebastian's mother. And just in case Mrs. Helmcken might be a shade prejudiced about her son's qualities, Douglas also obtained a reference from Dr. Graves. Persuaded, Douglas finally gave his consent to the marriage.

Excusing his preoccupation with the fair Cecilia, Helmcken explained, "Anyhow, all I had to do at this time was to attend the sick of the Company, also to strangers who came from the other side [the United States] for treatment. I really being the only surgeon for many hundred miles. They likewise used to buy various drugs, for which I had to account, but our stock was not very large then, and patent medicines existed not, save Turlington's Balsam and Juniper Peppermint. I might have made money out of these sick, but they really looked so poor, and no doubt often were, that I neglected to do so, but in process of time, I became a celebrity and had lots of patients 'from the other side.'"

Helmcken supplied all the Hudson's Bay posts in the area and neighbouring parts of the United States with such medications. The treatment was simple enough: an emetic as soon as a patient fell ill, followed by a purge as soon as he was weak enough. Dr. Helmcken used Turlington's Balsam for cuts, wounds, coughs, and colds. Fortunately the colonists were a robust lot, so he was not called upon too frequently to make what was often a week-long journey. (More than one pioneer doctor noted the interesting medical phenomenon that when there was no doctor within easy call, the people remained healthy. It was only when medical aid became more readily available that the general health deteriorated.)

As he was soon to be married, Helmcken had to think of building a house. Now that the doctor was to become a member of the family, Douglas wanted him to live as close by as possible. He presented the little doctor with an acre plot, right next to his own house. Helmcken had some misgivings, for this location necessitated a long walk to his office near the fort. He accepted, partly because it was free, and partly for Cecilia's sake. During his long absences, she would be close to her mother and other relatives.

The walls of Helmcken's house were built of logs, felled in the forest and squared on two sides by his French-Canadian contractors, though Helmcken had to beg oxen from the company to haul the logs to the site. He grumbled mightily over the steep expense and the slow pace of the carpenters. In fact the work was not completed in time, so that he and Cecilia had to live for a while in Government House, attended by an Indian couple whose wages were two blankets and one shirt per month.

The Helmckens moved into the house with its three rooms and kitchen shortly before their first-born came along, before even the doors had been hung. "Of course the boy-baby was a wonder, a light-haired blue-eyed fair little fellow. When he was about a month or two old we found him dead in the bed one morning." The Helmckens appear to have encountered the still mysterious phenomenon of the crib death.

"The anguish felt at this is indescribable," he wrote. "The poor little fellow was buried in the garden where the holly now grows."

Helmcken, at least, had his medical duties to distract him from the painful loss. Not infrequently it was exciting and dangerous work. As well as a steady business in prescriptions—jalap and calomel, ipecacuanha and tartar emetic for people, and Mustang Liniment for horses—and the amputations resulting from the accidents that were so common among settlers who were not familiar or careful enough with axes and adzes—he was also sometimes called out on non-medical business. Soon after Douglas had replaced Blanshard as governor, he conscripted the doctor and several other colonists to apprehend an Indian who had deliberately killed somebody's cow. The Indian lived in a village across the water from Fort Victoria.

Helmcken was placed in command of one of the boats, his men being armed with rusty weapons that, had they been fired, would have done more harm to their owners than to an enemy. At least one musket had been improperly loaded, with the bullet first, then the powder.

Luckily the colonists had no chance to fire their weapons, for as soon as they rowed across to the Indian village, the Indians rushed the boat and wrested the muskets from the doctor's crew. Helmcken was exceedingly alarmed. A great many Indians had sided with the cow-killer, and they were a frightening sight, "some blackened—all yelling—having muskets, axes, knives and what not, but the nastiest things were their long poles with sharp spears at the end—pointed towards *our* stomachs." Preferring discretion to valour, he rowed hurriedly back to the fort.

As Helmcken conferred on the shore with a distinctly displeased Mr. Douglas, the Indians opened fire across the water. As Helmcken's fright gave way to guilty fury, he proposed going back again and fighting it out; but Douglas calmed him down, though the governor insisted on walking along the shore slowly and deliberately, despite the bullets that were cracking overhead, to show the Indians that he, at least, was not to be intimidated. In the end, the 'Case of the Murdered Cow' was resolved peacefully, over a pow-wow.

Inevitably, Helmcken entered politics, partly because men of education and authority like himself were scarce, and partly because he was bored. He found frontier medicine an unchallenging occupation. He was persuaded to represent the Esquimalt and Victoria District, and in 1856 was returned to the Legislative Assembly unopposed.

Helmcken was immediately appointed Speaker of the House, presumably because, having many acquaintances but no intimates, he was thought to be objective. Just how objective he could be was amply demonstrated when, during a committee meeting, in an attempt to force through a motion he was particularly interested in, he argued forcefully on a point of order. He was just about to get his way when "some grey-haired old rat" suggested that the point of order should be referred to the speaker. The meeting then adjourned to the chamber—where Helmcken proceeded to render a judgement—against himself. The decision earned him hoots of laughter, then appreciative cheers.

He was just as judicial outside the House. Among his confrères were Dr. Ash, a clever, well-read man with a powerful physique and a quick temper, and Amor De Cosmos (real name, Bill Smith). They sat on opposite sides of the House, and on one occasion had a dispute so acrimonious that it was continued outside, on the James Bay bridge. Words proving insufficient to express their ire, they resorted to blows. De Cosmos always carried a stick. He used it on Dr. Ash's head. The latter was just about to throw De Cosmos over the bridge when Dr. Helmcken interceded and persuaded a crimson-faced Dr. Ash—his face bloodied from the encounter—to walk away from the fracas, up Bird Cage Walk.

Governor Douglas did not in the least appreciate Helmcken's peace-making efforts. That evening when he met Dr. Helmcken he said in his icily humorous way, "Mr. Speaker, are you aware that your authority ceases when out of the House? You had no authority to interfere, when gentlemen out of your jurisdiction wished to settle their little difficulties." Apparently Douglas disliked De Cosmos, and had been hoping to see him heaved into the briny.

In his *Reminiscences*, Helmcken said that he was to find politics destructive of domestic duties, but it could be conjectured that it was also destructive of those skills that develop after years of undistracted observation, percussion, palpitation, and smelling and tasting, in the search for the superficial signs and sounds, odours and tastes that lead to correct judgement. In her biographical sketch of Helmcken written in 1947, Dr. Honor Kidd commented, "As for the type of medicine he practised—it appears the doctor had come a long way from the painstaking and careful investigations of his patients that he carried out at Guy's Hospital in his student days." Citing one particular case she added, "The casual diagnosis and the therapy both seem a little fearsome today." But his patients remained faithful to him. "Perhaps," Dr. Kidd wrote, "John Sebastian Helmcken was not a good doctor, even by the standards of the times; his methods were rough and ready, and his diagnosis often arrived at by trial and error; but if medical success be judged by the esteem, confidence and love of patients, then Helmcken was outstanding in his profession."

The impressions of just one of those patients suggest that Honor Kidd's estimate was not unfair. It was written by Emily Carr, the artist. In the 1880s, she wrote, "When Victoria was young, specialists had not been invented—the Family Doctor did you all over. You did not have a special doctor for each part. Dr. Helmcken attended to all our ailments—Father's gout, our stomach-aches; he even told us what to do once when the cat had fits. If he was wanted in a hurry he got there in no time and did not wait for you to become sicker so that he could make a bigger cure. You began to get better the moment you heard Dr. Helmcken coming up the stairs. He did have the most horrible medicines—castor oil, Gregory's powder, blue pills, black draughts, sulphur and treacle.

"Jokey people called him Dr. Heal-my-skin. He had been Doctor in the old Fort and knew everybody in Victoria. He was very thin, very active, very cheery. He had an old brown mare called Julia. When the Doctor came to see Mother we fed Julia at the gate with clover. The Doctor loved old Julia. One stormy night he was sent for because Mother was very ill. He came very quickly and Mother said, "I am sorry to bring you and Julia out on such a night, Doctor." 'Julia is in her stable. What was the good of two of us getting wet?' he replied.

"My little brother fell across a picket fence once and tore his leg. The doctor put him on our dining-room sofa and sewed it up. The Chinaboy came rushing in to say, 'House all burn up!' Dr. Helmcken put in the last stitch, wiped his needle on his coat sleeve and put it into his case, then stripping off his coat, rushed to the kitchen pump and pumped till the fire was put out.

"Once I knelt on a needle which broke into my knee. While I was telling Mother about it who should come up the steps but the Doctor! He had just looked in to see the baby who had not been very well. They put me on the kitchen table. The Doctor cut slits in my knee and wiggled his fingers round inside it for three hours hunting for the pieces of needle. They did not know the way of drawing bits out with a magnet then, nor did they give chloroform for little things like that.

"The Doctor said, 'Yell, lassie, yell! It will let the pain out.' I did yell but the pain stayed in.

"I remember the Doctor's glad voice as he said, 'Thank God, I have got all of it now, or the lassie would have been lame for life with that under the knee cap!' Then he washed his hands under the kitchen tap and gave me a peppermint."

The knee is a particularly sensitive part of the body, so Emily Carr must have wished with all her heart that Dr. Helmcken had indeed used chloroform. After all, Dr. Gerald O'Reilly of Hamilton had used it thirty years previously in similar circumstances, when he discovered that a broken needle had become deeply embedded in the foot of his infant son.

The use of the anesthetic was then a recent development—the first public demonstration of chloroform had taken place only a short time previously, in 1847—so it could not have been an easy decision for Dr.

O'Reilly, especially as the baby was only a few days old. But O'Reilly, who had become a quick and expert surgeon over the years, was only too aware of how terribly an unanesthetized patient could suffer, even when the procedure lasted only ninety seconds. So he took the risk of administering the anesthetic to the then youngest person ever to receive it; and located and extracted the broken needle, in glorious silence.

How awed he must have been, by the merciful hush. It must have been the greatest moment in O'Reilly's professional life. At last he was able to cut and probe without that sick tension felt by so many surgeons in the past, like the Englishman John Abernethy, who was thoroughly rude to his patients before operations on their conscious, quivering bodies. He was rude partly because he thought that this would inspire their confidence, but perhaps mostly in order to cover up his own sympathetic anguish, as the patient shrieked and cursed, or prayed and wrenched frantically at the restraining straps. After such an experience, Abernethy would rush from the operating room and vomit.

13

Perspective: "Oh, I'm an Angel!"

"**P**AIN," SAID ALFRED Velpeau, a professor of the Paris Faculty, "is the inseparable companion of an operation." And so it had been throughout history.

Naturally there were many attempts to ameliorate the sufferings of those few who were desperate enough to risk a surgical invasion. Opium was used in Ancient Egypt by history's first woman doctor, Tefnut. Hashish or marijuana was used by the Hindus and Arabians, while the Greeks tried out henbane, hemlock, crushed marble, and vinegar, and even lettuce—after the death of her beloved Adonis, Venus was said to have flung herself into a giant salad in the belief that the lettuce leaves would act as a tranquillizer.

The mysterious mandrake root, which vaguely resembled the form of a man or woman, was popular in Imperial Rome as a genuine narcotic. It was still in use in the Middle Ages, though harvesting it was believed to be a highly dangerous procedure. We have it on good authority that whenever the mandrake was wrenched from the ground, the homunculus-shaped vegetable would emit such a frightful shriek as to drive its gardener into insanity. The herbalists of the day got over the difficulty by stuffing their ears with wax, or by attaching the root to the tail of a dog. The dog was then encouraged with a sharp stone flung from a safe distance to start forward, thus dragging the root from the loosened earth.

These remedies, though, were mostly soporifics, blunting only the edges of pain. If anything, the situation for the surgical patient grew steadily worse. During the Age of Reason (Shakespeare, Rembrandt, Copernicus), a Scotswoman, Eufame Macalyne, was burned at the stake, her crime being that she had attempted to seek relief from the pain of childbirth. Pain was good for the sinful soul. No doubt the appropriate passage in Genesis was intoned at her trial: "In sorrow thou shalt bring forth children." Had she the dialectics, she might have pointed out another passage in the same book, showing that God was an anesthesiologist. Before taking out Adam's rib, God had first caused a deep sleep to fall upon him.

The deep sleep was not to fall for a quarter millenium after Eufame's heresy. In the meantime, most people preferred to let cruel nature take its course, rather than be literally tortured to death on the operating bench. Pain could kill as surely as hemorrhage or infection. As late as the middle of the nineteenth century, hospital patients had little hope of going home alive after an operation. If they survived the trip across the Styx of purulence, surgical shock was likely to carry them off.

Some people preferred to anticipate the event through suicide. A few allowed optimism or desperation to sway their better judgement, like the patient of the French surgeon, Depuytren, who had a tumour of the lower jaw. As recounted by Philip Smith in his *Arrows of Mercy* the patient, who was thirty-nine, sat there, fully conscious, while the surgeon made an incision through the underlip, extending to the tongue bone. After another incision the jaw was exposed. Then from both sides of the gap pieces were taken by sawing the bone or by breaking off a piece of it with bone snippers, until the distance between the two sides was two and a half inches. "The soft portions of the jaw [werc] also removed where unsound, and blood vessels tied at the same time."

The operation lasted for hours. "And all that time, while those great gashes were being cut in his face and pieces of his jaw were being broken off, the patient was fully conscious. He died, as may be imagined, but not until thirteen days after the operation."

There were a few fortunate patients with a high pain threshold, or those like Tom, the old janitor of the first Toronto General Hospital, whose life had so accustomed him to discomfort that an operation was just one more ordeal, just another sample of life's vicious ways. In Tom's case, the discomforts had been those of the Royal Navy, which had fed him on weevils and maggots, forced him aloft in gale-force winds, flogged him at the grating with the cat of nine tails, and finally taken his leg at the Battle of Trafalgar. The ship's surgeon had cut it off at the hip. Ever since, Tom had put up with agonizing sciatica.

His was one of the last operations without an anesthetic to be performed at the old Toronto General on King Street. W. G. Cosbie reported, in his history of that institution, that old Tom "was not a very satisfactory janitor. He was gruff, and very deaf. On fine days he spent his time on the lawn under the trees with a long clay pipe in his mouth and in foul weather he retired to his room or somewhere out of sight and presumably continued to smoke. He eventually developed cancer of the tongue. Dr. James H. Richardson operated, removed the tongue with the ecraseur. Old Tom refused an anesthetic. He said that he had stood the amputation of his leg, so he could stand this. Which he did, giving a responsive groan at each tightening twist of the instrument until the tongue came off. When Dr. Richardson had finished, he placed the tongue on the table, turned to the students and said 'You see of what our sailors are composed.' The next morning Old Tom was under the trees smoking his pipe as usual." (It was many years before the ecraseur, the most brutal surgical instrument ever invented—it was employed without any preliminary tying-off of the lingual arteries—was succeeded by fast-cutting surgical scissors.)

Old Tom's fortitude was exceptional. For the most part, the suffering of the fully conscious patient was such that cannot even be imagined today. Writing to James Young Simpson, the discoverer of chloroform, Professor George Wilson described one such operation. It was on himself, the amputation of his foot at the ankle-joint. "I do not suppose," he wrote, "that it was more painful than the majority of severe surgical operations are.... Suffering so great as I underwent cannot be expressed in words, and thus fortunately cannot be recalled. The particular pangs are now forgotten, but the black whirlwind of emotion, the horror of great darkness, and the sense of desertion by God and man, bordering close on despair, which swept through my mind and overwhelmed my heart, I can never forget however gladly I would do so. During the operation, in spite of the pain it occasioned, my senses were preternaturally acute, as I have been told they generally are in patients in such circumstances. I still recall with unwelcome vividness the spreading out of the instruments: the twisting of the tourniquet: the first incision: the fingering of the sawed bone: the sponge pressed on the flap: the tying of the blood vessels: the stitching of the skin: and the bloody dismembered limb lying on the floor...."

Obviously the surgeons who would gain the greatest fame would not be the ones who were most painstaking but the ones who were fastest. The Scottish giant, Robert Liston, could amputate a leg in twenty-eight seconds. Even so, when these were amputations at the thigh, which they often were, two out of every three of the amputees died. When mesmerism and hypnotism came along, they raised hopes for a time that the magnetic eye of the healer might substitute for the almost useless narcotic, soporific, or depressant. But in mesmerism and hypnotism, concentration was necessary, and how could patients suffering from gangrene, wounds, or complicated childbirth be expected to concentrate?

Occasionally, surgeons found other ways of rendering their patients quiescent. Dupuytren's method was to address his patients so brutally that they fainted with shock. Unfortunately the method did not always work, as in the tumour case just described.

As it turned out, it was a substance whose effects had been known since the turn of the century that was to herald the age of the deep sleep. As so often happened in medicine, its significance went entirely unrecognized at the time by the profession or even by the great chemist who proved its value on himself. In 1800, Sir Humphrey Davy discovered and described the effects of a new gas, nitrous oxide. When he inhaled it he found it to be not just pleasant and reasonably safe but downright exhilarating. It produced an overwhelming desire to laugh. He called it "laughing gas." And in his *Research Chemical and Philosophical* he suggested that it might be used in surgical operations, possibly mixed with "oxygene" to make it safer to breathe.

To understand the significance of this proposal, it need only be said that nitrous oxide mixed with oxygen is still in use by anesthesiologists.

Yet though Davy's words were eagerly perused by scientists the world over, not a single member of the medical profession appears to have followed up his suggestion. Perhaps not too surprisingly, for though he had demonstrated the effect of the gas—he had used it to effectively stifle the pain of an aching wisdom tooth—Davy himself didn't really absorb the fact that he had taken the first step in the conquest of pain. He wrote nothing more on the subject.

Instead, it was an American tooth that was to revolutionize surgery. One December day in 1844, a Connecticut dentist named Horace Wells attended a lecture in Hartford where the hilarious effects of laughing gas were being demonstrated by a traveling lecturer, "Professor" Gardner Quincy Colton. Wells, a handsome fellow of twenty-nine, perceived something that nobody else appeared to have noticed: a member of the audience who had stepped up to the stage to make a fool of himself under the influence of the laughing gas, cracked his shins against a bench so hard that he should have cried out in pain, or at the very least winced, and rubbed his leg. He continued to lurch about in the Laughing Gas Follies, the audience hooting with merriment, as if nothing had happened. Wells was fascinated, and at the first opportunity, he questioned the volunteer about his injury. The fellow did not understand what Wells was talking about until he pulled up his trouser leg and found that his shins were bleeding. Wells speculated excitedly that using this gas it might be possible for teeth to be extracted painlessly. Intrigued, Colton agreed to come to Well's office the next day with a bladder of nitrous oxide.

Wells decided to make himself the guinea pig. This would not only be in keeping with the experimental tradition but might do him a lot of good personally, for he happened to have an upper molar that was bothering him. A fellow dentist would make the extraction. Accordingly, Wells sat in his own chair and breathed in the gas through a rubber tube. When he recovered consciousness a few minutes later he was overjoyed to find that the tooth was out. He had felt absolutely nothing.

"A new era in tooth-pulling!" he exclaimed, and immediately set about producing quantities of the gas for himself, from ammonium nitrate. Within a month, between December and January 1845, he used nitrous oxide several times on his patients. Though he was unsuccessful once or twice, he did not wait to analyse the reason for these failures, but enthusiastically publicized his discovery. In the process he suggested to as many surgeons as would listen that nitrous oxide would surely enable them to revolutionize surgery.

Surgery without pain? The idea was absurd. Velpeau knew what he was talking about. The two were inseparable. Wells was dismissed as a pain in the neck. But one doctor had the sensibility to listen attentively to the excited dentist, and to give the idea some thought, and that was Dr. Warren, New England's leading surgeon. He agreed to a public demonstration of the new method, to take place before an audience of students and doctors at the Massachusetts General Hospital.

Unfortunately, the student who volunteered to be the subject of the experiment emitted a groan at the worst possible moment, just as Wells was extracting the tooth. Wells was laughed out of the theatre, and speeded back to Hartford with shouts of "Humbug!"

The humiliation was quite undeserved. When history had sorted out the facts, it would show that Wells had really succeeded, for the student-volunteer was to admit afterwards that he had felt no pain whatsoever. Because he had not done his research, Wells was not properly aware, and therefore could not impart the knowledge to the audience, that it was possible for an anesthetized patient to cry out or thrash about even though he was genuinely unconscious.

Wells' part in America's most important contribution to medicine ruined his life. After the Boston fiasco he continued to use nitrous oxide on his patients, until a fatal case caused him to withdraw from practice. Later, when others insisted that they were the inaugurators of anesthesia, he attempted to establish his own claim, failed, and grew increasingly bitter. As the months went by, he tore himself apart with feelings of rage and frustration. At the same time he experimented more and more recklessly on himself with anesthetics. He undermined his health, as surely as John Hunter had ruined his health with his experiments in the laboratory of his body. Just three years after his first triumphant use of nitrous oxide, Wells abandoned his family in Hartford and went to New York. Soon afterwards he was arrested and imprisoned. In his bitter derangement he had dashed acid over a Broadway prostitute.

The tragedy ended when, after writing a poignant letter to his wife, he slashed open an artery—after first dulling his senses with an anesthetic.

As for Wells' rivals, one of them was a former pupil of his, an ambitious, energetic young man named William Morton. Morton had wanted to be a doctor, but his father could not afford the medical school fees, so he went into dentistry. Alerted by Well's discovery, Morton decided that there was money to be made out of painless tooth-pulling. "At this point," wrote Philip Smith, "there enters the story of the third man whose ruin was to be caused by his contribution to the discovery of anesthesia. His name was Charles Thomas Jackson, and he was known to both Wells and Morton as a chemist. He was also a respected geologist and a qualified physician—and an entirely unashamed poacher of other men's ideas." An example of which was Jackson's attempt to obtain the credit for Samuel Morse's invention of the telegraph.

One day when Morton asked this opportunist physician for a supply of nitrous oxide, Jackson replied that he had none available. He suggested that Morton should try sulfuric ether.

The effects of this volatile liquid were already quite familiar. Among college students, ether was the marijuana of the day. The students attended parties where a cheap jag could be obtained by sniffing it. Their "Ether frolics" were a popular pastime.

So Morton tried it out on his patients, and was delighted with the results. Being more interested in money than in scientific prestige, he attempted to protect his financial interest by disguising the substance with aromatic oils and giving it a new name, *letheon.*

Once again the surgeon, John Warren, was approached for a surgical demonstration at the Massachusetts General, in an operating theatre that would become famous as the Ether Dome. The patient was a printer named Gilbert Abbott, who had a tumour on the neck, near the angle of the jaw. It was thus an operation similar to the one performed in Paris by Depuytren twenty-seven years previously. Once again the operating theatre was packed with skeptical students and doctors, among them William Fraser, who would carry the news to Britain—if there was any news to carry. Fraser was a surgeon on the first Cunard liner.

It was almost another fiasco. Morton was late. By the time Dr. Warren had completed his summing-up of the case for the benefit of the students, Morton had still not turned up. "As Dr. Morton has not arrived," Warren said coldly, "I presume he is otherwise engaged." And he reached for his knife. "At that moment, Morton bustled in." He had decided that the ether would be better administered from a glass inhaler than on a handkerchief, and he had just come from the workshop of the craftsman who had fabricated the inhaler. "The glass globe contained a sponge saturated with ether and had two openings in the top—one to admit air and the other fitted with a tube to be put in the patient's mouth....

"Dr. Warren listened courteously as Morton apologized for being late and then told him: 'Well, sir, your patient is ready.' Morton was a burly man with a flowing moustache and on this day he was wearing a flamboyant patterned waistcoat in jaunty contrast with Warren's sober frock coat. His appearance evidently inspired confidence in Abbott, for the young man seemed unafraid as Morton told him how to take the tube of the inhaler in his mouth and breathe deeply through it. The secret 'preparation,' he said, would completely blot out the pain of the knife... Abbott followed Morton's instructions and took the tube in his mouth. Even though he was bound to the chair, his body twitched and his arms jerked spasmodically as he slipped into unconsciousness, struggles that were to become familiar to later generations of anesthesiologists. Morton held the tube in his patient's mouth until he was still and his breathing was deep and regular. Then, with a confidence verging on insolence, the unknown dentist told the eminent surgeon: 'Sir, *your* patient is ready.'

"The watching doctors and students craned forward in their seats. Warren grasped the tumour in his left hand; his right, with a practiced sweep of flashing steel, laid open the flesh. This was the hated moment his lifetime in the operation room had taught him to accept, the moment when the despairing screams would break over his head in a wave of protesting torment. This time, the screams never came. Swiftly he worked on in the unnatural silence, slicing around the tumor, separating it from the surrounding tissues, tying off the blood vessels, stitching up the wound. Once, Abbott stirred slightly and mumbled a few unintelligible sounds, but by this time Warren had almost finished. As the patient slowly returned to consciousness, the old surgeon bent down and asked him urgently if he had felt any pain. Not really, the printer replied— perhaps just a sort of blunt scratching on his cheek.

"John Collins Warren must certainly now have remembered that other demonstration months before. For he straightened up, faced his audience, and said with an echo of the jeers that had driven Horace Wells from this same room: 'Gentlemen, this is no humbug!'"

It was about ten-thirty on the morning of October 16, 1846, the official beginning of the end of the operating room agony. Yet like so many great moments in science which are often the sum of an accumulation of discoveries, it was not quite a clean-cut moment in the history of surgery. A Dr. Long of Georgia was the first to use ether as an anesthetic to remove a small cystic tumour, and he had a receipted bill to prove it: two dollars for the operation, twenty-five cents for the ether. That was four years previously. But Long has been assigned no influence on the historical development of surgical anesthesia, nor has he been given any share in its introduction to the world's operating rooms. As William Osler put it, "In Science the credit goes to the man who convinces the world, not to the man to whom the idea first occurs." And William Morton was the man who convinced the world.

As for the participants in this greatest moment in American medical history, their contributions were somewhat devalued by their subsequent behaviour. Morton and Jackson squabbled squalidly as to who should be the Father of Anesthesia, until Morton impoverished himself with his unscientific self-seeking. He died of a stroke at the age of forty-eight, while Jackson ended up in an insane asylum.

A few weeks later, ether anesthesia was used in London, where the renowned Robert Liston amputated the leg of a butler named Churchill. By the time he had finished, Liston was almost gibbering with excitement. "This Yankee dodge, gentlemen," he cried, "beats mesmerism hollow."

John Richardson, the Arctic explorer, was also quick to try it out at the naval hospital at Gosport. He had a considerable interest in ether. He had already tried it out as a cryoscopic local anesthetic (using ether to freeze the parts to be operated on).

While ethyl ether remained the favourite in North America, the British were to place more reliance on an alternative that had been discovered by James Y. Simpson. Simpson, professor of midwifery at Edinburgh University, had been searching for a long time for ways to mitigate the pains of childbirth, but with little result. By the spring of 1847 he had published a paper recording his use of ether in several cases. He was not entirely satisfied. Ether was expensive, needed a special inhaler, and had to be used in large quantities. It had an unpleasant smell, and tended to irritate the lungs.

Also, it was inflammable. The first time that the dentist Morton tried it, an assistant illuminated the patient's mouth by holding a lighted taper to it. The ether absorbed by the patient could have exploded. So for almost a year, Simpson continued to investigate other substances that might have the advantages of ether without the disadvantages.

One day a Mr. Waldie suggested that he might try a "curious liquid" that had been discovered simultaneously in France and Germany. Simpson obtained a quantity of it. It was named chloroform. But chloroform was just one of the substances he was testing with his two assistants, Dr. George Keith and Dr. Matthews, so he put it aside on a nearby table for several days.

Meanwhile the three doctors continued their usual procedure, which was to sit at the dining room table in Simpson's house and inhale the various substances they were investigating. The trio were extraordinarily fortunate that not once during their twelve months' trials did they breathe in any of chemistry's truly lethal products, though Dr. Simpson sometimes made himself ill, and on one occasion it took two hours to bring him round after he had sniffed a succession of mixtures.

"Then one evening in early November," according to Harvey Graham's *The Story of Surgery*, "after a long day's work, Simpson sat down with his two assistants and they continued their rather risky experiments. Several substances had been tried without much effect when Simpson remembered the 'curious liquid.' A search finally revealed it beneath a heap of waste-paper and empty bottles. The tumblers were filled with chloroform and the three men began inhaling again. Almost immediately three tired men became amazingly talkative. Some ladies of the family were with them and a naval officer, Simpson's brother-in-law. They were startled and delighted at the change that came over the three doctors, then suddenly horrified as one by one they became rapidly incoherent and then crashed to the floor.

"Simpson was the first to come round, to realize in a flash that this substance was better and stronger than ether. Then he heard an appalling noise, and rather dazedly turned round to see Dr. Duncan lying indecorously under a chair, jaw dropped, eyes staring, and snoring stentoriously. There were louder noises, and he saw that Dr. Keith who was under the table was making a tremendous attempt to overturn it and destroy everything within reach of his violent kicks. Simpson slowly returned to his seat, as did Dr. Duncan. Dr. Keith, defeated by the table, was the last to assume a normal position again. They knew that they had found what they had sought, and so more gingerly they tried the chloroform again and again. The ladies were persuaded to join in the festivities which continued hilariously till nearly three in the morning. One of them, Mrs. Simpson's niece, Miss Petrie, as she went under the influence cried out, to the great delight of the others, 'I'm an angel! Oh, I'm an angel!'"

The first of Simpson's midwifery cases to receive chloroform was a doctor's wife. She was so impressed that she christened her new daughter, Anaesthesia.

The first public demonstration of chloroform took place in November 1847. It was administered to a small boy, with Simpson acting as anesthesiologist for a friend of his, Professor Miller. Watched by a huge crowd of doctors and students, Simpson held a handkerchief soaked in chloroform over the boy's face until his wimperings and struggles had subsided into regular breathing. Whereupon most of one of the long bones in his forearm was removed. Two other difficult operations followed, in a wondrous silence broken only by the clink of instruments and an occasional comment from the surgeon and a murmuring from the students and distinguished visitors. Yet even though they were taking part in a revolution, not all of the onlookers grasped the significance of the event. Simpson would have to battle much opposition to the use of chloroform, from medical, moral, and religious quarters. (One of his opponents actually objected on grounds similar to those that had been used to sentence Eufame Macalyne to be burned at the stake.) But as the years passed, chloroform came to be unreservedly accepted in the operating room, especially after Queen Victoria agreed to its use during the birth of her son Leopold in 1853.

As it turned out, the critics of chloroform had more justification for their opposition than they realized. Though it was still being used in the 1930s, for instance by Dr. Macmillan in Cape Breton Island, the substance is now largely discredited. It was responsible for quite a few deaths over the years, causing sudden heart failure during the operations or destruction of the liver. But nitrous oxide still reigns, and even ether is still used in some parts of the world, although because of its intoxicating effect, it is not used in the more medically advanced countries.

While much of the anesthesiological credit goes to the United States, Canada was involved in two major developments, one of them the greatest advance in technique since the pioneer work of Wells and Morton. In 1923, W. Easson Brown, working at the University of Toronto, published a paper on the anesthetic capability of ethylene, which represented the greatest advance in gaseous anesthesia since nitrous oxide. And in 1942, Harold Griffith focused the world's attention on a substance that would change the whole course of surgery, a substance that for the first time would make anesthesia a precise science.

Harold's father, Alexander Griffith, was a physician and a practitioner of homeopathy (treating disease by minute doses of remedies that in healthy persons would produce symptoms of the disease, e.g., quinine, to treat malaria). He founded the Montreal Homeopathic Hospital—now the Queen Elizabeth—and his son Harold, who was born in 1894, had first-hand experience of it when he entered the hospital as a patient at the age of twelve. He had appendicitis.

Harold was delighted at the prospect of an operation—it would save him from having to write his school exams. He was not too happy the next day, however. "The ether was rotten," he confided to his diary.

At the beginning of the First World War he was twenty, and was about to start his second year in medicine at McGill University. He enlisted as a stretcher bearer, and won the Military Medal for gallantry under fire at Vimy Ridge. By 1917, the Royal Navy was desperately short of doctors and was offering responsible positions to anybody who could prove they had studied for three years at medical school. Griffith had studied for only one but felt that his medical experience at the front more than made up the difference. He persuaded his commanding officer to put his name forward. He ended the war as a surgeon on a destroyer.

When Griffith resumed medical studies at McGill after the war, anesthesia was still almost as crude a procedure as it had been at the beginning. It was certainly not a specialty. Quite often the job was given to any reasonably experienced student who happened to be around at the right time. Griffith tried to get as much experience as he could, not least because it was a paying job and he needed the money to help cover the cost of his tuition. He also assisted general practitioners by giving anesthetics for minor operations, such as tonsilectomies. As quoted by Philip Smith, he recalled the procedure used on children: "We would give them a whiff of ether, the doctor would force open their mouths and snip out the tonsils and then we would hold them over a bowl until they stopped bleeding." He had put over four hundred patients to sleep by the time he graduated.

Many of the patients resisted ether violently. Sometimes several orderlies were needed to hold a strong man down, not because he was unwilling to be operated upon, but because that was one of the effects of ether. It was problems such as these, and Griffith's deep concern for the patient, that made him particularly receptive to new ideas and procedures in the art, even if they were controversial. This attitude made Dr. Griffith a pioneer in the endotracheal technique, the insertion of a tube into the trachea so that in case of an accident, the anesthesiologist could supply the lungs with oxygen.

Griffith also insisted on modifying the normal urethral catheter, which was used, for instance, in draining the male bladder. To this end he wrote to the manufacturers in France, asking them for progressively thicker and thicker tubes. He had proved that these were superior to the normal catheters. (He also greatly intrigued the girls in the French factory, for the manufacturer's representative, on his next visit to Montreal, told Griffith that the girls were eager to find out more about these Canadian supermen who required catheters that were so much bigger than the usual size.)

Griffith was also among the first to try cyclopropane, a new anesthetic discovered at the University of Toronto in 1929 by G. H. W. Lucas and V. E. Henderson. By 1939, Griffith had used it more than five thousand times, without a single death on the operating table. "By this time, also, the stocky little Canadian anesthesiologist with the barrel chest and austere rimless spectacles—an odd contrast with his genial nature and lively sense of humor—had become a familiar figure at American medical meetings. He had no advanced academic honors and he represented no university or famous teaching hospital. But his obvious competence and wide-ranging knowledge of the technicalities of his calling had won him the respect and friendship of the leaders of his profession. And so, in 1940, when Wright began to seek someone to try out curare in the operating room, it was natural that among those he should approach would be Harold Griffith." Curare, the substance that Griffith was to introduce to the operating room to initiate "the greatest advance in anesthesia since its introduction to a pain-wracked world in 1846," is a black resin-like plant extract used by South American Indians as an arrow poison and the most sinister poison that nature has ever produced.

The Wright mentioned in the above quotation was Lewis H. Wright, an American obstetrician whose interest in anesthesia had led him into a pharmaceutical company, Squibb, as a representative and specialist in the subject. One of his company's drugs was Intocostrin, the first commercial preparation of curare. In 1940 it occurred to Wright that curare's effect on the muscles might make it a superior anesthetic. He was long familiar with the action of curare, for he had used it extensively in his youth as an instructor in physiology.

Unfortunately Wright was no longer in practice, and so had no opportunity to experiment himself. But, excited by the possibilities, he tried to persuade others to do so. They refused to take him seriously. They all knew the terrible effects of that legendary yellow liquid, derived from the bark of a South American vine.

Curare had first come to the attention of the European explorers in South America when it was carried into the bodies of the Spanish conquistadores on the points of the Indian arrows. Its effect was so dreadful as to inspire fearful speculation even among those who had merely heard of it. Three hundred years after the first European contact with curare, Claude Bernard, a French physiologist, carried out a series of experiments with the drug. Years later he was still writing about it with awe. "Within the motionless body, behind the staring eye, with all the appearance of death, feeling and intelligence persist in all their force. Could one conceive of a more horrible suffering than that of an intelligence witnessing the successive subtraction of all the organs that serve it, and thus finding itself enclosed alive within a corpse?" For that was the effect of curare. It paralyzed the voluntary muscles but had no effect on the ones over which there was no control, such as the heart. First the eye and facial muscles were paralyzed, then the lips, tongue, and vocal cords. Next the arms and legs became immobilized. Followed by the muscles of the chest and diaphragm; and when it was finally the turn of the lungs—sometimes after a full twenty minutes of helpless, silent terror— only then did merciful death intervene. All the time the poison was working, the victim knew what was happening, but could not communicate his frenzy of terror.

This was the substance that Wright wished to give to a patient? Some of his colleagues were appalled at the idea.

It was no accident, or impulse, or irresponsible bent for experimentation that caused Harold Griffith to act on the idea. His life and experience had created a receptivity. He could not fail to be influenced by his father's homeopathy, with its emphasis on natural substances. Whatever its hideous results, curare was certainly a natural product. Griffith's unborn sympathy was another motivation. He had always been deeply concerned for the operating room patients, wherever possible visiting them before-hand to comfort them. And in him there was also the drive of the original thinker. He had never been satisfied with the old anesthetics, which tended to poison the system, and recovery from which was often so distressful. Besides, he was expert in keeping his patients breathing through endotracheal tubes, which would surely combat the basic danger of curare, its paralyzing effect on the lungs. And curare did after all, have an antidote.

After all—why not? Curare's effect was well known. It relaxed the muscles, and that was precisely what was most needed in so many surgical operations. So, provided the patient could be kept breathing, it might just possibly be of tremendous help to the surgeon.

After he had studied the reports on the experimental use of the commercial version of curare, Intocostrin, Griffith was convinced of its merits despite the unfavourable opinion of every other anesthesiologist on the continent. On January 23, 1942, he selected a patient, a young plumber. In preparation for an appendicitis operation, the plumber was rendered drowsy by an injection of morphine, then lowered into uncons-ciousness with a mixture of cyclopropane and oxygen, and finally, as the surgeon laid open the flesh, he was given three and a half cc. of curare solution.

Griffith paused to assess the effect. "Would it work? Was the patient still breathing properly? Was his heart beating normally? Anxiously he eyed the rebreathing bag and the young plumber's rhythmically moving chest, felt his pulse, questioned the intent Enid Johnson [Griffith's assist-ant]. Everything seemed to be under control, so to make sure he would have the full effect of the curare he injected the rest of the dose.

"This was the critical moment. Griffith grasped the control wheel of the gas machine and gradually turned it to reduce the flow of cyclopro-pane. Peering into the now wide-open wound, he cut down the anesthetic to the point at which, in every operation before this one, the patient's muscles would have recovered their tautness, and the surgeon, his manipulation frustrated by their returning rigidity, would have asked for 'more relaxation, please.' Instead [the surgeon] worked on unconcernedly. Griffith's excitement mounted as his young colleague easily parted the strong criss-cross network of abdominal muscles with his gloved fingers, found the peritoneum—the membrane covering the internal organs— held it up with a pair of artery forceps and cut into it with his surgical scissors."

Curare had worked. Within a few weeks, Griffith had given curare to twenty-five other patients. "Eloquent, if inelegant, testimony to the new technique's effectiveness came during an operation to cut out the hemorrhoids of a man weighing two hundred and fifty pounds. Finding his probing impeded by the rigidity of the man's anal muscles, the surgeon requested more relaxation. Griffith administered Intocostrin and a few moments later asked the surgeon if there was any improvement. 'My God, yes,' the surgeon replied. 'I could drive a horse and cart in here now.'"

Griffith had initiated the greatest advance in anesthesia since William Morton created the loudest silence in history. Curare itself was to make a fundamental change in the philosophy and practice of anesthesia. From 1942 onward anesthesia became a true science.

14

One-Eyed MacKay and Others

ALBERTA'S MOST RENOWNED pioneer doctor was a one-eyed stoic by the name of William Morrison MacKay. He was one of Sir James Y. Simpson's pupils, and when he graduated from Edinburgh, the discoverer of chloroform was sufficiently impressed by the young man's qualities to recommend him for the post of surgeon to a Scottish parish. But perhaps Simpson was not quite influential enough to get him the job, or perhaps the parish was not to MacKay's liking, for he decided to practice elsewhere.

He was noticed to rather more effect by a representative of the Hudson's Bay Company, who, ever alert for likely recruits for the service, talked MacKay into a life of hunting, shooting, portaging, prescribing, and delivering babies and profit.

By 1867, the year of Confederation, when MacKay landed at York Factory on the shores of Hudson Bay, the company governed an empire that extended from Labrador to the Pacific. Over the next three decades, MacKay traversed thousands of miles of this territory, from York Factory to Fort Simpson on the Mackenzie River, to Fort Resolution on Great Slave Lake, to Dunvegan on the Peace River, and to Lake Athabasca, before taking up residence in Edmonton, just before the end of the century.

When MacKay started doctoring, there were very few white settlers between the Red River Colony and the Rockies, so that most of his patients were Eskimos and Indians. He proved to be ideally suited to the task of coping with the devastating epidemics among his charges: scarlet fever, smallpox, and typhus; and to the primitive conditions of the

Northwest. In time his ability to withstand hardship and fatigue became legendary.

Having himself experienced the skin-polishing heat of summer, the brain-numbing cold of winter, and the monotonous, slogging effort of travel in any season, he was all the more appreciative of the stamina of his fellow frontiersmen. He was particularly impressed by the skill and daring of the French Indian voyageurs. He once saw four boatloads of them sweeping downriver, heading for Trout Falls, where there was a sixteen-foot drop. Without faltering, the voyageurs shot over the lip of the waterfall in a headlong rush. When they reappeared in the thrashing waters below, they continued on, as if hurtling boats into space was as normal a procedure as lighting a campfire at dusk. MacKay was still gaping as they disappeared downstream with a jaunty flourish of their steering oars.

One of his trips with them was to the Mackenzie River via Norway House. There was a great deal of portaging to do. As described by H. C. Jamieson in his *Early Medicine in Alberta*, "For three weeks they toiled upstream, then over the height of land, then downstream, before reaching Norway House. The French voyageurs worked from dawn until sunset on a diet that an unemployed man on relief today would not consider fit for his dog. Pemmican, made of dried and partly pulverized buffalo meat mixed with tallow, was the food that appeased their gigantic appetites and supplied the energy for their strenuous work."

MacKay spent the winter at Norway House, which was where the voyageurs, the trappers, and the company clerks in their gray-blue capotes, silver buttons, and scarlet sashes, gathered from all over the territory to deliver their furs, collect their mail and barter goods, and exchange news, rumours, and gossip. By then MacKay had been in Canada for three years, and had learned how to make himself comfortable. Even Isaac Cowrie, a company veteran, was impressed when he met MacKay at Norway House and looked into his tent. MacKay had all his effects arranged, ordered, and stowed as handily as if he had spent his entire life in the tundra. Invited inside, Cowrie found an equally well-organized supper waiting for him, of ham, buffalo tongue, and wine.

After the meal there was the usual impromptu entertainment when one of the clerks brought out a concertina, and everybody joined in uproarious singsong until ten at night.

After seven years of soothing the feverish, binding the wounded, and prescribing the few drugs available to him—chiefly Epsom Salts, rhubarb, and gray powder—and of searching for a suitably self-sufficient wife, MacKay met and married Jane Flett. Being the daughter of a company factor, she was used to the loneliness of the vast land. Which was just as well, for her husband was often away for long periods. On one of his journeys, to combat an epidemic among the Indians at Great Bear Lake, he set out in the middle of winter, and did not return until spring.

Nevertheless, he made good use of his time when he was home. His wife bore him eight children, which must have kept her busy, sewing moccasins and deerskin clothes.

She became so expert at these tasks that once, when a company clerk was gored by a bull and suffered a large gash in the abdominal muscles, MacKay got his wife to sew up the wound, remarking that "You're better at this work than I am."

The remark was perhaps a rueful one. For the hard-muscled, self-sufficient pioneer doctor, the frontier life had many rewards, but for a true professional there was a massive drawback: his isolation from the world of medicine. He was short of instruments, materia medica, and the ready advice of colleagues. The greatest lack was that of up-to-date information. Occasionally he might receive a six-month-old medical journal in the mail, but for the most part he was isolated from news of the latest techniques, products, and discoveries. MacKay realized this most forcefully when he returned to Edinburgh on a visit in 1881. He was amazed at the revolution that had taken place since he had left home, particularly in obstetrics and surgery. Consequently he felt his isolation all the more keenly when he returned for a further sixteen years in the wilderness.

Still, this was the life he had picked, so he made the most of it. After all, it was not without its adventures. In a Scottish parish his farthest journey might have been to some outlying granite hovel, with the occasional shopping or professional trip to Edinburgh or Glasgow. Here a visit was likely to take him a thousand miles from home, by York boat, stern-wheeler, canoe, snowshoe, or dog-train—or even on skates. On one winter trip to Edmonton, a distance of two hundred miles, he skated nearly all the way. The skates were pieces of hard wood shaped to fit the soles of his boots, the blades being metal files. "On these primitive gliders the employees of the Company often enjoyed exercise on the northern water courses," notes H. C. Jamieson. But a two-hundred-mile skating journey on a couple of workshop files—no wonder Dr. MacKay's endurance was legendary.

Most of the Indian tribes that called upon the white doctor's services were friendly enough, though they still preferred their own methods, until these had been rendered impotent by the white man's diseases. The worst of these afflictions were the smallpox epidemics that periodically decimated almost every tribe from Nova Scotia to Vancouver Island.

It was not only the foreign diseases that brought cultural ruin even to such proud confederacies as the Blackfeet. Even the Blackfeet, who had so fiercely resisted the white man's treatment and trade, could not avoid the calamity brought on by the collision of a primitive culture with one represented by the traders and get-rich-quick merchants from south of the border.

The American traders began to irrupt into Canadian territory from Montana in the 1860s. The Blackfeet spurned them time after time, until the traders made them an offer they could not refuse: quick-firing rifles and "whoop-up jug-juice," a concoction of whisky, liquid tobacco, red pepper, ginger, and molasses, that amply justified its appellation as fire-water. For this lethal combination the Indians were prepared to trade not just furs but everything they owned, even their horses.

While the Indians grew more demoralized, the traders grew steadily more greedy and violent. It was their lawlessness that finally forced the federal prime minister, Sir John A. Macdonald, into establishing the North West Mounted Police.

With this semi-military force came the West's second wavelet of surgeons. Among the first were John Kittson, a McGill graduate, and his assistant, Richard Nevitt. Nevitt was based mainly at Fort MacLeod. The doctors were regular members of the force, with the non-commissioned rank of staff-sergeant.

As Albertans appear to have been careless with the early journals and records of their medical forebears—more than once Jamieson mentions the loss of such documents in his medical history of the province—we have to be content with sporadic details, such as Nevitt's, "I operated upon Kennedy's woman in Jerry Pott's house this afternoon and removed a large piece of dead bone from the humerus near the head."

Like the Hudson's Bay Company and the Mounted Police, the Canadian Pacific Railway also brought in its own medical personnel. "Railway construction in those days," wrote H. C. Jamieson, "was attended by accidents of major and minor severity and unsanitary camps invited fly-borne disease. The water supplies were often contaminated and long remained so. In consequence of this, medical men were required to look after the thousands of men on construction work. Recent medical graduates from the East were at first the only ones available, but in 1883 Manitoba having organized a Medical School, their graduates later took their places with the easterners and followed the railway west. As small centres of population grew into villages, many of these railroad doctors picked out a place where conditions promised a future home and a practice, left their positions, and became the nucleus of the civilian medical profession of the future province."

A nurse, Ellen Birtles, provided a few details of procedures in a Western hospital in the 1890s. She worked for a time in the first incorporated hospital, in Medicine Hat. "This being the only hospital between Winnipeg and Victoria," Miss Birtles wrote, "patients came from long

distances—Golden, Edmonton, Calgary, MacLeod, Lethbridge, Grenfell, Prince Albert, Saskatoon and many intervening points of the C.P.R.
A greater number of the patients were railway men and a greater part of
the work was surgery. Dr. Calder was a clever surgeon.

"At major operations the two doctors did the work, the matron gave
the anesthetic and the assistant was 'scrub-up' nurse. The sterilizing of
dressings, towels and instruments was done on the kitchen stove in
saucepans and steamers as sterilizers were unknown at that time, at least
as far as the North West Territories was concerned."

Ellen Birtles, a graduate of the Winnipeg General, later moved to a
small general hospital in Calgary. It was a former brothel. Bullet holes in
the front door suggested that it had entertained—or failed to entertain—
at least one frustrated client.

The Calgary hospital was under the command of a Mrs. N. Hoade.
Mrs. Hoade's antiseptic ideas were rather rudimentary. "She kept a
basin of carbolic solution in the entrance hall. All doctors coming into
hospital were supposed to disinfect their hands on their arrival. What
they did after that did not matter much. Her husband who acted as
orderly and general factotum saw to it that the patients took the medicine
ordered. For the more obstinate ones he had the threat of turning them
over to the local undertaker for treatment.

"Sometimes there were more than eight patients; the extra ones
stowed wherever a bed could be placed. On one occasion they were in the
corridor or in the room where meals were eaten. The latter could scarcely
be called a dining room, for it had to serve as an operating room....

"Miss Birles," Dr. Jamieson continued, "became matron after four
years of Mrs. Hoade's unconventional nursing. The new matron said
that it was very difficult working under the conditions that prevailed
then. Patients came and went as they pleased; to ask permission never
occurred to them. When one patient was remonstrated with, he said
'Show me your rules.' Of course there were none to show....

"The surgical instruments of the hospital consisted of a probe, one pair
of scissors and one dressing forceps. One mackintosh and a winchester of
carbolic acid solution completed the operating room equipment. No
towels, gowns, aprons or gloves were available. The doctor had to supply
these as well as instruments, suturing material, and whatever else he
required.

"Typhoid fever patients outnumbered all others in this as well as in all
early Alberta hospitals.

"The only assistance provided was an orderly and a woman who was
supposed to help with the nursing, and do the cooking and laundry as
well."

Alberta's first woman doctor was Etta Denovan, who came to Red

Deer with her doctor-husband in 1895. After about eight years she found the life too much for her, and moved to California. Just how hard the life was for a woman doctor can be judged by Dr. Mary Percy's description of a few day's activity in the Notikewin district, north of Grimshaw. "Wednesday I was out all day, got home at 12:30 a.m. very cold—it was freezing hard—to find a man waiting to take me to a case 20 miles away; so I had to repack my bag, snatch a biscuit or two, and start off again; they'd had to send for me to go on a saddle horse; as the trail was impassable to anything else—miles of it under water, and a couple of creeks to swim! When we were two miles from our destination a man met us and told us they wanted us in a hurry, so I did the last two miles of a 45-mile day at a dead gallop. Found the woman pulseless, cold and clammy, so it was a very good job we hurried. Stayed there till 6 p.m. (from 4 a.m.) and got in at 10 p.m., looked to the horse, made supper and went to bed. At 1 a.m. a man's voice outside my window—Could I go and see his wife?—he thought she had appendicitis—and the trail to his house was only fit for a horse. So I dressed, packed my bag, and off again. Sure enough, she was starting an appendix. I was arranging to take her down to Peace River to hospital, when another man arrived. Could I come at once to his wife? He had had to follow me over to this case, taking an extra hour, so we hurried on. Back home to fetch my bags, and then a 9-mile hurry up there. And here I've been all day, and look like being here most of the night.

"The rush continues. I've had 1½ nights in bed in the last 8 days, and have done 180 miles down here with an acute appendix. I'm just off to the hospital to give the anesthetic and then am off back to the battle. We've had another snowstorm, so we had to bring the appendix case out with a sleigh pulled by a caterpillar tractor! It was the only way. I kept her nearly unconscious with morphia, but oh boy you don't know how trying this rat-atat-a-tat of a caterpillar is until you've done seventy miles behind one."

The year of this pioneer moil: 1930.

While Alberta's progress toward the status of a province was relatively serene, tension elsewhere in the West was ready to snap into armed rebellion. As usual, whenever political passion and conflict arose, medical men were sure to be involved. One of them was Dr. John Schultz, another of those medical giants whose physique, if not his capabilities, almost guaranteed him a prominent role in the Red River Opera Company with principal tenor Louis Riel.

Schultz, who was scaled in proportion to a Scandinavian father, began his medical studies at Queen's University in Kingston, and completed them in Toronto, in the first year of the American Civil War. He set out for the West on the day of his graduation. In the Red River settlement he soon came to share the point of view of the "Canadian" party, a group that favoured union with Canada, and who strongly opposed the dominion of the Hudson's Bay Company.

"Wherever Schultz strode either the grass withered or the snow melted," wrote W. G. Hardy. Four years after the brawny doctor's arrival at the Red River, he had become the noisiest spokesman of the Canadian party. This, of course, did not earn him a living, so to keep his bellicose soul and outsized body together, and to maintain him in the comfort that a medical practice could not, he established a commercial enterprise with his half-brother, McKenney. The business failed, creating such acrimony between the partners that when McKenney tried to force Schultz to pay his share of the company debts, the doctor refused, and was promptly flung into jail.

Schultz's new wife, who was as aggressive as her mate, just as promptly organized a band of vigilantes, attacked the jail, subdued the guard, and set her husband free.

It was typical of the feeble administration in the country that not only did the rescuers go unprosecuted, but no real effort was made to enforce the law as it applied to the giant medico. It was not exactly a lesson in civic responsibility calculated to increase respect for law and order among the Red River settlers or the half-breed Metis, both of which groups were already highly skeptical about the advantages of Confederation. The Metis in particular were apprehensive that a rush of immigrants from Eastern Canada might end their light-hearted carousals and wild buffalo hunts. Inevitably, when Louis Riel, a trainee despot with hypnotic eyes and a gift of the gab, proved able to express the Metis resentment, they rallied behind him to defy the federal authority.

Our equally hot-headed doctor made things worse with a provocative gesture of his own. He fortified his house near Fort Garry (Winnipeg), crammed it with armed bunkies, and loudly defied the half-breeds; though when Riel appeared with four times as many followers and two cannons, the number of Schultz's supporters diminished considerably.

With his house surrounded, Schultz's enthusiasm for a counter-revolution also wavered. Choking with fury, he attempted to arrange terms with the rebel chief, but Riel refused to negotiate. Dr. Schultz surrendered. With his remaining supporters, he was escorted to jail.

Once again, Mrs. Schultz helped to spring her husband. On a January night in 1870, "the indomitable Dr. John Christian Schultz screwed a gimlet, smuggled along with a pocketknife given to him by his wife in a pudding, into the window casing of his cell. To it he tied a rope made by slicing the buffalo robe on his bed into strips. Then he squeezed his six-foot-four body through the window. Part way down, the gimlet pulled out, Schultz fell heavily into the snow, one leg twisted under him. He waited a moment, anxiously. The night was cold and Riel's guards were slack. Dragging himself to the wall, by boxes piled up, Schultz got over. Somehow, in spite of his injury, he staggered four miles through the snow and cold to Kildonan. There Robert MacBeth...though he was not even a particular friend of Schultz, hid him for four days while the red-blanketed horses of the Metis streamed by with orders to shoot the escaped prisoner on sight."

Dr. Schultz managed to get away to Ontario, where he helped to rabble-rouse the East against the Metis. He returned later to avenge himself on the Riel supporters, his ardour inflamed by his own poor showing at Fort Garry.

Riel's first rebellion might have made a passable if somewhat unglamorous musical comedy, possibly climaxed by the scene in Ottawa where Dr. Schultz, newly elected as a member of Parliament, discovers that his detested opponent, the outlaw Riel, has also been elected, and has actually had the gall to sneak into Parliament to sign the members' register.

The second rebellion, a few years later, was serious enough for the federal authorities to oppose him with a considerable military force. Its chief of medical staff in the field was another of the country's powerful medical men, in influence as well as in physique. At thirty-nine, Thomas Roddick was already on the way to becoming one of the most commanding figures in the medical and social world in nineteenth-century Canada.

Roddick, a native of Harbour Grace, Newfoundland, had begun his medical training at the age of fourteen, as an unofficial apprentice to a Truro, Nova Scotia, doctor. Three years later he decided to continue his studies in Edinburgh. On his way through Montreal, he presented a letter of introduction to George Fenwick of the Montreal General Hospital. While he was talking to Fenwick, the chief surgeon received news of a railway disaster at St. Hilaire. That morning a train filled with German immigrants had failed to stop at an open drawbridge over the Richelieu River. There were heavy casualties, with nearly a hundred dead.

Roddick volunteered to help. Dr. Fenwick was so impressed with the boy's emergency surgery at the site of the disaster that he persuaded the lad to stay in Montreal, and take his medical training at McGill.

Edinburgh, with its galaxy of great teachers, was then at the height of its fame, so the decision could not have been an easy one. On the other hand, the McGill School was on its way to becoming one of the continent's top institutions.

Roddick stayed. By the age of twenty-nine he was professor of clinical surgery.

"From the first," wrote a colleague, "Roddick brought a new spirit into the teaching of bedside surgery, becoming most skillful as an operator, and renowned as a teacher. He had a wonderful facility in diagnosis and treating fractures, and his bandaging was a work of art. His love for his work, genial manner, and innate kindness of heart endeared him to all the students."

A group of those students once paid him a remarkable tribute. While they were taking their final exams in surgery, Roddick entered the examination place, the old Molson Hall. Whereupon the students, despite the tension of the occasion and the importance of not wasting a minute of the available time, laid aside their pens to applaud their teacher for several minutes. The spontaneous demonstration was all the more remarkable in that it was Roddick who had set the examination paper.

At least one of his patients was not quite as respectful. While Roddick was standing beside the operating table one day, lecturing the students in the gallery, the patient, described by Roddick's biographer, H. E. Mac-Dermot, as a husky thug, leaned up on one elbow and delivered a piledriver that knocked Roddick cold. Possibly the patient was demonstrating one of the side effects of ether, or perhaps he was hoping to postpone the operation — which did, in fact, have to be postponed until the surgeon could be revived from *his* anesthetic.

At the time of the second Riel Rebellion in 1885, Roddick was a fine figure of a man. From the set of his powerful shoulders to the candid light in his heavy-lidded eyes, he emanated vigour and self-confidence. It was a vigour that was greatly needed in building up the army medical staff. He accomplished the task in short order, and by April 7 was ready to entrain for Winnipeg in the company of the commanding officer of N. 1 Field Hospital, Dr. Campbell Douglas.

The army commander, Fred Middleton, was already in the field with his five thousand men, and already following the army custom of considering all the alternatives and plumping for the least imaginative. He ordered Roddick to set up his medical organization at Swift Current and to use the Saskatchewan River as a line of communication to the front; though as Roddick soon discovered, the Moose Jaw trail provided a better route.

Further, Middleton, despite Roddick's increasingly exasperated promptings, was tardy about giving the order for the transfer of the field hospital to the front. It was April 23 before a hospital staff, under surgeon James Bell, was ordered to join Middleton's forces. But before Bell could get there, Middleton had bungled an attack on the Metis, at Fish Creek, and suffered fifty casualties.

Days later, Roddick learned that Bell had still not reached the vicinity of the battle. Bell's river transport, the steamer *Northcote,* had run aground. Aware that Middleton must now be desperately in need of his medical services, Roddick decided to go to the front without orders. Simultaneously Campbell Douglas volunteered to try and reach the front by river.

Taking four dressers and as much in the way of supplies as he could carry in a wagon, Roddick traveled overland by the Moose Jaw trail. Four days later he reached Saskatoon to find that Campbell Douglas had managed to get there ahead of him. Douglas had paddled a canoe two hundred miles along the South Saskatchewan River, a notable achievement that earned him a Mention in Despatches.

It was not his first award. A native of Quebec City, the redoubtable Major Douglas had earned the Empire's supreme military award, the Victoria Cross, for his exploits eighteen years previously, in the Pacific Andaman campaign. After retiring with the rank of brigadier, he settled on a farm near Lakefield, Ontario, until the prospect of further battles and adventures brought him to Roddick's side.

Dr. Campbell's account of his canoe trip was, as MacDermot notes, "a good illustration of the casual manner in which the campaign was regarded."

"One sunny morning in April," Douglas wrote in a magazine article, "we were sitting at breakfast in a caboose on the Canadian Pacific Railway at Swift Current, and were talking about an encounter that had recently taken place between a party of half-breeds and the force of Canadian Militia under General Middleton, and were discussing the possibilities of the 'Northcote' making her way down the river safely. A happy thought occurred to me. Why not go down the river in a canoe I had with me? I would be such an insignificant object that if there were hostile Indians along the bank I would probably pass without being seen. I would see what the river was like and how the steamer was getting on. After a little discussion with the General in command it was decided that I should start next morning.

"Then I set to work to make my preparations, not without sundry misgivings as to my reaching my destination, a sort of half regret that I had committed myself, and mental visions of wily Indians taking a pot shot at the solitary navigator and sending him to the happy hunting grounds to paddle his own canoe at his leisure."

Accordingly, Dr. Douglas set off for the river, thirty miles away—after his friends had requested a few locks of his scanty hair, "to leave as little as possible for the inhabitants of the country through which I was going to pass." He rode out in a buckboard supplied by Roddick, drawn by a deceptively mild-looking Indian horse. Halfway to the river, Douglas got down to make sure his collapsible canoe was still in good shape, after all the buffeting it had received on the corrugated, pot-holed trail. The horse immediately added some buffeting of its own. "No sooner was I engaged with both hands about the package than he humped up his back, kicked up his heels, and away went buckboard and pony at a pace I should never have dreamed of his being able to accomplish, leaving me standing holding onto my canoe package."

When Douglas finally caught up with the animal again, "He looked as sleepy as ever, and immediately coughed as if to hint that his chest was delicate."

Douglas reached the river the following morning and set off, paddling during the day and sleeping under the canoe at night. In due course he caught up with the *Northcote*, which was still grounded. He joined the rest of the medical personnel on board, and shortly afterwards the boat was warped off the sandbank. Almost immediately it became embedded in another sandbank. Finally Major Douglas grew tired of being warped from sandbank to sandbank, and set off again in his canoe. Consequently he was the first to reach Saskatoon, then a village of twenty houses and a small school.

He was soon joined by Dr. Roddick, who bustled about, organizing hospital accommodation for the casualties, including those from the Battle of Batoche, where Riel was finally defeated.

Roddick was the first surgeon in Montreal to apply the new antiseptic methods systematically, and in Saskatoon he took particular care over the sanitary arrangements for the wounded. He was tremendously excited over the results, and when Dr. Henry Chown of Winnipeg met him some time later, he was still marveling about it. "His one medical topic then," Chown wrote, "was the wonderful results they had secured in their operations after the battles: 'Hopeless cases recovered. Dead men were brought to life.' Compared to the results which they had been accustomed to secure in the Montreal General Hospital in similar cases they were amazing, and he could not stop reporting. Looking back now, this was evidently due to the aseptic atmosphere of the tent hospital. There were no germs there," Dr. Chown concluded, "while the Montreal General Hospital was saturated with them."

15

Perspective:
The Bloodstained Frock Coat

THE MAN WHO defeated the germs, Joseph Lister, was one of the students who had been present during the first act of that other revolution in the operating theatre, when Robert Liston amputated the leg of the London butler, Churchill, while the butler was under the influence of ether. Lister, a tall nineteen-year-old with a nervous stammer, had begun to study surgery shortly before the introduction of anesthesia. As a freshman he was naturally curious about the "Yankee dodge," but was even more anxious to watch the famous Mr. Liston perform one of his lightning operations. Lister wanted to see how Liston compressed the artery with his left hand while cutting with his right, or, if he needed both hands, by holding the bone saw between his teeth.

Anesthesia had ended the screams of terror and agony that resounded through the mid-century operating room with its instrument cupboard, sturdy wooden table, gas jet, and wash basin, but Lister was well aware of what happened afterwards, when the patient was trundled back to the ward. His way to recovery was barred by tides of inflammation, suppuration, erysipelas, or gangrene. Before anesthesia, two out of every three patients operated on died. Afterwards, one out of every three. These were statistics hardly calculated to encourage surgeons to undertake any but the least complicated knifework. So the art continued to be rough and ready. In Lister's school in London, University College Hospital, the senior surgeons got through the week's operations in just one afternoon, with plenty of time left over to change out of their bloodstained frock coats and dress for dinner. Closer to home, Dr. George Bingham, recalling his student days at the Toronto General, said that, "I can remember when a clinic consisted of a rabble of students following a professor about the fetid-smelling ward while he examined unhealed wounds with unwashed hands; then after lowering his olfactory organ to the reeking stump he would straighten himself up and declare to the class, 'gentlemen, this pus is laudable.' Yet the patients died just the same. I remember the preparation of a fashionable surgeon for a major operation consisted in turning back the cuffs of his Prince Albert coat, which was preferably an old one, and washing his hands in a very perfunctory way at the tap. The usual treatment for compound fracture was an amputation, otherwise the patient would die, as he often did anyway. I recollect that during one whole winter session the abdominal cavity was opened on only three occasions, with two deaths."

Richard B. Nevitt, then an intern at the same hospital, described how, before Listerism, "Instruments and basins were cleaned after the operation in the manner of a camper washing his dinner dishes, and then put away for the next operation. The silk and linen thread used for ligatures was cut to convenient lengths as it came from the shop and often passed through the buttonhole of my coat to be reached for use by the operating surgeons when required to tie a vessel or put in a suture. Scissors and probes were wiped on a towel or bandage and used again without special preparation. I carried in the upper pocket of my vest a probe, a pair of scissors, a pair of dissecting forceps and a scalpel and would only wash them in water if it was handy."

Dr. Nevitt also recollected that, "During an operation the favourite place for the knife when it was out of use was in the surgeon's mouth to prevent the danger of its edge being dulled by contact with the table."

There was one seemingly unanswerable question until Lister revised the medical catechism. Why was it that the simplest surgical operations were so very often followed by disastrous poisoning? Lister came to believe that putrefaction caused wounds to become infected, and that the process somehow resulted from their exposure to the air. Take, for instance, fractures. With a simple fracture, where there was no break in the skin, the patient recovered easily. If it was a compound fracture, with the bones sticking through the skin, the patient usually died of blood poisoning.

The answer seemed obvious enough. In the former case, the bones and tissues were protected by the unbroken skin, while in the latter they were wide-open to infection.

All the same, not all wounds exposed to the atmosphere became infected. Lister noted that a private patient operated on in his bedroom at home remained mostly uninfected, while in a hospital ward a patient's wound suppurated as often as not. Why should this be so, when the air to which the wound was exposed was identical in its gaseous composition?

Or was there something else floating in the hospital air that had not yet been detected?

The answer had been staring the surgeon in the face for years, but because the question had been addressed to obstetricians rather than to people like himself in general surgery, he did not see how the lesson applied. At the end of the previous century, a Scottish doctor, Gordon, had shown that puerperal, or childbed, fever, which killed as many as one out of every two women who had just given birth, was conveyed from one victim to another by "an atmosphere of infection," which was clearly transmitted by the midwives or other attendants. Unfortunately for Gordon, he did not present his facts convincingly, and therefore did not qualify as an originator under Osler's definition: "the credit goes to the man who convinces the world, not to the man to whom the idea first occurs."

Ignaz Semmelweis was the one who presented the facts clearly. His findings were promoted so forcefully by the American, Oliver Wendell Holmes, that the profession was finally forced to pay attention.

Semmelweis, a Hungarian, stalked two maternity wards in Vienna. One of them was used for teaching students. Three times as many women died in that ward as in the other, and the authorities had resigned themselves to the situation as an 'Act of God.' Semmelweis' attitude was that there had to be a rational explanation, and he spent most of his working hours considering it. One day at a post-mortem examination on a professor who had stabbed his finger during a dissection and died of blood poisoning, he noted that the changes in the body of the victim were exactly like those that took place in a woman's body after a fatal bout of puerperal fever. He asked himself the obvious question—obvious except that it had never occurred to anyone else—What was the connection between the dissecting room and the maternity ward? Simple. The students made their way directly from the one to the other.

Semmelweis considered the situation for several days, then placed a bowl of chloride of lime solution between the two wards, and ordered his students to rinse their hands in the disinfectant before touching any parturient woman. The mortality rate from puerperal fever declined spectacularly. Semmelweis then went on to show that *any* putrid substance could cause puerperal fever, not just the shreds and particles from cadavers conveyed to the female patients by the medical students. Any kind of poisonous material, such as pus, if potent enough, could be passed on to the women without physical contact. In other words, it could pass through the atmosphere.

Perhaps not so amazingly, in a time when men's minds were still barely ajar to new principles, years went by before Semmelweis's colleagues were prepared to accept his doctrine. Even the obstetrical expert, James

Y. Simpson, the discoverer of chloroform, scoffed at first, though to his credit he abandoned his opposition and became an enthusiastic convert once the facts of this major advance in midwifery were properly presented to him.

In the meantime, Joseph Lister was taking a different route to the solution of his surgical problems. He was discovering Pasteur.

Louis Pasteur, linked with the Englishman as one of the greatest of all benefactors of humanity, was a chemist who had brought to the problems of biology the same brilliant technique that Harvey had applied to the study of the healthy body. Through his studies on fermentation, Pasteur showed that the changes in fermenting acids were due to micro-organisms, some airborne, others to which the air was unsympathetic. He was struck by the similarity between putrefaction and the infectious diseases. As soon as he was provided with the opportunity to do so, he turned from chemistry to biology, and established by methods that could be ignored but not refuted, that putrefaction was caused by microscopic organisms which could be borne by particles of dust in the air.

With growing excitement, Lister read everything that Pasteur had to say on the subject, and it was both a revelation and a confirmation of what he had suspected for some time but had not been able to prove. There were profound truths to be learned from Monsieur Pasteur. The organisms not only sailed through the air. They rode along on skin or clothes. They were even capable of hitch-hiking on glass and metal. But. They could be roadblocked.

Lister later wrote to the Frenchman, "to tender you my most cordial thanks for having, by your brilliant researches, demonstrated to me the truth of the germ theory of putrefaction, and thus furnished me with the principle upon which alone the antiseptic system can be carried out" — a letter for which Pasteur was deeply grateful, especially as so many of his compatriots had still not grasped the importance of his work. When he received the letter, he had only recently finished explaining to the surgeons of the Academy of Medicine why they should pass their instruments through a flame before using them. The surgeons did not have a clue what he was talking about until he explained that fire destroyed the infection's organic dusts harboured in the minute crevices of the instruments.

(Such is the ultra-conservatism of medicine that the combined contributions of Pasteur and Lister were still being ignored during the Franco-Prussian War of 1870, about which Vallery-Radot wrote, "It is impossible...not to feel an immense sadness at the thought of the hundreds and thousands of young men who perished in ambulances and hospitals during that fateful year, and who might have been saved by Lister's method.")

Lister's initial method was to prevent the lethal organisms from gaining access to such wounds as abscesses, and those resulting from compound fractures. Obviously he could not destroy the germs by heating the wounds, so he searched for a chemical that would do the same job. He decided on an agent that was being used as a sewage disinfectant, carbolic acid. For his first case, a compound fracture, he prepared a dressing of lint soaked in carbolic acid, with a piece of tin fixed to it by adhesive plaster, to prevent the disinfectant from evaporating. But the acid was too violent. It caused sloughing, or death of the tissues. He obtained a purer sample of carbolic acid with an "almost fragrant" smell, and diluted it. The recovery of the patient was so startling that he considered publishing this case immediately, but as others followed he found that with modifications to his technique the results were even better. He extended the treatment to surgical wounds, such as treated abscesses that were formerly lethal, owing to infection. His first such case involved "a gentleman from whose arm I removed two days ago a tumour, deeply seated, and such as probably would have suppurated in a somewhat serious manner with ordinary dressing," said Lister, in a letter to his scientist father. "Besides the patient is accustomed to a bottle of port every day after dinner; not a very pleasant patient to have to do with. Well his arm is today as free from pain, redness or swelling as if it had not been touched, and he remarked today as I was finishing the dressing, 'I always understood that the dressing of wounds was a painful thing.' He, however, had not felt the slightest inconvenience from it. He is also today regaining the appetite which chloroform had abolished," Lister added, possibly referring to the fellow's leaning to port.

Lister's antiseptic treatment benefited not only the particular patient but the hospital as a whole. He was then working at the Glasgow Royal Infirmary. "Previous to its introduction, the two large wards in which most of my cases of accident and of operation are treated, were amongst the unhealthiest in the whole surgical division," he wrote in his *On the Antiseptic Principle in the Practise of Surgery.* But since the antiseptic treatment has been brought into full operation, and wounds and abscesses no longer poison the atmosphere with putrid exhalations, my wards, though in other respects under precisely the same circumstances as before, have completely changed their character; so that during the last nine months not a single instance of pyaemia, hospital gangrene, or erysipelas has occurred in them."

Lister had discovered a new principle requiring a fundamental change in surgical practice. A band of devoted disciples carried his doctrine to all parts of the world, but many of his colleagues at home simply could not or would not understand his discovery. They thought he was merely claiming to have pioneered in the use of carbolic acid. They pointed out that carbolic acid as a disinfectant had been in use on the European continent for years.

Among Lister's detractors was Sir James Y. Simpson, who was now trapped in the habit of controversy. When Lister read his revolutionary paper on the antiseptic principle at a British Medical Association meeting in Dublin, Simpson jumped up and made disparaging remarks about it. For once Lister, who hated controversy, allowed his irritation to show. He described Simpson's response as "feeble." But then Simpson's opposition was not objectively scientific. There was self-interest involved. Simpson felt that Lister's treatment was a rival to his own invention, "Acupressure," which also aimed at procuring healing without suppuration, acupressure being defined by Godlee as "a method of arresting haemorrhage by passing needles beneath the vessels. It dispensed with the use of ligatures; and thus did away with a fruitful cause of decomposition." But it was an inconvenient and risky method, and was not widely adopted.

This did not serve to increase Simpson's receptivity to Lister's ideas, or enlarge his own benevolence. He attacked both the antiseptic system and its inaugurator with considerable animosity, even to the extent of writing anonymous letters to the Edinburgh *Daily Review,* in which, once again, he focused attention on the means rather than principle, on the carbolic acid rather than the idea.

Lister was mortified and disgusted, especially as the attacks were coming at a bad time, just as a member of his family had become a patient. A beloved sister was found to be suffering from "a mortal complaint," which "could only be relieved by a dangerous operation not hitherto performed by anyone, and which no surgeon of the day would have felt justified in undertaking either with or without antiseptic precautions." With nobody else willing to operate on "darling B.," Lister was forced to do so himself. A friend who was present said that it was a fearful ordeal for him, though the operation was successful. All Lister would say was that he would not wish to do such a thing again.

Lister fought back against the medically obtuse in clear, scientific language, pointing out that carbolic acid happened to be the first antiseptic agent he had used, but that others might answer the purpose just as well. To prove it, he continued to experiment with new antiseptics in his home laboratory, working diligently among his flasks, retorts, spirit lamps and hot boxes, his chemicals and his microscope. In time he graduated to other acids, including one suggested by Charles Darwin, benzoic acid. But he continued to emphasize over and over again that an intelligent belief in the germ *theory* of putrefaction was essential if the antiseptic treatment was to be followed successfully. To convince his colleagues once and for all, he persuaded a group of obliging friends to urinate into four flasks.

It was to be the world's most famous urine. Lister's purpose was to show that if the germ-laden air did not reach the putrescible liquid, then the urine would not putrify. To this end, the long necks of three of the flasks were cleaned, after the urine had gone into them. The necks were then heated and bent over at various angles, while the neck of the fourth flask was cut short and left vertical. The contents of all four flasks were then boiled, after which the heat was withdrawn so that the air would rush into the flasks. After that the flasks were left undisturbed, except for procedures designed to reproduce the normal temperature changes that the urine would have been subject to had it been naturally exposed to the air.

After six months, the fluid in the three misshapen flasks was unaltered, while mould had grown in the one that the air could easily enter. "What is it, then," Lister asked, "that is essential to putrefaction of urine by atmospheric influence which the bent tubes have arrested? It cannot be any of the gases [in the air] but it may be, it must be, some particles suspended in them, some dust, which the angles of the tubes might arrest mechanically. And this conclusion, inevitable as it is from the consideration of the flasks with bent necks, is confirmed by comparison with the other in which the orifice, though narrower, was purposely so arranged as to afford a better chance for the introduction of particles of dust, and in which accordingly chemical changes soon declared themselves in the contained liquid."

The flasks became classical exhibits. Two years after the initial samples were provided, Lister personally carried the containers to Edinburgh on the train, nursing them in his lap, to the amusement of his fellow passengers. Though the contents whirled and frothed in the misshapen vessels, no putrefaction resulted, not even after the jolting they received over the cobbled streets of Edinburgh. They were to be exhibited to many generations of students. Four years after the experiment the fluid was still clear, "and in 1877 they survived a yet more dangerous journey south, and were shown to his class at King's College, London. it is believed that in the end they were accidentally destroyed by fire, but that the contents retained their clearness to the last." In the meantime, they had become a convincing illustration of the validity of the germ theory.

While he was occupying the chair of surgery at Edinburgh, Lister advanced the defences of the antiseptic principle. Instead of holding a last line of defence at the site of the wound, he developed a carbolic spray to surround the wound and kill the micro-organisms and fungi in the air. (The antiseptic disciples thought that the air was the prime source of septic infection, though the work of the surgeons Spencer Wells and Thomas Keith in making the formerly lethal ovariotomy operation a safe procedure by paying extremely careful attention to cleanliness—for instance, by boiling the sponges—showed that the air was not quite as dangerous as Pasteur and Lister had thought.) In any event, still pioneering into the mainly unexplored land of bacteriology (which would shortly show that the tissues themselves modified the growth of micro-organisms), Lister continued to develop a spray that would fill the air far and wide with tiny droplets of carbolic acid. The spray-producer, says Godlee, Lister's biographer, underwent a process of rapid evolution. "First a small hand spray, originally intended for freezing the skin, by means of ether, and known as Dr. Richardson's spray, was used; and Lister pointed out, in one of his papers, that by holding the india rubber ball and the bottle in one hand, it was just possible for the surgeon to manipulate the apparatus without the help of an assistant in changing a dressing. But this feat required an amount of ambidexterity not easy to attain. To get over the difficulty a foot spray was introduced, in which the bellows was worked by the foot, leaving both hands, if not the coordinating faculty, unoccupied. But both the hand and the foot spray involved so much physical exhaustion that they could only be used for an operation of even moderate length by providing a relay of assistants. The next model stood upon a tripod, and was worked with easily by a long handle. It was a cumbrous affair, which, as it could not be concealed from view in the brougham during its passage from house to house, became the object of mild chaff, and the possessor of an unflattering nickname—'the donkey engine.'"

A steam spray followed. It came in two sizes, one for prolonged operations, the other for short operations, or for changing dressings. The larger model produced a huge cloud of spray, like a very clean version of a London fog. Often a very wet fog, which was so numbing as to render the surgeon's fingers almost useless. In addition, the carbolized steam passed into the patient's lungs, which did not exactly speed his recovery. As if that were not bad enough, at the same time the combination of the operating room lamps and the chloroform vapour sometimes produced chlorine gas. Plainly, the anesthetic and antiseptic doctrines were not without their discomforts.

Still, the ordeal was considered a small price to pay for the results. Wherever antiseptism was practiced, death in the surgical wards became a rarity rather than a commonplace. Accordingly, the dense, stinging mist was endured in the more progressive of the world's operating theatres for several years, until less harrowing aseptic methods came along.

In Canada, "Listerism" caught on as slowly and with as much misunderstanding as in the rest of the world, despite the band of Canadian disciples that had surrounded Lister; among them were his house surgeon Malloch, from Hamilton, his clerk, from Toronto, and his dresser, from

Halifax. They were among the few who properly understood the master's methods. Two years after his return from Scotland, Malloch described, in the *Canada Medical Journal,* how he had opened an abscess under a piece of lint that had been dipped in a mixture of carbolic acid and linseed oil. The lint acted as a shield while he used the knife, which had also been dipped in the mixture. Afterwards he applied the carbolic dressing. The first recorded account of the use of the method in the Toronto General involved a fifty-nine-year-old woman who had had a facial tumour for sixteen years. As quoted by W. G. Cosbie, from the subsequent account in a medical journal: "The removal of the tumour was comparatively easy and after haemostatic control was established the cut surfaces were wiped over with carbolic acid in oil…and a strip of lint soaked in a similar solution was laid over the cut edges and kept in place by a few strips of plaster and a bandage. A week later it was noted that 'there had not been any suppuration, even in the course of the ligatures.' This patient left hospital in a month with a well healed wound but with facial paralysis."

Dr. Canniff, though, could not understand what all the fuss was about. After all, hadn't carbolic acid been used as a disinfectant for years and years? Canniff's views harmonized with those of Sir William Hingston, M.D., who had just stepped down from the position of mayor of Montreal, and who stoutly asserted that "he was not a believer in the germ theory, and yet he was daily in the habit of using carbolic acid….Surgeons nowadays, it seemed to him, were afraid of pure air. If the atmosphere was loaded with germs…would they not make their presence felt upon all occasions? In hospital practice, where there were unpleasant odors, he would employ it, but in private practice where plenty of pure fresh air was to be obtained, he would not think of using it."

These sentiments, expressed at a medical society meeting in Montreal, were opposed by another prominent member, Dr. Craik, who riposted that *naturally* the germs would not make their presence felt upon *all* occasions. "In Canada," he said, "at certain seasons and in certain localities, thistledowns might be seen in large quantities floating in the air, and being carried with it to reproduce themselves and contaminate healthy soil elsewhere. But it would be…absurd to argue that the air was always, and under all circumstances, loaded with thistledowns."

But, he snapped, "Dr. Hingston should not jump to the hasty conclusion that because he could not see the germs, they did not therefore exist. There were other kinds of evidence which ought to convince a reasonable mind."

Unfortunately Dr. Craik was not able to supply that evidence, prompting Roddick's biographer to observe that "It is curiously interesting now to look back on these discussions, and see how near and yet how far even Lister's followers were from the truth. There was really very little difference between Craik and Hingston in practise. The former believed in the 'germ theory' but was quite vague about it; the latter wanted more proof than could then be given him."

Thomas Roddick did much to convert Canada to Listerism. Even so, it was 1877 before he imported the full antiseptic works from Britain, including gauze charged with antiseptic, treated drainage tubes, and the carbolic spray that only a year later would start to go out of fashion in Europe, after a respected German surgeon attacked it in a paper entitled *Fort mit dem Spray!* From Roddick's first use of the spray, Montreal surgeons were quickly converted by Roddick's remarkable results, even though the carbolic spray led to many cases of nephritis (an inflammation of the kidney) among both patients and doctors, and even though there was a good deal of grumbling from such as the professor of anatomy at McGill, who claimed to have been nearly drowned by "that fellow Roddick and his spray."

But even the professor could not deny that Roddick was showing results unmatched by anyone else on the continent. During the two-year period before Listerism was adopted at the Montreal General, almost every single amputation performed proved fatal, as did nearly every breast amputation and tumour excision. It was next to impossible to protect a wound against that severe contagious infection of the skin, erysipelas, and blood poisoning was an everyday occurrence. Over a similar period following the introduction of Lister's method, out of sixty-four major operations, there were two deaths. And, wrote Roddick, "There is another remarkable fact which is well-worth recording, namely, that in the two years under consideration, there has not been a single dath from erysipelas."

It was only slowly that Roddick realized that the spray was really not all that valuable as an antiseptic technique, and that the situation had become a bit absurd, especially in places like Germany where they had developed such enthusiastic spray machines that the surgeons had to wade around the operating room in Wellingtons, and onlookers had to stand on chairs to keep their feet out of "a Niagara of antiseptic solutions." But then, bacteriological knowledge was still accumulating quite slowly, so it was still a while before it was appreciated that showering the patient, the surgeons, and his helpers, with a deluge of acid was not really necessary; that dry dressings with aseptic and sterilized materials could combat the widespread infective organisms just as well.

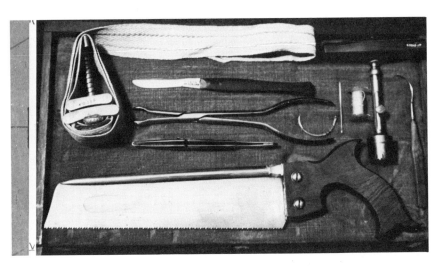

ABOVE: The military sur-
geon's kit. (Museum,
Academy of Medicine,
Toronto) RIGHT: Tiger
Dunlop, surgeon, scribe,
and swashbuckler. (Public
Archives Canada/C98796)

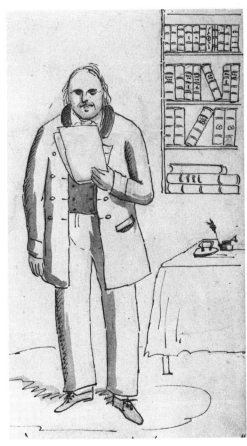

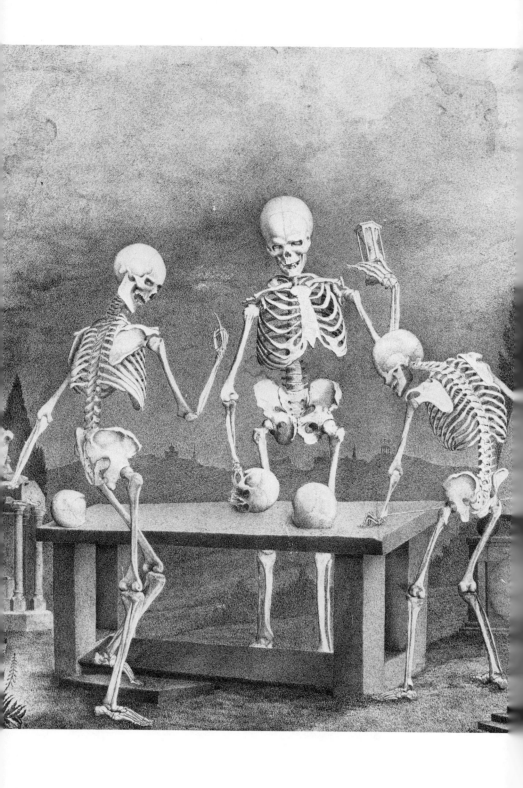

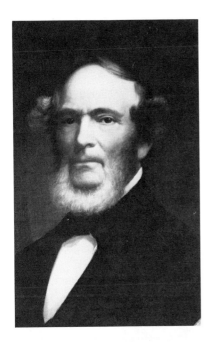

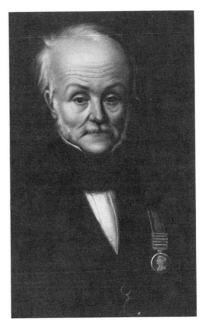

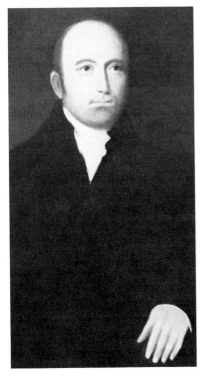

FAR LEFT: A nineteenth-century drawing by Dr. Norman Bethune (grandfather of the famous surgeon and adventurer) of the skeletons of three of his colleagues playing at log-gats in the cemetery. On the left is George Herrick, whose specialty is indicated by his right hand with index finger in the attitude of obstetrical examination. In the middle stands Christopher Widmer; the hour glass in his left hand is a memorial of his military punctuality. On the right is John King. (Museum, A of M) ABOVE LEFT: Charles Duncombe, rebel medico involved in the 1837 agitation. (PAC/C4500) ABOVE RIGHT: Christopher Widmer, one of English Canada's first establishment surgeons. (Museum, A of M) LEFT: John Rolph, teacher of medicine and rebellion. (Museum, A of M)

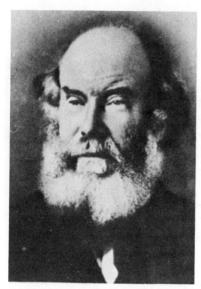

LEFT: William Tolmie, pioneer physician and fur trader of British Columbia. (Mitchell Press) BELOW: Post mortem 1898. The subject is Jefferson Smith, gangster, shot after robbing a Canadian miner in Alaska. (PAC/C52202)

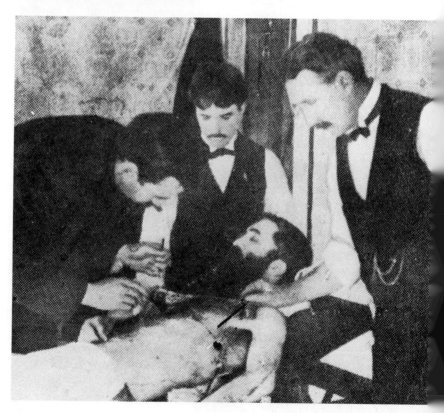

16

William Osler

D R. GEORGE LIVINGSTONE Peabody, attending physician to the New York Hospital and professor in the College of Physicians and Surgeons, a man of fine family connections and social standing, had studied extensively abroad; at Vienna, Prague, Leipzig, and other continental centres, and had met many promising men in the profession, but the one who inspired his warmest admiration was a man from Canada named William Osler, for whom a brilliant career was predicted. Osler had recently, at the age of twenty-five, gained a position at McGill University. Dr. Bryson Delavan, who was working with Peabody in a laboratory adjacent to the New York Hospital, heard a good deal about this Dr. Osler and was willing to appreciate anyone who had Peabody's approval, yet, "my first impressions far surpassed expectation."

"One bright afternoon while working in our laboratory, the door was suddenly opened and a picture was presented never to be forgotten by me," said Dr. Delavan. "In the full light of the room, framed in the doorway and with the dark background behind, there appeared in the verisimilitude of a portrait the presence of a particularly attractive young man, radiating the spirit of youthful buoyancy and delight, an expression instantly reflected in the countenance of his joyously welcoming friend. Never was there manifested more perfect sympathy of heart, mind and soul than shone from the faces of those two fine youths. My introduction to Dr. Osler proceeded at once, and the acquaintance begun from that moment was happily continued until the end of his wonderful life."

With no certain exception, everyone who met Osler responded with love to his unaffected warmth, his enthusiasm, his devotion to science and to the joy of life, and to his belief in his fellow man. "When he entered a room or a ward, even the eminent Francis Shepherd, who was not noted for effusiveness, agreed that "one could see how much he was beloved by all," while one of his students exclaimed, "How we respected and loved Osler in my class of '79 at McGill. How he worked for the students and made them a part of himself." And, said Sir Arthur Keith of the Royal College of Surgeons of England, "A future generation will never understand the love which Osler's own generation lavished on him, and the respect in which it held him. He was an outstanding figure in the medical life of his time, but it was not what he did for medical progress that made him great and loved. He was really great and truly loved, because his qualities and abilities made him the central pivot round which the social medical life of two continents turned."

Sir Arthur underestimated his contemporaries' ability to portray this remarkable man. To begin with, we see Osler vividly through their descriptions. "Among the earliest recollections I have of Dr. Osler," said Dr. Darey of Sioux City, Iowa, "are those of seeing him almost daily walking down McGill College Avenue when I was a High School boy. He always seemed to be in a hurry to get somewhere. As a boy I remember admiring his personal appearance with his high silk hat and his Prince Albert coat. He knew all the children on the street and always had a cheery word for them." From a Dr. Shultz of Montreal: "From the time I saw him, a small, alert, black-eyed intellectual looking young man, he gave me the impression that he was one of the most, if not the most, intelligent-looking man I had ever met. His whole appearance, his speech and his ways and manner, all seemed so easy, and indicated to my mind a very well-balanced man, mentally as well as bodily, with an exquisitely perfect control over his actions and movements." And from a Dr. Finney of Baltimore: "Well do I remember that eventful day, May 7th, 1889, when the doors of the Johns Hopkins Hospital were thrown open to the public. There had gathered a distinguished assemblage containing many notable personages, both lay and medical, representing the elite of the profession of the country, and the responsible citizens of Baltimore and vicinity. Among the prominent figures who were present was one on whom, perhaps more than anyone else, were focussed the attention and interest of the assemblage. That man, a rather spare figure, a little below the average height; dressed immaculately; debonair, with a flower in the buttonhole of his prince Albert; with coal black hair, just beginning to get a little thin over a high forehead indicative of great intellect, a flowing moustache, bright, piercing eyes in which lurked almost constantly a most engaging twinkle; a complexion rather sallow, yet suggesting good health and constitution; with quick and agile movement, indicating great nervous energy; and altogether giving the impression of a body under excellent control physically, endowed with great mental acumen and poise, and possessed to a marked degree of the sense of humor."

"I never saw a face like his," wrote Charles Emerson of Indianapolis, and went on to wonder if perhaps Osler's charisma was not overblown, the product of a fashionably excessive admiration. After meeting Osler again in Paris, Emerson had no further doubts. "He had not seen the hospitals of that city for several years," Emerson recalled, "and so visited several. We entered the outpatient department of one in the morning while the medical clinic was at its busiest. This occupied a large single room in which were crowded doctors, students and the patients, both those being cared for and those awaiting their turn. Four patients just then were being examined, each in a different part of the room and each surrounded by a group of doctors and students. No one there knew Dr. Osler; no one of them had any idea who this stranger was. He was not introduced; in fact, he did not speak a word; and yet from the time he entered the room it was evident that many of the doctors there were interested in him. As he moved about the examinations stopped, the groups opened and the doctors signified by gestures that he was welcome to examine the patients. He was there not over ten minutes. When I held the door open for him and Dr. Jacobs to pass out, looking back I noticed that all the work in the room had stopped and that many were following him with enquiring eyes as he passed through the door. Two evenings later the intern group of another hospital, which he had visited that evening, spoke of him frequently during the dinner with admiration, using such phrases as 'What a remarkable face,' 'What sympathy!'"

Dr. Emerson had been living among those French interns and was sure that they had known nothing of Dr. Osler's reputation, and knew that it was not the custom of French students to speak enthusiastically about any visiting doctors, especially foreign ones.

This extraordinary personality, this openness to his fellow human beings, drew children to him even more magnetically than it did his fellows and colleagues. "No one," wrote Edith Reid in *The Great Physician,* can appreciate his psychology unless they know him with children.... He was what few grown people are to children—of their own age; only he was their chosen Captain. The lithe form, full of vitality, the beautiful dark face so vivid, and the radiant eyes, were all sympathy for them; their pleasures, their woes, were his pleasures, his woes; everything in their lives was a part of him." When Osler moved to Philadelphia he wrote constantly to his young friends in Montreal, often sending presents or enclosing money from his meagre salary. When young Willie Francis, who was later to become a doctor himself, wrote saying how much he missed Dr. Osler: "It's myself that's longing to see you old boy!" was Osler's typically-phrased reply; and he went on to suggest that if Willie's skinny little body could not manage the journey, perhaps his spirit could. When Dr. Osler's friend Beatrice was ailing: "Are you better? My heart bleeds for you in seven places." When Willie was ailing, Osler prescribed on a postcard:

> I will to you speed
> If you truly me need
> But meanwhile apply
> Three or four crumbs of bread
> To the edge of your head
> If relief does not come
> While you spell the word thumb
> Take a hair of your mother
> Or sister or brother
> Cut it up very fine
> And take it in wine
> No head can withstand
> A medicine so bland
> The ache will just fly
> Like the glance of an eye.
> For advice thus by post
> My charges at most
> Are a dollar a word.
> *Signed, Mailliw Relso, D.M.*

On at least one occasion, his colleagues were greatly put out by his delight in the company of children. When a group of physicians boarded a transatlantic liner to attend a medical congress in Europe, they were thrilled to learn that the great Dr. Osler was on board, and looked forward eagerly to discussing medical problems with him. Not one managed to exchange so much as a sentence with him. Osler spent the voyage playing with the children on deck, refereeing their games and joining in the fun himself.

One of his students could have explained. "Dr. Osler frequently advised us to make friends of children, for, said he, 'That is the way to keep your own mind young.'" As for the children, in those days they looked upon adults as heavy, moral forces, and to meet one who could so heighten their world of imagination was a marvellous experience. The first time he met the children of his Montreal relatives he captivated them by vaulting right across their dining room table with effortless grace. Better still, understanding their need for routine and their joy in the repetition of a joke, he vaulted the table every time he came to the house.

His playfulness was not confined to children. At the University of Pennsylvania, when a society lady asked him whether he pronounced his name Osler or Ossler, he replied, "I will answer to Hi! or to any loud cry." During his first week there, the most pious and venerable member of the faculty invited him to church. When he came into the pew with his typical dancing steps, the old man asked him why he had not brought Mrs. Osler. "Mrs. Osler is a Buddhist, and would not come," Osler lied gravely.

His impish spirit, a hundred-proof blend of the totally serious and the consistently playful, was in the Oxford tradition (to which he would later contribute), and it was some time before his American colleagues got used to his bursts of frivolity. At a medical meeting in Washington, a reporter asked him to point out some of the important medical men who were present. Osler took his arm and pointed out Dr. Delafield, a famous New York consultant. Osler informed the reporter that that old fellow over there was crazy about baseball, but as he could not play on a regular team, "he got groups of street urchins to play the game with him on vacant lots." Delafield was not at all pleased when he read the story in the newspaper the next morning.

The place of this "greatest physician of his time," in the history of medicine is not easy to explain. His fame was not the result of any particular scientific achievement, not even his authorship of *The Principles and Practice of Medicine*. It is the sum total of many eminences, in research, bedside medicine, and teaching, and in his written contributions to science, literature, and history. But certainly, "No other Canadian of his time," wrote Fielding Garrison in the 633-page *Osler Memorial Volume*, "did so much for the good name and fame of his country in all lands as this kindly, benignant and most unrivalled physician."

Willie, or Bill, Osler took his dark colouring from his mother, Ellen Free Pickton, a Londoner who had been brought up by an uncle in Cornwall. A slender, pretty girl, Ellen had the olive complexion of the English Celts; so deep an olive that when she came out to Upper Canada with her clergyman husband, Featherstone Osler, and gave birth to her equally dark eighth child, William, the Chippewa Indians in the neighbourhood thought that the Oslers had taken over a papoose, and, according to Harvey Cushion's landmark biography of the physician, aroused fears in the family that the Indians might attempt to take back the baby.

Osler's father had led an adventurous life in the navy before becoming a missionary clergyman and establishing a parsonage at Bond Head, north of Toronto. William was born there in 1849, and was a family favourite from the start, with his beautiful appearance, his gypsy colouring and bright black eyes, and his nature, which was impulsive and mischievous, but affectionate enough to protect him from the consequences of many a foolish prank around the parsonage and the hundred acres that his father had so backbreakingly wrested from the forest of white oak and maple, basswood and beech.

Not that Featherstone and Ellen were over-indulgent. There was no corporal punishment, but regulations were strict; from early morning prayers to lights-out, with farm chores rigorously apportioned, and rough schooling, miles away in Bradford. The household books were mostly religious, with one well-remembered copy of the *Illustrated London News*, containing pictures of the Crimean War. But there were also "the happy spring days," Osler remembered, "when we went off to the bush to make maple sugar—the bright sunny days, the delicious cold nights, the camp fires, the log cabins, and the fascinating work tapping the trees, putting in the birch-bark spouts, arranging the troughs, and then going from tree to tree, collecting in pails the clear sweet sap."

When William was seven, the family moved to a new parish at Dundas, on the western end of Lake Ontario, near Hamilton. There he attended a grammar school which was run by a classical despot. The headmaster was one of the few who failed to succumb to the boy's vivid personality.

A number of japes contributed to William's downfall. In one he urged a gaggle of geese into the school and locked them in; in another, he unscrewed all the school desks and hoisted them out of sight through a trap door. Failing to appreciate the humour of either a classroom filled with geese or emptiness, the headmaster expelled him. Chattie, his sister, was the first to hear the news. She met him while he was riding home on the blacksmith's horse, and when he saw her he shouted gleefully, "Chattie, I've got the sack!"

Established in a new boarding school at Barrie, he was quick to team up with two other high-spirited lads, Ned Milburn and Charlie Locke. They were soon in trouble. Irked by the early lights-out policy of the school, the trio would sneak out the dormitory window after dark and cavort along the shores of lake Simcoe, which was about a hundred yards away . One night they made two mistakes in a row. They were caught stealing melons; and the person they were caught stealing them from was the local sheriff. The sheriff was excessively proud of his melons. The boys were gated for a week and forced to copy out every page of the Virgil textbook. In reprisal, William climbed onto the roof and blocked up the chimney, filling the school with smoke. The teachers called in the fire brigade, the Barrie Hook and Ladder Company.

One of the three boys, Ned Milburn, recalled their final trick before Osler moved on to his next school, in Weston. The prank was played on an American who had advertised for a wife. "In our Toronto papers O. noticed the advertisement and suggested the following plan—to answer the advertisement describing ourselves as a brunette and a blonde respectively—so that he could make the choice according to his fancy. We had some trouble in fitting ourselves out with girls' clothes, but with my sister's help we developed into pretty fair specimens of the genus girl.

"In due time the farmer arrived at the Grand Trunk Station where we had agreed to meet him, for the station, we knew, was badly lighted, which would be of advantage to us. All went well—we resisted his request for another meeting by daylight and asked him to make his choice there and then. He did so, and as he rather liked blondes his choice fell on me. I wonder at it, for O. made a beautiful girl with his clear-cut features and olive complexion. We never knew what became of the farmer—he left us, promising to return in a month, as this would give him time to fix up his house. I hope he got a blonde."

O's real education began in 1866 at his third school, Trinity College School, in the town of Weston (now a part of Toronto). There was a teacher there who would become one of the two vital formative influences in Osler's life. This was the Reverend William Johnson, known as Father Johnson because of his stubborn adherence to High Anglican ritual. He was the founder and warden of the school, and he was popular with the boys, unlike the headmaster, a man who, with long black whiskers and a busy hickory cane, was feared.

Johnson was an enlightened educator. He did not believe in stuffing facts and figures into his students as if they were roasting chickens, but in stimulating their imaginations, in particular encouraging them to understand the beauty and order of nature, as perceived through the microscope. William, used to the drudgery of syntax and sums, mnemonics and prosody, felt liberated. "Imagine the delight of a boy of an inquisitive nature," he said later, "to meet a man who cared nothing about words, but who knew about things—who knew the stars in their courses and could tell us their names, who delighted in the woods in springtime, and told us about the frog-spawn and the caddis worms, and who read us in the evenings Gilbert White and Kingsley's 'Glaucus,' who showed us with the microscope the marvels in a drop of dirty pond water, and who on Saturday excursions up the river could talk of the Trilobites and the Orthoceratites and explain the formation of the earth's crust."

"Father" Johnson also fearlessly discussed with his favourite pupils the materialist doctrines that were flooding from the inkpots of such men as Charles Lyell, Charles Darwin, and T. H. Huxley. If Johnson was unable to reconcile Genesis with geology, it did not affect William. He did not know enough to feel bewildered. Two months after entering the school, "with a red pocket handkerchief round his neck and a sling in his hand," he was firmly on course for a career in the church.

Johnson's influence on the boy's literary and religious perceptions was to guide Osler's pen and his moral course for the rest of his life. Johnson was accustomed to reading aloud to the boys in the parsonage, and often, to illustrate the beauty of the English language, he selected passages from the *Religio Medici,* which was written in 1635 by Sir Thomas Browne, physician and author. The majestic prose of *The Religion of a Physician* came to mean far more to Osler than its purely literary worth. As Cushing says, "it was an important thread which from this point weaves its way through Osler's story to the end; and the 1862 edition of the 'Religio', his second book purchase, to which he referred more than once in his published addresses, was the very volume which lay on his coffin fifty-two years later."

William's way to a career in the church, though, was not precisely circumspect. He had only been at the school for a short time when he was branded as a criminal in the pages of the Toronto Globe. "School Row at Weston," the headline read. "Pupils Turned Outlaws." "They Fumigate the Matron with Sulphur."

What happened was that the headmaster had taken on a housekeeper, an old woman who soon came to be heartily detested by the boys. One day the old girl drenched a pupil with a bucket of slops. Whether the incident was accidental or otherwise, it was too much for the boys. Led by William, they waited until the dreaded headmaster was out of the way and proceeded to mix a preparation of molasses, mustard, and pepper. They then barricaded the housekeeper into her room and stoked the schoolroom stove with the concoction, so that the fumes would pour through the stovepipe hole to her room, which was immediately above. To avoid suffocating, the lady promptly stuffed the hole with clothes, meanwhile hollering for help at the top of her voice. Her resourcefulness was to no avail, for the boys pushed the clothes aside with blackboard pointers, and when she responded by sitting on the hole, they poked at her as well, to dislodge the obstruction of *gluteus maximus.*

Though the culprits were duly chastised with the headmaster's length of Walpole hickory, the matron was not mollified, and obtained a warrant for their arrest on a charge of assault and battery. As a result, nine of the boys, including William, spent several days in the Toronto jail. They were effectively defended by the ringleader's oldest brother, Featherston Osler. He managed to persuade the magistrate to let them off with a reprimand and a fine of one dollar. Ellen Osler also reprimanded William, by mail; but being a mother, she enclosed two dollars and a postage stamp in the same envelope.

The incident did not affect William's scholastic progress, and in due course he was made head prefect of the school. Academically he was helped by an exceptional memory and powers of concentration. During an unsupervised "prep" period he could absorb himself in a textbook in the midst of the unseemliest uproar, by holding his hands to his head with his thumbs in his ears, until he had finished what he had set out to do, and was ready to add to the pandemonium. Athletically, though undersized, he was wiry, and proved to be a fine all-rounder, breaking the record for throwing the cricket ball at term-end sports. (The school was run on English public school lines, complete with *Boys Own Paper* terminology.)

Under the Reverend Johnson's tutelage William also became the school scientist. Johnson gave him considerable responsibility in the delicate work of grinding down and mounting fossil specimens and preparing biological specimens for the microscope, and the lad's name appeared more and more frequently in Johnson's natural history notebooks— *"crocodile scale ground by Osler, ground through—dry."* The friendship between the warden and his flashing-eyed pupil, based on their almost fanatic interest in microscopy, was such that Johnson took to visiting William at his home in Dundas during the summer holidays. Together they would scour the marshes for the polyps that William was now particularly interested in. His study of diatomaceae—minute, single-celled fresh-water creatures—was to form the basis of his first scientific publications some years later. During one of these field trips he discovered a variation from the ordinary species of polyp not noted in his zoological textbook.

Without realizing it, Johnson was simultaneously encouraging the boy to enter the church and busily deflecting him from it, into science.

On holiday at home in Dundas in 1866, Osler was not so absorbed in natural history as to be immune to the excitements of that summer, caused by the Fenian raids from the United States. The Fenian Brotherhood, a well-known secret society, had decided to liberate Ireland from its English oppressors by a typically Irish route, i.e., via Canada. Their plans called for an Irish army to occupy the Great Lakes region, while other units were to capture Montreal, which was thought to be somewhere in the hills of British Columbia. Canada would then be renamed New Ireland and converted to Catholicism and Guinness.

In June, a Civil War veteran named John O'Neill crossed the Niagara River at the head of a force of several hundred, and occupied Fort Erie. There O'Neill informed the villagers that they had been liberated from the British yoke. The villagers responded by giving the invaders some fried bread, then went about their business as if nothing was happening. Actually, nothing much was happening, apart from a confrontation between a company of militiamen and the invaders at Frenchman's Creek, where the inefficiency of one side was nicely balanced by the insufficiency of the other.

O'Neill soon realized that the Canadians were not quite ready for the Pursuit of Happiness, Hibernian Division, and went home, but in the meantime he had roused a good deal of indignation among the natives, who were outraged at the way he and his rapscallions had been allowed to wander about the countryside almost unmolested. As a result, there was a fair amount of volunteer militia activity that summer, and Osler took part in it, drilling a company of youngsters for the defence of Dundas, which was uncomfortably close to the border.

He was also thought to have had at least one love affair, for when he returned for his final year at school, his elder sister wrote to warn him against entanglements. There are no further details. Osler was generous with information in his medical writings, but miserly with details of his intimate affairs.

Despite his interest in biology and geology, Osler still had the church in mind when he went up to Trinity College, Toronto, in Confederation year. But his religious enthusiasm was waning. As early as a month into the arts course, one of his exercise books showed where his interest really lay. It started out determinedly enough with a Latin prose composition, but by November he was using the pages for notes on fresh-water polyzoa—*Genus I Epthemia: adherent, quadrilateral; valves circinate furnished with transverse caniculi*—and for a list of elaborately described specimens taken from Humber Bay, Grenadier Pond, the Thames (London, Ontario, of course), and Desjardins Canal.

Osler's interest in biology rather than in such theological exercises as explaining Eternal Life in its initial, partial, and perfectionist aspects, was further stimulated by the second great influence on his life in the person of James Bovell. It was an odd influence. In contrast to Father Johnson, who was a clergyman fascinated by science, Bovell was a scientist fascinated by religion. Born in the Barbadoes, he was forty-nine when he took Osler under his wing. He had a professorship in physiology and pathology, hospital appointments, and an extensive private practice. His chief medical claim to fame was a rather peculiar one. During a cholera epidemic in 1854, he argued in favour of milk transfusions in place of blood. He transferred the milk into the patient by means of a tube, an earthenware bowl, and a cow that happened to be grazing close at hand, near the cholera sheds. "Two patients, apparently moribund, showed immediate and dramatic improvement and both survived," reported W. G. Cosbie. "However, five subsequent patients did not have such a satisfactory result from the treatment."

At Trinity, Bovell's students regarded him with resigned affection. When he appeared before them, they never knew whether to expect a lecture on medicine or theology—assuming that he remembered to come at all. He ably maintained the tradition of the absent-minded professor. When one of his students fell ill, Bovell ordered him to return to his boarding house on Grosvenor Street and stay in bed until Bovell came to visit. Three days went by before Bovell remembered to do so. Greatly agitated, he collected Osler and rushed off to visit the patient—only to find that now he could not remember the number of the house on Grosvenor Street.

As it turned out, the student had recovered and gone out for a walk. On his return he found Osler scuttling from door to door, asking if there was a sick man inside, and Bovell pacing up and down outside, looking very distressed. On another occasion, Bovell lost his horse and buggy. It was finally located outside a house that he had visited the previous day.

Bovell lived on Spadina Avenue with his four daughters. From his first year at Trinity, Osler was a frequent visitor. He was responsible for keeping the professor's aquarium stocked with pond material likely to contain good specimens of algae, and getting a variety of zoological specimens for the professor. It is not known whether Osler was interested in any of the girls, but if he was, he allocated little time for dalliance. His weekdays were spent in intense study, and his weekends were spent at Weston huddled over the microscope with Father Johnson.

One of Bovell's daughters was certainly aware of Osler. When she married, she went to live on St. Patrick's Street, and soon after, when the rest of Bovell's family moved to the West Indies, Bovell moved in with her and her husband, Mr. Barwick. Osler practically moved in as well. Mrs. Barwick's granddaughter later described how Osler, who was about twenty in those days, "literally lived at our house. He adored grandfather and the latter loved him like a son—and they were both crazy about the microscope. Mother [Mrs. Barwick] says her life was a perfect burden to her with weird parcels arriving which might contain a rattlesnake, a few frogs, toads or dormice. She found quite a large snake meandering about the study one afternoon, and when she protested violently, the two told her she should not have been in there."

William also kept up his sports activities at Weston, and one of the students later described him at that period as a "lithe, swarthy, athletic, keen-eyed boy. I don't think I ever saw anyone with such piercing black eyes.... He had a peculiar forward inclination of the body as he walked, which caused his arms to hang slightly forward and gave them an appearance of being always ready to use. He was an excellent round-arm bowler, and a batter became distinctly conscious of the strength of the lithe arm, which seemed to acquire a great part of it from his determined and piercing glance as he delivered the ball. You may think it strange that I should enlarge upon this," Mr. Armour told Dr. Cushing, "but the fact that it is as distinctly impressed upon my mind after a lapse of fifty-three years as if I had seen it yesterday will indicate the strong personality that a boy of eighteen or nineteen possessed."

In 1868, William returned for his second year in arts. He had spent the summer gathering additional samples of algae from the waterways around

Dundas. He must also have come close to a decision about his future during that summer, for he had only been back at Trinity for a few days when he announced that he was transferring to medicine. His clergyman father was naturally disappointed, but did not stand in his way. What with his son's obsession with science, Mr. Osler must have been more than half-prepared for the decision. As for Bovell, though he was soon to take up a reciprocal heading by transferring from medicine to the church, when he heard the news he exclaimed, "That's splendid, come along with me."

Osler did so literally, for during the next two years the two "lived more like father and son than as teacher and pupil." From then on, Osler poured his redoubtable energies into his studies in the Trinity College medical department, particularly in its dissecting room, one of the few places where a Toronto student could obtain practical experience. At the same time he kept up his personal and scientific friendship with Father Johnson, who continued to receive from his former pupil such specimens and slides for microscopic study as the "Trachea of a mouse... beautifully stained."

Bovell was now the stronger influence on the youth; so extraordinary an influence that for decades to come, when Osler paused to gather his thoughts or to try out a new pen, he would often write the name of James Bovell on the margins of his writing paper.

A detailed knowledge of the structure of the human body is the basic requirement for any medical student, and Osler's knowledge was to be perhaps the most complete of any physician living in that century. The groundwork for his profound understanding of the body in sickness and health was laid during those two years at the School of Medicine. His prosector in anatomy recalled that he "spent more time in the dissecting-room than any other student, frequently bringing his lunch with him in order to get some extra time there. He did much of this work alone, working out problems of his own in his own way, without the aid of a demonstrator. There he pointed out the presence of the *Trinchina spiralis*, [a parasite of pigs] in the muscles of one of the bodies, which no one else had observed." Osler was later to write a paper on the subject.

Working so many hours alone, his nerves must have been under firm control, for dead-houses in those days were dreadful places. The medical school established a few years later in London, Ontario, was not untypical. It was in makeshift quarters, a cottage on the grounds of the Hellmuth Boys' College which had been taken over by the university. The dissecting room was in the former dining room. According to Edwin Seaborn, "it contained two tables, a few chairs, a pile of sawdust, a shovel in a corner, old coats and aprons on hooks along the walls. A trap-door in the floor led to the cellar where two large vats, filled with ancient wood alcohol and other things, permeated the whole building with their odors."

In time, the cottage, which already inspired dread and fascination throughout the neighbourhood, took on a sinister appearance, as if the ghastly activities inside were affecting the very foundations. "To prevent the peering of the morbidly curious, anxious to see the 'Cuttin' up Place,' its windows had been whitewashed on the inside, a useful if not ornamental expedient. Wagons came to it at night. Strange lights would appear and in a moment disappear. Even stranger noises, cries and groans, had been heard. More terrifying than the noises had been the noiselessness with which a bent figure would disappear into it carrying a heavy burden on his back. Teamsters disliked delivering fuel to it. One of them, unable to open a door in the absence of the janitor, in attempting to force an entrance through a window, came face to face with the cadaver of a Negro. He drove away incontinently and refused to return with his load."

There is no record of Osler undergoing an initiation into this netherworld, but if his introduction to anatomy was gentle, he was fortunate. In London, "After the first month's lectures on Anatomy had been delivered, dissecting was heralded by forcing the 'Freshies' to bring the bodies up from the cellar. On the appointed day fighting began with the appearance of the first freshman. The battles were always fierce and often prolonged, and did not cease until all the freshmen had been pushed through the trap-door. On opening the trap-door, steps, in the middle of which was a plank which led from the top step to the floor, were discovered. The students, one by one, were shot down 'the plank' while a guard, whooping and dancing on the door, stood guard. The first man might be down an hour. With matches, fag ends of candles and 'the hooks' they could spend their time 'fishing' in the vats. They presented a haggard, sorry plight as they came up at last, dragging up the cadavers by slippery arms and legs."

The initiation served the purpose of accustoming the students to the rigours of *mortis* in one ghastly trial, though the Western Ontario method was such that, as Dr. Seaborn observes, it was providential that none of those involved became a maniac "permanently."

It was hardly surprising that unrestrained hysteria would follow such an ordeal. "The students, by now in rags, with wild abandonment, overturned tables and chairs, festooned 'the remains' about the room, knocked down the stovepipes, and as a finale, poured pails of water into the coal-stove."

Sometimes even the most hardened preceptor or demonstrator was not immune to the atmosphere of these primitive surroundings. At the McGill Medical School, to which Osler would shortly transfer, most of the staff and all of the students were afraid to work in the dead-house at night. "Having occupied for two sessions the position of Prosector to the Professor of Anatomy," said Dr. D. C. MacCallum, who was a student at

McGill in the mid-nineteenth century, "I had to prepare, during the greater part of the session, the dissections of the parts which were to be the subject of the Professor's lectures on the following day. This necessitated my passing several hours, usually from nine to twelve o'clock at night, in the dismal, foul-smelling dissecting room, my only company being several partially dissected subjects, and numerous rats which kept up a lively racket coursing over and below the floor, and within the walls of the room. Their piercing and vicious shrieks as they fought together, the thumping caused by their bodies coming into forcible contact with the floor and walls, and the rattling produced by their rush over loose bones, furnished a variety of sounds that would have been highly creditable to any old-fashioned haunted house."

Such locations were to be among Osler's principal addresses over the next two decades. There is an extraordinary photograph of him in one of them, the mortuary of the Blockley Hospital, Philadelphia, taken in 1886. Osler was never a satisfactory subject for a photograph. The lens, aimed at an untypical repose, could rarely capture his handsome aura, could not even hint at the subtle force of his personality. The picture in the Blockley mortuary, showing him wearing an apron with his sleeves rolled up, examining with his bare hands a heap of human organs on a wooden table, captures just one element of his character: the intensity of his concentration. He was totally absorbed.

Osler considered a knowledge of morbid anatomy to be supremely important for an understanding of the clinical problems of his live patients. At Johns Hopkins in Baltimore, says Thomas McCrae in *The Influence of Pathology on the Clinical Medicine of William Osler,* "his 'clinics' in the autopsy room were if anything more interesting than those by the bedside. He reconstructed the history of events from the specimens and correlated it with the clinical history.... He often referred to the salutary lessons of the dead-house, and the benefit that might be gained from them," McCrae wrote; and, deepening our perception of the photograph: "There was never any difficulty in having him present at an autopsy and almost any other engagement would have to wait. He may have come as an onlooker but very often he was taking part before he knew it. It was always amusing to watch him when the pathologist was perhaps rather slow in getting on with the examination. He usually took hold of the work himself. His assistants were always watching to turn up his sleeves and cuffs, as he rarely thought of them and it was difficult to persuade him to put on rubber gloves. Nearly always he handled the specimens himself and was not content with merely looking at them. Dr. Barker has told the story of a physician in a Maryland town who commented on the fact that often he was unable to get Dr. Osler to come for a consultation with a large fee, but that he would always come to attend an autopsy in which he was interested."

By the end of his third year at Trinity, Osler had made the greatest discovery of his life. It was not a scientific discovery, but the realization that the secret of a satisfying life is work. He already had the capacity for sustained concentration on the tasks at hand. Now, on top of the usual practical and theoretical program, his workload included: visits to the jail, which aroused his special interest in aneurism; visits to the veterinary college for zoological study; the preparation of two articles on the microscope and on his diatomaceae, and the cutting of thousands of sections for microscopic study on behalf of his beloved friends, Johnson and Bovell. It was a workload that would have made the average student's last-minute cramming session seem lethargic by comparison. Even so, he was not satisfied with the opportunities that the Toronto school afforded. He found many of the lectures mechanical and uninspiring, and the doodlings in the margins of his lecture notes show it: *James Bovell M.D., M.R.C.P. James Bovell M.D. James Bovell M.R.C.P.* But the principal cause of his dissatisfaction was the clinical situation. In Montreal, the doors to the hospitals were wide open to the medical students. In Toronto, at the General Hospital, they were barely ajar, and even after the students had edged inside, they found many faults in the teaching they received.

The Toronto General was inadequate in other ways. It had a messy history. It had started out as a two-story building on King Street. By 1855 it was being scathingly denounced by an informed critic in the *Colonist* as a filthy place, reeking of moral pollution and favouritism. The matron, Mrs. Donnelly, was often drunk. The critic had seen one of the orderlies brutally treating a black patient. Another patient had been resuscitated by having a pail of water thrown over him. (The critic's principal ground for complaint was that the water had not been thrown on him "in a Christian spirit.")

The *Colonist* critic also made the point that the student instruction was utterly worthless, and the money spent on it would have been better cast down the drains—if there had been any proper drains.

Shortly after these disclosures, a fine new building in the French provincial style, with a central tower a hundred feet high, was opened on Gerrard Street, but the financial support for the new hospital was so miserly that by Confederation year, when Osler was entering Trinity, the hospital was forced to close its doors. It needed five thousand dollars to stay open, but the mayor and aldermen refused to pay up. It was ten months before the Toronto General opened again, and even then it continued to be so poorly supported that it had to restrict admissions to twenty-five public patients. All others were to be charged forty cents a day. And the nursing assistance remained as bad as ever. While the cook and the washerwoman received nine dollars a month, the nurses received eight. Consequently the hospital got the kind of nursing service it was paying for.

Meanwhile the backbiting continued, as well as the financial starvation. The trustees complained about the cost of supplying the patients with milk at 12½ cents, beer at 25 cents, and whisky at 85 cents a gallon, and about irregular attendance by the medical staff, though they disagreed about the dirty conditions which had been uncovered during a snap inspection. The trustees claimed that, "The discolouration and dirty condition of sheets, blankets and coverlids was not unreasonable, as the inspection was made on Thursday and the bedding was always changed on Saturday. It was felt that the sheets must not be tested by the standards of a private family or even of a jail or a lunatic asylum, 'because they were often stained by blood and ulcerous matter.'"

The situation improved a few years later when adequate funding came along, but in the meantime the facilities for students remained inadequate. It was the trustees who sold the tickets that permitted students to receive clinical instruction at the General—the medical schools had no control over that essential aspect of training.

So in the summer of 1870, Osler left for Montreal, to complete his degree course at McGill. Parting from his surrogate fathers was not easy, but Bovell, at least, made it easier for him. He left Toronto at the same time for Barbadoes, where he finally straightened out his allegiance by giving up medicine and becoming a clergyman of the Church of England.

The closeness of Osler's friendship with William Johnson and James Bovell was quite remarkable. Their common interest in science might have formed an enduring basis for friendship, but it does not entirely explain the depth of affection that existed between Osler and the two older men. Perhaps they became substitute fathers because the warmth of their communication exceeded that of the boy's real father. Featherstone Osler was not intellectually inferior—he had been elected mathematical scholar at Cambridge before being posted to Canada—and was sympathetic to Willie's aspirations, but there did not appear to have been much warmth of feeling between father and son. In Cushing's richly detailed biography, Featherstone is not caught out in any affectionate gesture. Nor is there any from William, though admittedly he tended to disguise his tender, sympathetic, and sometimes sentimental nature. When his father died, he wrote in a letter to an old friend, "Delighted! But you must stay a week at least. Plenty of room & a hearty welcome & I want you to meet Mrs. O. My father died two weeks ago—arteriosclerosis. Sorry to hear that you have had a cold—the trip will do you good."

Except in one respect, Osler found that conditions at the Montreal General Hospital were no better than those in Toronto.

The Montreal institution had begun with a bang. Soon after it was established, a member of the Quebec Legislature, Michael O'Sullivan, heard that Dr. William Caldwell, a staff man, intended turning the

General into a professional medical clinic. O'Sullivan immediately challenged Caldwell to a duel. He believed that the French tradition should
be maintained, that "patients should be served by nuns devoted to the
service of God, not by hirelings."

Possibly O'Sullivan thought that Caldwell, being a man devoted to
relieving suffering rather than adding to it, would decline the opportunity
to determine policy with pistols. Unfortunately for him, Caldwell not
only accepted the challenge but turned out to be thoroughly familiar
with firearms, as he was a former army surgeon. During the duel he
proceeded to place a bullet in each of O'Sullivan's legs, then cold-
bloodedly put the final bullet into his body. (The hospital itself later
revenged O'Sullivan by claiming Dr. Caldwell as a typhus victim.)

Half a century later, the building on Dorchester Street was a thoroughly rat- and coccus-riddled lodgement, grossly overcrowded despite
the addition of various wings. (Even one of the wings had a wing, the
infectious diseases hospital.) Much of the trouble was caused by an
abominable ventilation system. Even after ventilation pipes were added,
somebody closed the dampers — presumably to keep out the drafts. They
remained closed for years. When a "Lady Trainer of Nurses" finally
opened them in 1880, she was deluged in dust. In addition, some fiendish
designer had placed the toilets next to the shaft through which the meals
were hoisted to the male side of the hospital; meals which were shared by
the rats that cavorted around the wards and which not only ate the scraps
left by the patients but sometimes, according to Francis Shepherd, attempted to eat the patients as well.

As for the rich variety of smells, including the odours from the dead-
house, which was just under the windows of the wards, they were so
omnipresent that the olfactory organs of the hospital governors must have
been desensitized. Following one inspection they reported that they had
"failed to detect any bad odors." A member of the staff promptly
penciled in the margin of the report, "Try again. Better luck next time."

Even toward the end of the century there was much room for
improvement. Upon joining the hospital, the superintendent of nurses,
Miss Livingston, found that "there were no bed springs. Patients rested
on straw mattresses or blankets, which were laid on a framework of iron
pipes. Some were propped up on chairs. Typhoid fever patients were
forced to get out of bed and drink the milk left in saucers in the middle of
the floor, for cats. Dead bodies were wrapped in newspapers. Shrouds
and mortuary blankets were unheard of. Miss Livingston asked the
committee for shrouds and they said to her, 'How will we get them
back?'"

From Osler's point of view, none of that mattered in the slightest,
considering the hospital's towering virtue: that it did not merely tolerate

students, it welcomed them. From its first years, the Montreal General, closely affiliated to the McGill Medical School, had dedicated itself to the teaching of medical students, and by the time Osler had completed his final two clinical years, it had developed several first-rate teachers, including Palmer Howard, who joined Johnson and Bovell as an object of the boy's admiration and affection.

As for the McGill Medical School, it went without saying that it was the best in the country. Not that the domestic competition was all that keen. Even by 1910, an American survey concluded that, "In the matter of medical schools, Canada reproduces the United States on a greatly reduced scale. Western University (London) is as bad as anything to be found on this side of the line; Laval (Quebec) and Halifax Medical College (Dalhousie) are feeble; Winnipeg and Kingston represent distinct effort towards higher levels; McGill and Toronto are excellent" — a report that caused a good deal of resentment in the schools that had been criticized, though the report soon shocked them into doing better. The authorities at McGill, of course, needed no pat on the back from an outsider. By the time the report came out, McGill had only one serious rival on the whole continent, the Johns Hopkins Medical School in Baltimore.

Two years after obtaining his M.D., C.M., at McGill, Osler was back on staff as a lecturer in physiology, histology, and pathology.

From the start he attracted considerable attention as a student. After graduating, he added to his reputation through two years in Europe, and studies under the great pathologist Virchow, in Berlin. He had also worked for seventeen months at a laboratory at University College Hospital in London, where, according to Cushing, he made perhaps his most important contribution to medical knowledge, the discovery of blood platelets, the platelets being an element of the blood that play an important role in clotting. His sanguinary observations, which were presented before the Royal Society in London, caused some excitement at McGill, and strengthened the agitation to bring him back as a member of the staff.

So now here he was, a professor of the Institute of Medicine at the age of twenty-five. His young cousin, Marian Osborne, then living on McGill College Avenue, was enormously proud of him. "He was younger than many of those whom he taught," she said, "but he never seemed to have any difficulty with discipline. He was not a disciplinarian with anyone but himself, and his rule for others was the rule of love and understanding. While the students were waiting for their lectures, they used to sing their College songs. Some of the Professors would walk into the room with a frown and say, 'Silence, gentlemen,' as though they had been insulted, but the 'Baby Professor' would wait till the song was ended and then come in smiling with a jest or word of approval. How thrilled I used to be when the students came at night and sang their songs to serenade him. No cavalier that stringed his adoration to his lady love could have awakened more rapture in her breast than those college songs, shouted with hoarse delight, did in mine.

"When Uncle Bill first had to lecture it was a great difficulty for him, and my mother spent many hours in practice with him that he might train and pitch his voice so that it could be heard. He had trouble, too, in preparing his lectures and my Aunt, Miss Jeannette Osler, who lived with us, used to proof-read them with him and help him toward a literary style."

Osler never did become a great lecturer in the traditional, sonorous manner. When he was appointed to the chair of clinical medicine at the University of Pennsylvania, the students there attended his introductory lecture with anticipation, for his high reputation as a researcher, teacher, and pathologist, had preceded him. Pennsylvania was already noted for its eloquent lecturers, so it would be interesting to see what made Professor Osler so special. It was a shock when they first heard him. His speech was so halting it sounded affected. He sounded almost unsure of his subject. His manner suggested that he was just a student himself who had suddenly been stuck with the job of giving a lecture when the professor had failed to turn up. He spoke as if he were holding a *conversation*, for heaven's sake. It was not a good beginning. Some of the students scoffed at the "brilliant" new man. There was already some opposition from the student body and the faculty to the appointment of a foreigner to such a critical post, and there was a good deal of adverse comment around the university over the new professor's poor performance in the lecture hall; until his colleagues got to know him and were magnetized by his personality, and the students realized that his stumbling delivery was somehow imparting a lot of information, and that somehow, "W. O." was making the process of learning, especially in his bedside teaching, an enormous pleasure.

In Montreal, young Marian Osborne loved to go out with her relative, the young professor. With his alchemic awareness he could transform the most ordinary encounter into an adventure in human relations. "One day," she remembered, "we were walking down the street together. He found it difficult to walk in the accepted sense of the term, his nature seemed too buoyant to allow him to place one foot in front of the other as is done by more humdrum individuals. He would dance along humming or whistling. His was the true joie de vivre, which never left him in spite of work and sorrow and years. On this day we were dancing along St. Catherine Street hand in hand, when an old and very seedy-looking man accosted us and asked for money. Uncle Bill looked at him with his penetrating brown eyes and then said with a laugh — 'You old rascal, why should I give you money to drink yourself to death?'

" 'Well, Sir, you see it lightens the road going.'

" 'There is only one thing of value about you and that is your hob-nailed liver.'

" 'I'll give it to you, sir, I'll give it to you.' "

Osler laughed again, and handed over some silver, and then, seeing how cold the old fellow was, also gave him his overcoat, though Marian said that Uncle Bill had no money to buy another. But he got the coat back only two weeks later when the old man died, "and after it was thoroughly disinfected, it was as good as new." (The coat is now in the museum at the Academy of Medicine, Toronto.) Osler also got the hob-nailed liver. The beggar had insisted on willing it to the young doctor.

Osler was so hard up at this time, desperate for money to pay for the microscopes that he had purchased for his students — and one for Father Johnson — that he took on the dangerous but well-paying job of running the General Hospital's smallpox ward. It gave him plenty of experience, for he took over at the height of a virulent outbreak of the disease (the outbreak that culminated in the anti-vaccination riots in Montreal). Naturally another benefit attracted him besides the money: the chance to have hospital patients under his control, which would complete the clinical cycle at the post-mortem table on the patients who succumbed.

Almost inevitably, he contracted smallpox himself. Fortunately it was a mild attack that left, as he put it, his beauty unconsumed. The enforced bed rest also gave him a chance to catch up on the general reading of the classics that would help him to acquire a fluent literary style in later years.

Recovered, he continued his systematic studies as a morbid anatomist, and over the next few years published many papers on pathology. From the beginning he had understood instinctively that a minute study of the processes of disease was the only route for a successful clinician. His industry was rewarded when the position of pathologist to the General Hospital was created specially to make use of his talents and his prodigious capacity for work.

He promptly offered his students an opportunity that had previously been lacking, the privilege of working with him in the autopsy room at the General. One of the students, Beaumont Small, described Osler's instruction methods. Before the class met, Osler supervised the arranging and labeling of the specimens on trays. "Each specimen in turn was carefully discussed and all the important points clearly indicated. At the close of each case, questions were asked for and answered, the whole being most informal and conversational. The facts elicited in the autopsies were carefully correlated with the clinical histories and notes of the cases as taken in the wards. In order that his teaching should be of the greatest value to those in attendance he furnished each one with a written description of each specimen, and with an epitome of the remarks which he had prepared. There were always four pages and at times eight pages of large letter size, written by himself and copied by means of a copying machine; there were from 30 to 40 copies required each Saturday, so that the demand such a task made on his time must have been heavy."

The demands were not so heavy as to devalue the communication between him and his students, a communication encouraging, reassuring, or challenging on his part, admiring and affectionate on theirs. When one of his students scratched himself with a dissecting knife, Osler saw him turn pale with fright. He restored the student's confidence by musing aloud as to who would take the student's place when he was gone. During another autopsy he suddenly lifted out a mass of intestines, turned to a new student, Ed Rogers, who was watching with all the horror and nausea one would expect of a student present at such an ordeal for the first time and said, "Rogers, you prepare these for inspection." A typical Oslerian act, Rogers later recalled. "Superficially, it seemed all dry humor, the sort of practical joke for which he was celebrated, but in reality it was an initiatory test. The questions in his mind were 'What ability has this man to meet an unexpected and unusual situation?' 'What capacity for work has he?'"

"There was one pretty certain index to his feelings for others," wrote another student. "I never knew him to say harsh things about anyone, but if he did not chaff one or play practical jokes on him, that man was pretty certain to be inferior."

One of Osler's students was Tom Cream. He was not an inferior student in intelligence, and Osler must certainly have noticed him among the serried ranks in the lecture hall, for Tom was physiognomically distinct. All the same, the endeavors that made Cream noteworthy were not ones in which Professor Osler could take pride.

Cream entered McGill in the year of Osler's graduation, so Osler could not have been aware of him until his return two years later as a member of the faculty. By then, Thomas Neill Cream had established a reputation for stylish and extravagant behaviour. He was that great rarity, a rich student. His father, William Cream, had emigrated with the family from Scotland in the 1850s, and had settled in Quebec City and prospered there as a lumber merchant. He was well able to indulge his eldest son. At McGill, Cream lived above and beyond the call of fashion, attiring himself in flashy clothes and flashing jewelry. He had his own carriage and pair. But the ostentation did not cause resentment because Tom seemed to be a good fellow. He was interested in sports and music, and used a fine voice and courteous manner to ingratiating effect.

Perhaps, too, he earned a certain sympathy because of the marked strabismus of his left eye.

Still, he did not appear to be unduly self-conscious about the hideous squint, nor did it hinder his relationships with the opposite sex. All in all, Tom seemed to be an exceedingly interesting young man, dramatic, colourful, and generous with his father's money.

Perhaps too generous, for as graduation day approached, he found himself living well beyond his means. Presumably it was to rectify this state of affairs that one day he set fire to his lodging house on Mansfield Street.

He then put in a claim for one thousand dollars against his insurance policy for the loss of personal effects. To his annoyance, he found that the moral standards of an insurance company could be as debased as his own. Suspecting arson but unable to prove it, the company forked out only $350.

Another misfortune quickly followed. In 1876, while Osler was taking charge of the smallpox ward at the General Hospital, Cream was dating Eliza Brooks, the daughter of a Waterloo hotel keeper. When she became pregnant, he procured an abortion, but either his surgical skill or his antiseptic procedure was deficient, for the girl fell ill. Her father learned what had happened when the family doctor was called in to treat her. Mr. Brooks immediately went after the brand-new doctor with a shotgun, cornered him in the Ottawa Hotel in Montreal, and gave him the alternative of either marrying the girl or having his head blown off. Cream married Eliza the very next day.

A year later, Eliza was dead, officially of "consumption." But once again Cream felt he had cause for moral indignation when he claimed one thousand dollars from his insurance company and they offered only two hundred dollars.

After postgraduate training in Edinburgh, Cream returned to Canada and set up in practice in London; until one day in May 1879, the body of a chambermaid was found "half-sitting, half-reclining" in an outhouse close to Cream's office on Dundas Street. At the inquest it was established that the girl had applied to Dr. Cream for an abortion. Though he must have been under suspicion, nothing was proved against him and an open verdict was returned, to the effect that she had died of an overdose of chloroform, administered by persons unknown.

Cream then moved to Chicago where, from an office on West Madison Avenue, he soon built up a flourishing practice, specializing in abortions. He later claimed that he had dealt with fifteen such cases in a single establishment, a nearby brothel.

While in Chicago, Dr. Cream was twice accused of murder. Both of the victims were Canadian. On the first charge, of killing an Ottawa woman named Mary Anne Faulkner by botching an abortion on her, he was acquitted, but instead of making him more cautious, his release from justice seemed to have subconsciously affronted him. Though he plainly illustrated the reality of inherent evil, there appears to have been a moral residue in him leading to what the authors of *An Encyclopedia of Murder* described as a "capture wish."

In the second case he sent a telegram and a letter to the authorities in Boone County, Illinois, suggesting that a post-mortem examination be performed on the body of Dan Stott of Garden Prairie. Stott was a sixty-five-year-old Canadian epileptic, who had married a young girl in Illinois. In his letter, Cream accused the girl, Julia Stott, of murdering the old man with strychnine. When the body was exhumed, strychnine was indeed found in the stomach. Questioned, Julia told police that it was Cream's idea. She had been his mistress. He had suggested that she buy a bottle of medicine for her husband's epileptic fits, and feed it, suitably treated, to her husband. With Mr. Stott out of the way, they would then sue the drug company that had filled the prescription, accusing it of causing Stott's death with its faulty pharmacy. Dr. Cream, Julia said, had convinced her that they would collect a fortune from the drug company; after which they would leave the district and get married.

The police believed her and went after Cream. By then, presumably trying to combat his inner desire to be punished, he was living under a false name in a hotel in Belle River, Ontario. He was taken back to Illinois, found guilty, and sentenced to life imprisonment in Joliet.

In matters of murder, the law appears to have been almost as feeble in 1891 as it is today in America, for in that year, Cream was pardoned after serving ten years of the life sentence. By then he looked decidedly sinister, bald, cross-eyed, and hairy as a troll. And his release ended the lives of four prostitutes in England before he was hanged there a year later.

There has been an attempt to prove that Neil Cream was Jack the Ripper, but the arguments are not too convincing, not least because, whereas Jack ripped on the spot, Cream killed by remote control— feeding the prostitutes strychnine pills so that they would die when he was far from the scene.

In one of his essays, W. H. Auden argues that hostility to humanity underlies the pranks of the practical joker. Osler was a renowned practical joker. In Montreal, we see him calling on Mrs. Molson, the wife of a fellow member of the Terrapin Club, to ask her for a latchkey. He explains that they usually have trouble sobering-up her husband, Billy, and a latchkey would be useful in case they have to carry him home. (Billy was a dedicated teetotaler.) Also in Montreal, he corners a Boston pediatrician and his wife, and, with his usual straight-faced delivery, gives the proper Bostonians such a glowing description of a colourful district of Montreal named Caughnawauga that the visitors spend the rest of the day trying to find it. They never quite forgive Osler when they learn that wherever Caughnawauga is, it isn't in Montreal. Osler later victimizes another children's specialist, an extremely frail man named Jacobi. Osler informs the press, who duly print the information, that Professor Jacobi is a champion pole-vaulter and high-jumper. And in the Athenaeum Club in London, Osler is found to be reacting against the stuffy atmosphere by inserting bulky objects into the august members' back pockets while their attention is elsewhere engaged. Some of the victims consider such pranks delightful; others feel that Sir William—he has been knighted by then—is not behaving in a manner worthy of his eminence.

Even the meanest reputation-demolisher could hardly claim that these practical jokes, which were typical, reflect anything but, at worst, fashionable caprice. Fashions in humour change, and as the medical historian W. B. Howell points out, what is considered humorous in one age might be looked down on as evidence of arrested mental development in another. (Howell also mentions Wingfield-Stratford's theory which links the practical joking of mid-Victorian men with their cultivation of a profuse growth of hair on the face; he considers that both phenomena were symptomatic of an inordinate desire to be, or to appear, manly.)

The worst that can be said about Osler's jokes is that occasionally they put his friends to a lot of trouble in a cause that today would not be considered risibly worthwhile. For instance, in Baltimore, he went to see the actor Richard Mansfield in *The Parisian Romance,* in which the character Mansfield played dies of apoplexy. After the performance, Osler danced over to the hospital and informed the pathologists that there had been a fatality, a cerebral hemorrhage, and an autopsy would be required. The pathologists went to the laboratory and made their preparations. Some time later they telephoned the ward to find out what the delay was, and learned that they had been fooled—the death was purely theatrical. Osler had long since gone to bed—after taking the precaution of locking his door, in case the pathologists retaliated.

Osler's close friend and biographer, Harvey Cushing, maintained that Osler could thoroughly enjoy a practical joke even when he himself was the victim. However, the assertion is not entirely borne out by at least one incident when Osler called on a colleague, Dr. Welch, for some informa-tion on ergotism for his book *The Principles and Practice of Medicine.* Dr. Welch immediately took up a copy of a German medical journal and proceeded to "translate" a learned article on ergotism. "I pretended to read him a wonderful description of the disease," Welch wrote, "with startling statistics on its prevalence in south-eastern Europe and its relation to obscure nervous afflictions. He took a pad and jotted down the notes which I gave him. I recall that I gave him the figures for Roumania. He became greatly interested and said that he had no doubt that they were overlooking ergotism every day as a cause of obscure nervous diseases and that he would put Harry Thomas to work on it in the dispensary.

"Off he went with the material for a beautiful article on ergotism, which would have immortalized the 'Practise.' I did not really expect him to swallow it, but he did; and thinking it over I became uneasy, and early the next morning I confessed the hoax to him, and took him around a real article on ergotism. He never quite liked reference to the joke. It was not a very good joke and I am rather ashamed of it, but the facts really are as I have stated. Like most practical jokers Osler was easy to fool, or else he was so confiding that he did not think me capable of trying to fool him."

Surely Welch had no cause to feel ashamed. It was a very good joke, superior to most of Osler's, considering the quick-thinking, the inventiveness, and the exploitation of knowlege involved, not to mention the acting ability required to carry it off. But on the whole, Cushing's opinion that Osler's pranks "were merely an expression of his lively sense of fun," seems the closest to the truth. Osler's kindness of heart and the trouble he would go to even for chance acquaintances was just as truly a part of his character. In the year of the anti-vaccination riots in Montreal, while dining in his club, he met an Englishman who was in the city on business. Divining that the young man was lonely, Osler chatted to him then and subsequently. One evening he noticed that the young man seemed ill. Osler questioned him about his symptoms and immediately escorted him back to his rooms and put him to bed. He had smallpox. He died three days later. Osler wrote to the man's parents in England, to tell them about their son's passing, and to comfort them. He told how he had stayed with the young man up to his last moment. "He did not speak much, but turned round at intervals to see if I were still by him. About 12 o'clock I heard him muttering some prayers, but could not catch distinctly what they were.... Shortly after this he turned round and held out his hand, which I took, & he said quite plainly, 'Oh thanks.' These were the last words the poor fellow spoke. From 12.30 he was unconscious, and at 1.25 a.m. passed away, without a groan or struggle. As the son of a clergyman & knowing well what it is to be a 'stranger in a strange land' I performed the last office of Christian friendship I could, & read the Commendatory Prayer at his departure."

After quoting this letter, Cushing continues: "thirty years almost to the day after this letter was written, the newly appointed Regius Professor of Medicine in Oxford chanced to meet at dinner a Lady S—who, attracted by his name, said she once had a young brother who had gone out to Montreal and had been cared for during a fatal illness by a doctor named Osler, who had sent a sympathetic letter that had been the greatest possible solace to her parents: that her mother, who was still living in the south of England, had always hoped she might see and talk with the man who had written it. Later, on his way to Cornwall, Osler paid a visit to this bereaved mother, taking with him a photograph of her boy's grave, which he had sent to Montreal to obtain."

Osler loved the company of old men as much as that of the young. When he first joined the McGill faculty, he lived on Radegonde Street, opposite the old Haymarket, but shortly moved to 26 Beaver Hall Hill, where he befriended an old eccentric known in the neighbourhood as Don Quixote. His real name was King and he was a Shakespeare nut. He lived and breathed Shakespeare, and had amassed an excellent library on his subject, a library where Osler spent many a pleasant hour. One day the young professor received a Shakespeare concordance that he had ordered in Berlin. "My first thought" Osler recounted, "was, 'How happy Mr. King will be to see it.' I looked at it hurriedly, but with much anticipatory pleasure. On my return to the house, Mr. King who had just come in, was sitting by the fire and greeted me in his cheery way with: 'What's that you've got?' 'Something that will rejoice your heart,' I said, and deposited the work in his lap. The shock of the realization of a life-long dream—a complete concordance of Shakespeare, seemed to daze the old man. He had no further interest in me and not a word did he say. I never again saw my Schmidt's Concordance! For months he avoided me, but helping him one day on the stairs, my manner showed that Schmidt was forgotten, and he never referred to it again. The work went to McGill College with his Shakespeare collection. When in the Library in 1912 I asked for the first edition of Schmidt and was glad to see my book again after nearly forty years. This story is written on the fly-leaf as a warning to bibliomaniacs!"

Osler's friendship with his students extended well beyond the threshold of ward, lecture, and autopsy room. One of them was a tall, gangling southerner, Henry Ogden, whose parents had emigrated to Canada after the Civil War. Learning that Ogden was living a lonely life in an unpleasant boarding house, Osler persuaded his friend and landlord, Dr. Frank Buller (by then Osler had left his Shakespearian friend to live at Buller's place on St. Catherine Street), to take Ogden in as well; though Buller wondered if he had made the right decision when one evening he found part of a dead horse in his bathtub.

One of Osler's traits was that he inspired, or bullied, others to work as hard as he did. You knew you were a friend of Osler's when he began to load you down with work, and Ogden was one such friend. Osler, haunting the veterinary halls in Montreal as he had done in Toronto, was working on papers in comparative anatomy, and one day he sent Ogden to perform an autopsy on a horse that had died of some nervous ailment. Osler wanted the animal's brain and spinal cord. Ogden was only a first-year student, and accordingly had a terrible time obtaining the brain and backbone. It took him all day, but he finally managed to hack it free. When he got home, he proudly laid the trophies in the family bathtub. Unfortunately Osler was out, and the landlord was the first to enter the bathroom. When he looked into the tub he recoiled so violently that he almost demolished the opposite wall. After he had gotten over the shock he was furious, and Osler arrived home just in time to save both student and specimen from summary ejection. Dr. Buller was not pacified until Osler agreed to take the first bath.

In spite of being landed with a job that would have been a challenge even for a senior student, Ogden remained captivated by his professor, who actually treated him like a human being and an equal. He had been in the house for two or three days when Osler came bounding up the steps to visit him. "I happened to be sitting up in bed reading at physiology," Ogden said. "He broke out at once in praise of the habit of reading in bed, but heartily disapproved of physiology—only literature, never medicine. He walked across the room standing with his back to me, his hands in his trousers' pockets, tilting up and down on his toes, and inspecting the little collection of about twenty or thirty books I had ranged on two small hanging shelves; and taking down the 'Golden Treasury' came over, sat on the foot of the bed, and half-recited, half-read, interjecting a running comment, a number of the poems. Then tossing the book to me he said: 'You'll find that much better stuff than physiology for reading in bed.' That same evening, too, he spoke of Sir Thomas Browne and the "Religio."... His enthusiasm rose as he spoke and running downstairs he brought up his copy, pointed out and read several passages and then left me."

Osler's consuming interest lay in teaching, writing, and research, and, though he was invariably hard up, he made little attempt to earn a living from private practice, though he was perfectly entitled to do so. His consulting room on St. Catherine Street was not fit for patients anyway, it was so crammed with books and papers. Ogden and another student who shared the house with him remember only three consultations in his office—not counting those who arrived for an appointment but found that the doctor hadn't. One patient, though, was so important that Osler was actually waiting for him when he entered, wheezing and gasping. This was Peter Redpath, the "Sugar King," who was suffering from lumbago. Osler treated him by acupuncture. "At each jab the old gentleman is said to have ripped out a string of oaths, and in the end got

up and hobbled out, no better of his pain." Much to Osler's disappointment. He had been hoping to impress Mr. Redpath with his skill so that
the old man, suffused with gratitude, would immediately donate a
million dollars to McGill.

Osler was interested in criminal as well as horses' brains. A professor
Benedikt of Vienna had claimed that the topography of criminal brains
bore telltale irregularities. Osler was to prove him wrong, that the
irregularities in question frequently occurred in the normal brain; but in
the meantime, in order to examine the evidence for himself, he obviously
needed the appropriate material.

The timing was good. Two notorious murderers were about to be
executed, one of them at Rimouski, Quebec. To which town Osler
despatched the faithful Henry Ogden as his deputy. So once again the
lanky southerner found himself engaged on an alarming errand, this time
one worthy of a horror movie. He was forced to make his way into the
depths of the French countryside in ten-below-zero weather. To ease his
negotiations with the authorities at Rimouski a command of French
would have been useful, but Ogden's was decidedly imperfect. Then
followed the ghastly experience of witnessing an execution. But that
wasn't even the worst of it. After the execution he was required to
perform the autopsy and secure the brain. The boy had never performed
a human autopsy in his life, let alone handled the delicate and macabre
task of getting and disconnecting the murderer's gray matter.

On that occasion, Ogden must have wished that he had never met his
charming but extraordinarily demanding professor.

It was also during this period that Osler attempted to obtain the
famous stomach of Alexis St. Martin.

By the end of his ten years at McGill, Osler's name had become well
known on two continents, though he had not even established his reputation as a great clinician, nor was he even idly contemplating writing the
enduring *Principles and Practice of Medicine.* In Cushing's summary of his
accomplishments in Montreal: "He had stirred into activity the slumber-
ing Medico-Chirurgical Society; he had founded and supported a students' medical club; he had brought the Veterinary School into relation
with the University; had edited the first clinical and pathological reports
of a Canadian hospital; had recorded nearly a thousand autopsies and
made innumerable museum preparations of the most important specimens; he had written countless papers, many of them ephemeral it is true,
but most of them on topics of live interest for the time, and a few of them
epoch-making; he had worked at biology and pathology both human
and comparative, as well as at the bedside; he had shown courage in
taking the small-pox wards, charity in his dealings with his fellow physicians in and out of his own school, generosity to his students, fidelity to his

tasks; and his many uncommon qualities had earned him popularity unsought and of a most unusual degree."

Not least among Osler's contributions was to the prestige of the university. Almost from the moment he became a full professor, McGill Medical School underwent a renaissance that made it one of the two most famous medical establishments on the continent. Osler was not the only assistant at the rebirth. The progressive ideas of the older men on the faculty, particularly Palmer Howard, had resulted in several young men being promoted to positions of responsibility, including Thomas Roddick, George Ross, William Gardner, and Francis Shepherd, one of Canada's great personalities. Nevertheless, the ascending curve of McGill's contribution to medicine flattened out after Osler left, and it is significant that the same pattern occurred at Philadelphia and Baltimore during his sojourn at their medical schools.

The offer from Philadelphia came while Osler was in Europe during the summer of 1884. "The thought of losing you stuns us," Palmer Howard wrote to him, and made a desperate attempt to keep him by offering to establish a special chair of pathology at quite a good salary, sixteen hundred a year. But the chair was to be established at "as early a date as possible," which was not quite definite enough. Whereas the offer from the distinguished American university was not only firm but pressing, especially after Horatio Wood, a member of the Philadelphia faculty, went to Montreal to check up on Dr. Osler. Even though Osler was well known for his writings, Wood felt that the opinions of Osler's colleagues should be probed—not all medical reputations were thoroughly justified. Curiously enough, he went first to the French hospitals; but every one of the French physicians spoke highly of Osler. He then visited the Montreal General. He investigated no further. The young house-staffers were so enthusiastic about Osler that Wood saw no reason to interview any of Osler's colleagues on the faculty. He went home, totally converted.

At the same time, another investigator, Dr. S. Weir Mitchell and his wife were busily checking up on Osler in Europe. In their case, the testing apparatus was a cherry pie. As Osler put it, "Dr. Mitchell said there was only one way in which the breeding of a man suitable for such a position, in such a city as Philadelphia, could be tested: give him cherry-pie and see how he disposed of the stones."

Fortunately Osler disposed of them in the proper way—genteelly, in his spoon.

Even so, the professorship in clinical medicine was very nearly turned down, by default. It was Francis Shepherd who forwarded the offer to Osler from Montreal. "I had played so many pranks on my friends there," Osler confessed later, "that when the letter came I felt sure it was a joke, so little did I think that I was one to be asked to succeed Dr. Pepper. It was several weeks before I ventured to answer that letter, fearing that Dr. Shepherd had surreptitiously taken a sheet of University of Pennsylvania note-paper on purpose to make the joke more certain."

In his book, Harvey Cushing confesses uncertainty as to what lured Osler away from McGill. "A great career was assured in Montreal, whereas Philadelphia was an uncertainty in a land more foreign to him than England." Apparently Cushing had not heard of Osler's remark in the lecture room when, shortly before he was to leave for the University of Pennsylvania, Osler paced up and down in front of his students and started to utter the usual conventional expressions of regret at having to leave this august institution, et cetera—but then he suddenly stopped and said, "Gentlemen, there is no use talking. I must admit that I am leaving McGill for a larger field through *ambition.*"

17

Osler Abroad

A S THE UNIVERSITY of Pennsylvania was descended from the College of Philadelphia, which had been established decades before the Declaration of Independence, and considered itself the premier institution of learning on the continent, its authorities would not have been overly flattered had they learned how Dr. Osler had decided to accept their invitation to occupy the chair of clinical medicine. Osler, not at all convinced that Pennsylvania was any better than McGill, had flipped a silver coin in the air: heads Philadelphia, tails Montreal. It came down heads, but when he went to wire his acceptance he found he had left the silver coin behind, and had no other money to pay for the cablegram. This seemed to him to be a nudge from providence, and very nearly decided him to stay where he was.

The election of a rank outsider to such an important post caused perturbation at Pennsylvania, not least because it thwarted the ambitions of a number of quite worthy medical clinicians. Consequently the eyes upon him were sharply focussed. His unimpressive performance in the lecture room seemed to justify the misgivings, especially as he was replacing the famous Dr. Pepper, a gentleman of great dignity and elegance, who had polished his discourses over the years to a mirror-like brilliance. By comparison, Osler seemed stumbling. It was only gradually that the students found that they were learning at least as much from the rather odd Canadian's conversational delivery as from Dr. Pepper's silvery eloquence.

His apparent lack of dignity was somewhat harder to get used to. Instead of turning up in a fine carriage, he rode to work in a streetcar, and popped in by the back door, wearing, besides the *de rigueur* top hat and frock coat, funny socks and a flowing red necktie. These, together with his swarthy complexion and drooping moustache, made him look disturbingly strange and foreign. Americans tended to have a low tolerance for eccentricity of appearance or manner.

He warmed the faculty members with the radiation of his personality as soon as he got down to work in the medical wards of the university hospital. He electrified the clinical students with his investigative spirit. Within a month he was involving them in the original study and research that until then had been almost unknown at Philadelphia. He rigged up a small clinical laboratory under the hospital amphitheatre, and in this squalid space recreated the encouraging McGill atmosphere. As Dr. H. A. Hare put it, "It was as if Beethoven was playing in a hovel." The students, their disillusionment rapidly transformed into devotion, flocked to him, delighted by his flashes of gaiety — "Most in earnest when he was most in fun" — transfixed as much by his personality as by the revolutionary bedside teaching, which stressed the importance of methodically examining the patient and obtaining the fullest possible history of the case before beginning a physical examination, and the importance of tying-up the clinical symptoms with post-mortem findings.

"We did not learn the use of all of the drugs in the pharmacopeia from him," observed one of his students, Harry Toulmin. "If my memory is correct, he thought we could get along quite satisfactorily with six or eight drugs; while one of his favorite prescriptions was 'Time in divided doses.'"

This was another startling aspect of the olive-skinned newcomer. He would not tip his topper to pharmacology. His attitude verged on contempt. When Dr. Joseph Leidy II asked his advice as to whether this drug or that might not be useful in a particular case, Osler retorted, "Well, my dear fellow, if it will ease your mind a bit, put on a poultice." Osler was later to attack the profession quite savagely, castigating the kind of physician "who without physiology and chemistry flounders along in an aimless fashion, never able to gain any accurate conception of disease, practising a sort of pop-gun pharmacy, hitting now the malady and again the patient, he himself not knowing which."

Some people accused him of being a therapeutic nihilist. The accusation was not dispelled by a couple of papers on pneumonia and typhoid, in the first of which he spurned the drugs advocated by his fellows, such as antimony, alcohol, and quinine. He pointed out that of two groups of pneumonia patients, "the majority of the former die in spite of all treatment; the majority of the latter get well with any, or no, treatment."

How insouciantly Osler viewed the whole subject of drugs can be seen in the following memoir of Dr. Leidy. Sometimes a whole mess of drugs, but principally digitalis, were employed in heart cases, but Osler "came in to the hospital one day and said, 'Collect all the chronic heart cases who apply for admission to hospital, especially those with secondary symptoms. Let us see what results are to be obtained from absolute rest, no medicine but our usual *placebo* (Compound Tincture of Cardamon). In a short time we had some fourteen cases under observation, presenting a variety of secondary symptoms—oedema of the lower extremities, pulmonary oedema, bronchitis, dyspnea, etc. etc. Improvement was noted from the beginning, and some weeks later it was decided to utilize a group of the cases for class demonstration. At the first clinic Dr. William Pepper (Professor of Medicine) appeared at the door of the amphitheatre with two elderly physicians who were introduced to Dr. Osler; one I think was the oldest living graduate of the Medical Department of the University, who was visiting his Alma Mater for the first time in many years. Osler directed them to seats of honor in the front of the arena. The lecture began, and was followed in rapt attention by the students and the two patriarchal alumni. Osler dilated at great length upon the importance of absolute rest in bed—the bed-pan imperative, and then, with a merry twinkle in his eyes, 'Gentlemen, now as to therapeutics, we will continue with mm—mm—Comp. Tinct. Cardamon, five drops t.i.d.,' hesitating between each word. With that the two alumni took out their note-books and recorded Osler's specific for chronic heart disease. After the clinic I said, 'Doctor, that was a cruel shame, as the darkies say, to allow those men to leave without further explanation; they will be prescribing Tr. Cardamon to all their heart cases.' 'Ah! Leidy, bless your soul, think how many lives will be saved; only, *only* think of the deaths from the indiscriminate use of Digitalis.'"

Leidy never met anyone who was a greater skeptic than Osler, in this regard. Another doctor, Charles Burr, wrote censoriously that, "Osler had one defect as a chief. He neither knew anything about, nor cared anything for, therapeutics. He depended on rest, exercise, diet and quiet, digitalis, opium, iodide, and mercury and, above all, nature's medicine, time. Worse than this the average resident came out of his hands having absorbed an attitude of contempt toward all methods of healing the sick." But Joseph Leidy continued to defend the great physician. "A good deal of criticism has been made of Dr. Osler's skepticism in therapeutics," he wrote. "He looked upon drugs in many instances as double-edged swords. Those who followed his treatment, however, learned to know it was *sound;* certainly those of us in hospital who were confined to his limited therapeutic armamentarium, will attest to its efficacy, with results the equal of any attained by his severest critics."

Osler further surprised his American colleagues by making little effort to exploit his position by building up a private practice, though it was customary for professors to supplement their incomes in this way. They saw their private patients in regular afternoon office hours. Though as hard up as ever, Osler saw very few private patients, and then only by appointment. Mostly he spent his afternoons at the Blockley Hospital mortuary, adding to the amazing total of one thousand autopsies that he had performed in Montreal.

His lodgings and office on Fifteenth Street near Chestnut reflected this indifference to what could have been a lucrative income. If the private patient hoped to see the usual front in the form of gleaming brassware and showy furniture, he was in for a shock. Osler's office was a literary dump: books, pamphlets, notes, reports, and manuscripts scattered on every available surface, and heaped high on his desk, as if he were throwing up a paper barricade across the route to material success.

His manner toward the patient could sometimes be as cavalier as his treatment of the consulting room decor. As related by Edith Reid, one woman who managed to get an appointment with Osler, bombarded him with lightweight symptoms, including nervous thrashings in bed. The doctor responded to this particular point by remarking that he hoped her husband did not have to sleep in the same bed with her. At this frivolous response, the woman was most indignant, and upbraided him. Perhaps feeling that he had been a trifle unprofessional, Osler then made a careful physical examination, but after only a few questions he lost interest, went to the door and held it open for her, saying, "'I know your husband, Mrs. —, a fine chap, with a small income. There's nothing whatever the matter with you. Go home and do your own housework and see how much you can save your husband.' The woman said furiously: 'Do you mean to insult me? I see I have been foolish to come to you.' 'Not if you do what I tell you,' and he opened the door for her to go. She told the story, ending it with, 'The idea of calling him a saint! He looks like a Mephistopheles and I think he is terribly overestimated. He didn't know what was the matter with me and just bluffed.'"

Unfortunately Osler could be as nonchalant toward the patient whose trouble was genuine. A Dr. Lewis once called him in for a consultation over a private patient. Osler quickly agreed as to the pathology of the trouble—"and almost immediately lost all interest, and spent the rest of the time at the house in examining the books in the library." Which, though it might make the observer smile, did not amuse the patient in the least.

It seems likely that however much he needed their money, Osler was really not very interested in private patients, unless they were good for a donation to science, or had a particularly interesting problem, or inspired sympathy, as in the case of the Philadelphia lady who, in the opinion of her friends, was being disgracefully exploited by her son. To pay for his excesses she was having to neglect her fine house and hock her diamonds. Her friends urged her to stop sacrificing herself for her unspeakably selfish son. One afternoon she came to see Dr. Osler, and though she had interrupted him at a particularly busy time, he fussed over her and settled her in an armchair, and listened sympathetically as she mourned her lost youth and good looks. After a few encouraging words he asked if her son Tommy was still in Paris. The lady braced herself, expecting another tirade about her selfish son, but to her relief and joy, Osler merely remarked that Tommy was a handsome young scamp, and offered to send him a letter of introduction to some people he knew in France who had two delightful daughters.

The lady departed, looking years younger—and proceeded to infuriate her righteous friends by telling them on every possible occasion thereafter, about how Dr. Osler had given Tommy a letter of introduction to one of the most important and exclusive families in Paris.

Another of his patients was Walt Whitman. In his case, if Osler was impressed by the complaint and the human interest of its bearer, he was certainly not impressed by the poetry. Whitman might be a fascinating prophet-like figure with his fine head mantled with snowy hair and stalactited with flowing beard, but his verse was too strong for Osler's "pampered palate," which had been conditioned by Keats and Shelley.

During his few years in Philadelphia, Osler made a life for himself similar to the one he had enjoyed in Montreal. He dropped in unexpectedly on delighted friends and romped with their children. He joined societies and stimulated them with his neurological and pathological insights. He deluged medical journals with articles, including the results of his extensive research into the malaria-causing organism, "which put Osler in the first rank of the investigators of Malaria." And he continued to build an international reputation. Four years after coming to Philadelphia, he traveled to London to deliver the Gouldstonian Lecture. The subject, endocarditis (inflammation of the lining of the heart and its valves), was based on research undertaken at the Montreal General. "The work he had done with a young man in Canada was so fundamental that it remained always as a reference-book," wrote Edith Olivers. "His most valuable work on endocarditis was described in these lectures. They were based on over 200 reported cases and on much of his own experience at the Montreal General. Physicians have said that these lectures gave such a wonderful exposition of the pathology, clinical picture and diagnosis of endocarditis that they were unequalled in medical literature."

At the same time he was developing his bedside clinics, and continuing his studies in morbid anatomy. He was not quite as successful as he had been in Montreal in building up a collection of pathological specimens. The medical department at Philadelphia could not afford to buy glass

containers for even the rarest hearts or brains. Osler solved the problem
in a typical way. He started pinching chamber pots from the wards and
using the jerries, as he called them, as containers for his specimens.
Unfortunately one Saturday afternoon the caretaker came into the lab,
saw the row of jerries, took a look inside and in a fit of squeamish zeal,
cleaned out the lot.

In spite of his terrific workload, Osler still kept in touch with affairs in
Canada, making frequent trips to Toronto on medical business and for
the Easter and Christmas holidays (where an acquaintance noted that,
"He dances along the street singing as he goes—as of old"), and to
Montreal for occasional lectures and demonstrations. His mother, by this
time living in Toronto, missed him more with every passing year, and
literally counted the days until his return. After one brief April holiday
she wrote, "Willie's meteor-like visit was pleasant while it lasted, he left at
noon yesterday—he is lamentably thin. I do wish he had a nice wife to
attend to little home comforts for him."

Willie missed the family, the children, and his Canadian friends almost
as much. "It seems long since I have heard from any of you," he wrote to
Francis Shepherd, in a rare moment of melancholy. "I feel very like
skipping North on the 1st, for your introductory lecture. I felt rather
homesick. I still, at times, feel like a stranger & a pilgrim though everyone
is very kind and I have got on better than I could have anticipated." And
he was still writing James Bovell's name in the margins of his papers.

Osler had been at the University of Pennsylvania for only four years
when its provost, Dr. Pepper, began to suspect that he was in danger of
losing his top man. During the Congress of Physicians and Surgeons in
Washington in 1888, John S. Billings, the president of the congress,
seemed to be spending far too much of his obviously valuable time with
one particular delegate, Professor Osler. Of course, that was the usual
scene at such conferences. Somehow, people always seemed to be swinging
into Osler's orbit. At a medical congress in Berlin, Bryson Delavan
described how, "One noontime, adjourning from one of the sessions,
weary and in need of refreshment, I met Dr. Osler who, in his customary
exhuberance in no wise dimmed by the strain of the morning, like myself
was hastening to lunch. Catching me by the arm he at once plunged into
a lively series of questions as to what I had been doing at the Congress,
whom I had met, and how profitable I had found the meetings. Presently
another acquaintance appeared across the narrow street. Him also Osler
hailed and locking arms between us proceeded onward, drawing from us
a running fire of conversation and convulsing us with his witty remarks.
By the time we had reached the restaurant only a short distance away,
Osler had joined to our happy trio one by one, five other members, each
wandering along, all congenial friends and delighted to have been

admitted to our party and thus rescued from the fate of a lonely meal. Under the inspiration of his inimitable spirit the repast which followed, although the simplest of its kind, became a royal banquet, a bright memory throughout our lives."

So the fact that John S. Billings kept gravitating toward Professor Osler was not all that unusual—except that Billings was connected with Pennsylvania's chief rival, Johns Hopkins University. Alarmed, Pepper hurried over to see Sam Gross, an especially close friend of Osler's, to find out if he knew what was going on. Pepper confessed his dismay at the prospect of losing Osler. Gross was not at all comforting. "Well, Pepper," he said, "If the position at the Johns Hopkins is offered him what have we got in Philadelphia to compete with it?"

Osler was indeed being wooed by Johns Hopkins, and would be won over. For some time he had been concerned about the standards of medical education in the United States, and he believed that at Johns Hopkins he would be able to do something about it, instead of merely criticizing—as in one speech he delivered in Baltimore when he said that, "It makes one's blood boil to think that there are sent out year by year scores of men, called doctors, who have never attended a case of labor, and who are utterly ignorant of the ordinary everyday diseases which they may be called upon to treat; men who may never have seen the inside of a hospital ward and who would not know Scarpa's space from the sole of the foot. Yet, gentlemen, this is the disgraceful condition which some school-men have the audacity to ask you to perpetuate."

The speech must have caused some collar-wrenching among his listeners in Baltimore, for in that city there were no fewer than five medical schools—and four of them were turning out the kind of doctor he was describing.

Though American medicine had not started out with the advantages of the scientifically minded physicians of New France, or the well-trained army and navy surgeons scattered throughout the rest of Canada, its progress was quite similar to the Canadian experience. There were the same halting beginnings in a hostile environment, the same surge, because of a scarcity of trained men, of quacks and charlatans, leading to the sort of pressure first to regulate the profession, and then to establish decent standards of medical education.

In the beginning, medicine in the Virginia and New England colonies naturally reflected the English practice. There were the university-trained physicians, who were the elite. They preferred to theorize about disease rather than soil their hands by actually dealing with it. Most of the dirty work was left to the surgeons, who had learned their skills as rude apprentices or in the stinking hospitals of the time, and to the apothecaries, who prescribed the drugs and who took the place of the aloof physicians by the bedsides of the ordinary people.

The first truly significant figure in American medicine was Cotton Mather, of Salem witches fame, who was characterized as being intelligent and able, "but also vain, quarrelsome, excitable, moody, and a fanatical believer in witches." He entered Harvard when he was twelve years old. Even for Puritan times he was an exceptionally pious lad, and almost drove his fellow students crazy with his priggish sermons and exhortations to lead a better life.

Somehow Mather managed to survive to be ordained as a minister in 1678, but, having a bad stammer, he turned to the study of medicine, suspecting that a stuttering preacher would have a hard time making a living. Though he never established a regular medical practice, it did not stop him from giving advice to those who had. Some of his recommendations to his fellow physicians were quite sensible. "In 1718 he proposed that doctors treating 'distracted persons' employ baths, a type of therapy that is still used in some cases of mental illness."

It was perhaps just as well for his patients' peace of mind that he did not practice on a regular basis, for he saw sickness as a divine punishment for original sin. Still, he contributed a good many papers to the Royal Society on such useful subjects as snakebite antidotes, and sweat-inducing methods to alleviate fevers and difficult childbirths. Most remarkably, he promoted the germ theory to explain epidemics, long before the theory was actually proved. He was similarly in advance of his time in his positive attitude toward innoculation with smallpox matter.

The longer Mather lived, the more sensible he became. Taking a cue from a contemporary, Signor Baglivi, who was having much success in Italy by regarding the patient as a person rather than as a playground for the usual high-flown theories of the time, Mather came to understand the importance of attending to the patient's mind as well as his body. "Let the Physician," he wrote, "with all possible Ingenuity of Conversation, find out what Matter of Anxiety there may be upon the Mind of the Patient; what there is that has made his Life uneasy to him. Having discovered the Burden let him use all the Ways he can devise to take it of."

By the end of the eighteenth century, a movement to the American West was in full swing. At first the settlers in Kentucky, Tennessee, Ohio, Illinois, and Missouri, were well out of reach of all but the most adventurous Eastern medico, so they were forced to depend on their own efforts. Consequently the settlers did not flourish physically. According to T. V. Woodring, the settlers bore little resemblance to fiction's picture of them as stalwart frontiersmen. The typical pioneer was "wan with fever, gaunt, and spindle-shanked. His wife was scrawny and peaked; their children were sick and fretful." Even in surgery, self-help was not uncommon. When one frontiersman, Pegleg Smith, had his leg smashed by an Indian bullet, he proceeded to apply a tourniquet of buckskin thongs, then, so the story goes, he cut off his leg with a hunting knife. To complete the job he clamped off the spurting arteries with bullet moulds, and finally whittled himself a new leg out of a handy piece of hickory.

The few professional medical men were not much better-equipped than the amateurs. Though there was a profligate use of firearms, few frontier doctors had more than a handful or rudimentary tools to deal with the results. "At best, a physician might carry in his saddlebags a set of amputating instruments, a set of trephining instruments for penetrating the skull, a case of pocket instruments, and some crooked and straight needles. (It must be remembered that on July 3, 1776, there were only six sets of amputating instruments to be distributed among fifteen regiments of Washington's army.) Some early physicians carried a scalpel or incision knife for dilating wounds and a pair of forceps for extracting bullets." Even so, many doctors dealt with gunshot wounds quite effectively. In time they were even able to repair some of the damage caused by scalping. According to the authors of *The Story of Medicine in America,* "The procedure involved taking a pegging awl and thickly perforating the naked area so that granulation would occur and form a covering to the denuded skull before its investing fibrous membrane should die and exfoliate."

American physicians may have started out as gentlemanly theorists, but the urgencies of a savage, competitive environment soon converted them to the pragmatic approach that has so clearly moulded American behaviour. One of the West's most prominent practitioners, John Sappington, for instance, had the scientific courage to abandon the standard methods of dealing with malaria to champion the use of quinine as the only treatment that was necessary.

Malaria was one of the fevers that had wracked the frontier people all their lives, so an effective preventative was an important development. Even as a medical student, Sappington, an alert young man from Nashville, who had that clarity of observation that is the most vital talent of the scientific pioneer, was challenging the time-honoured methods of treating fevers by purging, vomiting, and bleeding the patient. After marrying and settling down with his family in a log cabin at Arrow Rock, Missouri, Sappington became convinced that such methods were uselessly debilitating, and when French chemists isolated quinine from cinchona bark in 1820, he was quick to adopt it as the sole method of treating malaria.

Though he used it effectively for several years, he could not convince his colleagues. They continued to drain their patients by means of the lancet, emetic tartar and the calomel purge. Sappington finally decided that if he could not gain any scientific profit he might as well try for the other kind, whereupon he "began the manufacture and sale of his 'Anti-Fever Pills.' These, at $1.50 for a box of twenty-four, were distributed by a regiment of drummers who traveled far and wide through the Mississippi Valley and into the Republic of Texas. Books and handbills as well as pills were distributed. The prescription for prevention was one pill three times daily. In ten years over a million boxes were sold."

By no means all of the country's medical endeavours were personalized in such ways. There were many pure contributions to medical science by such parents as Benjamin Rush, Father of American Psychiatry, Daniel Drake, Father of Western Medicine, and Ephraim McDowell, Father of Ovariotomy, who performed the first such operation on a Kentucky woman who thought she was ten months pregnant until McDowell delivered her of a twenty-two pound ovarian tumour. Nevertheless, an intensely competitive society nurtured an impatience not only with the ideals of medical science as being the rightful inheritance of mankind without considerations of profit, but an impatience with the science itself.

In the nineteenth century, numerous medical cults marched to the tempo of quick, concrete results. Thomsonianism was one of them, invented by Samuel Thompson of New Hampshire, whose formal training consisted of a short stint as an apprentice to a Dr. Fuller. At the age of nineteen, Thomson slashed his ankle, and under the care of the family doctor the wound got steadily worse, until at last, "The flesh on my leg and thigh were mostly gone and my life was despaired of." Thomson insisted on a remedy of his own, a poultice of comfrey root and turpentine. The wound healed. This inspired him to practice the healing art first on members of his family—it was claimed that he saved the lives of his wife and daughter—then, when the neighbours began to flock to him for treatment he decided to make a business of it.

The business, Thomsonianism, was based on ancient Greek teachings, which Thomson interpreted as meaning that all disease was the effect of one general cause: cold. Or, to put it another way, a lack of heat. His remedy was to "increase the internal heat, remove all obstructions of the system, restore the digestive powers of the stomach, and produce a natural perspiration." He used only two treatment aids, according to Marks and Beatty: "the botanicals, to which he had become attached at an early age, and external 'steaming,' a procedure developed to save his daughter."

He patented the system in 1813, and advertised it in the newspapers, and over the next thirty years it was widely used, particularly in the southern and midwestern states.

No doubt Samuel Thomson knew a good deal about roots and herbs, though, given his highly simplified regime, it seems likely that it was a natural gift for healing that made him successful, rather than his calorific endeavours. It was certainly not the essential knowledge of the workings of the body in health and sickness that a medical school would have provided.

Even if Thomson had attended a medical school, it is unlikely that it would have made him a knowledgeable doctor; not because he was incompetent but because most of the medical schools were. There were exceptions, such as the College of Physicians and Surgeons of New York, the Harvard Medical School, and the one in Pennsylvania, but in most cases the standard of admission was too low and the course too short. In 1846, three years after Thomson's death, medical instruction was so deficient that one of the societies set up to regulate the profession and certify doctors, the New York State Medical Society, felt impelled to call for a national convention to take action against the abuses and failures in the field. This was the first meeting of the American Medical Association. Even so, it was well into the twentieth century before many of the "disgraceful conditions" were rectified.

Toward the end of the nineteenth century, the brightest hope for the future lay in the proposed Johns Hopkins Medical School. Johns Hopkins was a Baltimore merchant who had made a fortune out of the agony of the Civil War. Aware that his life and deeds were hardly likely to impress posterity, he made sure that his name, at least, would rescue him from obscurity. He left his money to be divided equally between two institutions that were not likely to fail: a university and a hospital.

Construction of the hospital, set on a hill outside Baltimore, began in 1877, with John S. Billings as medical advisor. Billings designed it in a style perfectly suited to the original methods that Osler would introduce, the system of separate wards that had become familiar to Billings during his time as a surgeon in the Union Army during the Civil War.

Right from the beginning, everybody associated with the university was of exceptional merit, including the trustees, who, among other acts of wisdom, selected the best available man, Daniel C. Gilman, to head the new institution. In his turn, Gilman chose the best available staff—much to the annoyance of the local doctors, who were all passed over.

In less than a decade, the new university became a Mecca for the nation's most brilliant scholars. At the same time, Gilman was preparing for the opening of the new hospital, assembling another distinguished group of professors that included William H. Welch for the chair of pathology, "the first time such a post had been established on a full university basis," and William Osler, to take charge of the medical department as physician-in-chief.

The official opening of the hospital excited interest among the general public almost as much as among the fraternity. "It was a brilliant day," recalled Osler's first resident physician, H. A. Lafleur, in his *Early Days at the Johns Hopkins Hospital with Dr. Osler,* "and notabilities, medical and otherwise, from Baltimore and the principal medical schools of America were grouped under the vast dome of the administration building to witness the inauguration of what was confidently believed to be the last word in hospital construction and management for the scientific study and treatment of disease. There was a feeling of elation—one might even say of exaltation—that the structure which had taken twenty years to evolve, absorbing the energies and thought of so many able minds, had at last become a *fait accompli.* And to none more than to Dr. Osler was this a red-letter day. To blaze a perfectly new road, untrammelled by tradition, vested interests or medical 'deadwood'—best of all, backed by a board of management inbued with a fundamental and abiding respect for scientific opinion and commanding an ample budget—what more could the heart of man desire."

The medical school, which would embody the best features of medical education in Britain, France, and Germany, was still four years away, but in the meantime, Osler had plenty to do in the hospital, writing, researching, publicizing, ordering materials and a clinical laboratory, and building up his staff, with whom he was soon enjoying the usual good fellowship. Their meals together were luminous with discussion and banter. Osler, like most of his fellow chiefs, was still a young man, thirty-nine years old, and with a young man's eye for a gaudy cravat. His hair was thinning but his moustache was longer than ever, "the position of the ends of which seemed to vary with his mood," wrote Dr. Councilman, one of the pathologists, who continued, "At first, with the exception of Welch and Mall, we all lived in the hospital. . . . We breakfasted together, then each sought his particular duties, to meet again at luncheon. The luncheon hour, at which most of those working at the hospital gathered, was the most delightful of the day. Osler, Welch, Halsted, Mall, Lafleur, and with the usual visiting stranger, sat at a table in the end of the dining-room. The conversation was always lively and interesting; everyone sought to bring something to the feast. There was talk about work; jokes, and laughter. A favorite game in which Osler rather excelled. . . was to relate the impossible and to lead up to this so skilfully that the line between fact and fiction was obscured. It was very well for us who knew the game, but occasionally it would be played when the serious visitor was present and he often carried away with him striking information of new facts in medical science."

Councilman went on to mention that the exchanges between Osler and the pathologist Halsted were particularly delightful, but at least one of Dr. Councilman's exchanges with Osler must have been well worth overhearing. It occurred the day after Councilman was supposed to have gone to Philadelphia to read a paper on a subject (presumably pathology) in which they were all interested. Unfortunately, Dr. Councilman had mixed up the dates of his engagement, and missed the medical meeting by a full week.

Given the importance of the occasion to Councilman's reputation and career, the reading of a research paper to an assembly at one of the country's premier institutions of learning, his explanation that he had mixed up the dates does not seem entirely convincing. One could speculate that his memory lapse was subconsciously deliberate, because Dr. Councilman stuttered, and it must have been an uncomfortable experience for him to read a paper inevitably crammed with Greek, Latin, English, and German combinations and consonants.

Anyway, Councilman failed to deliver the results of his research. Thus he was not looking forward to meeting his confreres the next day. So naturally the first words Osler spoke next day were in the form of an enquiry as to how the paper had been received at Philadelphia.

Too embarrassed to confess his mistake, Councilman, in the quick-witted tradition of Osler's group, decided to bluff it out. He replied that the paper had received a tremendously enthusiastic response in Philadelphia. Osler then gravely asked for details on the subsequent discussion. With a flair and invention inspired by the chief, Councilman summarized the discussion at some length. "What did Wilson say?" Osler asked. Councilman, hurriedly assessing Wilson's conservative proclivities, decided that he had better number Wilson among the opposition. Accordingly he did his best to invent an opposing argument for Wilson. "Yes," said Osler, "Jim Wilson spent last night with me and said he immensely enjoyed your paper but he could not quite agree with you."

The Johns Hopkins Hospital evidenced originality in almost all its activities. A training school for nurses, the first time such a school was to be made an essential part of a hospital, was opened in the October of Osler's first year, 1889, under a Canadian nurse, Isabel Hampton. In the same month, the famous Monday-evening societies were started. "The first and third Mondays of each month were to be given over to the presentation of interesting cases, to the reading of papers, and to the discussion of problems in process of solution. The first meeting was held on October 22nd, with Welch presiding and Hunter Robb acting as secretary; and before this group of enthusiastic young people eager to advance knowledge and to control opinions by experimental tests, hardly a subject could be mentioned that did not lead to further work in view of the free and suggestive exchange of ideas. In the history of medicine there has never been anything quite like it: there was no need to drum up an audience for these meetings, and it is recalled that Reginald H. Fitz, who at about this time went down from Boston to learn something of the spirit of this new place which already was being so much talked about, likened the life to that of a monastery, with the unusual feature that the monks did not appear to bother their minds about the future."

As well as his clinical work—within a few months of its opening, the hospital had dealt with one thousand in-patients and eleven thousand out-patients—Osler was continuing his scholarly work, paricularly into diseases produced by parasites. It included his presentation to the hospital society of a rare case of *Filaria sanguinis hominis,* a minor example of his almost lifelong fascination with the parasitic diseases—now especially malaria—that had been aroused in Toronto while he was associated with Father Johnson.

His work in pathology, though, was dying away. During a medical occasion in Toronto round about this time, the profession in that city was surprised when Osler, whose name to them was synonymous with pathology, gave way to William Welch during the presentation on that subject. But of course, Professor Welch had been made the official university pathologist. So Osler stood aside, manifesting the generosity of spirit that pervaded the Hopkins group. "But his long apprenticeship in pathology had by no means been wasted," as Harvey Cushing pointed out. "It was unquestionably an ideal preparation for a clinician and gave him the rare ability to interpret his patients' symptoms in terms of the pictures which his long hours at the autopsy-table had indelibly stamped on his mind. So in the textbook he finally came to write, his pathological descriptions, drawn from his own experience, were regarded as the best part of his treatise and could have been written by no other clinician of the day, unless possibly by Fitz, who had had a similar training."

The publication of the textbook *The Principles and Practice of Medicine,* which was to become one of the most renowned of all medical works, was not the only major event in Osler's life in 1892; though his actions suggested that the other event was about as significant as a moose-hunting trip. He got married.

The appellation given the lady by one of Osler's friends as "the widow Gross," suggests a character out of a Restoration comedy. In fact she was a proper Bostonian by the name of Grace Linzee Revere, a descendant of Paul Revere, the colonial silversmith who had galloped from Lexington to Concord, waking people up with hoarse cries and thus making the War of Independence inevitable.

When Osler first met Grace she was the wife of his close friend, Sam Gross, the doyen of American surgery, whose death had been almost as much of a blow to Osler as to the widow, especially as it had occurred shortly after the death of another dear friend, Palmer Howard, in Montreal.

Osler had been determined at the outset not to marry until he was well established. Now, three years after Sam's death, he went to the lady with the proof that he was indeed established, the proof being a copy of the *Practice*. He tossed it into her lap with the words, "There, take the darned thing; now what are you going to do with the man?"

Naturally she was not so unwise as to tell him—at least, not until they were married.

In April, he was in Toronto to give his mother the news she had been hoping to hear for fifteen years. He hardly let anyone else in on the secret, though an exception was Beatrice Francis, the little girl to whom, when she was ill, he had confessed that his heart bled for her in seven places. Now he wrote to her: "Dearest Trixie: Do not laugh but be very sober and quiet when I tell you—stop that laughing—that I am going to be married. It is Mrs. Gross this time—You will love her I am sure—for your old Doctor's sake as well as your own. Your loving Uncle Willie.

The following month, "Osler took an early train to Philadelphia. There was nothing unusual in this, nor in the fact that in the course of the morning he called at 1112 Walnut Street, Mrs. Gross' residence. Here, 'unbeknownst' even to the faithful colored servants, Morris and Margaret, some trunks had been packed and sent by an express-man to the station at an early hour in the morning. Shortly before lunch, James Wilson dropped in, and finding Mrs. Gross and his former colleague sitting under a tree in the garden, remarked: 'Hello, Osler, what are you doing over here? Won't you have lunch with me?' 'No,' said Osler, 'I'll come in to tea. I'm lunching here. Why don't you stay?' This he did; and Wilson recalls that 'We talked lightly of Grand Manan which they knew; of St. Andrews and the salmon rivers, and moose hunting; of northern New Brunswick of which I had knowledge; and of the charming Canadian doctors, Osler's friends, whom we had met.' This dragged on between the two men, until presently Mrs. Gross asked to be excused, with the statement that she was going out and a hansom was waiting at the door; whereupon Wilson made his manners, pleading an appointment, leaving Osler, who said that Mrs. Gross would give him a lift as she was going in his direction. It was not until then that the devoted Margaret was told by her mistress that she was to be married at 2:30, and, darkey fashion, the faithful girl, overcome by the informal ways of 'white folks,' exclaimed: 'My Gawd, Mam, only a hansom! Lemmee go and fetch a hack.' Leaving their bags at the station they drove to St. James' Church, where the ceremony was performed, and having walked back to take their train, Osler sent this telegram to Wilson: 'It was awfully kind of you to come to the wedding breakfast.'"

In the available accounts of their relationship, there is nothing to suggest that the new Osler duo was derived from the accepted chemical combination of love. Osler's mind was too disciplined to admit love's illogical formulae, while Mrs. Osler no longer felt compelled to curtsy to romance; though at thirty-eight she was "a rather splendid creature, tall, with a proud, handsome, highbred face, large gray-blue eyes that were kind or quizzical or indifferent; a beautiful short Roman nose and an attractive mouth. With great feminine efficiency there was something of the nice boy about her—brave and downright and such a 'good sport.'"

She needed to be a good sport. Anyone who had earned Osler's affection was likely to be japed, and his wife was not excepted. As in the case of the pregnant society lady. Not given to gossip, Osler never spoke to Grace about his patients. This failure to confide worried her slightly—people might think they were not getting on. So one day he obliged by confiding that one of her friends was expecting. Grace was deliciously shocked, for the lady in question was over fifty. It was only when she attempted to commiserate with the friend that she learned that she had been hoaxed.

That Grace was fond of relating such stories herself says much about her quality, which was of the kind that had attracted Osler to her in the first place. Another of her stories against herself concerned a distinguished physician whom Osler had invited to lunch, after first warning Grace that the visitor was exceedingly deaf. When he appeared, he seemed, in fact, to be so deaf that even *he* had to shout, in order to hear himself. Mrs. Osler and the distinguished physician spent the entire meal bellowing at each other over the table. It was days before they learned that this was another of Osler's tricks. He had not only told his wife that the visitor was deaf—he had told the visitor that Mrs. Osler was deaf, as well.

One of Edith Reid's paragraphs admirably conveys the atmosphere of the Osler household at 1 West Franklin Street, Baltimore. One afternoon around a tea table crowded, as usual, with students and other visitors, Dr. Osler was holding forth enthusiastically on the insights of the Swiss philosopher, Amiel. As was his wont, he suddenly jumped up to fetch Mrs. Humphrey Ward's recent translation from his library. Then he rushed back to quote from it. During a pause, one of the women present said, "'Dr. Osler, isn't it amazing that the —s are getting a divorce?' He had his finger in the book searching for the line he wanted, and he looked up with such withering scorn that the offender almost burst into tears, and though the words were not audible, his lips seemed to be saying something like 'go to H...!' After the offending gossip left everyone laughed and Mrs. Osler said: 'I see nothing to laugh at—horrid manners—you were hateful to —.' Dr. Osler: 'She's a venemous little beast!' Mrs. Osler: 'It's not morals with you, Willie. You are just put out because she interrupted you when you were explaining your anaemic Monsieur Amiel.' Everyone laughed, Dr. Osler joining. 'I'll send her a box of chocolates,' he said. 'Oh, will you?' Mrs. Osler replied. 'You mean

I'll send her a box of chocolates and all the work you will do will be to write: "Nasty temper, forgive, read something in the Bible about Charity!" I know you, Dr. Osler.' 'You do! Here's my card,' and he scribbled a text from the Bible, tossed it on the tray in front of her and seizing one of his young students who was present dragged him off with him to his study. Mrs. Osler looked at the card and after reading it aloud, said: "Poor —, I am certain that she hasn't a Bible. She only subscribes to *Town Topics*, and I adore hearing all she has to say. I do wish Willie had let us hear about the —'s. Never mind, we'll find out." ' "

The Johns Hopkins Medical School—co-educational, yet—registered its first students in the fall of 1893. The entrance requirements astounded the fraternity: two years pre-medical training in biology and chemistry, the ability to read in French and German, *and* a B.A. or B.Sc. degree. (The qualifications were so steep that Osler remarked one day to William Welch that it was a good job they were in as professors, because they would never have gotten in as students.)

The school was in its third year before one of its three principal designers resumed his clinical teaching. By then, 1896, Osler's powers were at their mightiest. Even those who had known his work at McGill and Pennsylvania were awed by his electrifying effect on the students. He inspired them to use their five senses and their powers of observation to the utmost, and their ability, hitherto unsuspected by them, to advance science through original research. A few seconds of his communication with the students sounded like this: " 'Don't touch the patient—state first what you see; cultivate your powers of observation.' And there would be an informal running comment, practical, amusing, stimulating; with apt illustrations and allusions that served to fix indelibly on his hearers' minds the points of the lesson he desired to bring out. 'Strong, go to the library and bring me Vol. V of Guy's Hospital Reports, and you'll find an account of this one page —' &c. 'Jones, what have you read in French or German this week? Nothing? Well, report next time to the class from the last *Berliner klinische Wochenschrift* what Ewald says bearing on this subject —' &c. And meanwhile, to the mystification of one who might be looking over his shoulder, 'James Bovell M.D. James Bovell M.D. M.R.C.P.' is being scribbled across the blotter or pad beside him as he patiently awaits the response of some student laboring with a question." .

The question was frequently on one of the three principal killers of the day: pneumonia, typhoid, and tuberculosis. Osler was investigating them himself, producing paper after paper for publication or for reading at medical gatherings.

Osler's organization was as novel as his extraordinarily personal teaching, and a revelation to the Americans. It comprised his medical unit of up to a hundred beds, a large out-patient department and clinical laboratory close to the chief wards. Just as Dr. Cushing described the previous scene with the students, Dr. W. S. Thayer enables us to follow Osler on his daily routine: "At 7 he rose; breakfast before 8. At a few minutes before 9 he entered the hospital door. After a morning greeting to the Superintendant, humming gaily, with arm passed through that of his assistant, he started with brisk, spring steps down the corridor towards the wards. The other arm, if not waving gay or humorous greetings to nurses or students as they passed, was thrown around the neck or passed through the arm of another colleague or assistant. One by one they gathered about him, and by the time the ward was reached, the little group had generally grown like a small avalanche.

"The visit over, to the private ward. For the many convalescents, or the nervous invalid whose mind needed diversion from self, some lively, droll greeting or absurd remark or preposterous and puzzling invention, and away to the next in an explosion of merriment, often amid the laughing but vain appeals of the patient for an opportunity to retaliate. For those who were gravely ill, few words, but a charming and reassuring manner. Then, running the gauntlet of a group of friends or colleagues or students or assistants, all with problems to discuss, he escaped. How? Heaven only knows!

"A cold luncheon, always ready, shortly after one. Twenty minutes rest in his room; then his afternoon hours. At half past four, in the parlor opposite his consulting room, the clans began to gather, graciously received by dear 'Mrs. Chief,' as [Mrs.] Osler was affectionately known. Soon the 'Chief' entered with a familiar greeting for all. It was an anxious moment for those who had been waiting long for the word that they had been seeking with him. After five or ten minutes he would rise, and perhaps beckon to the lucky man to follow him to his study. More often he slipped quietly from the room and in a minute reappeared at the door in his overcoat, hat in hand. A gay wave of the hand, 'Goodby,' and he was off to his consultations.

"Dinner at seven, to which, impartially and often, his assistants were invited. In the evening he did no set work, and retired early to his study where, his wife by the fire, he signed letters and cleared up the affairs of the day. Between ten and eleven o'clock, to bed."

Where, in time, Edward Revere Osler was conceived, and who, on being born at the end of 1895 was described in Osler's casual fashion as "a strong and healthy specimen." Mrs. Osler, though, knew that her husband was far from feeling casual. "On New Year's Day," she wrote to the other Mrs. Osler in Toronto, "he told me in the most solemn manner that he had not kissed the baby yet, but was going to then. Before he left last night he said he had kissed him five times. He brings all his medical friends up to look at him."

Osler's trove of affection, amassed through his friendships, particularly with small children and old men of wisdom and experience, was supremely enriched by the arrival of his only child. Revere was to be the source of his greatest happiness, and his death on active service in the First World War, was Osler's most desolate sorrow; a grief concealed. "Dear MacAlister, So glad to hear that you are better. Harrogate is a great place for the *Prime viae ductus vitae.* I will write to the G. A. Hard blow today. News of the death of my boy in France. Fortunately his great friend was at the Casualty Clearing Station when he was brought in. He was a great lover of books and a son after my own heart. Yours sincerely W. O."

Given the way William Osler filled every minute of his day with work, work, work, his crowning achievement, the monumental *Principles and Practice of Medicine,* might not have been written if the B. and O. Railroad had not gotten into financial difficulties.

Millionaire Hopkins had invested much of his money in the Baltimore and Ohio Railroad, and it was these shares that had endowed the university. Following the slump of '87, the railroad ceased to pay dividends, forcing postponement of the construction work on the new medical school. Thus, for the first time since he had given up the frivolities of childhood for his studies with Father Johnson in natural history, Osler found that he had spare time on his hands. For the most part he had spurned general practice, his consultations took up a maximum of ninety minutes a day, and he could easily delegate much of the hospital work to his juniors.

In the whole continent, perhaps in the whole world, there was nobody more competent to write such a book. He had a knowledge of medical progress in nearly all departments, his base in pathology was rivaled only by that of the great Virchow who had founded modern pathology. He was steeped in medical history, and twenty years of writing had given him a clarity and style ideal for such a work.

The sole weakness of the book was said to be in therapeutics, "if a healthy skepticism concerning drugs may be regarded as a weakness." His distrust of "pop-gun pharmacy" was simply too profound for him to overcome. Having preached restraint in this regard — or joshed his juniors out of it — he could only feel annoyance with a public that continued to "wander off after all manner of idols, and delight more and more in patent medicine, and be more than ever in the hands of advertising quacks." Not to mention his disdain for other doctors who encouraged the public to worship the idol drug. Cushing quotes one revealing reaction to such views expressed in the *Principles and Practice* as, "Many specifics have been vaunted in scarlet fever, but they are all useless," and

"Pneumonia is a self-limited disease, and runs its course uninfluenced in any way by medicine. It can neither be aborted or cut short by any known means at our command." Cushing continues: "These are hard words for the neophyte but not for the experienced. Drugs, drugs, is the cry of the average doctor, and of the average patient too. But drugs are not all, and in many cases it is well for us to remember their uselessness as compared with other means. Weir Mitchell, in his little book on Doctor and Patient, says that, 'throughout the history of medicine, the really great physicians were peculiarly free from the bondage of drugs.'"

The book was for the most part written in the Johns Hopkins Hospital. The senior residents in medicine, surgery, gynecology, and pathology, all had separate studies and bedrooms, and Hunter Robb, one of the residents and assistant to one of the "Big Four," and Howard Kelly (the others being Welch, Halsted and Osler) had the best quarters, at the end of the corridor. So Osler asked Robb if he could use his rooms in the morning, to do his writing.

Dr. Robb said he would be delighted, and by the time he realized what he was letting himself in for, it was too late. "The first morning, he [Dr. Osler] appeared with one book under his arm accompanied by his stenographer, Miss Humpton. When the morning's work was over, he left the book on my library desk, wide open with a marker in it. The next morning he brought two books with him, and so on for the next two weeks, so that the table and all the chairs and the sofa and the piano and even the floor was covered with open books. As a consequence I never was able to use the room for fully six months. Oftentimes right in the middle of his dictating, he would stop and rush into my other room, and ask me to match quarters with him, or we would engage in an exchange of yarns. It was a great treat for me...except when he would court inspiration by kicking my waste-paper basket about the room."

Robb soon cured Osler of that. Getting tired of having his rubbish booted all over the carpet, one morning he filled the basket with bricks, carefully concealed under a top layer of discarded notes, old letters, rough drafts, and blotting paper.

Taking a flying kick at a basket of bricks might have provided Osler with a memorable quip, but maybe his mashed toes preferred to forget it. His version, scribbled on the flyleaf of Robb's copy of the *Principles* goes: "In the spring of 1891, I coolly entered and took possession of the working room of Dr. Hunter Robb—popularly known as the Robin. As in the old story of the Cookoo and the hedge sparrow I just turned him out of his comfortable nest, besplattered his floor with pamphlets papers & trash & played the devil generally with his comfort. In spite of the vilest treatment on my part he rarely failed to have oranges in his cupboard, chocolates &c (yum!yum!) on his table and ginger ale & 'Old Tom' on the sideboard."

The book was published the following year and was received on both sides of the Atlantic with "enormous approbation." It was a tremendous enterprise that, in style, perspective, honesty, and weight of knowledge, would alone have ensured Osler a well-lit corner in the gallery of great medical men. It proved to be based mostly on the work he had done in Canada, the climax to twenty years of microscopical, bacteriological, and chemical investigation. The book's symptomatology and diagnosis of disease was built on this foundation. And the dedication confirmed once and for all Osler's indebtedness: to William Arthur Johnson, priest of the parish of Weston, Ontario; James Bovell of the Toronto School of Medicine and of the University of Trinity College, Toronto; and Robert Palmer Howard, dean of the medical faculty and professor of medicine, McGill University, Montreal.

This phenomenally successful book was not only intrinsically valuable; it was to have a major influence on medicine in the United States, and to lay the foundations of the great twentieth-century achievements in American medicine.

Five years after the book was published, while Osler was holidaying at St. Andrews in New Brunswick, a member of John D. Rockefeller's philanthropic staff, holidaying in the Catskills, started to read the book on the recommendation of a visitor to his home, a medical student. Impressed by the student's enthusiasm and wishing to contribute more knowledgeably to their conversations, the Rockefeller man bought a copy of the *Practice* and, although he was a layman, he "read the whole book without skipping any of it.

"I speak of this," the staff man went on, "not to commemorate my industry or intelligence but to testify to Osler's charm, for it is one of the very few scientific books that are possessed of high literary quality. There was a fascination about the style itself that led me on, and having once started I found a hook in my nose that pulled me from page to page, and chapter to chapter, until the whole of about a thousand large and closely printed pages brought me to the end.

"But there were other things besides its style that attracted and intensified my interest.... To the layman student, like me, demanding cures, and specifics, he had no word of comfort whatever. In fact, I saw clearly from the work of this thoroughly enlightened, able and honest man, perhaps the foremost practitioner in the world, that medicine had—with the few exceptions above mentioned—no cures, and that about all that medicine up to 1897 could do was to suggest some measure of relief, how to nurse the sick, and to alleviate in some degree the suffering. Beyond this, medicine as a cure had not progressed. I found further that a large number of the most common diseases, especially of the young and middle-aged, were infections or contagions, caused by infinitesimal germs that are breathed in with the atmosphere, or are imparted by contact or are taken in with the food or drink or communicated by the incision of insects in the skin. I learned that of these germs, only a few had been identified and isolated. I made a list — and it was a very long one at that time, much longer than it is now — of the germs which we might reasonably hope to discover but which as yet had never been, with certainty, identified; and I made a longer list of the infectious or contagious diseases for which there had been as yet no cure at all discovered.

"When I laid down this book I had begun to realize how woefully neglected in all civilized countries and perhaps most of all in this country, had been the scientific study of medicine.... It became clear to me that medicine could hardly hope to become a science until it should be endowed, and qualified men could give themselves to uninterrupted study and investigation, on ample salary, entirely independent of practice.... Here was an opportunity for Mr. Rockefeller to become a pioneer. This idea took possession of me. The more I thought of it the more interested I became. I knew nothing of the cost of research; I did not realize its enormous difficulty; the only thing I saw was the overwhelming and universal need and the infinite promise, world-wide, universal, eternal. Filled with these thoughts and enthusiasms, I returned from my vacation on July 24th. I brought my Osler into the office at No. 26 Broadway, and there I dictated for Mr. Rockefeller's eye a memorandum in which I aimed to show to him the actual condition of medicine in the United States and the world as disclosed by Dr. Osler's book. I enumerated the infectious diseases and pointed out how few of the germs had yet been discovered and how great the field of discovery; how few specifics had yet been found and how appalling was the unremedied suffering. I pointed to the Koch Institute in Berlin. I pointed out the fact, first stated by Huxley I think, that the results in dollars or francs of Pasteur's discoveries about anthrax and on the diseases of fermentation and of the silkworm had saved for the French nation a sum far in excess of the entire cost of the Franco-German War....

"These considerations took root in the mind of Mr. Rockefeller and, later, of his son. Eminent physicians were consulted as to the feasibility of the project, a competent agent was employed to secure the counsel of specialists on research, and out of wide consultation the Rockefeller Institute of Medical Research came into being. It had its origin in Dr. Osler's perfectly frank disclosure of the very narrow limitations of ascertained truth in medicine as it existed in 1897."

Though Osler never parted in spirit from McGill — it was to that University that he left his treasured collection of medical works, now housed in the Bibliotheca Osleriana — it was Oxford that finally claimed him from Johns Hopkins. There he remained until his death in 1919, vivid to the last in personality and influence.

His accomplishments are so extensive that this limited account can be hardly more than a cartoon for the fresco of his life. In summary, he made enduring contributions to science through his work in pathology and epidemiology, and through his investigations into the blood platelets, heart disease, the malarial parasite, and tuberculosis. In his writings he illuminated the meaning of medicine and reaffirmed its international character. Above all, he revolutionized medical teaching in North America through his co-ordination of the work in the wards and laboratories with bedside teaching.

In personality and character he was magical. He transformed so many lives, from narrowness to generosity of spirit, from drudgery to inspiration, from a rudderless course to one guided by example, and powered by energies that might not otherwise have been exploited. He was the most fascinating, the most lovable, and the most inspiring of great men. In medicine and in human affairs his life spoke eloquently of his beliefs, even more so than his words: "We are not here to get all we can out of life for ourselves, but to try to make the lives of others happier."

It was not a bloodless ethic. Osler was a man with a passion for life through work and through a thousand friends, scholars, children, surgeons, patients, students, and old men. His was a passion containing a paradoxical element of inhibition. Osler understood the real as distinct from any fashionable sanity, that inhibition is not a harm but a safeguard against a debasing crudity in human relationships, that inhibition brings a beautiful subtlety to human relationships.

He was by no means perfect in any superficial sense. He was on a self-imposed probation for decades, to restrain a temper that could be quick and fierce. At a medical gathering he made a slashing attack on an administrator as an incompetent, and was hissed for it. He was eager for honours and the increased power they brought (he was not joking when he told the McGill students that he was leaving out of pure ambition). His appeal was not universal because he needed a personal, electric response before he could respond properly himself. And though his practical jokes were neither superficially nor subconsciously malevolent, they could on occasion be insensitive.

Two contrasting examples of his effect on others, both Toronto medical graduates who would contribute substantially to the reputation of the Johns Hopkins, are worth giving. First Lewellys Barker. "I remember very well my first contact with him. It was in 1891, toward the end of my year's internship in the Toronto General Hospital. A stray copy of the first number of the *Bulletin of the Johns Hopkins Hospital* had found its way to the residents' lounge and I was so impressed with the possible opportunities of work at the new hospital that I turned to a fellow-intern (Dr. Thomas Cullen) and said to him, 'I wish I could go to Johns Hopkins.' All young Canadians in medicine had heard with pride of Dr. Osler's successful career and of his appointment in Baltimore, and in a moment of courage that now looked back upon seems to have been close to audacity, I sat down and wrote directly to Dr. Osler, asking him whether there was any way in which a young graduate who had no money could find opportunity to work at the Johns Hopkins Hospital. In a few days came a reply, stating that he would be in Toronto soon and would see me. I shall never forget the trepidation with which a week or two later, at his summons, I called upon him at the house of a relative, nor the great relief I felt on meeting him, for he quickly discerned my anxiety and timidity, and by that magic that many have known and marvelled at, put me at ease and led me to talk in a way that surprised me, of what I should like to do. He then told me that it was his desire that at the Johns Hopkins there should be opportunities provided for young men who, like myself, desired to continue their studies after graduation and before entrance upon practice. Though he had no vacancy on his resident staff at the time, he thought there might be one later. In the meantime, he had been authorized by Dr. Walter B. Platt to select an intern for a three months' service (living and $30.00 per month) at the Garrett Hospital for Sick Children at Mt. Airy, Md. Would I care to take this position? If so, he would recommend my appointment. I was delighted of course, and accepted on the spot. Was not Mt. Airy near Baltimore? And, possibly, at the end of the summer, I could at least see Johns Hopkins Hospital and the men at work there.

"In the autumn, having saved $60.00 of the $90.00 honorarium, I found that I had ample funds to defray expenses in Baltimore for a month and still pay my way back to Canada. Dr. Osler invited me to go through the wards with him, or with Lafleur, daily, and there I saw and heard much of typhoid fever, malaria, and amoebic dysentery that was novel to me. He also introduced me to Dr. Welch, who assigned me a place in his laboratory and taught me to grow and study several strains of streptococci in which he was then interested. Dr. Councilman was diligently working in the pathological laboratory; Dr. Flexner, who had just been appointed Fellow in Pathology, was experimenting with diphtheria toxins, and Dr. Thayer, back from Europe, showed us Ehrlich's technique for staining blood-smears. That was a month of intense enjoyment to me, saddened only by the fact that it was but four weeks long. For there seemed to be no prospect of any position on the intern staff of the hospital; all the vacancies for the coming year had been filled.

"The last day of September came and with it a recognition that my purse contained but little more than the price of a ticket to Toronto. But on that very day, Dr. Osler summoned me again to say that one of his assistant residents had been compelled to relinquish his post and that I could have the place if I desired it. Though there was no salary, it included board and lodging in the hospital, and as he had need of 'help' in the way of gathering materials for the revision of an article on the anaemias, this would enable me, if I desired to undertake the work, to make a little money through the winter. I was thus suddenly and unexpectedly elevated to the seventh heaven of delight—all through the thoughtfulness and kindness of one upon whom I had not the slightest claim."

Barker's more vulnerable character had created an instant warmth of communication. Barker's friend, Tom Cullen, was a different character altogether: a streetwise rooster, tough, determined, and resourceful. He and Lewellys Barker were working at the Burnside, the Toronto General's lying-in hospital, when they discussed the revolutionary new hospital in Baltimore, and Cullen's version went as follows: "Lew and I had been having a wash-and-dress-the-baby race. When things were not so busy at the Burnside we used to run races to see who could wash and dress a baby faster. Lew usually won. I could never get below eleven minutes. This day when the race was over Barker turned to me and said, 'I'm going to Hopkins, Tommy.'

"I said, 'What's Hopkins, Lew?'

"He pulled a Johns Hopkins Hospital Bulletin out of his pocket and showed me the cover. It had the picture of the new hospital, open only about a year then. I studied the picture and looked through the bulletin a bit. Then I said, 'Shake, Lew. I'm going too.' But it wasn't quite as easy as that."

One reason it wasn't easy was that when Cullen in his turn applied to Osler for help, there was no rapport between them. So Osler made no attempt to find a vacancy for him at the Hopkins. Osler's opinion of Cullen is not known—he never spoke ill of anybody except in the rarest, most unguarded moments—but it was a long time before Cullen got over his unsympathetic feelings toward Osler.

Though a cool witness, Cullen's comments on Osler, possibly because of his reservations, are among the most interesting of all analyses of Osler's behaviour and motivation—especially his account of what Howard Kelly, chief of the gynecological department, had to say.

"I didn't know Osler well for a long time," Cullen recounted. "the fellows in his service, Lew Barker and Billy Thayer and August Hoch and Frank Smith were devoted to him. My chief, Dr. Kelly, who was closer to him than anyone at Hopkins, had the greatest affection for him. He was always pleasant to us who were juniors in other services, and that was all for quite a while.

"Osler was at his best in personal relationships. He had the greatest charm, but he had to feel some sort of temperamental sympathy before he could release it, and his sense of humour was apt to interrupt. I knew one

Baltimorean who never forgave him a trick he played on her when I was a resident. She was a nurse in training at the time; a probationer taking her duties very hard. Dr. Osler came into her ward one evening just as she finished preparing the evening medicines. He eyed the tray with the glasses and pills set out and ticketed, an impulse hit him and he picked them all up and poured the doses into each other."

The probationary nurse was very upset by this perhaps subconscious manifestation of Osler's therapeutic nihilism. Even years later she could not hear of Osler without a surge of indignation. Cullen knew how she felt because the nurse was the girl he married.

"Teasing was incurable in Osler," he continued. "all his life it got him into scrapes in all sorts of places with all sorts of people. The last one I heard of was in Oxford with the Archbishop of Canterbury. It would have made him more enemies than it did, except that it was never deliberate and he was always surprised and sorry when it offended. If he discovered that a trick or a joke of his had hurt anyone, especially if it had hurt someone defenceless, he would regret it sincerely, but he could never resist the impulse when it took him again.

"There was a little nurse I remember, who came new to the hospital and had never seen Dr. Osler until she met him in a ward one morning. She was carrying a bowl of broth with a napkin over it and Dr. Osler was with a group of physicians and the usual retinue of nurses and residents and interns. When they met, the impulse took him and he stopped, put his finger on the napkin and pushed it down into the broth. Then he got a surprise. The little nurse turned on him half-crying.

"'I don't know who you are,' she said, 'but I think you're the meanest man I ever saw.'

"Osler didn't say anything. What could he say? But shortly after he went home that day Mrs. Osler came to the hospital to find the nurse and apologize for her husband. I am perfectly certain that, until the girl flared up, it had never occurred to him that he was joking at the expense of someone who had no defence. It was a blind spot, and those who were fond of him allowed for it.

"Kelly could handle Osler in a teasing mood as no one else could; smile affectionately when Dr. Osler started to joke at his expense, and reach over and chuck him under the chin. The joke would end right there. The idea that he could be funny too always surprised Osler; I doubt whether he would have taken it as kindly from anyone but Kelly. There was a remarkable understanding between those two. Each seemed to know as much of the other's thoughts as of his own. I can remember as though it were yesterday one afternoon when I was bicycling down Broadway with Dr. Kelly, and he suddenly started to talk about Dr. Osler.

"'Do you know what Osler wants, Tom?' he said. 'He wants to go to

England and he wants to be knighted. How would you like to come to England with me and practice in Harley Street?"

"That was in '94, twelve years before Osler went to England, almost twenty before he got his title. I am sure Osler had not spoken of such a wish then. I doubt if he knew he had it. But Kelly knew; it was one of his intuitions; and he was considering the possibility of pulling up stakes in mid-career and going to England too, if Osler wanted to practice there. That is how deep the friendship went with him."

It seems only right that the last words on Osler should be by Harvey Cushing, a great contributor to American medicine, in neurology, in his own right. "What is more, behind his mask there lay a tender, affectionate, sympathetic, almost sentimental heart, whose emotions he had trained himself to disguise. There is a story told of how he offended some good people in the early days in Baltimore by humming a tune—as near as he could get to one—on leaving the sickroom of a man, evidently near his end, whom he had been asked to see in consultation. His attention was drawn to this lapse by the doctor who had called him in, with the hint that such unheard-of behaviour would make him an undesirable consultant, and he merely replied, in Uncle Toby's words: 'Tis that I may not weep.' It was not for want of thought that he whistled as he went. So, in his letters, when mentioning some sorrow, even that of the loss of his son, which, years later, broke him beyond words, whatever his inward feelings, he disguised them outwardly, and with the gesture of putting sorrow behind him he quickly turned to other things."

18

A Cheeky Gynecologist

A T THE AGE of twenty-seven, Tom Cullen, another of the enthusiastic band of Canadians who contributed to world medicine at Johns Hopkins, was sure enough of his own mind and methods to take on the great von Recklinghausen of Strasbourg over his findings in myomatous womb tissue (myoma is a tumour consisting of muscle tissue). The German pathologist was considered to be the supreme authority in the field. He was in the process of publishing the last word on the subject when Cullen, who was not one to allow his own observations to be blinkered by anyone, brought out his *Adeno-myoma Uteri Diffusum Benignum* in 1896, a paper showing "that such tumours were of endometrial origin and did not originate, as von Recklinghausen held, in remains of the Wolffian body." He was able to elucidate his points all the more clearly because he was using a new tissue-slicing device, the microtome, for making sections for microscopic study, while the Herr Professor was stuck with the old razor and starchy liver.

At first, Cullen's superior at Hopkins, Howard Kelly, was extremely doubtful. After all, the august German, the first to identify the typhoid bacillus, was a long-established pathologist, while the perky young Canadian with the generously curved nose was merely a lab instructor. Kelly "had read von Recklinghausen and he wanted to pull me out," Cullen told Judith Robinson, his biographer. "'You're wrong in your interpretation, Cullen,' he told me 'von Recklinghausen says...' But I had brought the evidence with me sectioned and mounted for examination.

"'I don't care a hoot what von Recklinghausen says,' I said, 'Look down the barrel of the microscope.'

"Popsy [this was Cullen's affectionate name for Kelly] looked and let me go on. I soon heard from von Recklinghausen and I answered him and we had a long and interesting correspondence on our subject. I sent him large sections of my tumours—the ones I had described in my paper—and it ended with something as near an admission of error as an old and famous Herr Professor could be expected to make; 'On all material points there is no difference between us.'

"There was a difference, of course, and the real reason for it was that von Recklinghausen had obtained his material from autopsies, after the changes due to death had occurred. I was working on living tissue, or on tissue so lately removed from living patients as to be the next thing. So I knew I was right."

Without being insufferable about it, Tom Cullen had known he was right since his youth. A bouncy self-confidence was the strongest element of his character. He was as sure of his worth as of his origins, despite the imposed humility of a religious upbringing from a Wesleyan preacher father, and a mother, Mary Cullen, who was the daughter of a Bible Christian minister, and despite beginnings of geographical anonymity. Tommy was born in 1868 in a town north of Belleville named Bridgewater, that had ceased to exist by the time the Reverend Mr. Cullen was transferred to the Richmond Street Church in Toronto.

After living in Demorestville, Sydney, Colbourne, Brighton, and other switches on the Wesleyan circuit, Toronto seemed to Tommy Cullen like the ultimate in urban sophistication. The provincial capital had a population of more than a hundred thousand. It had miles and miles of double-track street railways with horse-drawn cars. At night, bright pools of gaslight illuminated the telegraph-tangled streets. Even more brilliantly lighted were the splendid theatres, such as the Princess and the Grand Opera House. Best of all, there was the Canadian National Exhibition every summer, which, though not national nor an exhibition, nor even particularly Canadian, lifted the provincial spirits of citizens and visitors alike with its fairground hokum and colourfully seedy wares.

With its narrow, winding river, its islands and deep, twisting ravines, the city was a wonderful place to explore, especially the harbour with its crystal waters and whirring wildlife. The bay was only a block or so away from the parsonage. To Tom's relief, the parsonage proved to have a coal furnace, which meant that he did not have to spend his Saturday mornings splitting logs, but could continue his explorations, or go visiting, or card collecting. Most of the Toronto stores gave out business cards, and boys competed to see who could collect the most. The paste boards were prettily decorated. One store also gave away free bright red dinner pails. Tommy collected those as well.

Family feelings and loyalties were intense in those hard, challenging times, and not least among the ties that gave a child a sense of purpose in life were his contributions to meagre family resources. It developed a sense of responsibility. After his father and sister died of typhoid, Tommy would help to support his mother, brother, and four remaining sisters for twenty years. "I sometimes wonder whether all families have as strong a family feeling as ours," his sister Rose wrote from China forty years later. "When we were in Toronto, Tom used to travel nearly a thousand miles just to come home for Sunday dinner....Mother, with all her energy, unselfishness and will power could never have given us the education we had unless Tom had been back of her. Even when Tom was in Baltimore with only five cents in his pocket we looked upon his as the source of all our prosperity and the hope of the future. The greatest gift that any human being can give another is the chance to develop and grow and see life and understand it a little and this is what Tom has given each one of us."

The loyalty began when he was thirteen, with contributions derived from his first summer job at the Exhibition, where he mixed the lemonade for the sweltering multitudes ("Take six lemons and a barrel of water"). While attending Jarvis Collegiate he had a paper route, and handed over those earnings, too, to his mother. The hardest part of that job was waking up at three-thirty in the morning, in order to reach the mailing room of the *Mail* by four. He tried to solve the problem by tying one end of a piece of string to his person and hanging the other end out the window, so that he could be yanked awake by a friend; but returning revelers soon got into the habit of tugging at the string at midnight, so he had to think of an alternative.

He continued as a newspaper boy right up to his graduation as a bachelor of medicine.

He also helped out at the church, pumping the organ and lighting the gaseliers. As well as the normal services, the Reverend Mr. Cullen also held weekly class meetings, attended by people who were sometimes a little more concerned for their souls than the minister's rest. Sometimes they exuded the odour of sanctity until late at night. Mr. Cullen was too polite and patient to shut them up. One evening, Tommy did it for him. He turned out the lights at the meter in the basement, and as a result, the "holiness meeting" ended abruptly, "and about two hundred people came scrambling out in the dark."

"On the way home Father said, 'Boy, did you do it?' I said 'Yes. I knew you were tired.' He didn't say a word, just smiled."

Small moments like that are often the turning point in a relationship. It was the first time Tommy had really felt anything other than dutiful respect for his bearded papa. The smile began a new, warmer relationship between the two, a bond that was not affected even when Tommy began to supplant his father as his mother's principal aid in running the household. The minister was not a very practical man, while Tommy was alert to the realities of baulky furnaces, and the necessity of preserving food for the winter, and of maintaining a good supply of candles from the candle-moulder.

Until that moment on the way home from church, Tommy had felt much closer to the family physician, Leslie Sweetnam. Sweetnam was to become for Cullen what Father Johnson had been to Osler, his scientific inspiration. The doctor, a rugged young man with a well-thatched roof of hair, had become a friend of the family shortly after they moved to the city. His influence on the minister's eldest child lay in Sweetnam's passionate interest in the science of medicine. Until Tommy met Sweetnam he had been destined for the law.

By the time he had enrolled at the Toronto School of Medicine, the family fortunes were secure enough for Tom to keep what little money he earned at the *Mail*. Jaunty with self-confidence, he kept an alert eye open for opportunities to increase his capital. When he became a foreman stuffer—supervising the insertion of the supplements into the Saturday morning newspaper—he teamed up with two other lads and went in for land speculation, buying lots and selling them at a profit. The first deal went very well, and made him a fair profit. "The next one I bought by myself. It was at a camp ground and had a big hickory nut tree on it. I doubled my money on that deal. Some time later I bought an acre in an outlying district, sold it after I started medical shcool and paid my fees with what I made. That was the sum total of my land speculation. I stopped. I had come to the conclusion that a fellow who wanted to make a success of studying medicine couldn't waste time watching the real estate market."

Besides, he was upsetting his parents. Just after he had spent his savings on the down payment for a lot, his college fees fell due. For once he was forced to ask his father for the money. "Mother came to me next morning," he said, "looking very upset. She said Father had slept badly; he had been worrying about me all night. Not that he objected to giving me the money I needed for my fees but that he wondered how I had been spending the money I had earned. So I had to let go my secret and tell Mother about the lot instead of waiting till we sold it and surprising her as I had planned."

It was the last time Cullen was to put money above medicine, or to concern himself with his own financial well-being. Which was just as well, for even by the end of the century, his salary was one that a dead-house janitor might have resented. After fifteen years at Johns Hopkins he would be turning down far-better-paying offers, such as the one he received from Yale, to head its department of gynecology, because the move would have caused a hiatus in his assembly of scientific material. (The financial sacrifice would be greater even than that, for the resulting publications, with their costly colour plates and definitive scope would, over the years, cost him personally fifty to sixty thousand dollars.)

Though destined to become a skilled general surgeon as well as a specialist in gynecology, Cullen seemed at first to be more suited to the physician's role, though he was surprised when the results of the third-year examinations at the Toronto School came out. He was placed first in medicine, though his friend and classmate, Lewellys Barker, was easily the top student.

Lewellys had been placed second, but, "We all knew there was something queer about it," Cullen said. "Lew was the most brilliant student I have ever known. He had an encyclopedic knowledge of every subject in the course and medicine was almost his best subject. Yet there I was first in the list with Lew second. Dr. H. H. Wright, our professor in medicine, had been the examiner. He was a delightful old fellow but odd. I can see him now, walking along Gerrard Street to morning lectures, in a pouring rain, coat collar up, hat brim down, dripping wet but scorning the umbrella I had hurried to offer him. 'Never use 'em,' he said, as though umbrellas were a sign of moral weakness, and walked on.

"H. H. was a character and his lectures were first class. We all took care not to miss them. I confess that I occasionally slept through others. With a big breakfast on top of my newspaper route it wasn't easy to keep awake if the lecturer was dull, and there were back benches well out of sight where you could lie flat and have a good sleep. But I had no trouble keeping awake in Dr. Wright's lectures or in making good marks in his subject. Not better than Lew's though; the whole class knew that and so did the faculty.

"One of the other professors tackled Dr. Wright about it in a faculty meeting. 'Barker knows more medicine than Cullen,' he said. The old man agreed with him: "'I know he does but, damn it, I don't want a book. Barker wrote fifty-two pages, Cullen wrote eight.'"

According to a contemporary, Dr. Herbert Bruce, when the court of examiners discovered that Wright had not even read Barker's 'treatise,' they asked him to reappraise it. Under this tactful prodding, Wright read the paper and reversed his original decision, placing Barker first, Cullen second.

Bruce also said that at the Toronto School of Medicine, Barker was a better instructor in dissection than the official prosector. So much so that the junior students were willing to pay him a fee for his demonstrations. Everybody prophesied a great future for Barker. In fact he ultimately succeeded Osler in the chair of medicine at Johns Hopkins.

Cullen's standing in the third-year examinations seemed to confirm that medicine was his direction, but Leslie Sweetnam was keenly inter-ested in surgery, and once again his influence prevailed.

Sweetnam was not only a good surgeon, he was also one of the few who properly understood the Listerian principle in antisepsis and asepsis. By his final year in medicine, Cullen was living in Sweetnam's house as the doctors' student apprentice. Much of the work involved surgery in the home. Cullen's part in this was in the preparation: scrubbing, sterlizing, and draping an improvised operating table with carbolic-scented sheets. It took hours to make a bedroom ready for an operation, to assemble the towels and gauzes, the catgut in alcohol, the basins of disinfectants, and to boil the surgeon's instruments on the kitchen stove. When the operation was done, the student's task was to dismantle the operating room and, while Dr. Sweetnam and the nurse were caring for the patient, he would clear away the trappings of surgery, clean the instruments, boil them once more on the kitchen stove, and pack them in their cases.

Sweetnam used a reddish disinfectant, subiodide of bismuth. "I have helped him assemble eighty dollars' worth of ingredients at a time." Cullen recalled, "and make the powder in a big porcelain bath. All his patients were supplied with vials of it to dust on cuts and scratches and it was remarkable how quickly ugly cuts would heal with its use.

"I noticed when I became an intern that my preceptor was well ahead of several senior men on the surgical side in his precautions against infection. It was quite a shock to me, coming from my preceptor's training, the first time I saw a well-known surgeon put the knife between his teeth after making an incision, hold it there while he tied off a blood vessel and then take it out and go on with the operation. The older surgeons were finding it hard to take germs seriously and a good many of them didn't try. I was lucky to get my grounding in aseptic techniques under a man as meticulous as Sweetnam."

It was not to be Cullen's only experience of reactionary medicine. A few years later, during a trip to Europe to further his professional skill and knowledge, he was amazed when he saw a famous English surgeon performing an operation in his black Prince Albert coat, "with no more preparation than unbuttoning and rolling back the cuffs." He was even more baffled when he heard this brilliant—technically brilliant—colleague tell the students that bacteriology was "all poppycock." The year was 1893—a quarter century after Lister's "Antiseptic Principle."

"So much that was new was coming out of Europe in those days," Cullen recounted in his sharp, critical way, "you had to go over as often as you could. Seeing a man at work and getting to know him gives you the surest gauge of the value of his written work. I have read some very impressive papers by men with big reputations that I wouldn't give you two cents for, because I have talked with the man and know the way his mind slants, or else have seen him at work and know the kind of work he does. I learned things of the greatest value to me professionally each time we went to Europe but I sometimes think what was of greatest value was the chance I had there to measure the big men's reputations by the men."

In 1890, Tom Cullen, who had been a paper boy throughout his years in medical school, flung his last newspaper against the portals of the General Hospital. On the following day he entered the portals as an intern. It was the first time that good marks rather than influence were the qualifications for internship, and brand-new Doctors Cullen and Barker were among the six choices from the graduating classes of the Toronto School of Medicine and of Trinity.

A year later, Cullen went on to Johns Hopkins and Dr. Sweetnam was again his mentor. Sweetnam was a friend of the gynecologist-in-chief at Johns Hopkins, Howard Kelly. In the spring of 1891, Kelly came to Toronto for a medical association meeting, after which he intended taking off on a canoeing trip with Sweetnam. Before leaving, Kelly consented to operate at the Toronto General, with Hunter Robb as his assistant. Sweetnam came along to watch, along with several other local practitioners, some of whom shared their American colleagues' reservations about Kelly. Kelly, a thirty-three-year-old Canadian, had upset many of the older men with his daring obstetrical techniques.

As it happened, Tom Cullen was on duty in the operating room that day. "Lew was giving the anesthetic," he said, "and I was handling the instruments and Roland Hill had been brought in to help. I turned around to thread a needle and when I turned back found to my amazement that the operator had the abdomen open. Operators in the General often took ten minutes to get that far. After cutting through the skin, fat and fascia, they were apt to get lost in the muscles. Kelly and Robb working together used dissecting forceps as I had never seen them used. One man pulling each way, the cleavage between the muscles was seen at once and the opening in the abdomen could be completed without difficulty.

"I watched, fascinated, while Kelly went ahead and finished that operation and did the second, working with clock-like precision and at a speed I had not imagined possible. By the time he had finished, the course of my professional life was decided. Up to that afternoon I had intended to be a physician. From that afternoon I knew I had to be a surgeon."

Later that evening, Sweetnam introduced Tom to Dr. Kelly, and to his delight, Cullen was promised a place on Kelly's junior staff, the appointment to begin the following January.

He arrived in Baltimore months ahead of time. Now that he had decided on a surgical career, he knew he would need to know a great deal more about pathology. Accordingly, Kelly arranged for him to study under Professor Welch.

Cullen had one of those enquiring minds that had been converted to the scientific approach to healing, "the application," as Pasteur put it, "of the exact methods of chemical and physical research to the elucidation of the complex problems of disease." So he entered the advanced pathology laboratory at Hopkins, overjoyed at his opportunity to work there for nothing.

Unfortunately he may also have entered a little too brashly, for William Councilman set about deflating him with equal enthusiasm. The clash between Osler's stuttering friend and the cocky Canadian began over a lab specimen, an angiomatous tumour. It came from Howard Kelly's clinic, and Kelly had particularly asked for Cullen to section it, stain it, mount it, and study it. Councilman put him down. "C-c-cullen, you are not s-s-s-sufficiently trained," he snapped.

"Taking this rebuff with unbowed head," Cullen's biographer, Judith Robinson, continues, "the confident apprentice was presently allowed to report an autopsy, writing the findings to Dr. Councilman's dictation. The finished report brought new scorn on the reporter:

"'C-c-c-cullen, g-g-g-get a c-c-c-copybook and l-l-l-learn to write.'" Thus for some days, with indifferent success, the senior laboured to instil diffidence. The end of the schooling came suddenly. Cullen again reporting. Dr. Councilman was again performing an autopsy. He turned from consideration of an abnormal liver to question his junior:

"'Wh-wh-what's this Cullen?'

"The answer was prompt as ever. 'Miliary tuberculosis of the liver,' Cullen said.

"'T-t-t-tisn't,' Dr. Councilman replied. The autopsy continued. In due course the liver was frozen, sectioned, examined under the microscope. The examination revealed an unusual liver condition; miliary tuberculosis. Dr. Councilman put aside the frozen section. 'B-b-boys,' he said, 'L-l-l-let's go over to the ch-ch-church.' They went.

"'The Church was Hanselman's saloon, across the road from the laboratory. There Hopkin's men gathered to eat sandwiches, drink beer and pop, talk shop. No further mention was made of miliary tuberculosis of the liver, but Tom Cullen counted, from that day's visit to the church, his acceptance as a fellow-enquirer by William T. Councilman."

The following January, Cullen officially became part of the hospital when he was appointed to Howard Kelly's superbly equipped operating room. It was Cullen's job to give the anesthetic. He did little else for four months. After a while it got on his nerves. "They used a lot of chloroform then, and chloroform is tricky. I began to have a dream every little while. It was always the same dream; that I had gone to sleep giving the anesthetic and my patient had died. I would waken with a start and be greatly relieved to find myself in bed in the residence. Fortunately I didn't lose any patients on the table while I was on anesthetics, but it was close more than once. Three times in ten days I have had to turn a patient up by the heels and now and then I had to carry one along for three-quarters of an hour with no wrist pulse. Had I told Dr. Kelly the condition it would only have worried him; he was in such a predicament each time that he could not have stopped. But it got on my nerves. I was only twenty-three."

Obviously, anesthesiology was still a rude procedure. So was surgery. There was no plasma, blood, or other solutions for sustaining the patient, so a high operating speed was still essential, to pull him through with, literally, bare hands. Gloves were not yet in use. In Kelly's Operating Room, however, there was careful handscrubbing before an operation. Moreover, to the amused disdain of surgeons elsewhere, special clothing was worn. No frock coats with rolled-up sleeves here, but white cotton shirts, trousers, and caps under sterile gowns. Which not only caused disapproving gossip among the traditionalists who felt that such garb lacked dignity, but sometimes upset the patients as well. When Howard Kelly went along to interview a patient attired in this fashion, he found her rather more than usually embarrassed about discussing her intimate problems. As soon as he left, she rang for the nurse. "A nice kind of hospital this is!" she complained. "The cook has just been in and asked me some very impertinent questions!"

In due course, Dr. Cullen became the hospital's first instructor in gynecology, and over the next three years received exactly two hundred dollars for the work. He was content. "I have made up my mind what to do if I couldn't make ends meet; get a night job as a streetcar conductor. I was not going to quit Baltimore or the laboratory. The work was too interesting. When I began in '93 relatively little had been done in gynecological pathology anywhere. The field was unworked and we were among the first in it."

He examined all the tissue from Kelly's operating room. "Every now and then some rare picture would show under the microscope and we often found things that had never been noted before. Anything out of the usual was carefully studied and all the relevant literature read. If no similar case had been recorded, the complete history of this one would be written up, including the clinical data, the operation performed and the laboratory finds, and the full report would be published in the Hopkins Hospital Bulletin." These bulletins were already being eagerly read in medical circles in Europe as well as America, and they now began to make Cullen's name well known. One of his reports was on adeno-myoma of the round ligament, the first myoma of the type that had ever been diagnosed and removed. As a peace-offering, Cullen sent von Recklinghausen sections of the tumour. These were so graciously received that it increased Cullen's desire to meet the great pathologist. The opportunity came many years later. Cullen went to Strasbourg specially to meet von Recklinghausen. He looked forward tremendously to hearing the great man discussing his life's work in pathology, and in particular to hearing a first-hand account of his latest research into bone infection.

Instead, von Recklinghausen allowed him only a brief visit—and spent most of it showing off his new autopsy table—a table that Cullen was already familiar with, as it had been manufactured in Pittsburgh.

In 1896, Tom Cullen became Hopkins' resident in gynecology. At first, there were doubts among Dr. Kelly's associates concerning the wisdom of the appointment. After all, for the previous three years, Cullen had been involved only in the pathological side of the specialty.

The test of his surgical skill came after only a few days of his residency. "I had assisted Dr. Kelly in several operations," he said. "In one, which he left me to start while he saw another patient, I had got on so far when he came back that he told me to finish it while he watched. That gave me confidence, although I would hardly have chosen to meet an emergency single-handed so soon. But it came, and I had no choice."

The emergency came after an operation for the removal of a womb that contained a large muscle tumour. It was Kelly who operated but he "left me to close the abdomen, " Cullen recounted. "I did so and was in the dressing room and changed when I remembered that I had left my watch in the scrubbing-up room. The assistant went to get it for me, going by way of the operating room from which the patient had not yet been moved. In passing, he noticed blood on the operating table, stopped to investigate, found the patient was bleeding from below—a rare thing after such an operation—and sent for me.

"I threw off my coat, and put on a rubber apron, washed up hurriedly and opened the abdomen. Everything was in perfect order. So I opened the neck of the womb and there was the trouble. An artery in a most unusual position was spurting, the blood coming out below. I caught the bleeding vessel, closed the stump of the womb, closed the abdomen. The patient was breathing but had no pulse at the wrist. What a godsend plasma or a transfusion would have been—but we knew nothing then of those life-savers.

"The patient was so nearly gone that wherever she was given a hypodermic there was a slough. She was too weak to move back to the ward. For two days we kept her in a room adjoining the operating room, looked after her there and managed to pull her through.

"Next day, I remember, Dr. Kelly came over and said, 'Tell me about the case, Cullen.' I did and he patted my shoulder when I had finished and said, 'You will never have a harder case than that, Tom. There is nothing you can't do now. Go ahead.'"

He went ahead, operating intensively on women who were usually in poor shape by the time he saw them, because they did not come to him soon enough. This was mostly the fault of the medical profession itself, which did not publicize the danger of cancer. (In 1913, Cullen would start the first public campaign to check the mounting death-toll of cancer, and in the process would be denounced by the extreme conservative element in the profession as "unethical.") One result of the delay in obtaining treatment was that tumours were allowed to grow to a fantastic size. In the case of Mrs. McA. who lived in West Baltimore, Cullen helped to remove a tumour that weighed more than the patient. She weighed eighty-five pounds, her tumour, eighty-nine. The abdominal incision was four feet long.

It was cases such as this that made Cullen realize that a full-scale work on gynecological pathology was urgently needed, to help other doctors reach an early diagnosis in cancer cases. With his usual confidence he decided that he was just the man to write it. After all, he told himself, he had a considerable advantage; he had been closely associated with the subject on both the clinical and laboratory sides, and he had access to the most complete case records that then existed.

Cullen's book, *Cancer of the Uterus, its Pathology, Symptomology, Diagnosis and Treatment,* was the first of his four major works on gynecological pathology written over the next sixteen years. It was highly praised in Britain, but it was Dr. Councilman's nod that pleased Cullen most of all. "Kn-n-n-new you were writing a b-b-b-book, Tommy," he said. "D-d-didn't think it'd b-b-be this g-g-good."

Together with Cullen's other books and a host of original papers, it was good enough to make his name internationally known by the time he retired as chief of the department of gynecology at Johns Hopkins, and became an American citizen when the United States entered the First World War in 1917.

By then he no longer took himself as seriously as he had when he first breezed into Councilman's lab, as evidenced by the stories he told against himself, such as the one about the lady in the theatre who, failing to catch and hold her surgeons' eye, turned to her companions in the box, and said, "There's Dr. Cullen, and he doesn't recognize me. He'd know me well enough if I were in bed."

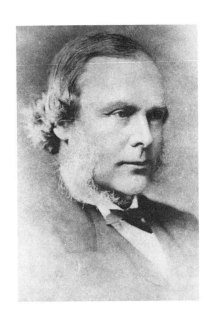

LEFT: Joseph Lister, father of the antiseptic method. (Museum, Academy of Medicine, Toronto) BELOW: The Lister spray. (Museum, A of M)

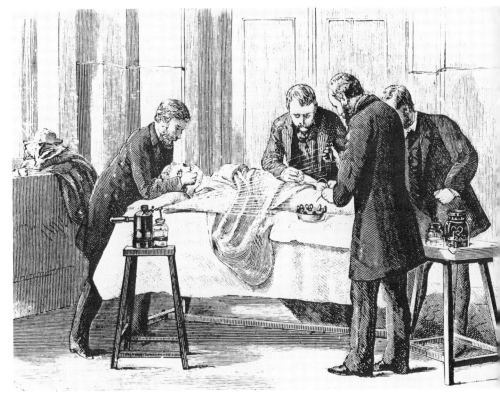

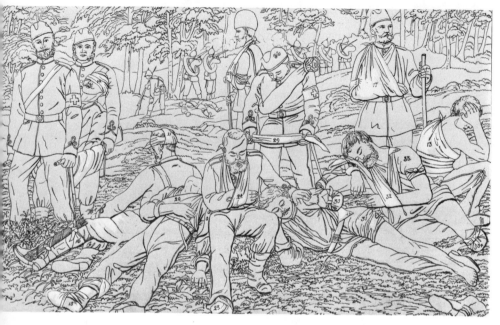

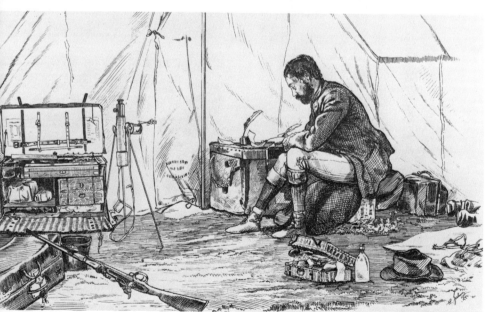

TOP: The Northwest Rebellion. On-the-spot sketch marking the application of the first bandages. (Public Archives Canada/C86543) ABOVE: Campbell Douglas, the Victoria Cross doctor who paddled to the Northwest Rebellion. (PAC/C62595)

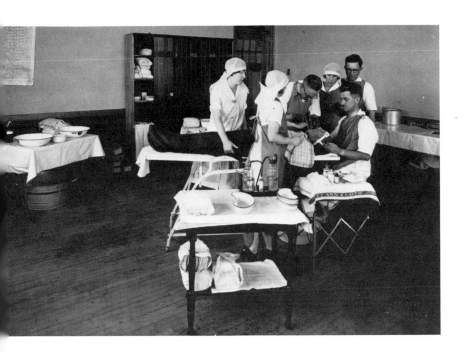

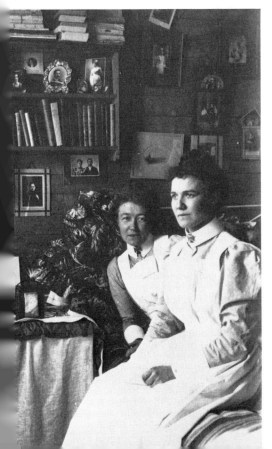

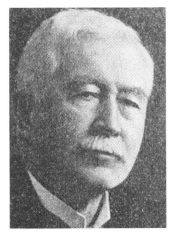

TOP: Travelling medical clinic in rural Alberta, 1920s. (PAC/C29449) LEFT: Nurses, Yukon Territory, 1900. (PAC/PA122795, P. A. Charlebois) ABOVE: Sir Thomas Roddick, the principal pioneer of the antiseptic method in Canada. (PAC/C22482)

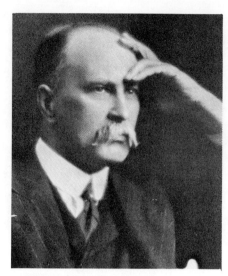

LEFT: Sir William Osler. (PAC/C7105) BELOW: A much more typical view of Osler. (Museum, A of M)

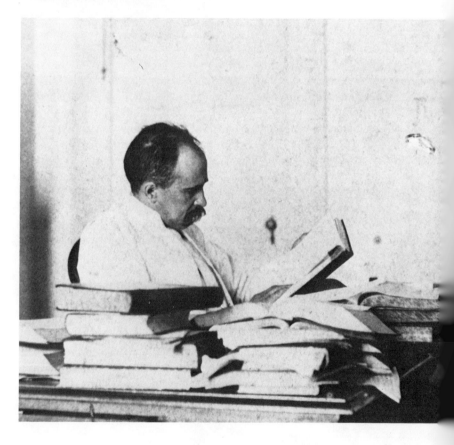

19

Marooned on an Ice Pan

MANY CANADIAN DOCTORS have worked without greed for gain among the people of other lands, particularly Africa and China, but the trade in good works has not been entirely one-sided. One of the most famous and enduring of all medical missions was Wilfred Grenfell's mission to Labrador and northern Newfoundland, whose forgotten people were so humbled by poverty that until Grenfell came they took it for granted that nobody from outside would care whether they lived or died.

Wilfred Grenfell had loved the company of fisherfolk ever since his childhood in the tiny fishing community of Parkgate in Cheshire, where he was born in 1865. Though the son of a local toff, he spent much of his time with the lowly fishermen, and went out with them as often as he could persuade them to let him join them, as they trawled and lined in Liverpool Bay, or seined for salmon in the estuary of the Dee. As a small boy he built a boat, the *Reptile*. It capsized in dangerous waters at least once, Wilfred's seamanship being as defective then as it was later, off the wild shores of Labrador.

He was often daring, but was not inhibited by family 'safety-firstism.' His mother, who came of a long line of soldiers, valued courage, and merely attempted to guide him away from a purely reckless course. She was not entirely successful either with her son or with her husband. When Wilfred was seventeen, his father suddenly gave up his serene way of life as a classical scholar, clergyman, and headmaster of a small private school to become chaplain to a hospital set in a London slum. The shock to Wilfred's parents, of an abrupt transition from pastoral Parkgate to the appalling slums of the East End, must have been considerable. Whatever

215

Mrs. Grenfell thought of the move, the clergyman was presumably sustained by a strong social conscience inherited from his forebears.

Presumably, too, it was the new environment that influenced Wilfred in his decision to enter medicine. He graduated in 1888 from the medical school of his father's hospital, the London Hospital. Apparently he was not a particularly gifted doctor. His hero and chief influence, the celebrated surgeon Frederick Treves, though a close friend of Wilfred's, had described him the previous year as being an indifferent student. But the work that Wilfred now entered did not call for great talent, but for an average ability allied with caring and compassion. For, now as socially conscious as his father, this fervent, boisterous doctor joined the Mission to Deep Sea Fishermen, a religious organization which had been set up to ease the harsh condition of the toilers of the North Sea.

In 1892, the Mission learned of the plight of the fishermen and their families in Newfoundland and Labrador, and that year they sent their young medical superintendent, Dr. Grenfell, to see what he could do about it.

The organization's method at home was to send missionaries among the fishing fleets, to help the men lead a better life, materially as well as spiritually. They found, though, that in Britain's oldest colony with its population of 140,000 and its own responsible government, this approach was not feasible. The Newfoundland vessels, schooners, and flat-bottomed dories, did not gather in fleets, but scattered themselves widely over the Newfoundland Banks and so were not accessible to evangelism.

The fishermen of Labrador, however, could be more easily helped. Every summer, as soon as the coastal waters were free of ice, as many as thirty thousand people sailed to Labrador from St. John's, to join the regular inhabitants of that harsh, dramatic land. Together the summer people from Newfoundland and the Anglo-Saxon inhabitants of Labrador (who called themselves Liveyeres because they "lived here"), combined to work the coastal fisheries, using huge fishing nets that trapped the cod just off shore.

It was the unholy conditions under which these fishermen and their families existed that was to translate Grenfell's religious theories into impulsive, driving practice. Temperamentally the youthful doctor was ideally suited for the rescue operation. He had a particular affection for fishermen. He was warm and understanding when comfort was needed, rough-tongued and aggressive when faced with primitive behaviour. Evangelically fervent, he was also imperfect enough to make him lovable, with an exuberant and reckless spirit and a hefty share of that intolerance so necessary to the true Christian. Above all, he had the excess energy that invariably powers the man of genius.

The boisterous doctor with the blue-gray eyes and the smile that came naturally to a boyish countenance, fell in love from the start with the misty vistas and the violent contours of the land, not least because his first view of it was so dramatic. The moment his hospital and supply ship, the *Albert,* appeared off St. John's, he saw his first whale, his first iceberg, and his first flaming capital. It was as if the three happenings had been specially arranged to enthral him. The whale heaved to the surface close to the ship like a smooth rock in a dipping sea. A moment later a gigantic iceberg slowly overturned with a reverberating boom, swashing an oily wave toward the ship. While in the background St. John's slowly burned to the ground.

The fire had been started by a carelessly disposed match, and by the time it was out, the wooden homes of eleven thousand people were gone. The fire was intense enough to have destroyed even the stone cathedral. Thus, quite unexpectedly, Grenfell found his relief supplies needed in what had been the only comfortable settlement along the entire two thousand miles of his new domain.

When he sailed to the islands and tickles of Labrador, Grenfell's senses were almost overwhelmed by the contrast between the stark beauty of the land with its twisted shapes of granite, limestone, and marble, the subtle shades of the mosses behind the brilliant red dots of berries, and the degradation of its inhabitants. He was filled with exultation and anger.

The beauty of the landscape varied with the seasons. The conditions under which the people lived remained constant. "I think that I must describe one house," Grenfell wrote in his autobiography, "for it seems a marvel that any man could live in it all winter, much less women and children. It was ten feet by twenty, one story high...made of mud and boards, with half a partition to divide bedroom from the sitting-room kitchen. If one adds a small porch filled with dirty, half-starved dogs, and refuse of every kind, an ancient and dilapidated stove in the sitting part of the house, two wooden benches against the walls, a fixed rude table, some shelves nailed to the wall, and two boarded-up beds; one has a fairly accurate description of the furnishings. Inside were fourteen persons, sleeping there, at any rate for a night or two. The ordinary regular family of a man and wife and four girls was to be increased this winter by the man's brother, his wife, and four boys from twelve months to seven years of age. His brother had 'handy enough flour,' but no tea or molasses. The owner was looking after Newfoundland Rooms, for which he got flour, tea, molasses, and firewood for the winter. The people assured me that one man, who was aboard us last fall just as we were going South, starved to death, and many more were just able to hold out till spring. The man, they tell me, ate his only dog as his last resource."

J. Lennox Kerr, in his biography of the famous physician and surgeon, wrote that, "Grenfell was horrified by what he found among these people. He saw men going out to fish in crude, unseaworthy boats built by themselves, short of fishing gear and unable to get credit for more. Women came to the Albert with their bodies scarcely covered with garments made out of old flour-sacks; children went barefooted and almost naked, crawling on the vermin-ridden floors of the huts and in the open in torn and dirty vests. They were often cruelly exploited by itinerant traders from New England and Canada who cruised the coast, and Grenfell heard of one man who received tobacco worth seventy-five cents in Newfoundland for a fox-skin that would fetch 35 to 40 dollars in the outside market. Some of the traders established along the coast asserted seigneurial power over the people, even forbidding marriages and dictating a man's movements."

Grenfell's first impressions of Labrador influenced all his subsequent actions. Late in the evening, when the rush of visitors was largely over, "I noticed a miserable bunch of boards, serving as a boat, with only a dab of tar along its seams, lying motionless a little way from us. In it, sitting silent, was a half-clad, brown-haired, brown-faced figure. After long hesitation, during which time I had been watching from the rail, he suddenly asked:

"'Be you a real doctor?'

"'That's what I call myself,' I replied.

"'Us hasn't got no money,' he fenced, 'but there's a very sick man ashore, if so be you'd come and see him.'

"A little later he led me to a tiny sod-covered hovel, compared with which the Irish cabins were palaces. It had one window of odd fragments of glass. The floor was of pebbles from the beach, the earth walls were damp and chilly. There were half a dozen rude wooden bunks built in tiers around the single room, and a group of some six neglected children, frightened by our arrival, were huddled together in one corner. A very sick man was coughing his soul out in the darkness of lower bunk, while a pitiably covered woman gave him cold water to sip out of a spoon. There was no furniture except a small stove with an iron pipe leading through a hole in the roof.

"My heart sank as I thought of the little I could do for the suffering in such surroundings. He had pneumonia, a high fever, and was probably tubercular. The thought of our attractive little hospital on board at once rose to my mind; but how could one sail away with this husband and father, probably never to bring him back. Advice, medicine, a few packages of food were only temporizing. The poor mother could never nurse him and tend the family. Furthermore, their earning season, 'while the fish were in,' was slipping away. To pray for the man, and with the family, was easy, but scarcely satisfying. A hospital and a trained nurse was the only chance for this bread-winner—and neither was available."

It was a land where even the most minor ailments went untreated. "The successful removal of a molar which has given torture for weeks in a dentistless country, gains one as much gratitude as the amputation of a limb," Grenfell observed, and went on to describe a case where part of a boy's jaw had died because his toothache had been neglected. The damage—necrosis—"had to be dug out from the new covering of bone which had grown up all around it.…

"Deformities went untreated. The crippled and blind halted through life, victims of what 'the blessed Lord saw best for them.' The torture of an ingrowing toenail, which could be relieved in a few minutes, had incapacitated one poor father for years. Tuberculosis and rickets carried on their evil work unchecked."

The appalling conditions the people lived in, bred, in Grenfell's words, "illiteracy, backwardness, ignorance, and superstition." His cases reflected this state. He described a visit to a boy of sixteen who lay dying of hip disease. "The indescribable dirt I cannot here picture," wrote Grenfell. "The bed, the house, and everything in it were full of vermin, and the poor boy had not been washed since he took to bed three or four months before. With the help of a clergyman who was travelling with me at the time, the lad was chloroformed and washed. We then ordered the bedding to be burned, provided him with fresh garments, and put him into a clean bed. The people's explanation was that he was in too much pain to be touched, and so they could do nothing."

Though they owned almost nothing, the Newfoundland and Labrador families still managed to live in debt, through an iniquitous "truck" system that was made possible by a state of mind induced by hopelessness. The St. John's traders gave credit to the families in the form of the barest essentials, fishing gear, and food. In return, the traders were entitled to handle the fisherman's entire catch—a catch whose value was determined by the traders. There was no appeal either from the price that the trader put upon the catch at the end of the season, or upon the value of the goods they had supplied at the beginning. No human beings can resist for long situations where unchecked power can be imposed, and the traders were no exception. They exploited the fisherfolk as if they were not human beings at all. The merchants built grand mansions atop the St. John's hills. The fishermen and their families went hungry during the winter months. Assuming they had survived that long. In one area off eastern Newfoundland, a few months before Grenfell's arrival, forty out of two hundred fishermen were lost in one storm.

Incensed by a system that was responsible for much of the sickness abroad in the land, especially among the Liveyeres, Grenfell persuaded some of the settlements to form co-operatives, so that the profits of their labour would be apportioned among themselves, instead of going to greedy traders. This interference would earn him the lifelong enmity of the St. John's merchants, and through them, members of the Newfoundland government.

Throughout his first two summers in Labrador, Grenfell traveled up and down the coast in the mission vessels, handing out clothes to the miserably clad women and children, and treating them for the pains and discomforts they had stoically borne all their lives. But many of the family heads would not submit to treatment if it meant stopping work for more than a few minutes. The men knew that if they could not use every daylight hour for fishing, their families might be starving by Christmas.

This situation grieved Grenfell most of all. He had done missionary work in the East End of London, where idleness was not an uncommon cause of distress among families, but here the men worked like slaves, and were still little better off by fall, after they had settled up with the traders.

Spiritual guidance was also part of the doctor's responsibility, and he organized church services at every settlement and outport. His religious attitude was narrow, at least by today's standards. He never traveled on the mission ship on the Lord's day, and approved of the piety of one Labrador fisherman who saw an iceberg drifting toward his trap but made no attempt to save the net, his livelihood, from being torn apart because the iceberg had picked a Sunday to do it. But even as he sermonized on the ship's deck, he was increasingly aware that material enlightenment had become his first priority.

Not that Grenfell's homilies were ineffective. At first the fishermen shifted about uncomfortably as he urged them up the steep slope of Christian devotion. Gradually he began to get through to them. His manner owed nothing to the professional sincerity of the regular clergyman. His was an urgency of belief that charged him with love and concern for the men and their families. It was an entirely genuine emotion. His religious star had guided him into the Mission in the first place, and from his very first days at sea he had felt a profound affinity for deep sea fishermen. He enjoyed their company, and admired their strength of character. He dressed like them. When he was not wearing his old, worn tweeds, he clumped about in serge trousers, guernsey, and squelching sea boots. The Labrador men returned his affection. "With him," Kerr wrote, "they never felt uncouth or deficient, for he accepted them as they were, sat with them at their tables, ate their kind of food, and joined in their conversations as naturally as their own mates. They were the people he loved." He put on no airs, was always ready to pitch in, to scrape paint or lend a muscular shoulder, when he wasn't tending to their injuries or listening to their troubles, or making things a little more comfortable for their families, or asking their advice on nautical matters.

As he sailed up the coast, calling in at every settlement to dispense medicine and comfort, rumours about the real doctor flew ahead. Most of the rumours were skeptically received. The kind of help he was offering was so outside the experience of the people that many of them refused to believe that there was a doctor coming who wanted nothing but to ease, to comfort, and to give. Most of the fishermen resisted the incredible stories that were being told. They did not want to be let down by the reality. He couldn't possibly be as good as people said he was. They didn't want to be thought credulous. John Sidey, a missionary living in northern Labrador, described the humble discussions that he overheard and took part in. Throughout the summer, he and his people had been hearing about this mission ship and it's doctor and crew. "'Them are goodmen whom ever they be,' said one, while another expatiated, with all a sailor's delight to sailors equally delighted, upon the size and rig and sailing powers of the vessel, until we were all hoping she would pay us a visit. The probability of this latter question was very freely discussed among our fishermen, who, now the season was well-nigh over and no more fish to be caught, were to be found daily sitting about in small groups, smoking and talking with that peculiar gravity which belongs to the Liveyeres of the coast.... Would she come here? Many shook their heads. 'No.'"

But the ship came, and Sidey was to become one of Grenfell's most devoted admirers after he saw the vigour and energy with which the doctor burst into the hovels to treat too many cases of scrofula, typhoid, tuberculosis, and the nutritional disease, beri-beri, and to hearten the sick and enlighten the ignorant and scold the unhygienic. Grenfell's affection for the fisherfolk was so evident, so plain. He could often be sharp with words and airy with plans for others to follow, reckless with his own safety and autocratic with traders and bureaucrats, but there would never be any doubt that he loved and admired the seafaring people, and wanted to give them the kind of life he felt they deserved.

Grenfell was deeply affected by many of the afflictions he was called upon to treat because they could so easily have been cured if normal medical care had been available. He met one fisherman whose wounded foot had turned gangrenous, and who had persuaded his two young daughters to try and amputate it with an ordinary knife. He could imagine the agony of the father and the trembling terror of the daughters.

On another occasion, anchoring in one spot off the coast between two of its typical desolate islands, he was asked to see a girl who had been cooking and mending for a group of men in one of the tiny summer fishing huts. She was being looked after by an old captain who, suspecting typhoid, had wisely ordered the rest of the men, who were handling fish for human consumption, to keep well away.

The captain had fed her as best he could, but, presumably out of delicacy, had refrained from washing her, or changing the bedclothes. She had lain in a bunk in a dark corner of the hut, burning with fever, encased in filth, for two weeks. Grenfell must have been able to smell her almost as soon as he landed on the island. Even in a clean patient, typhoid, which indeed was what she had, is a malodorous disease. As Grenfell examined her in the faded daylight that glowed reluctantly in the hut, he saw that she was very pretty; and that she was dying. Looking down on her, he became aware that the elements seemed to be contributing a symbolism of their own. Though it was a summer afternoon, the sky suddenly became ominously dark, and tendrils of fog wisped into the fetid hut.

With the captain's help, Grenfell set about the "augean task" of washing and cleaning her feverish body, though he knew she had only hours to live. It was night before they had finished, by which time another anxiety had overtaken the captain. His trap boat, with six men aboard, including his sons, was now long overdue, and the fog off the dangerous coast was dense. "The skipper had stayed home out of sympathy for his servant girl," Grenfell wrote, "and his mind was torn asunder by anxiety for the girl and his fear for his boys.

"When night fell, the old captain and I were through the hardest part of our work. We had new bedding on the bed and the patient clean and sleeping quietly. Still the boat and its precious compliment did not come. Every few minutes the skipper would go out and listen, and stare into the darkness. The girl's heart suddenly failed, and about midnight her spirit left this world. The captain and I decided that the best thing to do was to burn everything—and in order to avoid publicity, to do it at once. So having laboriously carried it all out onto the edge of the cliff, we set a light to the pile." And thus quite unintentionally ensured that the girl had not died entirely in vain, for the blaze of bedding provided the crew of the trap boat with a beacon in the fog and darkness, to guide them back to shore.

In Labrador, burdened with Victorian morality as well as aging toil, the lot of young girls must often have been hideous. When Grenfell was called to a large schooner one morning, he found that one of the two girls who did all the cooking and cleaning on board, had also been providing sexual relief for the fishermen with the time or energy for it. One of the girls had given premature birth, and had been lying feverishly in her bunk for days, with willing but feckless assistance from the crew. Grenfell, seething at Newfoundland society's apathy toward what he considered to be a scandalous employment of girls on board the schooners, wrapped her up and transferred her to his boat, and took her to the nearest Moravian station. (A Moravian Church mission had been doing what they could do for the Eskimos in the area for a hundred years.) He was able to combat her illness, but he could not cure her shame. She told him, 'I want to die, Doctor; I can never go home again.' A few days later he buried her on a lonely headland.

As well as dirt and ignorance and the organized prostitution on the Newfoundland schooners, Grenfell also had some strange superstitions to combat, mixed with the quack remedies that had grown up in a doctorless society. Some of the fishermen used decapitated animal heads as weather vanes. The head of a fox or wolf was suspended from the ceiling, in the belief that it would twist the way from which the wind was going to blow. One old chap confided that he never got sea boils because he always cut his nails on a Monday. Another believed that a haddock's fin bone was a charm against rheumatism. Green worsted tied around the wrist was a cure for hemorrhage, while Protestants and Catholics alike wore amulets around their necks, little sacks containing prayers written on scraps of paper. "One old woman treated the grippe that broke out and ravaged the coast regularly with nine lice swallowed every third day for nine days. A favorite cure for abscesses was a mixture of white paint and herbs mixed into a poultice. The tooth of a dying deer worn round the neck was accounted a cure for fits, and liniment was drunk as treatment for chest diseases. Charms were worn by many, and time after time, Grenfell was asked to 'charm' away a pain. He grinned and waved his hand and said, 'Meenie Mini Mo,' then got to work properly."

Until Grenfell, these were the defences against the diseases that racked the people, including tuberculosis, which was rife among whole families, and scurvy, which was supposed to have been vanquished two centuries previously. As far as some local midwives were concerned, Lister or Semmelweis might never have lived—childbed fever carried off a large proportion of their patients. William Morton or Sir James Y. Simpson went similarly unacknowledged. Grenfell's first operation on the coast was on a woman who had an agonizing tumour of the leg. She refused an anesthetic, "as she did not believe it was right to be put to sleep." Five men had to sit on her, during the operation, to hold her down.

Gradually, however, as Grenfell's work showed results, confidence in charm and amulet wavered. The attitude toward professional medical aid changed, not least because of the total faith people had in their boisterous, bullying, loving doctor.

The stoicism of the fishermen was not so easy to overcome. Grenfell once found himself hunting around in the dark holds of a ship for patients suffering from snow blindness. "I never went round without a bottle of cocaine solution in my pocket for the snow-blind men, who suffered the most excruciating pain, often rolling about and moaning as if in a kind of frenzy, and to whom the cocaine gave wonderful relief," he wrote. Even so, when he called out into the dark corner and recesses of the hold, "Is there anyone here?" there was no answer, until a sound or movement betrayed their whereabouts. It was if the victims were saying, "Don't bother, we're not really worth it." Or perhaps it was shame, because they were idle. A day away from fishing might mean a week without food in winter. As for the loss or even the temporary incapacitation of a limb, that was a calamity. One father of eight children had his hand over the muzzle of his rifle when it went off, practically blowing his hand to pieces. To stop the bleeding he plunged his hand into a barrel of flour and then tied it up in a bag. By the time Grenfell saw him, the arm was poisoned way up above the elbow. "He preferred death to losing his right arm," Grenfell wrote. "Day and night for weeks our nurse tended him, as he hovered between life and death with general blood poisoning. Slowly his fine constitution brought him through, and at last a secondary operation for repair became possible. We took a chance on bone-grafting to form a hand; and he was left with a flipper like a seal's, able, however, to oppose one long index finger and 'nip a line' when he fished." As for the skin graft, Grenfell and a fellow doctor supplied the material from the palm of Grenfell's hand and the skin of his colleague's back.

That fisherman was lucky. Others were not as fortunate, and as the years passed, Grenfell found himself having to care for increasing numbers of dependents whose money-earning parent had died. In his time, he was to rescue, support, or place with others, hundreds of children who might otherwise have died. For some of them he was too late. His most famous case was that of an Eskimo boy named Pomiuk. Hearing that an Eskimo boy was dying in a tent in some inlet far up the Labrador coast, Grenfell and a companion searched for two days among thousands of bolders at the foot of the stupendous cliffs near Nachvak. He finally located the tent and found a boy of eleven, lying naked on the rocks nearby, with a broken thigh bone that had never been set properly. Normally a laughing, happy child, Pomiuk's face was drawn with pain. The wound was infected, and there were terrible sores.

As the doctor put it, "The Eskimos were only too glad to be rid of the responsibility of the sick lad, and, furthermore, he was 'no good fishing.' Grenfell carried the boy back to the ship, washed him (a unique experience that the boy found terrifying), treated his wounds and fed him his favourite dish, raw walrus meat. On the way south, discovering that Pomiuk had never received religious instruction, Grenfell took him to the Moravian missionaries, who baptized him in the name of Gabriel Pomiuk. By the time the ship reached Indian Harbour he was once again a happy, sunny child, though the condition of his leg gave Grenfell cause for concern.

While looking after him, Grenfell came across the boy's most treasured possession, a letter from a clergyman at Andover, Massachusetts. It contained a photograph of the letter-writer, and when the doctor showed it to Pomiuk and looked at him enquiringly, Pomiuk said simply, "Me even love him."

Grenfell wrote to the clergyman, Charles Carpenter, to tell him about Pomiuk. It seemed that Carpenter had been a missionary in Labrador at one time, but had met Pomiuk at, of all places, the Chicago World Fair.

In 1890, one of the Fair promoters had come up with an original idea for an exhibit, an Eskimo village, complete with huskies, an igloo, and naturally, Eskimos. Accordingly, the promoter journeyed north to recruit the real thing. Pomiuk's foster father—his real father had been murdered when Pomiuk was a baby—was one of the Eskimos who were tempted by the promoter's promise of riches in the form of the coins that the World Fair audiences were expected to toss to them. The foster father took the boy with him. At the Fair, Pomiuk proved to be such a delightful eight-year-old and so dextrous with the dogwhip, which he used to flick the promised coins toward his companions, that he became the hit of the show.

One of the World Fair visitors was the Reverend Charles Carpenter. He had a special interest in people from the land where he had been a missionary, and visited the Eskimo village every day. He made friends with Pomiuk, talking to him in a halting mixture of English and Eskimo. By the time Carpenter's visit to Chicago was over, the two had become warmly attached to each other, and Carpenter promised to write when Pomiuk got home, and enclose a photograph.

Pomiuk must have had great difficulty in getting home. It was typical of Victorian society that, while fluttering financiers and hardened matrons could be reduced to gushing tears by sentimental woes, they could be remarkably obtuse where real hardship was concerned. When the promoters of the show had finished with their band of Eskimos, they took them back only as far as Newfoundland. How Pomiuk managed to get across the strait of Belle Isle, between Newfoundland and Labrador, and make his way back to Andover, Labrador, is not known, but it seems to have occurred to nobody that dumping an eight-year-old boy two thousand miles from home might be considered a trifle unfeeling.

The Reverend Mr. Carpenter had often wondered what became of Pomiuk. Now, when he heard of the boy's misfortune, he wrote back to Grenfell, "Keep him. He must never know cold and loneliness again." And offered to publicize the case in the *Congregationalist* to help Pomiuk financially.

Grenfell wrote again. He had intended lecturing in Canada that winter. He wondered if the lecture tour might be extended to the United States. Carpenter took the hint and invited him to Boston. There the doctor's personality and the dramatic and wrenching stories he had to tell about the people of Labrador did the rest. It inspired the generous American help, in treasure and in the volunteer work of their idealist nurses, surgeons, and college students, that was from thenceforth to be the principal support of the Grenfell Mission. "Grenfell," wrote J. Lennox Kerr, "was what many Americans aspired to be, a man of vision and a man of action. His mixture of strong masculinity and strong faith was in their pattern and understanding."

He appealed particularly to the youth of the country, and though many of them had great difficulty in finding the fare for the journey north, nevertheless they went, to work without pay at every kind of job from gathering fuel to acting as anesthesiologists (still mostly a matter of holding down struggling chloroformed patients). Grenfell offered the Americans not sermons but Christianity in action—adventure.

As a lecturer, Grenfell was far from being a sonorous orator, but his almost palpable energy and his instinctive sense of drama had a jolting effect on audiences on both sides of the Atlantic, not least because his talks occassionally strayed into a sentimentality that appealed to Victorians, as when he dwelt on the death of Pomiuk. Pomiuk had been rescued just a little too late to save either his leg or his life. In one of his speeches in England, Grenfell read a letter from Pomiuk in which he described his last Christmas. "Me got a nice time at Xmas, sweets and a cake. Lot of little girls and boys got a tea. It makes them laugh to look at Xmas big tree. Sister got Tommy and me jack in box. I opened box. I very frightened and made people laugh very much.... I want a letter bye and bye, please. Me like to see you next year....*Aukshenai*, Dr. Grenfell, very much, Gabriel Pomiuk." Grenfell had his audiences fumbling for their hankies over that one. But also their pocketbooks.

The reception in Canada was almost as enthusiastic as that in the United States. Even by the end of his second season in the north, he was making a triumphant tour across the country from Halifax to Vancouver, and in the process making friends with such diverse personalties as Sir Donald Smith of Canadian Pacific fame, and Dr. Roddick. The former contributed substantially to the cost of a new hospital ship. By then, Dr. Grenfell had become a legend in Labrador. He was constantly surprised by the loving reception he received at the coastal settlements, and even his hatred of strong drink was accepted, albeit ruefully, as Grenfell slowly drove out the booze traders. Naturally the traders hated him. He eroded their rackets, including that of barratry. There had been many suspicious but uncheckable shipwrecks on the Labrador coast, and Lloyd's of London, having no representative on the coast, had asked Grenfell to act as their agent. The adventure appealed to him, and on his first investigation he travelled eight hundred miles north in vicious November weather to check up on a claim involving a ship, the *Bessie Dodd*, that was said to have been wrecked at Smoky Tickle. When Grenfell got there he found that the barquentine, after loading a cargo of dried fish at a trader's wharf, had traveled only a few feet before running aground on to a nice sandy beach, and was practically undamaged. The ship's master had sold both the ship and the cargo to the trader for eighty dollars. The master and the trader had claimed $170,000 from the insurers.

Dr. Grenfell was to face many vindictive and false accusations from traders, their newspaper lackeys, and their allies in government, but he never lost the affection and loyalty of the people. By 1899 his coastal journeys had begun to take on the trappings of a royal tour, with flags and guns firing and reception committees escorting him between lines of smiling fishermen and their families. He had inspired the building of hospitals where none had previously existed, of co-operatives where for the first time the fishermen were sharing in the profits of their own work, and of orphanages for children who had been voluntarily or involuntarily abandoned. Most of all, he inspired hope and the beginning of health and self-respect among the people. He gave up material success to accomplish this, and subjected himself to physical hardship. It was hardly suprising that the fisherfolk loved and admired him. He returned the feelings both to the people and to their land. Labrador, with its subtle shades and tortured rock, edged with the lace of Atlantic foam, held a beauty for him unrivaled even by the velvet slopes of his native Cheshire.

The people's regard for Grenfell was all the stronger because of his foolhardiness. He fancied himself as an expert mariner, though it was often sheer good luck that brought him safely ashore. During his second tour in 1893 he had transferred from the *Albert* to a frail, forty-five-footer, the *Princess May* , which, with its narrow beam and two-foot freeboard, should not have survived a week off one of the most dangerous coasts in the world. Grenfell captained it through three thousand miles of mostly unsurveyed waters, through storms, one of which was severe enough to damage even the mother ship, and which resulted in his being reported lost at sea by the newspapers. By the time he returned to St. John's, the boat was a wreck, the steam pipes leaked, the propeller shaft wrenched out of true, and it seemed a miracle to the fishermen that it was still afloat.

His seamanship at Battle Harbour with a far better boat, the brand-new *Sir Donald,* inspired similar amazement. After conning the flag-bedecked little vessel through the rocks and islands between Battle Harbour and Great Caribou Island, Grenfell, puffed up with pride at having negotiated the difficult waterway and wishing to celebrate his arrival with an impressive entrance, called for full speed ahead. With a long drawn-out grinding rumble, the boat ran aground. Flushed with mortification, the doctor had to row for help to get the boat towed off the reef.

His bouts of vagueness added to the legend. The fishermen related them with relish, though they were not much appreciated by a lengthening list of dignitaries, who might find themselves invited several hundred miles to such places as St. Anthony to view the doctor's splendid new hospital, only to find that he had forgotten about them and had gone off to visit the site of yet another grand scheme for the betterment of his people—or to break up a still. His hatred of drink was his greatest intolerance, causing a character in one of H. G. Well's novels to remark, "Doctor Grenfell was a very good man, a very good man, but he made brandy dear, dear beyond the reach of the common men altogether on the coast."

Another aspect of Grenfell's vagueness was his habit of bringing children to the orphanage at St. Anthony without making a note of their names or being able to remember where he had found them. He could also confuse one patient with another. At one isolated harbour, a Liveyere came on board for medicine, and after examining him, Grenfell went below to make up the medicine. When he reappeared on deck, he handed the medicine to a fisherman, who looked a trifle surprised but unhesitatingly paid the twenty-five-cent fee. Just as the man was leaving, another man came up and asked for his medicine. Realizing that he had given it to the wrong person, Grenfell hurried after him, but having paid the fee, the man refused to surrender the mixture, admitting that though he was not ill, he "guessed that it would suit his complaint all right."

The doctor's orientation on land was sometimes not much superior to his compass-work at sea. On one sick call, traveling across a winter landscape on a sledge with a nurse and his driver, he came to a bay with a direct run of seven miles over sea ice. He was halfway across when fog drifted in from the Strait of Belle Isle. When the lumpy nature of the ice suggested that he might be approaching the sea edge, the doctor ordered the driver to stay where he was and not to move, then went ahead on foot to explore through the fog. Finding nothing, he shouted over his shoulder to the driver—whose voice answered from barely inches away—in front of Grenfell. Angrily, Grenfell asked the driver why he'd moved—they might all have gotten lost. "Haven't budged an inch," the driver answered, while the nurse heaved with laughter as she realized that the doctor had explored in a perfect circle.

It was Grenfell's impatience, though, rather than his somewhat deficient navigation, that brought him close to the death that had been prophesied for him time after time by the head-shaking fishermen. On Easter Sunday in 1908, when he was returning to the hospital at St. Anthony in northern Newfoundland after taking morning service, a boy ran up to say that he was wanted sixty miles to the south. Two weeks previously, Grenfell had operated on a young man for acute bone disease of the thigh, but his relatives had not looked after the wound as instructed, and now he had blood poisoning and was seriously ill.

Guessing that the leg would have to come off at once, Grenfell decided to leave immediately, despite anxious warnings that it was an exceedingly bad time of year to travel alone. Airily he swept aside all objections and set off with seven of his best dogs and Jack, his pet spaniel. At the hospital, Dr. Little and Jessie Luther (a Bostonian occupational therapist who had been helping the wives and daughters of the fishermen to earn extra money for their families by hooking rugs, carving wood, and making clothes from skins), watched with foreboding until he reached the ridge of a range of hills. He turned to wave before disappearing from sight.

Grenfell was already well known in the English-speaking world. He had publicized his work in several books and in numerous magazine articles, including one started specially by his Canadian supporters, and an American author had written two books about him. In Canada, according to Kerr, "he had almost ambassadorial status, his hosts the Governor-General or the governors of states." Theodore Roosevelt had invited him to lunch at the White House, and Edward VII to Buckingham Palace. Now, his adventures over the next two days were to make him known throughout the world.

He had no difficulty in negotiating the first twenty miles of his journey behind an eager dog team, with his pet retriever scampering joyfully alongside. Mushing through the slush, he reached Lock's Cove by late afternoon. There he stayed the night. During the night a high wind arose and the thaw changed to a freeze-up. Once again he was advised to wait until the weather settled down, but, even though he had now spent many seasons in the far North, he had still not learned to treat the weather with the respect that was its due. He insisted on pushing on to reach the sick boy. Well at least, they warned him, he should be careful to go around the bay on which Lock's Cove was located, and not try any short-cuts across it.

Naturally, with his reckless spirit and excessive confidence, that was just what the doctor attempted, even though the elements were more unruly than ever. The wind was from the sea and was bringing in fog and rain. In addition, as he described it later, "The sea, rolling in during the previous night, had smashed the ponderous layer of surface ice right up to the landwash. Between the huge ice-pans were gaping chasms, while a half a mile out all was clear water."

At first he stuck obediently to the shoreline, but when he had a mere four miles to go, he noticed that the island in the middle of the bay had preserved an ice bridge. He decided to take a short-cut over the ice bridge. He thought the ice looked safe enough, because, though it had been smashed up by the sea, it had been packed tight again by the wind. "Therefore, without giving the matter a second thought, I flung myself on the komatik [sled] and the dogs started for the rocky promontory some four miles distant."

Grenfell was only a quarter mile from this objective when he realized that the sledge was traveling not over firm ice but over sish ice—floating snow packed together by the wind. The dog-drawn komatik started to sink. In order to avoid being entangled in the traces, Grenfell hurriedly slashed at them with his knife, freeing the dogs.

They managed to reach a piece of frozen snow. It was at that point that Grenfell realized that he might have only a few minutes to live. The island of packed snow was being driven seaward. Once in open water it would very rapidly break up.

He had one chance to escape death. Twenty yards away there was a larger and firmer pan floating in the sish. If he could reach it he might postpone for a time the death which now seemed inescapable.

Unfortunately Grenfell could not induce the dogs to swim across, though he kept throwing them into the ice-sheathed water and shouting at them. "Perhaps it was only natural that they should struggle back," he wrote, "for once in the water they could see no other pan to which to swim. It flashed into my mind that my small black spaniel which was with me was as light as a feather and would get across with no difficulty. I showed him the direction and then flung a bit of ice toward the desired goal. Without a second's hesitation he made a dash and reached the pan safely, as the tough layer of sea ice easily carried his weight. As he lay on the white surface looking like a round black fuzz ball, my leaders could plainly see him. They now understood what I wanted and fought their way bravely toward the little retriever, carrying with them the line that gave me yet another chance for my life. The other dogs followed them, and all but one succeeded in getting out on the new haven of refuge."

By the time Grenfell had joined the dogs on the ice pan, he was soaked and knew that he would soon die if he could not obtain protection from the wind. He tried cutting down his long boots to the feet, using the leather to protect his back from the wind, but by midday he saw that he would have to take extreme measures. He was drifting out to sea, while landward the immense pans of arctic ice were crashing and grinding against the cliffs with such ferocity that obviously no rescue was possible. If he could not save himself by his own efforts he was done for. And those efforts, if he was to live for at least one night, must involve a painful sacrifice. Accordingly, in a scene made all the more dreadful by his cold-induced clumsiness and the terror of his canine companions, he slaughtered three of his beloved dogs.

That night, four men were out on the headland, cutting up some seals that they had taken the previous fall. Just as they were leaving for home, one of them thought he detected something unusual, far out on the ice. They hurried home to tell one of their friends, the only one on that stretch of coast who owned a telescope. He abandoned his supper and hurried to the lookout on the cliffs, and just minutes before darkness fell, he was able to make out the figure of a man on a tiny bobbing ice pan, miles away across the turbulent, slob-iced sea. He guessed immediately who it might be. It was a standing joke among the fishermen that whenever the weather was at its foulest, the doctor was sure to be out in it.

There was nothing they could do that night. The fishermen made plans for a rescue operation the next morning. They did not believe for a moment that the doctor would survive the night in the bitter cold on a crumbling pan the size of a kitchen floor.

By nightfall, Grenfell had skinned the three dogs and wrapped their fur around him. "The carcasses of my dogs I piled up to make a windbreak, and at intervals I took off my clothes, wrung them out, swung them in the wind, and put on first one and then the other inside, hoping that the heat of my body would dry them. My feet gave me the most trouble, as the moccasins were so easily soaked through in the snow. But I remembered the way in which the Lapps who tended our reindeer carried grass with them, to use in their boots in place of dry socks. As soon as I could sit down I began to unravel the ropes from the dogs' harnesses, and although by this time my fingers were more or less frozen, I managed to stuff the oakum into my shoes." His will to survive was intense. All the same, while he worked, he contemplated using the knife on himself if the wind drifted him much further out to sea. Suicide was preferable to such a slow death. By nightfall there was nothing else to do, so he cuddled up against his biggest surviving dog, drew the bloodstained pelts over him and, helped by the rocking motion of the pan, went to sleep. "One hand being against the dog was warm, but the other was frozen, and about midnight I woke up shivering enough, so I thought, to shatter my frail pan to atoms. The moon was just rising, and the wind was steadily driving me toward the open sea. Suddenly what seemed a miracle happened, for the wind veered, then dropped away entirely, leaving it flat calm. I turned over and fell asleep again. I was next awakened by the sudden and persistent thought that I must have a flag, and accordingly set to work to disarticulate the frozen legs of my dead dogs."

Lashing the bones together with harness rope, he was ready, when dawn came, to wave at the shore with his makeshift flagstaff, a grisly, crooked pole that grew even more crooked as the warmth of the rising sun thawed the bones. Even now his sense of humour did not desert him. "I could not help laughing at my position, standing hour after hour waving my shirt at those barren and lonely cliffs." For he did not really believe that anyone was watching, or, with heaving ice pans covering the bay, that a rescue attempt was possible.

Possible or not, it was attempted, despite the very real danger that the rescue craft might be caught and crushed between ice pans. Led by Captain Read, they finally reached Grenfell's pan after several narrow escapes, by dragging the boat onto the ice before the pans closed on it. When the fishermen saw their doctor clearly, they were shocked. He had turned to an old man overnight. His face was a strange dark red, his eyes vividly bloodshot. At first he just peered at his rescuers solemnly out of semi-snowblind eyes. It was the first time they remembered his greeting them without a joke. When he finally started talking he couldn't stop apologizing for having risked their lives. Then he began an interminable account of what had happened. He was still talking when he reached the hospital at St. Anthony, until they finally sedated him.

It had all been quite unnecessary. The boy whose life he had been intent on saving was brought to the hospital the next day in a boat without the slightest difficulty, the ice having cleared the coast entirely.

Grenfell was quick to seize any opportunity to publicize his work, and the book that resulted from the adventure, *Adrift on an Ice Pan* became an international best-seller, and brought in gifts and subscriptions to the Mission from all over the world.

It also brought him a wife. Voyaging across the Atlantic the following spring, to receive honorary degrees from Harvard and Williams College, Grenfell caught sight of a fellow passenger, a young lady who, in the company of a Chicago banker and his wife, was returning from a motor tour of Europe and Algeria. Grenfell's gaze sharpened. She was truly beautiful, but what particularly attracted him was a wide, firm, and determined mouth that suggested a decided force of personality, and a pair of steady eyes that other men might have considered just a little too intelligent and challenging.

Having only four and half days in which to woo her, he set about this delicate task by marching up to her and attacking her as a society parasite. He told her that she should do something with her frivolous life. Affronted by his impertinence, she asked him how he dared criticize her in this fashion without even knowing her name. He replied that maybe he didn't know what it was now, but he knew what it was going to be: Mrs. Wilfred Grenfell.

That she accepted this oblique stroke of a proposal was evidently not due to his fame, for she confessed afterwards that she had heard of him only once, vaguely, while she was at Bryn Mawr College. She had been invited to attend a lecture to be delivered by some missionary or other named Grenfell, but she had declined, thinking that she would be subjected to a boring spiel by a doddering old do-gooder.

Anne MacClanachan's willingness to take up missionary work caused a sensation in her society circles. A bluestocking heiress, she had been brought up in Chicago's fashionable Lake Forest district, and her friends and the newspapers wondered how long she would last in the frozen North. One newspaper published a photograph of what was supposed to be her new home, a hideous log hut. Whatever it was—Kerr says that it was a deer-herder's shelter—it certainly was not her new abode. Grenfell's friends at St. Anthony had aimed at giving their doctor and his young wife the best residence on the coast. They had built a fine two-storey dwelling which was protected on three sides by a glass porch and which had the most efficient electrical, heating and plumbing system available.

Many of the doctor's friends also wondered how the tall, graceful young lady with the drawing-room voice would take to their harsh environment, though they gave her an impressive enough reception. When she stepped off the mail steamer at St. Anthony she was greeted with rifle shots and booming signal guns, bursting flares, flapping flags, barking dogs and cracking whips, and two long lines of fishermen and their families standing silently under a bedsheet banner reading, "Welcome to our noble Doctor and his bonnie bride."

The bonnie bride seemed to have no doubts about her ability to cope. "The morning after her arrival, she was borrowing an apron and directing the furnishing of her home with a cool and composed authority. She was demanding a cook and solving the problem of a leaky roof in a manner that made the mission staff realize that a new personality had arrived. They were to find, in the months that followed, that Mrs. Grenfell was not only capable but fully conscious of being consort to one who was almost a king in the northern land, and intended to make this clear."

She immediately set about making her Englishman's home a castle, and, anticipating the honour that would soon be conferred on him, making her husband its knight. The locals were soon discouraged from dropping in in their usual casual manner. They would have to wait for an invitation.

"That summer," Kerr continues, "Grenfell carried his wife on board the *Strathcona* to show her his beloved Labrador and introduce her to his friends along the coast. She stood up to the experience courageously, but with little enjoyment. She did not share Grenfell's pleasure when he was presented with barrels of half-rotten whale meat for his dogs, or enjoy being shipmates with piles of fried and salted fish. Her idea of social entertainment was not sitting in a smoke-filled tilt or being entertained by somewhat odorous fishermen on board their schooners. Grenfell gave little thought to food, but he had a fondness that his wife could not share for the glutinous mess that is boiled cod's heads, and Labrador's favourite 'browse,' soaked ship's biscuit mixed with cod and served with crisped pork fat."

She felt much more at home in London, hobnobbing with the aristocracy that then fluttered so many American female hearts. "Her appearance and manner were regal, and she lived up to them. She could tell a Customs officer who asked if she had any spirits to declare, 'My husband does not allow strong drink in his colonies.' Her affection for, and pride in him, was maternal, despite being twenty years his junior, and very often in acting to protect him from spending his time and energy she offended his old friends."

In time she took Grenfell over completely, even managing to curb his sartorial eccentricity. Until he met her he was as likely as not to be wearing odd socks, or a horrible old suit. When he received his degree from Harvard he was wearing brilliant tweeds and yellow shoes under his splendid Oxford gown. Gently, Mrs. Grenfell urged him into a top hat and tails, making him look ridiculous to his friends. But he put up with it because he adored his young wife.

She was also to steer him away from the real work of the mission, now that it was a going concern. The many doctors and nurses and volunteers who now staffed the four hospitals and the nursing stations and orphanages that Grenfell had founded in Labrador and northern Newfoundland, could, she felt, carry on without his help. Which was true enough. Many of the doctors, notable surgeons and great specialists, were professionally far more competent than Grenfell. Anne felt that Wilfred would be of more use to the mission if he exploited his talents as a publicist — preferably as far from Labrador as possible. "Alone he would have been content to carry out his lecture engagements without any special flourish, staying wherever he found a room and avoiding so-called Society or irritating ceremonies. His wife had other ideas. She took charge, and the Grenfells travelled in state, the handsome and regal Anne commanding the private homes and hotels where they lodged. Hosts and hostesses found themselves swamped by Grenfell's restless if stimulating presence, his wife's royal appropriation of their homes. Telephones were monopolized, rooms taken over for secretaries or for Grenfell to write. Wherever they were pulsed with their energy and presence....She used her own and her husband's high social positions to attract the snobbish, flatter the aspiring leaders of provincial Society, and with Scottish shrewdness...found out who were the wealthiest and saw to it that they were given prominence."

A female American anthropologst once observed that men are superior to women in all respects save one: men are too easily trained. Grenfell liked being trained. "Nearly ten years have rolled away since our marriage." he wrote in his autobiography. "The puzzle to me is how I ever got along before." He did not, of course, see it as training exercise. In his *Forty Years for Labrador*, he likened his wife and himself to a large camel and a cow that he once saw in Egypt, pulling a plough together. "I felt like the smaller partner," he explained, "grateful for redoubled capacity."

He did not record what his wife thought about being compared to a camel.

Three years later, the Grenfell Mission had developed into such an empire of hospitals, nursing stations, seamen's schools, institutes, orphanages, hospital ships, and various commercial endeavours, that the supporting associations were forced to reorganize. The British Mission to Deep Sea Fishermen was not at all happy about the doctor's involving them in all kinds of expensive schemes, often without even consulting them. Moreover, his work was now on behalf of the Liveyeres and the Newfoundlanders on land, rather than the fishermen who were the mission's chief concern. In Canada, Grenfell's principal supporter, Miss Greenshields, was trying to hold fifteen separate Grenfell committees together, while the Grenfell Association of America, which was supplying much of the money and nearly all the volunteers, was increasingly aware that formal order was needed to bring all the haphazard efforts together. Out of these separate concerns emerged the International Grenfell Association, which is still functioning, and commemorating the name of one of the most selfless, generous, and lovable medical man who has ever lived.

20

The Magnetic Dr. Shepherd

WHILE WILLIAM OSLER'S spirit could never be captured by a photographer, Dr. Francis Shepherd never took a bad picture in his life. There is a photograph of the two friends, taken when they were together at McGill, standing side by side against a studio backdrop, painted to represent a rocky bay. The photograph does not flatter Osler. He looks as if he has just dismembered the parlour maid, and expects to be severely reprimanded at any moment. Shepherd, on the other hand, looks as if he has just come from the parlour maid's bedroom. There he stands, confident, self-assured, bold as a buccaneer, with just a hint of the chilly personality beneath. You can't help wondering what he might have had to say about that painted backdrop behind him with its muddy look and unlikely rocks. Shepherd was a discerning art lover. By the time he became dean of the medical faculty, he had accumulated a magnificient collection of Dutch paintings. One can easily imagine him directing some humorously sarcastic remark to the photographer about his studio backdrop—probably with no more effect than on the occasion when he chose a painting for the Art Association of Montreal, and it was rejected when one of the council members threatened to resign if the Association was so foolish as to pay $18,000 for a work by some dauber named Manet.

Shepherd's own backdrop was one of imagination, enterprise, and wealth. His father, R. W. Shepherd, who had come out to Canada as a boy in 1830, was a pioneer in the development of water transportation along the Ottawa River. He was a steamship master by the age of twenty-two. In 1846 he joined forces with two other businessmen, one of them being Sir George Simpson, governor of the Hudson's Bay Company, to form a shipping firm. With R. W. in charge, the company rapidly expanded until it controled a sizeable fleet of vessels for transporting passengers and freight, or for such specialized tasks as towing barges and rafts along the river.

Mr. Shepherd later went into land transportation as well, becoming part owner of the Carillon and Grenville Railway Company.

Having achieved a great deal himself, Mr. Shepherd expected great things of his son, Francis. He was not to be disappointed. Francis John Shepherd, born at Como near Montreal in 1851, not only had the right autocratic attitudes and a sharply outlined and forceful personality, he would become distinguished in three important fields: anatomy, surgery, and dermatology, as a scientist, practitioner, and teacher.

By the time the handsome lad with the impertinent eyes and stubborn mouth was ready to attend high school, the family had moved into a large residence on Beaver Hall Hill in Montreal. There Mr. Shepherd and his wife entertained the urban nobs, the officers of the most fashionable regiments, and the merchants who were growing rich off them. One of his acquaintances was Prince Arthur, and Mr. Shepherd often mentioned the fact in a suitably off-hand way that he had treated the future Duke of Connaught to his first sleigh ride.

The prince made no great impression on Francis, but he clearly remembered the young lady he saw walking up Beaver Hall Hill without a crinoline. He confessed himself shaken to the core by his first sight of a skirt closely moulded to female flanks.

The young lady who made Francis gape may have been even more shocked at what her skirts had to drag through. Sewage. Visitors to Montreal in the sixties were enthralled by its majestic contours when seen from a distance, and delighted by the grace and gaiety of its garrison-town society. But when they were forced to manoeuvre past open sewers and through choking, pulverized-limestone streets, or along ankle-wrenching boardwalks, that was another matter. The young lady was likely to end up with her hems sodden with the trickling effluence from ten thousand cesspools, or dusted with windblown ashes and limestone, or the powdered essence of rotted garbage, her lungs shrinking from the miasma of wooden drains, and her eyes from the sight of slums where typhoid, dysentery, and smallpox were the next-door neighbours. A contemporary report described the city as "a huge charnel house in which the very air we breathe teems with sickness, suffering and death."

Montreal did have a board of health, but it was composed of volunteers who knew nothing about sanitation. They simply did not understand the association between open cesspools, putrefying garbage, and foul water, and the epidemics that smothered the city every stinking summer. As a result, the city had, it was said, the highest death rate of any place in North America.

Apart from that it was a delightful, cosmopolitan town with an abundant supply of medical men in their obligatory silk toppers and frock coats, and with a medical school to be proud of. Despite its limitations, the school was probably the best on the continent. Other institutions in Canada and the United States considered that a doctor was fully qualified after three years' instruction, or in some cases after only two years. McGill demanded a four-year discipline.

Even so, when Shepherd began his medical carrer in 1869, McGill Medical School still compared unfavourably with the best of the European schools. The quality of its lecturers, as summarized by Shepherd's biographer, W. B. Howell, gives a hint as to why this was so. Shepherd's professors included W. E. Scott, a big, good-looking man with a bluff manner, who "was an indifferent teacher. He took his lectures word for word from Erasmus Wilson's *Anatomy*, and made no attempt to illustrate them by drawing on the blackboard. Occasionally he passed bones about the class or had a dissected subject in front of him as he lectured. He never went into the dissecting room. The demonstrator of anatomy — there was only one — was William Fuller, who had been a painter by trade before he became a doctor. He was without any gift for teaching and managed the dissecting room, according to Shepherd, in a haphazard way. The time spent by the students in the dissecting room was devoted to exposing the muscles, arteries, veins, and nerves of the neck and extremities. It was not obligatory to dissect the brain, thorax, or abdomen. It was customary to toss up to decide who should clean out the abdominal viscera so that the pre-vertebral muscles could be seen. The examination in anatomy took place at the end of the third year and was both written and oral. At the oral, which lasted only a few minutes, no dissections or specimens were shown....

"The institutes of medicine included physiology and pathology, and were taught by a solemn old Scotsman, William Fraser. He had the broadest of accents and on account of the way he pronounced the word 'communicate' was known among the students as 'Old Commoonicate.' His lectures were taken from Todd and Bowman's *Physiology*. The edition he used in Shepherd's time had been published more than ten years before. There was no practical physiology, there were, indeed, no laboratories of any kind at McGill when Shepherd was a student. Once during his course, a young house-surgeon at the Montreal General Hospital, Thomas G. Roddick, brought a microscope to the college and showed the students the circulation in the frog's foot, to their intense interest. The subject of pathology was disposed of during the last week of the course in the institutes of medicine by a few lectures on 'inflammation.'...

"The chair of chemistry was occupied by Robert Craik, a bird of plumage somewhat brighter than that of the other members of the flock. Handsome, agreeable, and very much a man of the world; he lived in a big house and owned a farm near Montreal where he bred race horses and prize cattle. He died poor. Craik was a good lecturer, he could not only teach, but could perform experiments successfully before his class."

Another of Shepherd's teachers was Gilbert Girdwood, who taught practical chemistry. His lectures were somewhat disorderly affairs because the students could hardly hear a word he said. He once made the mistake of turning his back on his audience to write a formula on the blackboard, whereupon one of the students threw a galosh at him. It hit the blackboard inches from his head with a squelchy thud. "Girdwood is said to have thrown down the chalk, pulled off his coat, and offered to fight any man in the class. In view of the fact that in his younger days he had been a noted athlete, there was nothing particularly attractive about the offer and no one accepted it." Still, Shepherd came to appreciate Girdwood's kind and fatherly ways.

"The course in materia medica was given by the Reverend William Wright, M.D., a clergyman of the Church of England, who had been in general practice for many years before he took Holy Orders.... He had a sarcastic tongue and a retentive memory; and used to devote a large proportion of his lectures to matters of no great importance. He would expatiate at great length on such subjects as the adulteration of gum acacia, the therapeutic properties of liquorice, and the views of the natives of West Africa on the value of calabar bean as a means of establishing the guilt or innocence of persons accused of evil-doing.... Dissatisfaction with the course in materia medica existed for years among the students and culminated in 1883 when they refused to attend Wright's lectures.... Wright was unable to see that there was anything wrong with his lectures; but believing himself the victim of persecution on account of his being a clergyman, resigned his chair. One of his peculiarities was a fondness for long words. Upon one occasion in his old age, being ill, he sent for Shepherd, who asked him when he noticed the first symptoms of his ailment. Wright's answer was: 'I was essaying to reach church for early service one tempestuous snowy day, when I had a retrocession of blood to my chylopeoietic viscera.'"

The outstanding man on the faculty was Osler's mentor, Palmer Howard, who was a fine teacher and a well-informed one. By extensive reading of medical publications he kept himself up to date on medical developments and passed them on enthusiastically to the students.

There is little record of Shepherd's years as a student. He provides few personal details in his *Reminiscences*. Dr. Howell speculated that, given Shepherd's chilly reserve, blunt speech, and "a certain spirit of mockery," he was not likely to have been a general favourite with his fellows. All the same, his friendships with, among others, William Osler and George Ross were enduring.

Ross was as difficult in his way as was Shepherd. Like many men of small stature, George Ross was intolerant, and his fellow students were wary of his slashing tongue. He was no more easy-going when he went to work at the Montreal General Hospital. Still, his colleagues were prepared to put up with his sharp, impatient manner because he was a superb diagnostician. Once, when a patient who was covered in pustules was admitted to the hospital, there was considerable uncertainty among the staff as to what was wrong. Some suspected smallpox, others pemphigus, or a number of other diseases. The medical superintendant, Dr. William McClure, finally went to Ross and asked him to see the patient. Ross refused, saying that the man was not his patient. Besides, he was off-duty. Damn it, he was entitled to *some* time off, surely. McClure persisted, and finally wheedled Ross back to the hospital. There Ross asked McClure to read the case book. McClure obliged. "Read it again," Ross snapped. McClure did so. Ross then strode into the ward, hauled the bedclothes away from the patient, looked him over and asked him if he had any running from the nose. On receiving an affirmative, Ross turned to the superintendant. "Glanders, McClure. Good morning." And marched away. McClure hurried after him, mumbling, perhaps a trifle defensively, that after all it was so easy for Ross to make such a lightning diagnosis, as he had probably seen many such cases. Ross shot back, "Ten years since I saw my first case of glanders. This is my second. Good morning."

After graduating, Shepherd, furnished with money and letters of introduction from his well-connected father, took a brief vacation in the United States before sailing to Europe to further his education. In the States he was entertained by admirals, Civil War generals, and by President Buchanan in the White House. He also went out with a Richmond belle, Miss Tirplett. He was not aware that she was engaged to a particularly hot-blooded southerner. It was fortunate for Francis that he did not become too involved with the beautiful blonde. Shortly after he parted from her, the fiancé fought a duel with another gentleman who had attempted to squire her around. That rival was killed. But Miss Tirplett's fiancé was himself lamed for life, whereupon the lady married somebody else. Shepherd presumably felt that there was a moral there, somewhere.

In London, with several fellow graduates of McGill, Francis settled down at St. Thomas' Hospital in preparation for the Royal College of Surgeons exams. He practiced dissection under Professor Rainey, who always wore a top hat and a frock coat in the dissecting room, and who taught Shepherd much "about the anatomy of parts I had never dissected or even seen, at home." He also studied under Seymour Sharkey, with whom he became lifelong friends, and under Sir John Simon, "a funny little round man who carried a number of pairs of colored spectacles about with him, and was continually changing them." Nearly every Saturday, Sir John operated on cases of ovarian tumour, but, "I never saw one recover," Shepherd remarked. (Lister's teachings had not yet been absorbed in London.)

Shepherd and several fellow Canadians studied at other hospitals as well as St. Thomas', among them the Stamford Street Skin Hospital, where his interest in dermatology originated.

By no means was all of Francis' time spent in study. He had a lasting interest in the arts, and in London he frequented the galleries and theatres, an impressionable young man trying to conceal his naiveté behind an impassive worldliness and his inexperienced face under a bushel of beard. "During the winter of 1873 we saw many fine plays at the theatres," he marveled. "Irving was acting in *The Bells*. This was before he took up Shakespearian plays and acted with Miss Ellen Terry. I liked Irving better then than later, when his stage settings were finer and he had more mannerisms. Miss Terry was acting in one of Charles Read's plays at Queen's Theatre, Long Acre. The play was, I think, *The Lost Heir*; she acted a boy's part quite wonderfully, I thought. That winter was remarkable for the Robertson plays, acted at the Prince of Wales Theatre by a noted company which included Marie Wilton, Hare, Squire Bancroft, and others. *School* and *Caste* were two of the most popular of the new plays. They created quite a revolution in the taste of theatre-goers, and the players acted as if they were at home, visiting, or on the street; not mouthing, attitudinizing, or ranting, but everything was natural, simple and apparently ordinary. The theatre world was taken by storm.

'During my spare time in London I went often to the National Gallery. At first I did not like Turner, but one day, looking through a door at one of his pictures, his greatness was suddenly revealed to me, and after I went frequently to see them. Of course I admired the English school, the Hogarths, Reynolds, Gainsboroughs, Constables, etc. I also admired the Dutch painters, especially Rembrandt."

He also marveled at the disorderly ways of a friend of his, a former fellow student, whose life was so different from his own ordered existence. "When I arrived in London in the fall of 1873, I came across a medical student, Paddy W—, whom I had known in Montreal. He was installed in lodgings with two other McGill men. He came originally from Newfoundland, was very popular and never passed his examinations, though he was able to coach everyone else. The secret came out later: when his father died, the will required that Paddy be paid £500 a year out of the estate for his medical education; his own share meanwhile accumulating. So he never passed his examinations and was still being educated at the expense of the estate. At times Paddy was hard up, and we all knew this by noticing the absence of the grand double-barreled microscope under a glass case in his sitting-room. Although the instrument had no lenses, still it was very imposing and he could always pawn it for £ll. When flush again he always redeemed it, and when we saw it restored to its old place of honour we knew everything was all right. Several of us at odd times met Paddy in out-of-the-way places walking with a lady, but he never recogized us on these occasions, and swore that it was a case of mistaken identity, denying that he had ever been near the place where we thought we had seen him. One day we were rowing up the Thames by Twicken-ham, when we saw, lolling in a deck-chair on the lawn of one of the villas by the river, a person who looked remarkably like Paddy W—. When our boat came abreast of the house, this individual suddenly disappeared into it. Nevertheless, we landed, went up to the house, rang the bell, which was answered by a smart housemaid, and asked for 'Mr. W—.' 'Oh,' she said, 'Captain W— lives here,' mentioning a name rather like that of our friend. We asked to see Captain W—, and were ushered into the drawing room, where lo and behold, we saw our friend, who could not then deny his identity. We spent a pleasant hour or two, but we did not see the lady. Paddy used to disappear at intervals for days and we never knew where he went.

"After a time the heirs of his father's estate, getting tired of educating him, got a law passed in the Newfoundland legislature to break this part of the will, and soon after my return home in 1875, I heard that Paddy had passed all his examinations with flying colours. Next I heard that he was going to be married to a charming young lady with money, but alas! a day or two before the wedding was to come off, Paddy was found dead from an overdose of a laudanum. At the inquest it is said that no less than three women claimed him as their husband. It was thought that one of them had threatened him with exposure if he carried through his marriage with the last love, and as he could not face the music, he put an end to himself."

After obtaining his M.R.C.S. in London at the age of twenty-two (the achievement can be measured by the results at the Royal College of Surgeons exams where, out of thirty-two candidates, only three passed), Francis continued on to Marburg in Germany, for further education in anatomy, surgery, and how the other half lived. The other half, the German students, lived a life that seemed to be dedicated mainly to beer. Francis, his handsome face buried in the undergrowth of his beard and his quiff of hair suppressed under a top hat, attempted manfully to keep up with the marathon tavern carousals of the student nights. "The entertainment lasted well past midnight and many of the older students drank from twenty to thirty litres of beer. Whenever the 'Fuchse-major,' or senior student in charge of the freshmen, drank, the freshmen had to do likewise. If he emptied his beer mug or tankard they had to follow his example, and then turn the mug upside down to show him they had emptied it. On special nights the 'Fuchse' (freshmen) could elect their own 'Fuchse-major'; and they always elected me when I was present because I could never drink more than six 'druge' of beer, and I did that with an effort.''

He also joined a dance club before learning that women members had the right to choose their partners. One hefty Valkyrie with massive bones and a powerful embrace took a fancy to Francis and began hurtling him around the dance floor on every possible, if not conceivable, occasion. Francis took to skulking in the crowd, but somehow she always managed to find him and sweep him off again in her arms.

(Tom Cullen also had an unusual time of it while furthering his education in Germany. Early one morning he was sitting around with a group of *Füchse* in Göttingen when someone called out, *Auf die Mensur!* Without further warning, his fellow students, who a moment before had been learnedly discussing surgery and strangulated hernias, jumped up and started hacking at other students with their long, curved swords. One of the men to whom Cullen had been chatting returned with so many wounds that it took thirty-six stitches to close them. "The whole procedure," Cullen said, "was *Unsinn*-madness.')

In between guzzling sessions and terpsichorean bear-hugs, Shepherd "attended Jager and von Arlt on the eye, Gruber and Politzer on the ear, Schenk on the microscope, Lange on anatomy, Hebra and Neumann on the Skin, Billroth and Dumreicher in surgery, Brucke in medicine, Rokitansky in pathology, and Meynert in neurology...and took courses on the nose and throat from Schroetter and Schnitzler, and special courses in medical diagnosis in the wards. I had operative surgery courses from the assistants of the surgeons, special courses in practical anatomy from Zuckerkandl, afterwards professor of anatomy at Graz. I had practical courses in pathology from Jundrat and in gynecology from Karl Braun, and also attended the children's hospital at St. Ann.''

It was in this fashion that an ambitious student in the 1870s attempted to fill in the gaps in his North American education.

Back in Montreal, Osler, noting Shepherd's M.R.C.S., began quietly lobbying on his friend's behalf. He wrote to Shepherd in Marburg to sound him out about an appointment on the McGill staff.

Whenever anyone received a letter from Osler, the recipient invariably found himself being forced to work harder than ever. Shepherd was no exception. Osler advised him to concentrate on his practical anatomy. Shepherd must have done so to Osler's satisfaction, for a few months later he wrote again: "My Dear Shepherd, I am delighted to be able to inform you that at a meeting of the Faculty last evening you were appointed demonstrator of anatomy, and allow me to offer you my sincere congratulations on the occasion."

Inevitably, Shepherd was urged to work harder than ever. "Could you not send Fenwick a paper—or letter—on Anatomy in Vienna?" Osler nudged. "It would take very well if you did." And added, a few lines further down in the same letter that, "I am going to pickle some brains for my own use this summer and will try to get some for you." He also urged Francis to take a course on the microscope.

Upon his return to Montreal to take up his duties at McGill and set up in general practice, Shepherd found himself in the peculiar position of renting rooms in his former home on Beaver Hall Hill. By that time the family had moved to Dorchester Street. It was lucky for Francis that his father was able to subsidize him, for during his first year as a practitioner, he earned less than a hundred dollars. His problems were not just the usual difficulties of a young man setting up in practice and getting known by the profession and trusted by the patients; his personality barred the way. "He had none of the qualities which lead quickly to success in medicine," wrote W. B. Howell. "He was tactless and appeared unsympathetic. He had abrupt manners and a 'you-be-damned' manner. He made no attempt to ingratiate himself with his seniors, who probably looked upon his independence as the result of bumptiousness." Worse still, he seemed to be treating his job at the university as if it were worthwhile. The older men were quite taken aback at the idea of an anatomist actually taking anatomy demonstrations seriously. They had always looked on the position as merely a stepping stone to better things. But Shepherd was one of the new men, intent on imposing on McGill the scientific methods he had studied abroad.

"He instituted a system of grinds which made it impossible for the students to scamp their dissecting," says Dr. Howell. "The cranial, thoracic, and abdominal cavities were no longer taken for granted. Scott [W. E. Scott, professor of anatomy] who had had nothing to move him out of his rut for twenty-five years, resented the new methods. There was friction between the two men, but Shepherd, young, energetic, and aggressive, bore down all opposition." He demanded, for instance, that examination in his subject be held every year instead of merely at the end of the third year. The faculy refused. McGill was going through a slump, and they feared that if the course were made more difficult, enrolment would decline still further. Shepherd insisted that anatomy was far too important to be treated in a perfunctory fashion. A year or so later he had his way. To the surprise of many among the faculty, Shepherd's higher standards, along with a number of other improvements, brought in not fewer students but many more.

As a result of Shepherd's emphasis on the importance of anatomy, production in the dissecting room increased. This worsened an already difficult problem, the supply of raw material. Subjects for dissection were hard to obtain. The province had had an anatomy act of sorts. After they died, indigents were supposed to be handed over to the inspector of anatomy, but there was no penalty if the authorities in the hospitals and poor houses failed to do so. Most of them preferred to bury the pauper dead, "a procedure," Howell says, "which satisfied their craving to perform a humane act at no expense to themselves, and gave them the pleasant feeling that they were doing something to baffle heartless medical students. That in putting obstacles in the way of medical men getting a knowledge of anatomy they were doing a disservice to their fellows was a consideration of no importance at all. The only charitable institution in Montreal which carried out the letter of the law was the Montreal General Hospital."

Accordingly, Shepherd had to depend on French-Canadian students, who paid their fees and other expenses by body-snatching, mostly from the cemetery off Côte des Neiges. After they had dug up the body, they would first strip it, in order to avoid a charge of theft if they were caught (the body by itself was not considered to be property), and then heave it onto a toboggan, wrapped in a blanket. Occasionally the students would shoot down Côte des Neiges on the same toboggan, and hope that it did not overturn at the bottom and deposit the cargo at the feet of some lady, gentleman, or gendarme.

Unfortunately if the snatch was discovered, the first place the affronted relatives tended to look was the dissecting room, and as Dr. Shepherd was the man who faced prosecution if the evidence was found on the dissection table, he had to attend court a number of times. The fine was fifty dollars.

The province finally put some clout into its anatomy act after the convent scandal. The convent concerned was located just outside Montreal. One winter, an epidemic of typhoid broke out, and several of the nuns and their charges died. As the ground was too hard for burial, the victims were placed in a vault until the spring thaw.

Such vaults, however, were the favourite targets of the resurrection men, for they ensured a maximum haul with a minimum of effort. From these storehouses, the students might bring Shepherd as many as a dozen bodies at one time. For a reasonably fresh subject they received as much as fifty dollars, with no questions asked.

Unfortunately, there were circumstances in this case that nearly undid the body snatchers. The first was that many of the victims were the daughters of American citizens, and Americans had a tradition of bringing home the deceased for burial. The second circumstance was that the parents arrived before the bodies could be delivered to Shepherd,

C.O.D. When the parents found the coffins unoccupied, they stirred up an international scandal that so alarmed the students that, cursing their bad luck, they hid the bodies in a snowbank. The students were thoroughly annoyed at the interfering Americans. After all, they were not doing the job for fun; they needed the money to help pay their tuition fees and living expenses.

However, it was not entirely a dead loss. When the outraged American parents offered a reward for the recovery of the bodies, the same students promptly dug them out of the snowbank, returned them, and claimed the reward.

The incident, though somewhat upsetting, achieved a great deal for the cause of medicine in Quebec, for it led to amendments to the anatomy act. Henceforth if deceased indigents were not handed over to the inspector of anatomy, the hospital or poorhouse authorities could be fined. From then on, the dissecting rooms were reasonably well supplied.

In 1883, when W. E. Scott died, Shepherd became professor of anatomy in his stead. He was now reaching the height of his powers as a teacher. He emphasized over and over again to the students the importance of a sound knowledge of anatomy, and he used his lectures, not as an alternative to dissection but as a supplement to help the students grasp the connection between their work in practical anatomy and the overall discipline it served. A few months after his appointment he was also made attending surgeon to the General Hospital, and though operations there were few and far between—until "Listerism" ensured a reasonable chance of surviving, patients still entered hospital only as a last resort—Shepherd's now-profound knowledge of anatomy gave him the confidence to undertake delicate and dangerous operations that most surgeons would have found excuses to avoid. One of his operations, reported in the Edinburgh *Medical Journal,* was on a three-day-old baby with an imperforate anus that was causing the meconium (a mass that accumulates in the bowel during fetal life, that is supposed to be discharged in the normal way shortly after birth) to be passed through the urethra. As summarized by Dr. Howell, "He dissected up two inches above the skin of the perineum before reaching the bowel, which he brought down and sutured to the skin." The operation on the miniature patient was successful.

At the same time Shepherd was running a dermatological clinic, and engaging in a Canadian version of the *Auf die Mensur!* with Miss Rimmer, the superintendant of nurses. Rimmer had a habit of slashing with the saber of her tongue at people who displeased her, and nearly everybody was afraid of her. She was not a trained nurse but an English gentlewoman of means who had arrived in Montreal merely on a visit, accompanied by her maid, Agnes Murray. When her beloved brother died, she decided to dedicate herself to helping others. She so impressed the hospital board with her character and noble ideals, that despite her lack of training, they decided to try her out as lady superintendant when the previous incumbent, Miss Machin, resigned under mysterious circumstances, along with four of her nurses. Or possibly Harriet Rimmer bullied the board into giving her the job. In either event she did well, not least because she encouraged a much better class of women to take up nursing at the General.

Though worthy and suffused with high ideals, Miss Rimmer appeared to be one of that dreadful regiment of Victorian Englishwomen whose attitude suggested that the rest of the population was composed of incompetents or scoundrels, or, in some cases, incompetent scoundrels. One source described her as being well liked, but the source could not have consulted all of the medical staff, for she treated them with contumely when they did not stand up to her. But she met her match when she slashed at the attending surgeon. Dr. Shepherd, not one to shrink from combat just because his adversary was a woman, riposted on their first confrontation over the hospital supply of antiseptic gauzes, oiled silk, and other protectives. When she arbitrarily refused to supply his outdoor clinic with a sufficient supply of these materials, he demolished her with cold, cutting effect, pointing out that he had a right to the materials, and she had better not stand in his way, or else.

He not only got what he wanted but in the process earned her respect and friendship. "Miss Rimmer managed everything and everybody," he wrote many years later. "She was able to get her own way with both doctors and committee of management. As regards to the doctors, she would find some irregularity or contravention of hospital rules which gave her power over them; and she used it. At this time doctors sometimes charged hospital patients and also took house-surgeons with them to help at operations. All this was against the rules. I myself took care to have my skirts particularly clean, so that she could never make any complaint against me."

She became increasingly friendly with the handsome bearded surgeon, and would have nobody else attend her when she fell ill. She continued to interest Shepherd right up to the end, revealing on her death bed a streak of humorous vulgarity that until then had been carefully buried under monumental respectability. She spent her last hours telling him dirty stories. When he hinted that her anecdotes did not seem entirely appropriate to such a solemn occasion, she replied that even worse was to come. "I am keeping my worst till the last," she said.

Francis Shepherd could be as cold and cutting in print as in conversation. Along with scores of papers on such subjects as exophthalmic goitre, melanotic sarcoma, congenital hypertrophic stenosis of the pylorus, hydronephroma, blastomycotic dermatitis, bronchocole, cholecysten-terostomy, exploratory laparotomy, and feigned eruptions, he covered, on behalf of *The Canada Medical and Surgical Journal,* such meetings as that of the Ontario Medical Association in Toronto, during which he reported that, "About twenty papers and reports were read, most of them by country members. None were of special merit. In fact, as a rule, it may be said that the papers were rather below than above the average.... Discussion was rather discouraged than otherwise. Papers were rapidly read, one after the other, and no opportunity for discussing them was offered. The acoustic properties of the hall were such, that unless the reader of the paper had a remarkable clear delivery, or the listener remarkable sharp ears, very little could be heard."

Shepherd's reviews of medical works were often filled with ungrudging condemnation. "This little work," he wrote about a pop volume on how to treat hemorrhoids by injecting carbolic acid, "... is meant to show how much better the author's mode of treatment is for the patient than that adopted by most surgeons. All that is contained in it of use to the profession might easily be compressed into a medical journal at no great length. The padding consists of the weakest kind of anatomical description of the rectum and the blood supply, a great number of prescriptions and 'sure cures' and reports of cases cured by his method of injection.... The language is not very choice or scientific.... The book is cheaply got up, the chapters are short and the margins wide, the print is large and the illustrations unobjectionable." About another book on fractures and dislocations by T. Pickering Pick, he wrote that, "The teaching of the book, as a whole, is such that a student will not be led far astray." Which could not have greatly increased T. Pickering Pick's sales.

The handsome devil with the chilly, autocratic eyes, rarely concurred with anybody if he could find grounds for disagreement. He was always sure that he was right, and his self-confidence often came close to an arrogance expressed in humorous sarcasm. But his training was thorough, and the men who worked for him invariably went on to distinguished careers of their own. "Were we to estimate Shepherd's power to judge men by the calibre of his demonstrators," Howell wrote, "we should believe that he had rare judgement. I am inclined to think, however, that it was his demonstrators who chose Shepherd. Clever and hard-working young men gravitated towards him just as naturally as the stupid and the lazy kept away from him. He paid his demonstrators little or nothing; he worked them hard; he gave no praise and no thanks; they knew that if they fell below his standard he would get rid of them without compunction. They gave him, in return not only their devoted service, but, to a considerable extent, their trust and affection."

It was Shepherd, his friends, and those who worked for him who contributed so much to the renaissance of McGill in the eighties and thereafter; men like Ross, Roddick, Gardner, and Osler, the Leonardo of the Renaissance.

One of Shepherd's close friends, William Gardner, was typical of the group in his will to succeed and his enjoyment of the process of succeeding. When Shepherd knew him, he was a dapper fellow, with a Scottish accent that had survived an upbringing in the Quebec countryside, and a bursting pride in the figure he cut as a respected young professor. He dressed in a natty frock coat and a carefully brushed top hat that changed colour with the season, from black in winter to gray in summer. Gardner had triumphed over poverty and prejudice, educating himself as he toiled on the family farm, with a plough handle in one hand and a book in the other. "William had no one to coach him in the Latin necessary for his matriculation into McGill, so he and a friend prepared themselves by studying the Latin parts of the pharmacopoeia in conjunction with a Latin grammar. After graduating he had settled in Beauharnois, but the road to success in practice was blocked by the village priest, who told his parishoners that if they went to Gardner for medical advice he would refuse them the sacrament." In Montreal, however, despite intense competition from a dense population of medicos, he soon built up an extensive practice. He became professor of medical jurisprudence around about the time that Osler joined McGill, and years later was appointed gynecologist to the Montreal General.

People often wondered how Gardner and Shepherd managed to get on so well together when they were so totally different in character. Gardner was as mild and accommodating as a salicylic cream dressing. Shepherd was as sharp and glittering as a scalpel. The physical contrast was just as marked, especially when they walked along the street together, Gardner, small, plump and slow, bald of head and red of moustache, trotting a little absurdly alongside Shepherd's establishment figure that supported an aggressive, bearded, skeptical-eyed head. Presumably it was their similar interests, especially their informed appreciation of art, that transformed their acquaintanceship into a lasting friendship. In this the inevitable practical jokes figured, such as the one that Gardner played on Shepherd while they were sightseeing in Russia. Venturing one day out of his Moscow hotel without a passport, Shepherd was arrested and taken to the police station. There his attempts to identify himself were greeted with skepticism that his ignorance of the language in nowise ameliorated. But when Gardner was summoned by a British consular official to vouch for the prisoner, Gardner took one look at Shepherd, who was naturally looking a trifle discomposed, and shaking his head, announced that he had never seen this man before in his life—and left Dr. Shepherd to fume in custody for another hour before handing over

Shepherd's passport to the authorities, who, being Russian officials, were not in the least amused by the antics of the *Nyemski*.

Mostly Gardner and Shepherd confined their japery within the walls of the various clubs they belonged to, including the Medico-Chirurgical Society, to which Osler had contributed such notable papers on pathology. One of Shepherd's friends in the Society was John Reddy, a tall skinny Irishman with curly black whiskers. "He had been a house-surgeon in the Meath Hospital," Shepherd wrote in his *Reminiscences*, "and told us much about that celebrated institution, and what he did there. Among other tales he told us that when he was there he had pulled 5,000 teeth. He had a large practise and was a very successful midwife. He had great faith in the diagnostic powers of George Ross. When Ross was house-surgeon at the General, Reddy on entering the hospital would ask him what new cases there were. On one occasion Ross said that there was a new case of pneumonia in a corner bed in Ward X. On going the rounds, followed by some clinical clerks and dressers, Reddy stopped at the door of this ward, and suddenly starting back, pointed to a man in a corner bed and said, 'What do I see? A man with a flushed face, rapid breathing, distressed look — surely a case of pneumonia.' Ross pulled Reddy's sleeve and said in a low voice: 'Not in that corner, the other.'"

In 1887, Shepherd made another visit to Europe to review the work of others in anatomy and surgery. In general he was not too impressed by European progress in the interim. In surgery he found that the Scots had retrogressed, the English were old-fashioned, the French backward, and the Germans reckless.

The trip had not started out too well, either. A day out of New York, his ship the *Britannic* was rammed by another liner, the S S *Celtic*. On reaching Dublin, Shepherd told his hosts all about it over dinner at Trinity College. "When we first saw the *Celtic* I was below the bridge. She immediately reversed her engines, and we went full ahead. It was an exciting moment. I ran back and saw the *Celtic* strike, or rather, walk into us immediately behind our engine-room, carrying away, as she fell back, all the bulwarks, mizzen-shrouds, three boats, and everything down to the main deck. There was really no great shock, merely a grating sound. The bow of the *Celtic* seemed to melt away like brown paper. She drifted astern and then the panic commenced. I saw our ship was stove in and in a serious condition, so I went below and got my great coat and flask of brandy, which I thought might be useful. When I came on deck again I saw the great amount of wreckage and several dead bodies under the debris. These people had been leaning over the rail or were sleeping behind the bulwarks and had not seen the ship approaching. I did all I could to comfort the women and keep order. I did not manage to secure a lifebelt for myself. The captain was not on deck at the time of the collision, but was playing poker, and when he came on deck could not maintain order. There was some awkwardness about getting the boats ready and lowering them, the ropes being stiff and the blocks rusty. Some of the male passengers tried to get into the first boats lowered and a few of them succeeded, but the officers provided themselves with pistols and then better order was maintained. The boats went off loaded with women and a few cowardly men. One boat on the starboard side had been appropriated by five men. For the first twenty-four hours there was considerable tension among the passengers. There were many injured. I spent the night after the collision operating upon them and sewing up their wounds, the ship's surgeon giving chloroform. The day after the collision the hole in the ship's side temporarily stopped with tarpaulin and sails, and we steamed slowly back to New York, where we arrived in a couple of days, accompanied by three ships which had overtaken us and which stood by."

On hearing this story, one of Shepherd's dinner companions at Trinity College asked, "What will they do with the captain? Hang him?" Whereupon another guest, the Irish wit John Pentland Mahaffy said, "Oh, no, they will only suspend him."

Shepherd was particularly shocked when he reached Edinburgh, the birthplace of antisepsis, to see the wards filled with patients with septic wounds and fever. It seemed that the moment Lister had left for London ten years previously they had almost instantly started to neglect his findings. The situation in London was hardly better. Though Lister was busy improving his methods still further at King's College Hospital — by then he had abandoned the spray and was using iodoform and eucalyptol gauze in his dressings — there were still too many reactionaries around, like Mr. Lawson Tait. During an address that Tait had made to the Canadian Medical Association in Montreal three years previously, the famous surgeon had poo-poohed the whole concept of Listerism. "I had practised all the details in their ever-varying form, as recommended by Mr. Lister, from 1866 onwards," he announced in his bellicose fashion, "and gave them all up one after another as I found they disappointed and hindered me. Finally I gave the spray and its adjuncts a long and complete trial — a trial far more careful in its detail than anything I ever saw elsewhere, extending over three years. I have published in detail," he ended, "the disastrous results."

William Gardner, however, who had invited Tait to stay with him while he was in Montreal, had heard that Tait's antiseptic trials were suspect. Gardner, giving his impressions of Lawson Tait to W. B. Howell, described the stout, bull-necked, heavy-drinking Tait as saying "that if he could get enough germs he would use them as a dressing for his abdominal wounds. He used to say he would as soon put his hands into the abdomen as into his pockets." Gardner added that he saw some of Tait's patients after operations, and "it was very noticeable how many of the wounds were suppurating. Many surgeons thought he was dishonest in the records he published. It was said that he hustled patients out of his hospital if he thought they were going to die."

In Germany, Shepherd found that "German surgeons thought nothing of a case if they could not operate upon it; in my opinion they often operated unnecessarily and sometimes recklessly." In France, "the Parisians seem to think that everything worth knowing can be learnt in Paris, and that there are no surgeons outside Paris," it seemed to him that they had failed to grasp the principles of antisepsis.

Shepherd's own reputation as a surgeon was secure enough, especially after one particularly difficult and dangerous operation at the Montreal General. It roused considerable interest when he described it to the C.M.A., the Canadian Medical Association, formed in 1867 to promote the interests and raise the professional standards of its nation-wide members. "My experience in this operation (herniotomy) has been small," he admitted, "but some months ago I operated on a very formidable case, the details of which I shall venture to mention. A blacksmith, aged fifty-two, had an enormous irreducible scrotal hernia on the left side, from which he had suffered for many years. The tumour had become so large that he could not wear trousers or follow his occupation. He was, besides, a rather corpulent man, and a hard drinker. I performed the operation for radical cure of hernia on the 25th of April last (1888). The sac was dissected out and opened, and the contents reduced with the greatest of difficulty. The sac contained all the small intestines, the transverse descending colon, and the sigmoid flexure, together with a large mass of omentum. Nearly two pounds of the latter were excised, and it was only by suspending the patient by the heels (a suggestion of Dr. Bell's) that I was enabled to reduce the protruded bowel. The intestines had not been in the abdomen for years, and that cavity now seemed too small to contain them; and when after an hour and a half's exertions the intestines were all returned, the abdomen was as tense as a drum. The sac was excised and the stump fixed to the intestinal ring according to Barker's method, and the canal closed by suturing the combined tendon to Poupart's ligament. The patient made an excellent recovery and is now pursuing his occupation as a blacksmith, with comfort. I saw him a week ago and there was not the slightest tendency to a return of the hernia."

If Francis Shepherd was ornery in ward and hospital corridor, he was the very prototype of the petulant maestro in the operating theatre. It was quite common for him to hurl instruments to the floor if they dissatisfied him; (or perhaps it was his use of them which dissatisfied him). Sometimes he even threw them out the window. His assistants could never be sure what he would be up to next.

He kept his senior nurse and his house-surgeon off-balance throughout one entire summer by constantly asking for instruments that had not been laid out. One day in desperation they sterilized everything right down to the obsolete ecraseur, and laid out every instrument, ready for the most improbable demand. Whereupon, in the middle of the operation, he asked for a triploid. Not only did they not have a triploid on display—they had never even heard of it. Shepherd gave them hell for this glaring omission. Later, when they asked him what a triploid looked like, he replied that he had no idea, he'd never seen one. He just happened to have noticed the name in a medical journal.

On the other hand, if anyone else in the operating room did not behave according to his standards, his exasperation was quite unrestrained. He never thanked anybody, or alloted them even a smidgin of praise. The only way his assistants could be sure he approved of their work was when he had nothing to say.

There were many surgeons who were more brilliant at the operating table than Dr. Shepherd. "Shepherd was too good a surgeon to be a brilliant operator." His surgery was not perfect in an artistic sense. It was, however, fast and accurate, and in the long run that was better for his patients than the work of *some* surgeons he could mention, who would rather do an artistic job and see the patient die than do a necessarily rough job and see him safely out of the hospital.

He was just as fast in the consulting room of his residence at 152 Mansfield Street, Montreal, to which he moved with his wife Lilias in 1889. It was said that more than one patient was operated on in there with scissors or scalpel before they knew what was happening.

With its bookcases, pictures, and ornaments, the consulting room was a reassuring place to his few patients. Apart from an old-fashioned monaural stethoscope, there were no instruments in sight. His medical record was a shabby calf-bound ledger, his operating table an old sofa. There were probably more social visitors to the house than patients. To the amazement of his young surgeons and demonstrators who were invited to dinner, the doctor whose cold eye and sarcastic humour had so often made them tremble in the wards, proved to be quite a kindly host. Perhaps he behaved in an agreeable fashion because he was happy in his home, with its walls crowded with the superb paintings that he had collected over a lifetime, and in the company of his young wife. The only tragedies in his life were the loss of his wife in 1892 and, like Osler, the death of his son in the First World War.

Shepherd had married Lilias Torrance when he was twenty-seven, a girl he had known since her childhood at Como, and their married life, which produced three children, was said to be completely happy. "Lilias Shepherd was a woman of unusual charm," said Dr. Howell who knew them both. "They were a notable couple, both of them with good looks above the average, and an air of distinction; his abrupt manner, and habit of speaking his mind regardless of consequences, made him a foil for her gentleness and tact."

Otherwise, the worst Shepherd had to bear in his life was the loss of the anatomical specimens he had collected over thirty years, when the McGill Medical Building was badly damaged by fire in 1907.

Despite his sharp speech, destructive humour and contrary ways, Shepherd earned the greatest admiration from his students as well as his friends. "From the moment when Shepherd walked with his quick, firm step into the amphitheatre, until his lecture was over, all eyes were fixed upon him and followed his every move. It was no effort to give him attention; rather it was an effort to withdraw attention from him. He was nearing middle age; his height about the average; his figure erect and well built; his face strong and resolute with regular features, for he was a good-looking man. His moustache and pointed beard were beginning to turn gray. He was fluent without art, and entirely free from self-consciousness. His lectures were interspersed with accounts of interesting surgical cases which showed the practical application of what he was teaching and were illustrated by excellent drawings on the blackboard. His gift for drawing was innate; he had at one time thought of cultivating it by taking lessons, but an artist whom he consulted, told him that they would be more likely to spoil his powers than to improve them."

Naturally, faced with a person of such authority, the students behaved themselves. On a rare occasion when one of them didn't, Shepherd asked the student to stand up. Then he told the young man to sit down again. Some time passed before Shepherd suddenly stopped in the middle of his lecture. "I see you are all wondering why I asked Mr. Blank to stand up," he said coldly. "I just wanted to find out if he is still wearing short trousers."

Though he never tried to conciliate the students, never encouraged them with mere praise, was brusque, demanding, and often humiliatingly critical, and "plucked" more of them than did any other professor, their admiration was very nearly as great as that felt for Osler in his day— partly because, like Osler, he could communicate his intense interest in medicine. "In after years," wrote his biographer W. B. Howell (who was a medical student under Shepherd), "he remained more vividly in their minds than any other member of the teaching staff. To this day, when two or three are gathered together and exchange reminsicences, it is generally 'Frankie' Shepherd who is most discussed."

By the age of fifty, Francis Shepherd was at the apogee of his powers and at the top of his profession. Next to Osler, he was the best-known Canadian doctor outside Canada, and a dominant influence at home, in the Medical School, and in the hospital. "His opinion on anything that concerned anatomy, surgery, or skin diseases was conclusive." His wide interests in fields outside medicine and his conversational skills ensured him a prominent place in society as well, even though he was often indiscreet. His forceful opinions quite frequently disconcerted his hosts. In his capacity as president of the Art Association, he once told off the governor-general for getting his facts wrong in a speech about the new art gallery on Sherbrooke Street, mortifying Earl Grey to no real purpose. In spite of which, he remained on a select list of guests who could be invited to Government House in Ottawa without utterly disgracing themselves. He also remained atop the invitation list of people worthy of meeting the most notable visitors to Montreal. Among these were Nansen of the North Pole and Amundsen of the South Pole, Lord Roberts, V.C., of Indian frontier fame, and Winston Churchill, who, during a speech in Montreal illustrated by lantern slides of scenes from the Boer War, was asked by Dr. Shepherd, "How is it, Mr. Churchill, that all the colonial troops in South Africa seem to be Canadians?" "Oh," replied Mr. Churchill, "those troops will all be Australians when I get to Australia."

One of his good friends was William Van Horne, whom Shepherd first met when the great man was chief engineer of the C.P.R. Shepherd found him fascinating and genuinely talented—he could read a newspaper held on a level with his eyes, but to one side, while he looked straight ahead. Van Horne's refusal to admit ignorance on any subject also amused his medical friend. Shepherd was always trying to catch him out. The opportunity came while they were touring Cuba together. (Like so many Canadian medicos, Shepherd traveled widely, maintaining the tradition of the Boswellian Grand Tour, and extending it far beyond Europe.) In Havana, immediately after a tour of a tapioca factory, he went to Van Horne, who had not joined that particular tour, and asked him if he knew how tapioca was obtained. Van Horne replied authoritatively that it was derived from the palm tree. Having just learned all about the cassava, from whose root tapioca comes, Shepherd was just about to confound him when Van Horne, sensing that the cocky doctor was about to crow, made some excuse and darted into the next room where an encyclopedia was available. The stout little man was back in less than three minutes with a great deal more information on tapioca than Shepherd had absorbed, even though he had just seen it being made. Van Horne was not only a quick thinker but a speed-reader.

"Though remarkably shrewd in many ways," Shepherd said about the railway pioneer, "he was simple in others. He was very susceptible to flattery about his knowledge of art and his own artistic efforts. He was a beautiful draughtsman. He painted pictures, but they were not as good as his sketches. They were hard and wanting in colour, though he had a fine colour sense.... He was fond of picking up old pictures and giving them a name. Many of these names he changed several times."

Toward the end of Van Horne's life, Shepherd tried to persuade him to leave his collection of pictures to the Montreal Art Gallery, but he refused. Shepherd blamed this lack of public spirit on "the bad example of many of the rich men of Montreal who had magnificent collections."

Van Horne also refused to leave his collection of geological and paleontological specimens to McGill University, though in this case his reason for snubbing that Canadian institution was slightly more understandable. As a youth, Van Horne had been passionately keen on education, and to this end liked to visit museums on his only day off, a Sunday. Unfortunately the McGill museum was under the influence of Scottish Presbyterianism, and closed its doors on the Lord's day. So, still in a huff umpteen years later, Van Horne left the collection to the University of Chicago.

Shepherd was also acquainted with many of the famous and infamous outside Canada. J. Pierpont Morgan was one. He first met the banker at the opening of the new Harvard Medical School in 1906 when Shepherd was to receive an honorary degree, his second Ll.D., the other having been awarded at Edinburgh the previous year. Shepherd was placed next to Pierpont Morgan because they were supposed to have a common interest in art. "I soon found he knew nothing about art," Shepherd snapped. "He professed to like only the Italian primitives and the early English, such as Gainsborough, Reynolds, etc." Giving up on the subject of art, Shepherd next tried to interest the billionaire in medicine, but Morgan failed to live up to the doctor's standards in that area, as well. At one point, Morgan asked Shepherd, "Why don't they invent something, a new cure, and patent it?" He thought all antitoxins should be patented and be of profit to the discoverer. I told him that this would be considered unprofessional and that we were working for the good of humanity. He seemed to think this was all bosh."

The following year, Morgan invited Shepherd to view his magnificent library in New York, but when he arrived, Mr. Morgan retired to another room "to receive his subjects, suppliants, or whatever you may call them, and sat in a chair, smoking a long cigar and working at his letters. We had to go through this room to the muniment room, where his valuable parchments and manuscripts were kept. Through the door I could see the line of humble vassals being disposed of. He treated them all like dirt. After hearing each one, he gave a grunt or snort of dismissal. Sometimes he would ejaculate a brief 'No.' He did not look up, but went on opening his letters. When we had finished seeing his library possessions we approached him, and he sat up and said 'Good bye.' It was the last time I ever saw him."

In the final twenty years of his life, honours were heaped on Francis Shepherd. His distinction in medicine was due almost as much to the man himself as to his work. All eyes tended to turn in his direction when he appeared. To a large extent his personal magnetism was a product of his faults. They added to his richness as a character rather than impoverishing it. He was vain, egotistical, argumentative, and believed that he understood art, medicine, and life better than practically anyone else. He was as independent as a cat, as contrary as a wolverine, but in the light of his work in surgery and dermatology, these were forgivable faults. As for his eminence in anatomy, somebody once asked another anatomist, J. D. Cunningham, why it was that McGill graduates who visited Edinburgh always seemed to know their anatomy so much better than men from other universities. Cunningham's reply was simply, "You don't know Shepherd."

21

Women in Medicine?
Certainly Not!

No WONDER "JAMES" Barry had to become a transvestite to get into medicine. According to Hyginus, even the enlightened Athenians did not permit women (or slaves) to engage in medicine. Which infuriated the handsome and talented Dr. Agnodice. She was a pupil of Herophilus (the greatest authority in Greece on the anatomy of females, their difficulties and diseases). Herophilus had inspired in Agnodice a profound interest in obstetrics, and she was determined that the law should not prevent her from offering her services to those female patients who found it embarrassing to be intimately examined by males. Accordingly, when she went to Athens to establish a practice she adopted male attire. Naturally her female clients soon learned that Agnodice was a woman, and her practice grew rapidly. This so aroused the jealousy of her male colleagues that they brought charges against their unnaturally successful competitor, claiming that "he" must surely be corrupting female patients wholesale. At her trial, Agnodice faced a fearful dilemma. If she did not reveal her sex and thus show that she was incapable of taking advantage of her patients in the way alleged by her accusers, she might be found guilty; but if she did reveal it, she would be accused of contravening Athenian law. Adopting the latter course as the lesser evil, she exposed herself, and was accordingly found guilty on the substitute charge.

Happily, a number of her influential friends came to her aid, lobbying their husbands so effectively (possibly in the Lysistrata manner, by withdrawing those favours that were likely to lead to Agnodice's services as an obstetrician), that the law was repealed and Agnodice was pardoned.

Whether Hyginus's account was accurate or not—as a historical researcher he was an excellent pope—the situation underlying it, the resistance to the idea of women as medical practitioners, was real enough. Even the wise and tolerant Hippocrates could not see women in medical schools. His oath read (and still does): "I will impart a knowledge of the art to my own sons and those of my own sons and those of my teachers and to disciples... but to none others."

Still, there was the occasional breakthrough in continental Europe. Women were admitted to one or two medical schools in Italy as early as the fourteenth century. One of them, Laura Bassi, became a professor of experimental physics at the University of Bologna, though her chief claim to fame, according to male historians, was that she was the teacher of one of the great men of physiology, Spallanzani. And, as already noted, Mundinus' anatomical assistant may have been a girl, Alessandra Gilliani.

In seventeenth-century America, a physician named Margaret Jones managed to set up in practice, but her example could not have encouraged other women, as she was the first person to be executed in the New England colonies.

The trouble was that she was so effective a physician that the Puritan Fathers had become suspicious. The condition of those of her patients who refused to take her medicines invariably worsened. So it was obvious that she was a witch. Suspicion deepened when the colonial governor, John Winthrop, had her forcibly examined. According to his account, she proved to have "an apparent teat in her secret parts as fresh as if it had been newly sucked." The final proof came when a jailer, peeping in at her as she sat on the floor with her clothes up, saw a child run out of her and into another room. Before he could summon a witness, the child had vanished. And what more proof was needed that she was a witch when, following her execution, a tempest arose in Connecticut, "which blew down many trees."

By the nineteenth century, a few women were studying medicine and doing clinical work in hospitals in France and Switzerland. Even Russia had a woman graduate by 1869, though admittedly the czarist authorities were not aware of it until she had received her degree. Her talents and intense desire to learn had so overcome the prejudice of the professors and students that they helped her to conceal her sex from the bureaucracy until it was too late for anything to be done about it, though for a while the Russian government prohibited any more women from attending university.

Resistance in the English-speaking countries was even more stubborn. Women could handle the nursing side and midwifery, but medicine was out. It was a strictly male preserve. Asserting that a woman did not have the mental capacity for medical studies, the author of an obstetrics textbook published in Philadelphia in 1848 noted that, "She has a head almost too small for intellect but just big enough for love," a comment that must have caused even a few males to writhe with embarrassment.

The English-speaking pioneer in the struggle to give women a place in medicine was Elizabeth Blackwell, an Englishwoman who accompanied her family to the United States in 1832 when she was eleven years old. Encouraged by her father, who was exceptional for the time in his belief that girls as well as boys deserved a proper education, she set out to realize her ambition to become a doctor by extensive reading, and, with the money she earned, by engaging private tutors. As soon as she felt she was ready, she applied for admission to a number of universities, and finally was accepted by a medical school in Geneva in upstate New York. But, her application was signed with her initial E, rather than with the full name, so that the authorities there were not aware that she was a woman until she turned up for classes.

The faculty were considerably taken aback when E. Blackwell, Esquire, turned out to be a little lady, wearing a simple dress and a shy yet determined expression. Still, they did not reject her out of hand. They left the decision to her fellow students, probably hoping that the students would do the job for them. Instead, to everybody's surprise the all-male student body, in a fit of idealism, accepted her. The faculty were all the more amazed because the boys were a particularly unruly lot. There had been many complaints from the citizens of Geneva about their riotous behaviour.

During lectures they were sometimes so boisterous that the professors could hardly be heard. Yet, according to one who was there, "Her entry into the Bedlam of confusion acted like magic on every student. Each hurriedly sought his seat, and the utmost silence prevailed. For the first time a lecture was given without the slightest interruption, and every word could be heard as distinctly as if there had been but a single person in the room. The sudden transformation by the mere presence of a lady, proved to be permanent in its effects."

Elizabeth faced a number of problems during her years at the school. In one incident involving the professor of anatomy, she was asked to skip his lecture, which dealt with "a delicate subject." "When Elizabeth wrote him a note objecting to such squeamishness over a "scientific subject," writes historian Edythe Lutzker, "the truth came out—it seems that this subject had indeed been made somewhat 'indelicate' by the professor's customary inclusion in this lecture of some dirty jokes. The professor admitted his shame over his former conduct, and Elizabeth was invited into the lecture room. She was given a standing ovation; and never again was there any question about her attendance at all lectures on all subjects."

Elizabeth graduated from the Geneva College of Medicine in 1849 with the highest marks in her class. But she had to travel to Paris for her hospital training.

The struggle for women in medicine was infinitely more fierce in Britain. The resistance ideology being summed up by a Dr. Bennet, who in a letter to *The Lancet*, wrote that women "as a body...are sexually, constitutionally, and mentally unfitted for the hard and incessant toil, and for the heavy responsibilities of general medical and surgical practise."

The most notable pioneer in Britain was Sophia Jex-Blake. Like Elizabeth Blackwell, she was an English girl who began her medical studies in the United States as a nurse at the Hospital for Women and Children in Boston. Inspired to become a doctor, she tried to enter the Harvard Medical School, but there being "no provision for the education of women in any department of this university," she returned home. Failing to break into any of the schools in England, she turned to the University of Edinburgh, considered to be the most liberal institution in the British Isles.

Sophia and four other women who applied for admission learned otherwise. They faced no fewer than five lines of defense: the Medical Faculty, the Senatus, the General Council, the University Council, and the Royal Infirmary. As soon as one position was overwhelmed by the determined ladies, the opposition fell back on the next. Yet Sophia overcame four of these august bodies by her infuriating stubborness and refusal to listen to reason—her opponents' conception of reason, that is. But when the girls attacked what they hoped was the final line of defense, the royal infirmary, the smouldering hostility of the student body flamed up into the shameful Surgeons' Hall riot.

It was so alarming an experience that even thirty years later, whenever she visited Edinburgh, one of the women involved preferred to go miles out of her way to avoid the gates of the Surgeons' Hall.

Sophia's jutting-jawed obstinacy, as well as her courage, can be discerned in her description of the scene that November day in 1870, that was to arouse the indignation of the press, and, indeed, of the whole world, and which did nothing to enhance Edinburgh's reputation as a centre of learning. "As soon as we came in sight of the gates," Sophia wrote, "we found a dense mob filling up the roadway in front of them, comprising some dozen of the lowest class of our fellow-students at Surgeons' Hall, with many more of ths same class from the University, a certain number of street rowdies, and some hundreds of gaping spectators, who took no particular part in the matter. Not a single policeman was visible, though the crowd was sufficient to stop all traffic for about an hour. We walked straight up to the gates, which remained open until we came within a yard of them, when they were slammed in our faces by a number of young men who stood within, smoking and passing about bottles of whisky, while they abused us in the foulest possible language, which I am thankful to say I have never heard equalled before or since. We waited quietly on the step to see if the rowdies were to have it all their own way, and in a minute we saw another fellow-student of ours, Mr. Sanderson, rush down from Surgeons' Hall and wrench open the gate, in spite of the howls and efforts of our half-tipsy opponents. We were quick to seize the chance offered, and in a very few seconds we have all passed through the gate, and entered the anatomical class-room, where the usual examination was conducted in spite of the yells and howls resounding outside, and the forcible intrusion of a luckless sheep, that was pushed inside by the rioters. 'Let it remain,' said Dr. Handyside, 'it has more sense than those who sent it here.' At the close of the class the lecturer offered to let us out by a back door, but I glanced round the ranks of our fellow-students and remarked that I thought there were enough gentlemen here to prevent any harm to us. I had judged rightly. In a moment a couple of dozen students came down from the benches, headed by Mr. Sanderson, Mr. Hogan, Mr. Macleod, and Mr. Lyon, formed themselves in to a regular bodyguard in front, behind and on each side and encompassed by them, we passed through the still howling crowd at the gate, and reached home with no other injuries than those inflicted on our dresses by the mud hurled at us by our chivalrous foes."

The girls were harried, taunted, and threatened for days afterwards, but even worse than the behaviour of the students was that of certain professors, who had done much to stir up hatred against the five girls by their consistently demeaning comments in the lecture halls.

In Canada, the prejudice of centuries had begun to soften by the 1890s, though the attitude to females in medicine was still such as to instil a want of confidence even in such redoubtable women as Bessie Efner and Elizabeth Matheson.

Bessie Efner came from a long-established American medical family. She was enthralled with medicine, and had assisted her father in his practice for many years. Even so, it was not until a neighbour suggested it that she dared to consider becoming a doctor herself.

Since the age of thirteen she had been mixing medicines, folding little papers for powders, helping her father to bandage the injured, and holding the kerosene lamp when some injured person came for help at night; but the idea of a girl becoming a doctor seemed preposterous, until the friendly neighbour, who had observed her interest over the years, urged Bessie to enter medical college. Bessie was startled. "I had thought about it so much, but never had the courage to discuss it with anyone else, not even with my father. And so when she suggested that I study medicine, I reached out, took her hand, and said, 'Mrs. Benson, do you really mean this? Do you really think that I could become a doctor like my father?'"

The general opposition to women doctors had begun to weaken by the time that Bessie Efner attended Sioux City School of Medicine in the very early years of the twentieth century. Even so, she and one other girl student found that though their male classmates, "were chivalrous enough to pretend that they were accepting us on equal terms,... I'm sure many of them considered us a nuisance that had to be tolerated. They called us hen medics, a term that students commonly apply to women doctors. This had a somewhat derogatory connotation because the male students and people in general regarded women unfit for the medical profession."

It was even more difficult for her after she had graduated. "I was a doctor like other doctors. I had completed the same course of medicine the men in my class had taken, and in all modesty I can say that I considered myself as competent as any of them. But I was a woman. Every young doctor has to contend with the social prejudice against the youthful practitioner. People quite naturally prefer to entrust their bodies and their lives to more experienced doctors, who have earned some confidence by their past performance. But in addition to being a young, inexperienced doctor, I was a woman. I was the first woman doctor in that community to venture into the field that from time immemorial had been the prerogative of men."

After she hung out her shingle, she first had to contend with the village gossips. People would watch to see who went into her office—and more particularly, when they came out. She could not afford to examine any male patient under ninety years of age for more than a few minutes without the risk of igniting a prurient imagination. In her relations with men, whether they were patients or otherwise, she had to perform a balancing act between an abyss of over-familiarity and the sheer drop of un-American reserve. In self-defense she was forced to dress up in the outward trappings of respectability by joining the local Methodist Church, singing circumspectly in its choir, and religiously attending its Sunday school.

Her first patient was a young farmer from out of town. When Bessie opened the office door he looked around, searching for the doctor, meanwhile explaining that his wife was about to have a baby.

Bessie, whose shingle sported only her initials, B.L., explained that she was the doctor.

"'You—you—the doctor? Well, I'm looking for a real doctor, like other doctors.'

"'I am a real doctor like other doctors.'

"'Is there no other doctor in town?'

Bessie replied courteously that the nearest alternative practitioner lived many miles away. "This was before the day of the automobile," she explained, "and for a moment the young man stood, and I could see that he was trying to calculate the approximate time it would require to drive there and back. Then after some hesitation and as though resigning himself to the inevitable he said, 'Very well, then, come out, my wife is in immediate need, she cannot wait much longer.'

Bessie's reception by the young farmer's wife was not too encouraging either. "When I arrived I found a typical young farmer's wife in the first stages of childbirth. But as I stepped in to the room, the expression in her face changed into one of disappointment. She was anxiously waiting for the doctor and instead a strange woman walked into her room." However, the attitude of both parents changed after Bessie had delivered a healthy infant—a boy.

The case that established her reputation and began to lessen the local prejudice against hen medics was also the one that restored her confidence in herself. "A transient worker had been imbibing too lustily in one of the local saloons," she remembered, "and on the way back to the place of work, his horse had become frightened and staged what the farmers call a runaway. The man was thrown from his buggy and dragged for some distance and then left lying unconscious in the road. Some passerby found him and brought him to my office. He was covered with dirt from head to foot and bleeding from many cuts and bruises.

"He himself was still in a drunken stupor and unable to give intelligent answers to the questions I directed to him. An examination showed that he had sustained a double fracture in his right jaw, besides cuts and bruises in his face and other parts of his body. The external wounds were soon cleaned and dressed. But what to do about the jaw puzzled me. To put on an ordinary cast was impossible. To bandage up the jaw without some device to hold the fractured bones in place was also not feasible. I could recall no similar case described in our text books. But something had to be done immediately. After a careful study of the case I decided on trying an experiment. I pulled one of his molars to provide an opening so that he could be fed by means of a tube. Then I brought the edges of the bones together, which I had to do by touch alone, without the aid of the fluoroscope or X-ray. These costly instruments were not yet available for the individual practitioner. Then I wired the upper and lower teeth together in such a way that the jaw was held firmly in position and the teeth in perfect alignment. Finally I reinforced the whole with a firm bandage around the chin, jaw and head."

She was delighted when the old drunk got his face back without the slightest deformity, and became a walking advertisement in the community for her skill.

One of the problems of a doctor in an ankle-length dress was that her own sex started to come to her in increasing numbers to plead for abortions. Bessie could not be sure that they were not being sent by her male colleagues, either to get such patients out of their offices or to set a trap for her.

Another problem was her vulnerability to bullying. She described what happened after she had delivered a woman of her twelfth child. During the last stages of his wife's pregnancy, the husband went to a local whore and contracted gonorrhea. Then, refusing to wait even until his wife had risen from the confinement bed, he made love to her and infected her.

The infection brought on a dangerous fever, and Bessie, suppressing her fury, told the husband that his wife would have to go into the hospital immediately if her life was to be saved. "But instead of showing any concern or shame as one would expect, he became abusive and vile in his language, blaming me for the trouble and saying that I had neglected his wife, and threatening that he wouldn't pay me a cent, and even more than that, he would sue me for malpractise.

"I knew that if I had been a man as big as he was, he would never have talked to me as he did.... But he did not even stop with that but went about in the community spreading slanderous rumors about me and blaming me for the condition of his wife."

Unable to floor him as a male doctor might have done, Bessie could only stop him from ruining her reputation by threatening him with a lawsuit.

"But a young lady doctor had other difficulties to contend with which would not affect her male counterparts in the same degree," Bessie said. One was the limitation of her physical strength in handling the traditional horse and buggy. The other was that her work made her more than usually vulnerable to assault. She described one such ordeal. "A severe thunderstorm had prevented me from leaving my office at the usual time one evening," she recounted, "and compelled me to remain there until quite late that night. On my way home after the rain I had to pass a livery barn. Livery barns in those days were sometimes known as the rendezvous of the rough element in the community, and sometimes transients would do some odd jobs around them for a night's lodging in the hay.

"I had to pass this barn every day and had never experienced the slightest annoyance. But this time the hour was very late, and the streets were completely deserted, the roads were muddy, the sidewalks dark, and the lights in the homes had already been extinguished.

"As I approached the barn, I noticed a dark figure in the background, partly hidden behind the trunk of a large tree. He remained motionless as I approached.

"I hesitated for a moment, but where could I go or what else could I do but go on?

"I accelerated my pace and grasped more firmly the instrument bag which I always carried with me for possible emergency calls. When I had passed the spot where I had seen the figure, I could hear a man was beginning to follow me. My heart began to beat furiously, I could almost hear it.

"I increased my gait still more, but as I walked faster so did the man behind me.

"Unless one has had a similar experience, he cannot understand the paralyzing terror that grips one under those circumstances. One feels as he does in a horrible nightmare, when in his dreams he is pursued by some frightful monster but is unable to move or to escape.

"The race between me and this unknown assailant continued for some time. I thought it was hours, but it was probably only a matter of minutes. I began to notice that the distance which had separated us was getting smaller and smaller, and despite all my efforts I was losing the race.

"At the moment when the man was close enough to reach out and grab me from the back, something gave me an impulse to stop. I turned abruptly, raised the heavy instrument bag in my right hand to the level of my head, and in a commanding voice which to my own surprise sounded as though it came from somewhere down deep within me, I said:

"'One more step forward and I will knock you down with this instrument bag.'

"The man halted, hesitated for a moment, stared at me while I kept my arm upraised and ready to strike, and then slowly began to back up, and finally he turned around and disappeared in the darkness from which he emerged.

"The man had probably watched the light in my office window. He evidently knew that I had to pass there sometime that night to go back to my boarding place and had been waiting for me to pass.

"I was calm and in complete self-control until I reached my room. But once I had closed the door behind me and had a feeling of security, a violent reaction set in, hard to understand or to explain. My calm gave way to a near hysteria. I began to sob and tremble in all my members, and it required considerable time before I had regained complete self-control."

Among other benefits marriage to a Lutheran pastor finally gave Bessie was the protection she needed from gossips and rapists. Shortly after the wedding, she and her husband moved to Pincher Creek in Alberta, which in the Eighties was being rapidly opened up for settlement by the building of the Canadian Pacific Railway. (A C.P.R. doctor, R.G. Brett, would become a lieutenant-governor of Alberta.) Following an offer by the government and the railway of free homesteads of 160 acres, there had been a scramble of immigrants into the territory, many of them Lutherans from Germany, Russia, Austria, Hungary, Poland, and other European countries. As their home churches had made no provision for the spiritual welfare of the flock in their new homeland, Lutheran bodies in the United States had undertaken the work, and Bessie's husband was one of these missionaries to Western Canada.

The move to Alberta was another painful adjustment that Dr. Bessie had to make to a way of life that she found shockingly different from the one she was used to. Canadians were "more European than American and distinctly British in character, with all that this implies," she noted darkly. The living accommodation was almost as much of a shock. The parsonage in Pincher Creek was a log house without central heating and with no insulation—in a territory where the winter temperature sometimes plunged to fifty below zero. The cellar of the house was no more than a hole in the ground. There was no indoor plumbing, and water had to be carried from a spring in the nearby hills.

Even her husband's second parsonage, in a residential area of Edmonton, had no central heating, though there was electricity and indoor plumbing.

As for the city streets, many of the sidewalks were of wooden construction, bordering roadbeds gouged with deep, hard ruts in winter and a sea of black, clinging gumbo in spring.

Still, Edmonton impressed Dr. Bessie with "its many colleges and theological schools," and as a medical centre serving a huge area of surrounding countryside.

The parsonage also served a considerable population of Lutherans. It was an open house for any homesteader, farmer, coal miner, or tradesman, complete with wife and children, and for young Lutheran ministers and spouses who were visiting the city for medical or dental care. Inevitably, some of the visitors took unfair advantage of the hospitality. In one case, Bessie's husband found a young woman living in desperate circumstances in a backstreet apartment house. He brought her home for Bessie to look after until the woman was able to return to her work as a nurse. Said Bessie, "She had not been in our house very long before I discovered the real cause of her trouble. She was not sick at all, as she pretended, but I found to my horror that she was a narcotic addict in an advanced stage. But now we had her in our home, and there was nothing we could do about it. There was no other place to which to send her. We could not put her out on the street. And there was no way to get rid of her unless we turned her over to the police. We naturally hesitated to do that.

So I cared for her for several weeks, though I myself was suffering much from a serious sinus ailment at that time.

"Then one day she made the mistake of taking an overdose of whatever drug she was getting. She went into a coma, and so we had to call a doctor [Bessie had not been licensed to practice in Alberta], and he notified the police and had her moved to the hospital. While she was there, I discovered that she had stolen various articles from me during her stay, among them a new pair of gloves my husband had just given me for my birthday, some of my best linens, and other articles."

Another Bessie, Elizabeth Scott, born in 1866 on a farm near Campbell-ford, Manitoba, was also encouraged to enter medical school on the promptings of a woman friend, Ellen Bilbrough. A pretty and impetuous girl with a delicious figure and decidedly stubborn lips, Elizabeth had left her job as a teacher in Manitoba to come East and help Miss Bilbrough in her charitable work. Ellen Bilbrough was an English gentlewoman who had built Marchmont House in Belleville, to care for boys and girls from the slums of Glasgow and Manchester, and prepare them for a useful life in Canada.

Elizabeth's liveliness, intelligence, and sympathetic attitude toward the slum girls in her charge, impressed Miss Bilbrough, and one day she took the girl aside and suggested that she was capable of better things than the voluntary work she was doing at present. "Because you're a woman, you think that such work is your fulfilment," Miss Bilbrough said, and went on to suggest that Elizabeth should aim higher. In fact, if she were interested in a medical career, she, Miss Bilbrough, was prepared to support her for one year at the Women's Medical College in Kingston.

Elizabeth was so overwhelmed by the generosity of the offer that she could barely stammer her thanks. But the reaction of her friend John Matheson, was disappointing. His was the usual attitude to women in medicine. When she wrote to tell him the exciting news, he wrote back that she should "abandon this difficult, foolish course for a woman," and suggested that she should marry him instead.

His letter very nearly ended their friendship forever.

John Matheson, nicknamed John Grace, had begun life as a lively and eager child. He had earned the nickname at the dinner table at home in Kildonan in the Red River colony, where he was always so noisy with chatter and excitement that his father had to shut him up with the words, "John—Grace." The words were repeated so frequently, that the rest of the children had started to call him John Grace, and the name had stuck.

At fifteen he was teaching school as well as handling a major share of the farm work. He was still teaching at the age of twenty when his father died and his mother remarried. Her new husband was a greedy farmer who had married for money. John was kicked out. From then on, he had drifted about the plains like tumbleweed.

Elizabeth had met the restless and disillusioned wanderer when she was nineteen, and it was obvious that he had fallen instantly in love with her. But she was not ready to marry, and besides, though he was a fine-looking six-footer, alert, vigorous and intelligent, and extremely popular with everyone he met, he was eighteen years older than she was, and had no direction in life except an erratic course from one frontier town or railway construction camp to another in the territory of Saskatchewan. Elizabeth had seen too many examples of that kind of aimless and often drunken existence when she was at school in Winnipeg, and she wanted none of it.

Still, she had kept up a correspondence with him, borne along, however unwillingly, on the tide of his love for her. Her letters, he told her, were all that made his life meaningful.

But now his own letter had come between them. It was only after he had written again, giving in to her ambitions and imploring her to continue writing to him, that she resumed the paper-thin friendship. All the same, his letter had made her more certain than ever that she could never love him in return.

The school Elizabeth attended in Kingston, the Women's Medical College, was affiliated with Queen's University. It had begun in the disorderly way that seemed to be typical of Ontario medical schools, through an anti-feminist revolt. A couple of years after the first half-dozen women were admitted to Queen's in 1880, the male students delivered an ultimatum to the faculty, announcing that if the women remained, they would not. They would transfer immediately to Trinity in Toronto. The faculty responded by creating a separate Women's Medical College. From then on, though the women might attend classes in chemistry and botany at the university, the classes in medicine were to be held in rooms on the top floor of the Kingston City Hall.

Despite this partial segregation, the girls still had to put up with a lot of rousting. The male students tended to pick on Elizabeth's friend, Mary Birmingham, in particular. The other girls, including Elizabeth, made special efforts to remain inconspicuous by being the first to take their places in the front row of the lecture theatre, but Mary was invariably late. She paid for her tardiness with an intimidating demonstration. "At Queen's," writes Elizabeth's biographer, Ruth Buck, "she [Mary Birmingham] would pause for a moment, alone at the top of the steps of the theatre, before she began her calm descent in the silence that always fell. If the professor had begun his lecture, that too would wait, for every head would turn to watch the lovely girl. Then the rhythmic stamp of the men's feet would begin, growing louder and louder, keeping time with each unhurried graceful step she took, only the soft colouring of her face giving the least indication that she heard them.

"One day, however, as she took her place beside Elizabeth, she murmured something; and a man behind tapped Elizabeth's shoulder. 'What did Miss Birmingham say?' The answer was unhesitating. He stood at once, turned to face the tiers of students, raised his arm for their attention, and declared solemnly, 'Gentlemen, Miss Birmingham says NUTS.'"

That young man and his friends, and probably most of the professors, still believed that women were incapable of intense and prolonged study. Accordingly, the girls had to work far harder than was really necessary, in order to prove the fatuity of this argument. Elizabeth was fortunate that she had her brother Tom with her, to sustain her belief in herself. It was Tom, in fact, who had urged her to come east in the first place, to help Ellen Bilbrough.

During her year at college, Elizabeth lived in the same boarding house as Tom and three of his friends. Her brother's support made a great deal of difference to Elizabeth, and was no small factor in her achievement in the spring examinations when in one exam alone, in botany, she received 100 percent.

The association with the four boys also had an effect on her appearance. She had her dark brown hair cut like a boy's to de-emphasize her sex. Actually the style made her look prettier than ever, and she kept it for several years.

Unhappily, she could not overcome the disadvantage of being a girl in the matter of summer employment. Unlike the men, there was no way for her to earn enough money during the summer to pay her way through the second year. Moreover she had no reserves; she had used up the miserable savings she had accumulated from four years of teaching in Manitoba, and Miss Bilbrough could not support her any longer. Elizabeth had to face up to it: her medical studies would have to be abandoned until she could save enough money to see herself through to graduation.

Elizabeth was about to commit herself to another job when she heard that the Presbyterian Board in Toronto were appealing for teachers for their mission in central India. The contract was for seven years, which would surely enable her to accumulate the necessary funds. So with a heavy heart at the prospect of a seven-year hiatus, she applied, and was accepted.

The news was a considerable shock to John Matheson. It had been bad enough when she had put thousands of miles between them by coming east to work for Miss Bilbrough, but even worse when she apprenticed herself for a further period to Minerva, goddess of medicine. Now she was talking about leaving the country entirely, and for seven years.

He was appalled. If she went, he wrote, he would lose her forever. He begged her to forget the whole idea, he could not bear it, his life would be useless without her. And to show how much she meant to him, he announced that he was prepared to pay for her entire course at Queen's, if she would even *consider* marrying him when she graduated.

It was not a tactful proposition to a proud woman, and her answer was cold and final. His importunities had upset her once too often. She had promised to go to India, and that was that, and now their friendship was at an end. If he wrote again she would not answer. She did not want to hear from him again.

This reply reduced John Matheson to despair. He had been saving as much money as he could in anticipation of the day when Elizabeth would finally consent to marry him. It had not seemed an impossible desire. Although his beard was now graying, he was still handsome and stalwart, hard-working, well liked because of his wit, his gift for mimicry, and his reputation as a story-teller, and he knew he had the ability that was only waiting for the conjoinment of a loving partner. But what was the point now? So, as Elizabeth sailed for India, he went back to roistering, to dancing Red River jigs in tavern company, to a wild life of poker-playing, horse-trading, and whiskey-smuggling. He started to give away what little money was left over from his reckless ways to almost anybody who wanted it or needed it. He had finally given up.

As it turned out, Elizabeth was back in Canada within two years, her health half-ruined by the fevers of India. But perhaps the experience had done more damage than that. The East sometimes had a debilitating effect on the will as well as the body, and the Elizabeth who returned to the farm that her family was now living on, in Tyner, North Dakota, was not the strong, stubborn girl who had shown the men at Queen's University that she had as much talent, application, and intelligence as any of them. Even though it was not her fault that she had had to give up the mission work in India, —the Presbyterian doctors had insisted on it for the sake of her health—she felt disillusioned and discouraged. So that when John Grace, now in New Westminster, B.C., ventured to write and express his joy at her return and tell her that Jesus Christ had reformed him, she give in, and wrote him back the first words of love she had ever uttered to him.

His reply was ecstatic. "My darling, my darling, how much happiness I owe that letter, how proud a man I am to know that you came out of the trial as a *woman* and showed me love that is not sentimental dross, that is worth a man's life, worth waiting for these six years. God bless you and keep you safe, and bring you speedily to me, your lover till death."

When they met in Vancouver, Elizabeth suggested hesitantly that perhaps now she could return to Queen's—a friend had broached the subject of a loan, which would enable her to graduate. But John's reaction was so intense at the idea of yet another separation from her, that her already faltering determination collapsed completely. In the words of her biographer and daughter, Ruth Buck, "Now she told him that she would not return to Medical College, not ever. She would be content and happy simply to be his wife, and she would marry him as soon as possible."

John, by then doing small contracting jobs for the railways, had been converted to religion. "With some companions, he had been wandering along streets in the roughest section of New Westminster, looking for any idle amusement. They came, in the same spirit, to a meeting held by two Methodist revivalists from Toronto. And in that crowded hall, John Matheson had experienced the amazing force of true conversion."

After the marriage, the reformed roisterer volunteered for mission work, was taken on by the Anglican Church and sent to the St. Barnabas Anglican Mission at Onion Lake on the Fort Carlton-Fort Edmonton trail, in the depths of Saskatchewan. There, John's fluent knowledge of the Cree language made him particularly effective. The church ordained him a few years later.

Now a married woman, Elizabeth lived for four years in reasonable content. Gray's *Anatomy* was laid aside forever, she believed, in favour of the grammar textbook; for she had taken up teaching again, in the schoolhouse that her husband had built for the Indian children, and, in due course for her own children.

For a while after their marriage, Elizabeth had felt somewhat disturbed by John's conversion. In his religious zeal, it seemed to her that he was striving too earnestly for piety, falsifying his real nature—perhaps, partly, to impress her with his worth. But now she needed no further proof, and was quite relieved when in time his true self reasserted itself: the robustious, life-loving character that had earned so many friends throughout the northwest and British Columbia.

By the time he amassed enough trading goods to make a trip to Edmonton worthwhile, John had thoroughly reconciled his religious beliefs with his robust outlook. (The trading trip, with bales of fur and bags of seneca root—used in medicine as an expectorant —was on behalf of the Mission. Like the Hudson's Bay Company, which required its surgeons to minister to the account book as well as to the patient, the church also liked its ministers to double as traders.) Consequently, on his arrival in Edmonton, the river men were able to reconcile his roistering past with his missionary present without too much surprise or dismay.

The reaction of one of John's friends was not untypical. She was the wife of the superintendent of the North West Mounted Police. He met her while he was on is way back from Edmonton with his river scows, and stopped off at Fort Saskatchewan. When she saw him striding up the street: "Matheson! By the living lights—John Grace" roared the jolly lady. "Haven't seen you in years. Come on in for dinner. What're you doing now?"

"Working for the Master," he replied with a cheerful reverence.

"Fine—bring him along too," she roared.

Even by 1895, Elizabeth had not been jarred out of her complacency. A doctor was desperately needed in the Indian reserve and surrounding communities, but she refused to let it trouble her. Even several fatalities that might have been prevented could the doctors have come quickly, and been sober, did not rouse her. Until one day, when an Indian named Ayimihos (He Who Knows Misfortune) came to her with a gangrenous foot. Though amputation was essential, she refused to do it.

The Indian looked at her. Was it not true that she had studied for one-third of the time required to make a white medicine woman? Elizabeth repeated in her halting Cree that she did not have enough experience. She did not dare to operate.

The Indian stared at her uncomprehendingly. Desperate she turned to her husband and cried, "Explain to him that I cannot do it, that he must go to Battleford, or get Mr. Mann to send for the doctor."

Ayimihos said something contemptuously in Cree, and turned away. "He says you are a coward," John Grace said quietly. "He will not wait for a doctor to come. He will not go to Battleford. If he must die, it will be here amongst his own people."

The next day, Ayimihos did the amputation himself with the aid of his son, using a hunting knife and a carpenter's saw. But the mutilated stump festered, and gangrene again appeared. Once more Ayimihos appealed to Elizabeth for help. Once again her courage failed her, and she told him to go to a doctor. Again he cut and sawed off the end of his own leg. Somehow, with few antiseptic precautions and no anesthetic, he survived the ordeal.

Elizabeth stubbornly turned her thoughts back to her teaching, her children, and her household duties. She was genuinely happy in her work for the mission. Besides, she had promised to give up medicine when she married John, and it had been the right decision. The mission work was so extensive that they had had to take on an extra helper, Annie Phillips, a charming and intelligent girl in her early twenties. Annie had brought energy and evangelical fervour to the work of the mission. The fact that the girl was obviously in love with John Matheson did not cause Elizabeth any real concern. She was confident that he loved only her. As for her love for John, it had, if anything, increased over the years.

Anyway, she had two little girls to bring up, so she had not the slightest reason to feel guilty over the Ayimihos incident. If she were justified in feeling anything, resentment over the disturbance to her routine was surely more appropriate.

But shortly after the incident, John asked her to go for a walk with him into the hills that overlooked the mission at Onion Lake. When she sat at the crest of the hill, he asked her if she agreed that Annie was capable of taking over Elizabeth's share of the work.

At first, Elizabeth could not understand what he was getting at, until he finally came out with it. The mission desperately needed a doctor. It was true what Ayimihos had said, that Battleford was too far to go for medical aid. It was her responsibility to their joint work that she should go back to college.

The irony of the situation left her first speechless, then dismayed, then bitterly angry. It was John who had protested in the first place at the idea of her taking up medicine. It was he who had finally dissuaded her four years previously from resuming her studies. Now, just as she had adjusted to the new heading, as she had settled into a peaceful, meaningful routine, he was forcing her back onto her original course, a course that would now be infinitely harder to follow, because she had lost seven years; the seven years when her mind was at its most receptive.

She couldn't do it. Why should she give up everything that had grown so dear to her, her household routine and her work with the Indian children and her own two lovely little girls—and she suspected, a third child on the way—to submit herself to the grinding toil of memorizing ten thousand names of parts, to months of fatigue in ward and operating theatre? Not only that. In suggesting that Annie, a mere domestic who had left school at fourteen, could replace her at the mission, John was devaluing her own contributions to the work. She felt bitterly hurt and resentful.

They quarreled, their voices competing with the wind at the top of the hill. But her resentment showed that she had given in. John had made the position clear. Whether she liked it or not, he was determined, for the sake of his beloved mission, to send her back to college.

It was decided. She would go to Winnipeg, and stay with her husband's younger sister. The two girls would stay at Poplar Point with an aunt.

Her resentment was now joined by a cold stubbornness. She knew she was pregnant again. If she had to return to college, there was no point in putting it off. Another lost year would only make things all the harder for her. So she said nothing to John about the expected child until it was too late to change the plans.

Elizabeth was accepted readily enough at the new medical college in Winnipeg. She received credit for her first year at Kingston and also for two second-year courses in chemistry and botany that she had completed seven years previously. But her morale was not improved when she found that she was the only woman attending the medical school that year.

Despite her mental and physical discomfort—Elizabeth's third child, another girl, would weigh-in at eleven pounds—she passed the term examinations at Christmas. "She then went to see Dr. J. R. Jones, the lecturer in obstetrics, who was acting Dean. When she said that she would be withdrawing he surprised her by trying to dissuade her. She was a good student, he told her. Had anyone made the year difficult for her as a woman? He knew that that had been the experience of women in other colleges. His concern amused her, and she laughed. 'I wasn't expecting to have to tell you, Dr. Jones, that I am seven months pregnant.'"

After this third daughter was born, and left with another foster mother, a Mrs. Stewart of Saskatoon, Elizabeth, who had been unutterably lonely as the only woman at the Winnipeg school, decided to take her third year at the Ontario Medical College for Women in Toronto. (The college in Kingston had closed down in the meantime.) Elizabeth was seriously ill by the time she arrived in the Ontario capital. The abrupt separation from her baby had brought on a recurrence of an old complaint, mastitis, and one breast was swollen and painful. When Dr. Wishart, the registrar of the college, examined her, he insisted that she was not fit to continue her studies. She insisted that she had to. She told him, "If you knew my husband, you would understand. The work we are doing means everything to him, and I cannot fail him. I don't think I could forgive myself, nor could I return to him a failure."

"Without her knowledge," said her biographer, "Dr. Wishart wrote to John Matheson, urging him to recall her, advising him that she was not well enough to undertake such work. He was answered with a telegram, referring him to Luke 9:62: 'No man, having put his hand to the plough, and looking back, is fit for the kingdom of God.'"

John Grace could certainly not be considered a weak man where his wife was concerned. As it turned out, Elizabeth slowly recovered under Dr. Wishart's care, and after successfully completing her third year, she returned to Saskatoon, to claim her third child from Mrs. Stewart. The baby, Letitia, had been handed over to this perfect stranger when, on their way through Saskatoon, Elizabeth and John had camped on the river bank and John had gone up to the lady's house to get water from the well. Mrs. Stewart had been entranced by the baby, and had pleaded with Elizabeth to let her look after it while Elizabeth was at medical school. Mrs. Stewart seemed a perfect foster mother.

Now Mrs. Stewart showed reluctance to surrender the child. When Elizabeth called in the evening, Mrs. Stewart said that Letitia was asleep and shouldn't be disturbed. Early next morning she would not co-operate in encouraging the little girl to adjust to her real mother. Though the stagecoach that Elizabeth had to catch was leaving shortly, Letitia was still in her nightdress. Mrs. Stewart told Elizabeth that she wanted to keep the child until Elizabeth graduated.

It was plain to Elizabeth that the woman considered her an unnatural mother who had been willing to abandon her children in order to become a doctor. Mrs. Stewart was determined to save Letitia from such a dreadful woman. A miserable scene followed, the foster mother pleading, the mother adamant. Further delaying tactics followed. Mrs. Stewart had dumped all of Letitia's clothes in a tub of cold water outside the house. She claimed that she had been about to wash them out, but the clothes were clean, some of them still in neat folds. In a cold fury, Elizabeth wrung out the garments and bundled them together; and walked away with the wet clothes under one arm and the struggling, screaming child under the other.

"The stage was waiting for them. Elizabeth set the child on the high seat of the democrat, and climbed up beside her. Letitia was quite silent now, a small withdrawn person, making no response to the friendliness of the driver, nor to her mother's efforts to interest her. Nothing in Elizabeth's experience or studies could have indicated to her that a child, to whom no harshness or unkindness had been intended, could still suffer shock in this second disruption of all that was familiar to her.

"When they made their stops along the trail, Letitia would not walk, but only crept; and Elizabeth, knowing nothing of such regression was vexed with a stubborn child. 'She has turned against me,' was all that she could think. 'Will it be the same with the others? Have I lost them too?'

When they got home, after some hesitation, Letitia responded warmly to her father. But John Grace had little sympathy for his wife. He thought that she was being too impatient with the child. Elizabeth felt disquieted, frustrated, and more alone than ever.

Her final year in medicine was an ordeal of grinding study and further ill health, but in April 1898, she received her degree from Trinity College.

The triumph seemed only to plunge her deeper into torment. When she arrived home she found that her position at the mission had been usurped by a presumptuous Annie Phillips. Elizabeth was rended with jealousy, and it did not help in the least that the jealousy made her despise herself. She felt utterly useless. Nobody seemed to need her anymore, not her husband, nor her children, nor even the people who were supposed to have needed her so desperately. She set up a dispensary and waited for recognition as a doctor, but it did not come. The Indians preferred their own medicine men, and the employees of the government, the Hudson's Bay Company, and the Mounted Police still telegraphed to Battleford for medical aid, distrusting a woman doctor.

She found she could no longer regard her husband with the same unreserved love and affection. He gave most of himself to the work of the mission. He had laid down a course for her as if she were a hospital ship and he a fleet commander, but now they both seemed rudderless. And he was getting old. He was fifty, his hair was turning white. "Where was the eager response to every challenge, the ready wit and laughter, the former happiness of their work together?" John wondered. And Elizabeth could only ask herself the same questions. Had those attributes too been taken from her, assumed by another, so that her role could be only a secondary one? Or had she really changed? Was it the company of young students interested in their work but sharing the normal interests and dreams of youth, that had wakened this yearning in her for a life of her own, not this negation, this constant, demanding absorption in the lives of others?"

Toward the end of the year of her graduation, pregnant again, sick and in despair, Elizabeth got out of a sleepless bed one morning and crawled to the dispensary, intent on killing herself. She had just enough strength left to resist the final humiliation of suicide. Miserably, she went back to bed on hands and knees.

Slowly, as her work and responsibility as a doctor increased, she began to regain a sense of purpose, and her black depression lifted—just in time for her to face the final challenge to her self-respect, from the College of Physicians and Surgeons of the Northwest Territories.

One of the purposes of the college, which had been created in 1888, was to licence medical practitioners to practice in the northwest. Those deemed to be qualified were not required to sit the examination set by the college. Many men with British degrees successfully took advantage of this concession.

Elizabeth, however, though a graduate of the second most-esteemed medical school in the country, was informed that she would have to come to Calgary to sit the examination.

She was not particularly surprised. She had met too many medical big-wigs who resented a woman's intrusion into what they considered to be a strictly male profession. She was furiously angry all the same, especially as she understood that two men who had graduated with her from Trinity, and who were currently practicing in the territories, had been registered without such an examination.

She refused to submit to this rank discrimination.

Fortunately the College of Physicians and Surgeons were not yet prepared to make an issue of it, probably because she was the only doctor in the district along the Fort Carlton-Fort Edmonton trail, and so was not in direct competition with any of their registered men.

Perhaps they were also hesitant to act against her because another official body had recognized her. When smallpox broke out in her area in 1901, the commissioner of health for the Northwest Territories had appointed her as their agent to combat the outbreak.

As the years went by and the local population increased, other doctors began to compete in the area, and Elizabeth knew that she would have to regularize her position very soon. Accordingly she reapplied for registration. Once again she was told that she would have to submit to an examination by the college, to see if she were competent to practice in their territory—this after she had been practicing in it for five years.

Resistance to a medical bureaucracy was not unprecedented. There was a doctor in New Brunswick, for instance, who was busily fighting the New Brunswick Medical Council on the same issue at the same time. He was "a most independent doctor who had trained in the U.S. and moved to New Brunswick where he steadfastly refused to register and pay the $1.00 annual fee," wrote W.B. Stewart in his *Medicine in New Brunswick*. "For years, the next order of business following the minutes was 'what the hell are we going to do about Dr....?'" Who, in spite of being prosecuted by the Medical Council, fined, kicked out of his job as Chairman of the Board of Health, ordered to resign from the Community Hospital, and hit with sundry other punitive measures, continued to dodge the Council until finally he capitulated, took his examinations, paid his fee and registered, twenty years later.

Elizabeth was a woman of considerable strength of will, but her sense of duty was too strong now to permit her the luxury of stubbornness. Muffling her pride she gave in, but after so many years she was not likely to pass the examination without a refresher course, so she decided to take her fourth year again. Making the now all-too-familiar arrangements for her children, including her fourth child, a boy, she registered at the Manitoba Medical College.

Once again, Elizabeth was the only woman in the class, but she was now much more confident in her relationships with others, and this time she was not lonely and disheartened, but stimulated by the company of others in the profession. Every morning she arose at four to study, to attend to her baby before leaving him with his Indian nurse, and to walk to the college at McDermott and Kate, or to the clinic at the hospital, across a stretch of open prairie.

At the final examinations she had one more difficulty to face: Dr. Chown. Henry Havelock Chown was one of the country's most famous surgeons and teachers. He had joined the staff of the Manitoba Medical College three years after its founding in 1883, and later became professor of surgery. When Elizabeth met him, he was dean of the college.

He was also a graduate of Queen's, a university not then noted for its tolerance toward women in the profession, and Elizabeth's encounter with him for her oral examination in surgery was not propitious. To begin with, she was in an angry mood because as she was going into the examination room, a fellow student had, in a hurried whisper, given her the answer to one of the questions. Elizabeth, confident in her ability, was thoroughly annoyed by the gratuitous advice, and was still in that mood when Dr. Chown asked his first question. Ignoring her fellow student's whispered advice, she started to "diagnose by the process of elimination, rather than give the only obvious answer."...Dr. Chown stopped her. Impatiently, he directed her to other cases, each of which she was certain she diagnosed quickly and correctly."

When the list of graduates was posted she was stunned to find her name not on it.

After composing herself, in a manner that later inspired her student friends to present her with a bunch of roses, she went to the dean.

"'I've come to ask if I may have a hood for graduation?' His surprise was evident. 'But you are not graduating.' 'You are mistaken, Dr. Chown. I am already a doctor, and I am convinced that I have actually passed every test here. You must know that my work has been satisfactory.'

"He stood up. 'That's what others say. There's a faculty meeting now, and I'll bring the matter up. I can't say that I'm in favour of women in Medicine. This is a man's profession.'"

But when he returned from the meeting, his manner had changed, and he now addressed her with respect, as Dr. Matheson, and gave her the hood.

As soon as she returned home, she applied for the third time for registration in the Northwest Territories.

Incredibly, the answer was the same. She would have to sit for an examination in Calgary.

Whatever Elizabeth felt, it was too much for John Matheson. "'Call their bluff,' he snapped, and wrote the cheque for her fifty-dollar fee."

Her registration came by the next mail. Sixteen years after starting her course in medicine, Elizabeth Matheson was finally officially recognized as a doctor.

22

King Murrough of Manitoba

A S THE WEEKLY train from Winnipeg wailed into town, Dr. Murrough O'Brien gazed out the window for the first view of his new home. He had seen enough of the West by 1897 not to expect too much in the way of urban sophistication, so he was not surprised to find that, in spite of its grandiose name, the town was little more than two rows of squat, frame buildings along a single street — no doubt named Main Street. Dominion City, population 300.

There seemed to be about four shops altogether. Plus two hotels, a livery stable, a lumber yard, an agricultural implement dealer, a couple of blacksmith shops, and a Chinese laundry. The owner of the laundry had probably been imported originally to work on the railways. Wooden sidewalks lurched along both sides of the single street of sun-baked mud, but where the business section petered out, so did the boardwalks.

The rest of the scene was of prairie grassland, with the Roseau River scrawled across it. He could see no telephone lines. Well, that was probably a good thing. If people needed him in the middle of the night they would have to come and fetch him, and thus supply him with free transportation.

A fair proportion of the population was waiting for him as the train grinded to a halt with a wincing screech of metal. The delegation included George Agnew, one of the town merchants, who had corresponded with Dr. O'Brien, and Dave Phillips, the owner and editor of the local newspaper, who was also a hardware merchant and tinsmith.

As Dominion City's first doctor stepped down from the coach, surrounded by wisps of steam, the crowd looked him over critically. He seemed a bit old to have recently graduated from the Manitoba Medical College. Still, maybe that wasn't such a bad thing. Last sort of person they wanted was some twenty-one-year-old youth, still wet behind the ears. Which would have made O'Brien very wet indeed, for he had extensive ears. They stuck out even further than his big nose.

The editor took in the newcomer's short, broad-shouldered figure and aggressive chin, and decided that he looked tough enough for the job. But to make sure he asked, "Do you take a drink?"

On receiving a cautious affirmative from the doctor—cautious in case this was a test question from a rabid temperancer—the welcoming committee led the way to the bar of the Queen's Hotel— *"Good Accommodation for Man and Beast"*—and Murrough O'Brien was suitably launched on his medical career.

Next day Murrough plodded down Main Street, looking for a place to hang up his shingle which Dave Phillips had kindly offered to design for him. The shed at the rear of Lim Yee's laundry looked as if it would fill the bill—a five-dollar bill, which was about as much as he could afford to pay for a month's rent.

Having negotiated with the grinning laundryman, Murrough quickly collected a few items of furniture, including some shelving to support a pair of coal-oil lamps, and two old kitchen chairs, one for the client, one for himself. Additional shelves were hammered to the walls to support his drugs, ointments, and five basic surgical instruments, including dental forceps. Next, the cracker-barrel that George Agnew had given him was rolled in. It was a perfect stand for a washbasin. Fortunately there was no need to spend money on window curtains. There were no windows in the hut.

Ready for business, Murrough had only an hour or two to wait before his first customer walked in. As the man was holding his face and complaining about an aching tooth, the diagnosis was simple enough. However, it was so dark in the hut that Murrough could hardly see into the patient's mouth. So they moved outside, and he extracted the tooth in the sunlight, with the patient clinging to the kitchen chair and the Chinese laundryman, who had come out to watch, interestedly following the doctor's every move. Thus Murrough earned his first fifty cents as a G.P.

There being no further business that morning, he repaired to the Queen's for lunch. There he met, in the words of O'Brien's biographer, Robert Tyre, "a thin, bony female of spinsterish aspect who responded with great sociability when George [the hotel proprietor] made the introductions."

As is the way with people who believe that any social encounter with a doctor entitles them to a free consultation, a lady asked if there was anything he could do about her chronic cold feet. After she had rejected his suggestion that a blood tonic might help, Murrough facetiously suggested that she should get herself a husband, adding, "They're wonderful for cold feet."

It seemed to him that the spinster's reaction was a trifle excessive — almost as if she thought he was proposing himself for the role of foot-warmer. He thought no more about it, and went back to his shed to wait for the next client, who turned out to be a mother whose baby had fallen off a cow.

That case having been dealt with satisfactorily, Murrough attended to his third patient that day, a powerful-looking fellow who was complaining with some justification about an egg-sized abscess on his right forearm. This case also proved to be slightly out of the ordinary, for the moment Murrough applied his lancet to the abscess, the patient's left fist jerked up by reflex action and connected with the doctor's jaw. Murrough went down with a crash that almost shook his office apart.

As compensation for his swollen cheek, Murrough felt amply justified in adding a fifty percent surcharge to his fee, bringing it up to three dollars.

His second day as a medical practitioner was no more propitious. He had hardly settled into his outhouse office and neatly set out his dental forceps, dressing scissors, thermometer, obstetrical forceps, and hypodermic syringe, when Lim Yee capered up, simpering and exhibiting his teeth. Lim Yee had come to congratulate the doctor on his forthcoming marriage. He had heard all about Dr. O'Brien's proposal to the local schoolteacher.

After he had gotten over his surprise, the physician angrily corrected the Chinaman on this point, and told him forcefully not to spread any more dreadful rumours like that. But it was too late. The news was already all over town, Lim Yee explained, that the new doctor had offered his hand, and various other extremities, to the schoolteacher in the Queen's Hotel, and, presumably after another night of cold feet, she had decided to accept.

The next visitor, Dave Phillips, confirmed it. He had come along to find out if Murrough and the lady had set a date. He would like to put it in the paper. In mounting frustration, Murrough attempted to disillusion the editor, but Phillips seemed to think that the doctor was trying to weasel out of the engagement.

It was not until Murrough roared that he would cut his throat rather than marry "that blathering bag of bones," that the editor, no longer able to keep a straight face, confirmed that, though the spinster was indeed spreading the word that the doctor had proposed to her, she had been pulling that stunt for years, so far without success.

A further cause for Dominion City hilarity occurred when Murrough delivered his first baby and it turned out to be mentally defective, the embarrassment in this case being that the parents had named the baby after him.

Like Elizabeth Matheson, it had taken Murrough an exceptionally long time to graduate; only, in his case it was entirely his own fault, the consequence of stiff-necked pride when, failing his finals in London and too proud to ask his father for a second chance, he emigrated to Canada.

The trouble was that the O'Briens were not used to failure. Theirs was an important family, directly descended from a king who had ruled in Ireland half a century before England was conquered by the Normans. Even the fifty-seventh king of Thomond, after whom Murrough was named, could not be considered a failure. True, when confronted by the rampaging Henry VIII and presented with the choice of losing either his crown or his head, King Murrough O'Brien preferred to surrender the former. But, there was no dishonour in that. No O'Brien ever lost his head in an emergency. Besides, ex-King Murrough was compensated with two lesser titles, Earl of Thomond and Baron Inchiquin.

By the time our Murrough was born in India in 1868, an English-oriented tradition was firmly established. The boys went to the best schools, then on to Oxford, Cambridge, or the Royal Military College at Sandhurst, and thereafter were expected to render high service to the state, and to accumulate as many laurels and titles as was consistent with honour and duty; while the girls were expected to marry men of suitable pedigree and accomplishment. (Murrough's two brothers amply maintained the tradition, one climaxing a distinguished career in the army and the civil service by becoming an author, while the other became governor of Malta.) Murrough managed to conform to this mould right up to his final year at St. Mary's Hospital Medical School, where he studied under a galaxy of well-known medical men. They included Braxton Hix, the discoverer of fetal movements, Sir William Broadbent, heart specialist and physician to Queen Victoria, Arthur Conan Doyle, who came down from Edinburgh to lecture on forensic science— Murrough understood that Dr. Conan Doyle also wrote stories for the *Strand Magazine*—and a visiting professor from St. Bartholomew's who was passionate on the subject of venereal diseases. "Scorn bad women, gentlemen," he could thunder at the students. "Remember, the pleasure is momentary, the position ludicrous, and the expense is damnable." Then adding, with an emphasis that seemed about to have an element of personal outrage to it, "I say *damnable*, gentlemen!"

Throughout his medical training, the young student with the Dumbo ears and redoubtable nose, lived a life of ease and some privilege. His father in India was deputy commissioner of the Punjab and provided

Murrough with a handsome allowance that enabled him to travel abroad in style and to attend the races at Ascot in the proper attire. He had his own valet. He had rich relatives who were happy to treat him to Drury Lane or to dinner at their private clubs, or introduce him to other established figures. One such was Sir Peter Edlin, a magistrate whom Murrough was to meet again in less sociable circumstances. One afternoon, Murrough picked up a girl in Piccadilly Circus, "a piquant young thing sporting a gay parasol, and being especially vulnerable after a tiring session in the dissecting-room, I acknowledged her smile with one of my own. Well, maybe I did smile first. At any rate, we got the preliminaries over with and set out arm in arm for a stroll."

Murrough thought she was a well-bred young woman, even if she did giggle alot—until she met another young woman with whom she was acquainted, but not on a friendly basis. The two of them ended up kicking, biting, and tearing at each other's hair, not to mention some fancy fencing work with their parasols. As no O'Brien had ever been known to leave a battlefield in flight, Murrough joined in, and was promptly arrested by a Bobby, who marched all three of them to the Bow Street quod—where Murrough found himself up before the magistrate with whom he had been dining only a few days previously.

Luckily, Sir Peter was a good sort. Pretending not to recognize the great-nephew of Lord Inchiquin, he merely fined him a quid, and then invited him to tea.

There was much more disapproval a year or so later when Murrough failed his final examination in surgical pathology. At St. Mary's Medical School this meant that he had to take his fourth year over again. But when he wrote to India, asking for another year of remittances, he received a considerable shock. His father curtly refused.

Though he could easily have obtained help from other relatives, Murrough, bitter and humiliated, turned away from the family. Shortly afterward, he received a letter from a fellow student who had fled to Manitoba in similar circumstances. He told Murrough that there was a pretty good school out there; the Manitoba Medical College. Murrough promptly packed his bags and sailed for Canada, his shame at letting down the side cleverly disguised as affronted pride.

In the summer of 1890, Winnipeg was still a raw frontier settlement. The Riel Rebellion of five years before had not helped to encourage outside investment and a suitable supply of immigrants; which made the little town's possession of a full-fledged medical school all the more surprising.

Four years elapsed before Murrough was able to accumulate enough money to attend this school. His first job, as a porter in a hotel near the railway station, did not advance his ambition much, as it was an unpaid position. It was also a rather dangerous one. He had been working there for only a few days, emptying spittoons and lugging drunken customers up to bed, when he was awakened one night by the hotel's proprietor, who ordered him, as a former medical student, to see to the woman in "Number Seven." She was offending the rest of the clientele with her moans of pain. Murrough, who was sharing an alcove under the stairs with the hotel buckets and mops, pulled on his trousers and, naked to the waist, reluctantly followed his employer to Number Seven, where the groans were coming from. The proprietor unlocked the door, shoved Murrough inside, and then hurriedly departed, in case it was something serious.

The patient, a whisky-reeking blonde, was twisting about on the bed fully dressed. When Murrough asked her what the matter was she indicated that she had terrible pain in her stomach. Murrough was just in the process of loosening her skirt when the lady's husband came lurching into the room—and an exceedingly large and aggressive-looking spouse he was, too. Seeing Murrough, naked to the waist, disheveled and wearing no shoes or socks, fumbling about with his wife's skirt, the bruiser demanded to know what he was up to. At which point the blonde on the bed clutched at her lower body and delivered the worst line of dialogue she could possibly have uttered in the circumstances, to whit, "It hurts." Immediately the husband started to advance on Murrough with apparently murderous intent.

Somehow Murrough felt that given the circumstances—the dialogue, the lady's moans and clutchings, and his own disheveled and half-naked appearance, and the fact that the outraged husband was advancing on him—he was not in a good position to convince the husband that he was a medical man. And so, recollecting that no O'Brien had ever fled a battlefield without good reason, he flung himself through the nearest exit, the second-floor window, and landed outside in a heap of dung. Whereupon, deciding that hotel work was not his cup of tea, he proceeded immediately to Portage la Prairie.

After a stint as a ploughman behind "a seedy-looking ox," he worked for a while for the Manitoba-Northwestern Railway, until a ferocious fight with a bullying construction boss got him fired. That winter was spent in farming, at Reaburn, Manitoba. It was while he was there that his father, presumably regretting his hasty response to the bad news from St. Mary's, wrote to him, offering to finance him in a farming career if he would settle down at it properly.

His timing could not have been worse. Among his chores, Murrough had over three dozen pigs to look after. Though naturally clean animals, pigs are as prolific in manure as in progeny, and Murrough was thoroughly fed-up with cleaning up after them. In fact, he was quite disenchanted with farming altogether. So he declined, telling his father that it was still his intention to continue in medicine.

It was their last exchange of letters. Three years later, while has was out riding near Delhi, the deputy commissioner's horse threw him over a precipice.

Thereafter, Murrough worked as a dog teamster, hauling fish between Lake Manitoba and Reaburn, as a teacher in a half-breed settlement, as assistant to the druggist, then to a vet, and as an actor in the Caroline-Gage Theatrical Company. This last, though it enabled him to see a good deal of the country, hardly brought him a dollar closer to a medical diploma. But he could not resist the adventure. "I took low comedy roles," he told his biographer, "and in between the acts I went out front to sing popular music hall ditties with the idea of keeping the audience quiet and peaceful. This was a precarious assignment. Most of the time my vocal efforts were well-received, but occasionally they provoked a hostile reaction. Audiences of those days always seemed to be equipped with things to throw—vegetables and ripe eggs. At the first sign of hostilities I would duck behind the curtain, and the prettiest girl in the company would be sent out to look helpless and frightened and thus win the sympathy of the audience and cool its urge to heave things."

He joined the company at Portage la Prairie. From there it moved to Brandon, where he was tried out as Bumble the Beadle in *Oliver Twist*. On one occasion when he was playing this role, a cowboy who felt that Mr. Bumble was giving Oliver a raw deal, came after Murrough with a gun. Fortunately, a policeman in the audience intervened and calmed the cow-puncher. After the performance Murrough learned that his saviour was Inspector Francis J. Dickens, the son of the author of *Oliver Twist*. Which suggested to Murrough that Charles Dickens' son was not entirely dissatisfied with his performance, otherwise he would surely have let the gunman go ahead.

The tour ended abruptly at Banff, Alberta, when three-quarters of the company came down with typhoid. It was only after he had spent a further two years as a coal miner and as a doctor's dispenser at Canmore, British Columbia, that Murrough was able to save enough money to take himself back to Winnipeg and get through at least part of the course at the Manitoba Medical College.

Winnipeg at the time was still a raw, frontier town that seemed to be composed mostly of mud. Years previously, Murrough's first impression of it had been of its black, muddy streets. It had changed little in the meantime, except that there seemed to be more mud than ever. The first two asphalt pavements, on McDermid off Main, and on Assiniboine Avenue, were still five years away. A few stretches of roadway were covered with gravel—half-heartedly, because the gravel soon disappeared into the gumbo—and in the shopping areas there were a few blocks of pavement created from sawed-off tree trunks, six or eight inches deep. Otherwise, it was boot-squelching, skirt-lifting country.

One of the principal problems of the mud was in parking a horse. Horses were usually hitched to a fifteen-pound weight, which was attached to the bridle by a strap. The horse was anchored by dropping the weight onto the ground. If there were a few dry days, there was no difficulty in upping anchor again, but if it rained it sometimes took the muscle power of a policeman to haul the flatiron out of the muck. But as least the mud was well-lit. Every street corner had a brilliant arc light with a carbon terminal.

As for the police, they were a striking feature of Winnipeg in the 1890s. The city had ambitious height requirements for its gendarmerie, and not one of them was under six feet five inches tall. In winter when they donned their buffalo fur coats they must have attracted many a nostalgic glance from the Metis buffalo hunters.

As for the buildings, there were several quite impressive structures, including the new Winnipeg City Hall, the Manitoba Hotel, the McIntyre Block, and the city's first apartment building, the Assiniboine Block. The Medical College, however, was not one of them. It was a two-storey brick building three blocks from the General Hospital, and its facilities were severely limited.

Nevertheless, it had high standards, and an exceptional faculty that included Henry Chown, surgery; R. M. Simpson, medicine; Robert Blanchard, anatomy; Gordon Bell, bacteriology and pathology; and A. H. Ferguson, clinical surgery. To Murrough's dismay, the faculty after considering his history of ditch-digging, hog-calling, coal-mining, acting, portering, and drifting, informed him that he would have to take his entire medical course all over again.

Murrough accepted the verdict resignedly, and got down to work; to enough effect that the dean later credited him a year for his time spent at St. Mary's.

During most of his three years at the Medical College, Murrough shared a cheap room with a fellow student in a rooming house on Notre Dame Avenue, which was also the abode of three harlots. He would board there, until he graduated, living, as he told one startled Winnipeg matron, off the avails of prostitution. He had too contrary a sense of humour to explain that the contributions of Sadie, Rose, and Celeste, were entirely gastronomic, in that they had taken an interest in the welfare of the two students when they saw how poor they were, and had taken to feeding them bacon and eggs, jam and pastry.

His mischievous remark to the Winnipeg matron led to no further trouble from that quarter except a refusal to invite him back again, but the remark he uttered during a medical association dinner could have led to much worse trouble. The main speaker of the evening was a Protestant clergyman, who droned on at such length that finally Gordon Bell, the professor of bacteriology and pathology, muttered to Murrough, "O'Brien, tell that old fool to shut up."

The remark was merely an exasperated letting-off of steam, but the said O'Brien, who was alcoholically vulnerable to suggestion, immediately jumped to his feet and bawled, "Shut up, you old fool!"

Naturally Murrough was on the carpet the next day, before the dean, Dr. J. Wilford Good, an ear, nose, and throat specialist. He was also an eye specialist, both ophthalmologically and in staring down unruly juniors. As Murrough stood before the dean, "the blue eyes pierced Murrough now and the dry voice said, 'You are a tactless creature, O'Brien. Your London training, no doubt. Out here we show more respect for the Cloth. And besides, it's good business. First thing a smart doctor does when he goes into practice is make friends with the local clerics. As you go through life butchering patients with your knife and annihilating them with faulty diagnosis, you will need that friendship. You would be surprised, O'Brien, how often the soothing, flattering phrases of a funeral oration assuage the grief of relatives and turn their thoughts away from law suits.'"

(The unpredictable dean was worthy of a portrait study himself. One day—it was while a newly graduated Murrough was working for him as an assistant—Dr. Good walked out of his office without a word to anyone, and failed to return the next day. Or the next week—or the next month. Three months went by before the ear, nose, throat, and eye specialist reappeared one morning, to explain that he had been to India to watch a cataract operation.)

As the finals approached, Sadie, Rosie, and Celeste grew increasingly concerned that in his neglect of food and sleep, their high-spirited protégé might fail the exams again. In this they were showing more solicitude for Murrough's welfare than any of his family had ever done. They cooked nourishing meals for him, and as the vital week approached tried to get him to go to bed at a reasonable time so that he would be fresh for his Minervan labours. Murrough, however, was not the least worried about the outcome. After all, he had taken the course twice over. He knew his stuff so well that he felt he could write a hundred pages on any given subject.

Which was why he very nearly failed a second time. When he came to write the paper on medicine, he got so involved in putting down all he knew about scarlet fever, that when the bell went, he found that he had answered, voluminiously, exhaustively, less than half of the exam paper.

He was in despair at the prospect of another year of poverty and sacrifice when he was called in by the professor of medicine, and asked to explain why, with his record, he had been able to answer only three of the eight questions. Dr. Simpson was particularly disappointed in him because Murrough had been a noteworthy student. Only a few weeks before, Murrough had diagnosed correctly a case that according to Tyre, had been puzzling the Winnipeg fraternity for two years. The patient was then in the General Hospital, and Simpson had asked Murrough to trot over there and compile the man's medical history. When Murrough returned, he informed his professor that he believed the patient had leprosy.

Simpson had looked at him in amazement. *Leprosy?* In *Manitoba?* Unheard of. The rest of the faculty had been just as skeptical when they were called in to hear the student's diagnosis. However, to make sure, Dr. Bell had taken smears and sent them to McGill and the results had confirmed the diagnosis.

Now, in Dr. Simpson's office, Murrough had to do some very fast talking to convince his professor that he really knew his stuff. To his intense relief, he finally succeeded; and shortly afterwards, in the spring of 1897, more than a decade after his first freshman year, Murrough O'Brien received his diploma.

Spurning invitations from various respectable quarters, he rushed back to the boarding house on Notre Dame Avenue to celebrate with Sadie, Rosie, and Celeste, and to wake up the next morning with probably the worst hangover of his career.

In Dominion City, Dr. O'Brien settled down into what at first was a practice circumscribed by the tiny population of the town and its sur-rounding areas. He invested in a bicycle, and with the bag that the three girls had given him as a farewell present slung over the handlebars, he cycled contentedly, even under the fierce prairie sun, along the dirt roads, attired in a tweed jacket, knickerbockers and canvas shoes, and with a straw hat tilted forward on his bony head.

His practice expanded slowly, though after a few weeks he was able to afford a horse and buggy. Soon, too, he was able to abandon the windowless outhouse when Lim Yee, disgusted by the local housewives' habit of washing their own clothes and boiling their own sheets, gave up and moved out of the house. Murrough took over the entire building, and divided it up into office space and living quarters.

Patients were few and far-flung, but Murrough was content. He looked forward to the time when he would be able to open his own hospital. Not for a minute did he regret turning down his mother's offer. Her faith in him had been restored by the news that he was finally a respectable medico, and she offered to set him up in a good practice in England or India.

Her faith must have faltered again, when she received his reply. He wrote back to indicate that his years of wandering the Canadian West had given him a love of the land and its people, and here he would stay, however unfashionable the practice, however restricted the tiny population of Dominion City.

It was not to remain restricted for long. That August, it became an eastern European boom town. Under the sponsorship of the Dominion Government, thousands of Galicians, Ruthenians, and Ukrainians, started to flood into the municipality to establish homesteads on the flat, dusty lands. Appointed by the government to look after the immigrants, Murrough suddenly found himself responsible, not for a few hundred patients but for four thousand.

The conditions that many of the immigrants were prepared to put up with, in order to establish themselves in their new country, were often appalling. Robert Tyre described Murrough's first encounter with an immigrant family. The doctor was awakened early one morning by a knock on the door that almost shifted his house off its flimsy foundations. Shuffling downstairs in his red flannel underwear, Murrough was told by the man at the door, simply that "Baby coming."

When he arrived at the man's house he found that "The baby had made a partial emergence and then stuck. The woman had lain in that condition for five days and the husband, without neglecting his farm work, had come in occasionally to make a new attempt to dislodge the dead infant. He had delivered all her other children, ten of them.

"It was a typical immigrant's home on the prairie—a one-room shack with dirt floors and a sod roof. The bed where his patient lay stood high on pine blocks and under it were a number of boxes filled with children. Two hens sat on eggs in a box at the foot of the bed. Two geese doing the same thing occupied a barrel at the head of the bed. Six young pigs were penned in one corner. Two calves were tethered in another corner. The stench was awful. The dissecting room of Murrough's old medical school in London was a rose garden in comparison.

"The woman's condition was dreadful. She lay in a state of coma and she was septic to an extreme that made the doctor's stomach squirm. Her pulse was so faint that he couldn't count it. She was, in short, just about ready to go out."

When the ghastly business was over, it was obvious why the birth had gone wrong. "The dead infant was a twenty-pound monstrosity—a cyclops. It had a single eye in the centre of its forehead and a skull with temporal and occipital bones unformed."

After remaining with the woman for twenty-two hours, during which period he bullied the husband into removing the livestock, shoveling out the filth and washing the children, Murrough left, not believing for a moment that the woman would survive five days from such a poisonous experience. He couldn't believe it when he came back the next day and found that the wife, "though pale and still very weak, was nevertheless up and around. The pigs and calves were back in the house and the children looked as dirty as ever. The household was back to normal."

Though the federal government had taken over financial responsibility for the health of the hosts of immigrants to Manitoba, it was limited to severe illness and major surgery only, so that Dr. O'Brien's income did not rise in anything like direct ratio to the size of the practice. Some patients could not pay, others would not. One of his debtors was an "old hag" of a widow who was always waiting down by the gate every time the doctor passed, in order to lure him into a marital snare, using her vague pains as bait. When he refused to mount to her bedroom to examine her chest, she riposted by refusing to examine his bill for service rendered, as, in her opinion, he had not satisfactorily rendered it.

Consequently it was some time before he could afford more sophisticated surgical equipment, and he often had to improvise. "On one midnight gallop to a sod shack on the prairie he found a Galician woman suffering the tortures of the damned with an abscessed antrum [in this case the *sinus* cavity]. The woman's cheek was inflated like a balloon and the measure of her agony was shown by the bloody grooves which the nails of her clenched fingers had ploughed in the palms of her hands. Morphine was one of the staples Murrough carried with him, but he decided against its use since he would need the woman's full co-operation in the job that had to be done. He reasoned too that the extent of her suffering was such that any pain he caused her would make no difference.

"This was an instance where he had to fall back on make-shift tools, and the patient's husband looked his amazement when he was ordered to produce a two-inch nail and a hammer. With the woman settled in a chair and the unwilling husband holding a lantern, the only light the shack possessed, Murrough pulled the first molar on the left hand side of her upper jaw. Then, holding the nail in position in the empty socket and praying that the patient would not pass out on him, he drove it up through gum and jawbone to the abscess. As drainage of the infection began, relief was almost immediate and with a sigh of pure gratitude the woman staggered across the room to her bed and fell fast asleep.

"The beaming husband thumped the doctor mightily on the back, and then hurried outside to return in a few seconds clutching a young chicken, plucked and drawn, and a bag of eggs—payment for the doctor."

On another occasion he used a pair of hairpins to save the life of a young girl who was in the last choking stages of diphtheria. After making a hurried incision in her throat down to the windpipe, he bent two hairpins into the shape of fish hooks and used the hooks to keep the flesh of the wound open. To complete the operation he chased a goose round the farmhouse until he could pluck out a few of its feathers, so that he could use the quills to clear the mucous.

Diphtheria, like whooping-cough, scarlet fever, and typhoid, was still a rampaging killer, though in 1898, help, in the form of a diphtheria antitoxin, was only weeks away. In one household alone, O'Brien arrived to find two members of the family dead, while a third died ten minutes later, and a fourth fifteen minutes later. Even so, when the antitoxin became available and he tried to convince the town fathers of the benefits of inoculation, "I couldn't get it through their thick heads," he said. "Every time I asked for authority to enforce inoculation of the residents of the town and municipality, they fussed and fidgeted and said it would be better to wait for a while.

"Well, they waited too long. One of the worst outbreaks of diphtheria occurred early in the summer of 1898 and the casket-maker had to hire two helpers to keep pace with the demand. Among the victims were children of the reeve and four of his councillors. Authority was given me then to begin a campaign of immunization.

"I didn't have much trouble convincing most of the people that the prick of a needle was a much pleasanter sensation than the strangling grip of diphtheria. However, there were a few who flatly refused to take the inoculation. One fellow met me at the door with a rifle in his hands. I did not argue the point. Another time I was chased out of a yard by a woman wielding an axe.

"We took strong measures to make these rebels capitulate. Their homes were put under quarantine and special constables were appointed to see that they did not leave their yards. The resistance lasted only a day or two and then they meekly agreed to take the needle."

A few years later, Murrough himself became a councillor, but not for long. During outbreaks of typhoid and smallpox, he infuriated the other part-time politicians by insisting that the town council bear the patients' medical expenses and provide food for families while they were under quarantine; otherwise they were unable to fend for themselves. He won, but when he went after the job of reeve, he was defeated as an "Apostle of Extravagance."

One significant aspect of life on the prairies at the turn of the century was the traveling medicine show. In Manitoba as in the rest of the country, entertainment was mostly a do-it-yourself activity, so that almost any organized presentation was looked forward to, greeted, and afterwards talked about for days with naive delight and simple enthusiasm. So the small medicine show that arrived during Murrough's second

August in Dominion City, brought settlers to the town from distances as far as horses, carts, feet, and bicycles could comfortably manage in one day.

Murrough was as interested in the show as everybody else, but in his case it was not the entertainment, or the sign reading "Purveyor of the Only Genuine Secret Indian Herbal Remedy" that enticed him to the caravan, but the other sign: "Teeth Pulled Painlessly." One of his choppers had been aching for a week, and he did not trust the only dentist in town (himself), to remove it.

The theatrical company included the med man himself, attired in a stovepipe hat and a professional-looking cutaway coat, and an Indian girl in a doeskin jerkin and skirt. Her part in the proceedings was to dance to the rhythm of a skin drum, which was being thumped by a "seedy-looking Indian." The purpose of the drum was not only to supply the rhythm but to drown out the moans of the patients as their teeth were extracted. As Murrough discovered when he sneaked in the back way. The dentist "sat me down on a stool and picked up his forceps. But before he used the instrument on me, he banged it sharply on the bottom of a tin pan. Evidently this was a signal, for almost immediately the Indian on the platform began to make a hell of a noise with his drum.

"The extraction hurt like the devil, but otherwise it was a pretty good piece of work. After the tooth was out, the fellow tapped the tin pan again with his forceps and the booming of the drum subsided. It was painless dentistry as far as the ears of the crowd outside were concerned.

"The show stayed with us for two days before it moved on to Emerson. Some of my patients who had plunked down a dollar for the herbal remedy swore it did them more good than any of the preparation they'd got from the medical profession. They were probably right, too. A fancy Latin prescription concealed many a bottle of pure bilge. I'll say this for the secret Indian herbal remedy—it made damn' good harness polish.

"Just the same," Murrough added, with the cynical honesty that did not hinder him from looking after his own interests, "I made up my mind there would be no more medicine shows allowed to sell their wares in Dominion City. A doctor can't afford to have his pills and potions discredited by itinerant medicine vendors. Legalized medical mumbo-jumbo is pretty tame stuff alongside a native tom-tom and a dancing squaw."

The story of such North American patent medicines as the *Secret Indian Herbal Remedy* was a continuation of the common peoples' ancient search for organic maintenance or relief from the vindictiveness of the flesh. The medical con men of Canada and the United States were merely bringing the story up-to-date with quackish advertising and show bezazz. At least their recipes for health did not contain the disgusting ingredients that had fouled the pharmacopoeia of the past.

Mixtures like the one that Dr. O'Brien found useful as harness polish had been on the North American market since colonial times. As early as 1692, the Boston *Almanac* was advertising an antidote to "Griping of the Guts and Wind Cholick." By the end of the nineteenth century, patent medicines and other nostrums were an eighty-million-dollar business, hugely profitable for the times.

In 1906 the Sears Roebuck catalogue listed twenty pages of such preparations and treatments, and a single corner of a contemporary newspaper offered the following products to a public that must have been either extremely short of doctors or highly mistrustful of them: *Kurakoff*, good for diphtheria; *Sarsonarilla*, safe for scrofula; *Kidney-Wort*, a sure cure for all diseases of the liver; the *African Kola Plant*, a guarantee against asthma; Dr. Case's treatment for *Catarrh* ("a terrible disease"); *Flanigan's Double Battery*, *"The best-known cure for Paralysis, Rheumatism, Neuralgia, heart, Nerve and all* blood diseases"; *Sapanule, triumphant over inflammation, and also cures "Wounds, Sprains... Piles, Erysipelas, Milk Leg...."*; the Health *Jolting Chair* for dyspepsia and constipation; *Pulvermacher's Belts and Bands* for spinal disease "and other chronic diseases of the Head, Chest, Liver, Stomach, Kidneys and Blood"; and various treatments for opium and morphine addiction, cancer, and lack of oxygen.

If by chance any of these failed, there were always alternative brands of sarsaparillas to turn to, or the celery compounds, or the balms, pectorals, balsams, inhalants and powders, flowers, embrocations or cordials; or the soothing syrups, eye salves, expectorants, family drops, emulsions, resolvents, cough drops, and slippery elm lozenges.

Sometimes the traders in the brews and pastes were cautious enough to avoid the word *Cure*. Invariably their regimens and dosages were vague enough to ensure that the purchaser came back for more within days— or hours, if, during temperance outbreaks, the remedy contained alcohol. Medicinal alcohol, of course.

Patent medicines and the like were extensively advertised in the newspapers and periodicals, but though the advertising magnified the demand, it did not create it. It was already there, huddled in the breast of all but the most sensible citizens. People were strangely impervious to common sense where their health was concerned. A fellow or his mistress might be shrewd and canny to the extreme when buying a horse or a bolt of muslin, but when it came to safeguarding their health, they became inveterate gulls, susceptible to the wildest claims and the most dubious testimonials.

Though the concoctions and appliances reached the market mainly through advertising in journals and on billboards, fences, and barn roofs, the medicine show, such as the one mentioned by Dr. O'Brien, was an effective supplement. Canadian medicine men were by no means backward in the field of pharmacological evangelism. Notable among them were James Doan of Doan's Kidney Pills fame, "the well-known Druggist of Kingsville, Ontario, who had inherited his secret remedy from 'Aunty Mary Rogers of the Canadian Quaker Settlement,'" and Thomas P. Kelley, named by his biographer, son, and namesake, as the King of the Medicine Men.

Kelley maintained that his prescriptions had real merit. He claimed that in nearly every town he played, the drugstores continued to order and sell his remedies for years after. "Sure I stretch the truth a bit when I lecture on the value of my remedies," he said, "but on the whole my tonics, oils and salves are equal to any you will find on the average drug store shelf. I am not saying they are any better, but certainly they are good remedies put up for me by a reputable patent medicine firm."

In Canada, Kelley said, they were made up for him by the John R. Cressy Company of Dundas Street West, Toronto. He never went in for "mixing up a batch of slum in the back room." He was referring to the method used by lone pitch doctors who concocted their medicines daily, as needed. One of them, Violet Blossom, "Queen of Female Pitch Doctors," manufactured her *Tiger Fat* and *Vital Sparks* in her hotel room. First she melted the Vaseline base in a bucket over a gas jet, and added gum, camphor, menthol crystals, oil of eucalyptus, turpentine, and oil of wintergreen. Next she shaved solid paraffin into the mixture to make it set. While the brew was still hot, it was poured into little tin boxes, and labeled as being good for eczema, ringworm, rheumatism, and cold sores. As for her *Vital Sparks*, described as "God's Gift to MEN," it was made of buckshot candy, which was prepared by throwing it into a bureau drawer. After water had been sprinkled over it, it was thoroughly shaken—by whipping the bureau drawer back and forth—until the candy was damp. Finally powdered aloes was dusted over the pellets, and presto, another batch of potency pills was hatched.

As for the medicine show itself, according to Doc Kelley, it was purely and simply a business enterprise, "an unusual way of getting goods before the eyes of the public, and...run on the legit by most of the med-men I know."

The average medicine show had seven to ten performers, and its tons of prop boxes, stage, tent, trucks, and medicine cartons were transported from town to town by freight cars. The shows were free, the nostrums paying for the productions, with, in Kelley's case, plenty of greenbacks left over for investment in Florida real estate.

A good-looking, twenty-one-year-old with a rapid patter, Kelley, who

was born at Newboro, Ontario, set out with his first medicine show in
1886. This was the Shamrock Concert Company, with himself as a
wire-walker, Ed Thardo as a contortionist, Al Lacy as the minstrel show,
and Jock McCulla, said by Thomas P. Kelley Jr. to be the funniset of all
medicine show comedians, despite his "almost maniacal hatred for the
stage or any form of entertainment."

Kelley's principal product was the New Oriental Discovery. Later he
developed the Shamrock Nerve Tablets, Shamrock Liniment, Shamrock
Corn Sale, and an electric belt for lame and weak backs.

By his second season in the show-hungry countryside around Toronto,
he had large audiences flocking by wagon, buggy, and horse, to gather in
front of the medicine show platform with the brown backdrop, the stage
illuminated by gasoline torches, to listen to the opening patter that
Kelley was to employ for forty years. "Good evening, Ladies and Gentlemen," he would begin. "And now if you will all gather in a little closer
where you can see and hear better, we are going to start up our grand free
open-air entertainment. Tonight, as on every other night, we have
comedy acts, novelty acts, and surprises. You will see the Magic Supper of
Zodiac, the Disappearing Pony, the young lady on the high wire and the
smallest monkey in the world, which I will take from my vest pocket.
There will also be two solid hours of side-splitting comedy; you will laugh
till you are blue in the face. Later you will have an opportunity to
purchase my remarks that will give you long life, strong bodies, good
health and.... Yes, that's it, gather in closer, folks. Step up a little closer."

At the right moment, with the audience's appetite whetted for more,
Kelley would reappear in his swallow-tail coat, brocaded white vest with
gold chain, black trousers, and patent leather shoes, his clear, handsome
face a sincere orange colour in the light of the gasoline flares, and deliver
his pitch. "Now is the time to buy the New Oriental Discovery," he
would crisply project. "It does you good when you take it and right from
the time you take it, but be sure you do take it in time. Not tomorrow, not
next week, but tonight. Remember, it is a mighty poor time to lock the
stable after the horse is gone. When the old man Death comes around and
knocks at your door, you've got to open it. You can't say, "Go away, come
back next month and I'll talk to you." When old grim Death knocks on
your door,thou must open it and nothing will prevent his eventual call.
But my New Oriental Discovery can build the stone wall of health that
will stave off the old boy for years. So buy it now, use it tonight and live to
see your great grandchildren flocking around you."

The sale followed. As described by his son, "Doc Kelley's three
performers hurry out into the audience, each with a carton of New
Oriental Discovery, while several hundred hands are raised, each holding
a silver dollar. 'Sold another, Professor,' shouts one of the performers,

making a speedy return to the platform, to hand over the dollar and return to the crowd with another carton and a 'Who is next, who is next? Ah, this intelligent man wishes to buy himself an additional twenty years of health for only a dollar. There you are and thank you sir.' From elsewhere in the audience comes more of the 'Sold another, Professor.' So it goes on for the next fifteen or twenty minutes with Doc Kelley on stage, applauding the assembly for their good judgement in buying his herbs."

Over the years, in addition to the Shamrock Show, Kelley organized some pretty big traveling productions, including Kelley's Lady Minstrels, Kelley's Coloured Forty, Kelley's Dixie Cotton Pickers, O'Grady's Tenants, and The Swamp Girl. Ever on the alert for new ideas to increase the sale of his remedies, in 1894 he inaugurated the Most Popular Baby Contest. One seventy-one-year-old man who had married a young slip of a girl, was so proud of his achievement in fatherhood that he bought five hundred dollars worth of tonics, herbs, oils, salves, soaps, and pills, to collect the nomination forms that accompanied them and make sure that his baby would win, and thus publicize his virility. (He won.)

Doc Kelley also seized on the tapeworm as a fearful means of worming extra plunks from the body of his audience. This was the Shamrock Tapeworm Remover, "a formidable concoction of pea soup and bitter taste," retailing at seven dollars a bottle, which, even by today's pharmaceutical pricing standards, was an astonishingly high charge. But if there was reluctance to shell out such a sum, Doc Kelley's frightening spiel was more than likely to overcome it. It was also visibly efficacious. As soon as he had collected enough tapeworms from his "patients," he had them placed in glass jars and preserved in alcohol, "with a label on each jar giving the date of the occurrence as well as the address and name of the individual who had been relieved of the enclosed parasitical trophy. As the number of the jars increased, every night before the beginning of the Big Free Fun Show, Doc Kelley would have twenty or so of the jars placed across the front of the stage. This was about the best form of advertising he could hope to get, as the jars always aroused the interest of the crowds arriving at the show lot."

Doc Kelley may have believed in the honesty of his products, but many of his rivals would have been hard put to defend them against an analytical chemist. One of the most famous patent medicines, for instance, was Peruna. According to its manufacturer, Dr. S. B. Hartman, it was an absolute cure for catarrh, which he described as the base of all disease. In truth, Peruna was merely an excuse to tipple. A bottle of the stuff contained half a pint of alcohol, one and a half pints of water, cubebs for flavour and burnt sugar for colour.

The first funeral chimes for the patent medicine body were rung in 1905, a few years after Dr. O'Brien determined to keep traveling med shows out of Dominion City. In that year, Samuel Hopkins Adams began a series of exposures in the weekly magazine, *Collier's*, on what he called the Great American Fraud. He denounced the products as expensively useless and the producers as thieves and murderers, backing up his attacks on a total of 264 concerns and individuals with enough proof to speed a pure food and drug acts bill through the Senate. Though his exposures did not kill the nostrum industry, at least it forced the med man to list the ingredients in their medicines.

By his second winter in Dominion City, Murrough O'Brien had added two valuable items to his surgical equipment, a sterilizer (or glorified double-boiler) designed by him and built by his friend Dave Phillips, and a U.S. army portable operating table. The latter was a great improvement over the microbe-crawling kitchen tables in the sod huts and shacks of his surgical patients. Murrough had purchased the table after seeing it advertised in an American medical journal. It was army surplus, and had been used in the Spanish-American War.

It came in handy for one of his most pressing operations. A fifteen-year-old girl, daughter of a neighbouring farmer, had been suffering for years from a chronic dislocation of the kneecap. The loose rotary motion of the bone would not support her weight so that she kept falling. The parents had taken her to several doctors, and in time, to Dr. O'Brien. After studying the problem, he recommended that they take the girl to Winnipeg for an operation by a specialist. They did so, but the surgeons there refused to attempt the operation, considering it too delicate and of doubtful value. When the farmer and his wife brought the girl back to Murrough, he decided to try a cast. However, he was not hopeful about the outcome.

When the cast was removed, there was no change. The girl could not walk more than a few steps without collapsing. When the parents pleaded with Murrough to attempt the operation that the Winnipeg specialist had refused, he protested that only a specialist could handle it. They pleaded with him. Why should he not try it himself, if they and the girl were willing to take the risk?

"Murrough finally agreed to it. He found the prospect both challenging and frightening. It was surgical pioneering in a field where he had no business to be. He gave himself two weeks to prepare for the operation, and step by step he carefully charted the surgical procedure. Particularly welcome at this time were the services of a young graduate, Dr. Maxwell Wallace, who had come down from Winnipeg to work with Murrough before staring out on his own."

It was done on the army operating table, in a bedroom in the farmer's house, and it took about two hours. "Murrough first made a circular incision below the disabled knee joint, and then a V-shaped opening on either side of the joint. Working through these apertures, he cut and shortened the ligaments to tighten them." He then once again put the knee in a cast. When it was removed, the girl immediately walked without mishap from her bedroom to the kitchen. Shortly afterwards, he delivered a paper on the subject at a meeting of the Canadian Medical Association in Winnipeg.

Murrough was just as good with animals. "The thing a country doctor had to be wary of," he said, "was getting a reputation for being a good man with animals. Once you got tagged with this reputation you got more calls to the barn than the house...

"The fleeting fame I got out of the kneecap operation was nothing compared to the renown that came my way for the job on the dog. This particular dog was no ordinary member of the canine family. It was a prize setter insured for fifteen thousand dollars and owned by an American. He brought it up to compete in the Manitoba Field Trials and a short time before the tests got under way the animal developed an abscess behind one eye."

As in the case of the kneecap girl, the owner tried specialists — veterinarians — all over Winnipeg, but they would not risk an operation. Somebody suggested that he try O'Brien over in Dominion — he was known to be crazy about dogs. Murrough obliged, and was so successful that when he sent the owner a bill for fifty dollars, the American sent back five hundred; a wonderful change for Murrough, who as often as not, never got paid at all, not even in trussed chickens.

Murrough's work was nothing if not varied. He mended morale as well as kneecaps and prize setters. One operation for depressed spirits was performed on a seventy-two-year-old woman, one of the first patients in the hospital that he had opened in 1901, in a converted house with three two-bed wards and an operating and delivery room. After the removal of an ovarian cyst, the old lady should have made an excellent recovery, but she remained listless, wouldn't eat, and didn't seem to care whether she lived or died. At the end of two weeks, the doctor despaired of ever getting her out of the hospital, when he chanced to meet a farmer, who wondered in passing if the old lady was missing her pipe. Murrough immediately returned to the hospital, dug out one of his old corncobs, primed it and took it along to the old woman. "I never saw another patient respond so quickly to treatment," he remarked. "Granny took the pipe the way a hungry baby takes a bottle, and when I left her she was puffing contentedly and grinning all over. I found out afterwards that she had smoked a pipe for fifty years."

Murrough also mended romances. One of these involved a girl whose well-off parents had better prospects in mind for her than the the boy she adored, a poor store clerk. He was a nice lad and in his love for the girl, he had the sympathy of the entire community. The parents remained obdurate. The girl grew thin and forlorn, hardly eating or sleeping. Her mother continued to insist that all her daughter needed was a pick-me-up.

Murrough diagnosed the case to himself as "frustrated love characterized by acute heart distress," and was just about to tell the mother that there was nothing a doctor could do about her condition, when it occurred to him that maybe he could fix it. "I composed a prescription and sent the girl over to Matt Irvine's to have it filled. I wanted her out of the way. When I was alone with the mother, I sat back, folded my hands, and tried to achieve the gravely subdued manner of a doctor who must impart distressing news. For the success of my little scheme I was counting on the mother's dignity and social pretensions. I chose my words carefully....

"'The examination of your daughter,' I said, 'reveals an unexpected and unfortunate condition. This condition, of course, accounts for the loss of weight.' I let this sink in and then hurried on when I saw a question forming. 'It is not for me to suggest what should be done in these distressing circumstances, but obviously the easiest way out for all concerned would be a quiet wedding performed as soon as possible.'

"Evidently she saw no further need to ask the question. She rose and said primly, 'I thank you for your tact and understanding, Doctor.' This was my cue to offer one more piece of advice. 'Your daughter is in a highly emotional state and for the time being at least I would strongly advise that you do not discuss this matter with her. This is especially important if an early wedding is contemplated. The consequences might be serious if you upset her and—master stroke—you know how people gossip in a small community such as this.'"

After that, Mother could hardly wait to fix a date. Murrough felt a trifle guilty about laying aside the doctoral gown to free the wings of an unscrupulous Cupid —but not guilty enough to rectify the unfortunate misunderstanding. "Two months after the wedding," he related to Robert Tyre, "the bride's mother called on me. I had been expecting her. Her attitude would not be described as friendly. She came right to the point. What, she demanded, had I found wrong with her daughter when I made the examination? I looked surprised. Had I not made myself clear? If not, I was sorry. I had found extreme nervous tension, a condition that sometimes brought on a serious emotional breakdown. With a smile that was very, very frigid, she said, 'It was so clever of you to think of marriage as a cure, doctor. What treatment do you prescribe for the same condition in married women? Divorce?'"

A year after opening his own private hospital, the thirty-four-year-old doctor attended his own wedding over at the Anglican church at Emerson. He was doing well enough by now that his nineteen-year-old bride, Margaret, was able to move into a new six-room house, where Murrough also located an office.

Not content in 1903 with the two houses in town, and carried away by an illusion of prosperity (the money owed him by his patients), Murrough built a lavish residence on the south bank of the Roseau River. "We moved into the new house in late summer and for a while the number of my office patients increased tenfold. Most of them didn't have a damn thing wrong with them. They just wanted an excuse to look the house over, and the big attraction was the indoor toilet. Some afternoons during the first week in the big house, the traffic to the bathroom was so heavy that I found it quicker to go outside behind the stable."

The move was not a success—his mother moved in as well. Perhaps unable to supress feelings of guilt that he had not done well by O'Brien standards—his marriage to the daughter of a Canadian Pacific express-man was not the least of his social transgressions—he may have been trying to impress his mother, when he invited her and his sister Eileen to live with him and his wife, his dogs, his cat, his goat, his fleas, and his Chinese cook. But Mary Oclanis O'Brien, who looked like Queen Victoria, and worse, behaved like her, was still not impressed. She considered all the territory west of Montreal a benighted wilderness. Used to the role of *mem-sahib*, she was appalled by a democracy that expected her to hobnob not only with social inferiors but even with people of other races. "We had trouble at dinner the first night she arrived," Murrough said. "She pretty near burst with indignation when she found that she was going to dine at the same table with my hired man and an elderly Galician who had come to see me about a bladder condition." She snubbed Margaret and most of Murrough's friends, and she got Sam the cook fired when, shortly after her arrival, he dished up a stew whose ingredients excited her squeamish curiosity. Accordingly, Sam who knew only about seven words of English, was called in and asked the secret of his culinary artistry. The chef thought for a moment then told them: "Cat". Murrough had to purge the whole family, when they suddenly realized that the household moggy had been missing for two days. Actually the cat turned up later with three kittens, so they never did find out what was in the stew.

Mrs. O'Brien stood the Wild West for four months, then thankfully departed. Murrough's last glimpse of her was through the train window, as she stood there upbraiding the conductor.

By 1905, Murrough's mansion was overrun with animals and debt. The animals included horses, chicken, cattle, Jimmy the pig, and forty wolfhounds. As if there weren't enough beasts around "O'Briens's Folly," he went out after others. While other western doctors soothed their autonomic nervous systems with line and reel, Murrough went wolf-hunting. His enthusiasm for the sport became so well known that an American outdoor magazine published an account of his activities. "The Manitoba Field Trial Club selected Arnaud, Manitoba as their running ground last season largely upon the advice of Dr. O'Brien of Dominion City," the article ran. "The country presented the proper diversity of grass and stubble, birds were plentiful and the same grounds will probably be used for this year's event.

"The trip to Manitoba is a long one, but it is well worth the while if only to have the pleasure of meeting the genial doctor, who is one of those open-hearted, enthusiastic young Irishmen with an inherent love of sport. He probably located at Dominion City, Manitoba, because there he found a way to combine business with pleasure. His medical practice takes him on long trips over the country and many of these he makes on horseback, accompanied by his great pack of wolfhounds, and between them they manage to account for many of the wolves that infest the country.

"One winter the doctor fitted up a sort of toboggan that would slide over the crust of snow without breaking through, hitched to it a couple of half-broken prairie bronchos, and he and Mrs. O'Brien started out wolf-hunting. His pack finally started one, the horses caught the enthusiasm of the chase and away they went in one wild, hair-raising helter-skelter, during which Mrs. O'Brien was spilled from the toboggan. The doctor, however, had no time to stop, but kept on after the wolf. After a long chase the dogs finally made a kill and the doctor in discussing the race added, 'Do you know, I had a devil of a time finding the little woman.'"

Wolves, though, did not bring in an income, and the house which cost a fortune — twenty thousand dollars — gobbled up what little the patients contributed. "Before I was rid of the house," Murrough said, I'd scarcely a pair of breeches to my name. The Methodist preacher termed it the madness of youth — which made me somewhat an elderly youth, for I was thirty-five the spring I got the itch to build myself a castle. Hindsight is always easier than foresight, as many a doctor has discovered after the autopsy, and in the wiser after-years it was easy to fix the blame on O'Brien pride and bullheadedness."

A local economic disaster finished him off in 1907. The Manitoba field crops failed owing to lack of rain, and his financial affairs, which were not well-ordered in the first place because he would not make his debtors pay up, collapsed entirely. "In one six-month period," he said, "I took in just twenty-nine dollars in cash." He sold as much of his livestock as he could, and gave away many of the dogs, but it still wasn't enough. "My scale of fees during this cashless period underwent some modification. Appendec-

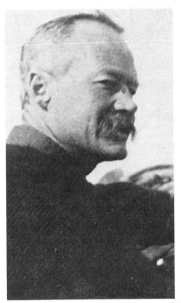
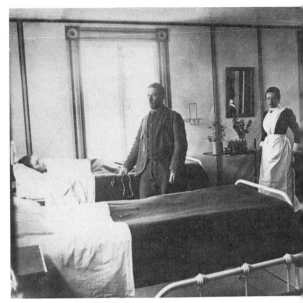

ABOVE LEFT: Wilfred Grenfell. (Public Archives Canada/C68717) ABOVE RIGHT: Volunteers in the Grenfell Hospital, St. Anthony, Newfoundland, 1906. (PAC/C4745) BELOW: The Grenfell Hospital at Battle Harbour, Nfld. (PAC/C65039)

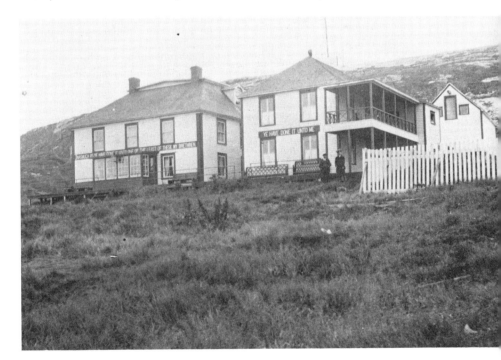

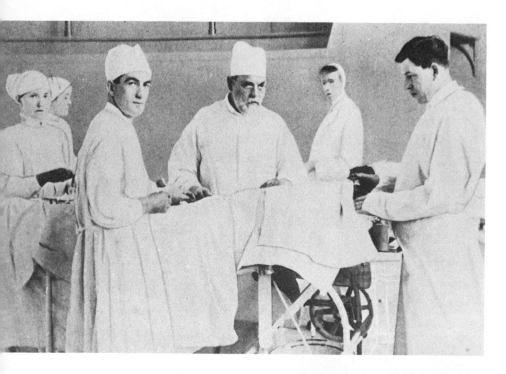

ABOVE: Dr. Francis Shepherd operating at Royal Victoria Hospital, Montreal, about 1909. RIGHT: The magnetic Dr. Shepherd. (Museum, Academy of Medicine, Toronto) TOP FAR RIGHT: Students at Trinity (University of Toronto) and their work, about 1900. (Museum, A of M) LOWER FAR RIGHT: Calgary General Hospital nurses some years after the converted-brothel days. (PAC/C25671)

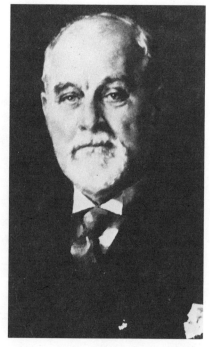

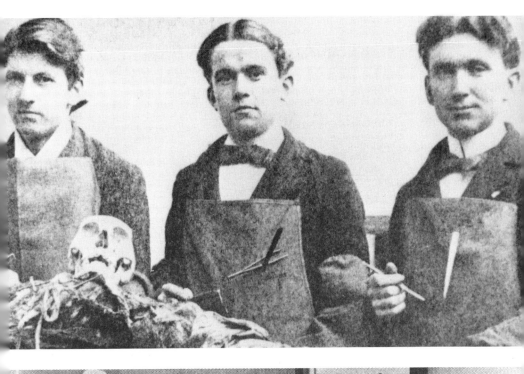

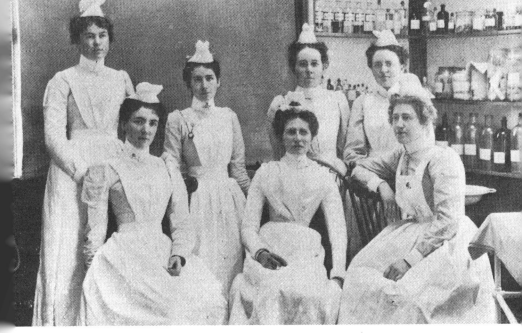

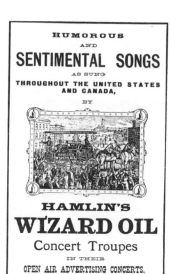

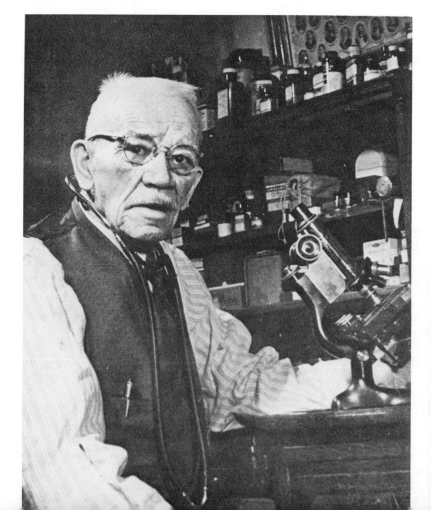

LEFT: Cover of a song book from a travelling medicine show. (Museum, A of M) BELOW: Murrough O'Brien. (Robert Tyre)

tomies were bartered for a side of beef or a load of hay; tonsillectomies brought me a leg of pork or half a dozen hens. I delivered babies for a bushel of potatoes and a sack of cabbage, and I treated a gonorrhea case for a load of poplar slabs. I amputated a fellow's toe one day and he offered me a choice of eggs or turnips. I took the turnips. Margaret was making a lot of soup at this time. I took the rump of a deer, out of season, for curetting a uterus."

Murrough finally left Dominion City for Winnipeg in 1909, unable to straighten up under the burden of debt that his failure to collect his fees had heaped upon him.

Murrough O'Brien died in North Battleford, Saskatchewan, in 1955. Apart from his army service during the First World War, he spent his whole life as a country doctor, and remained to the end a vividly distinct personality.

The achievements of great men and women in the arts, sciences, and technology undoubtedly swell a nation's prestige. But it is the persons of independent outlook, the eccentrics, the intensely individual, who give distinction to a society. It is the lack of that determined individuality that tends to starve the Canadian identity. In his autobiography, David Niven, the actor, mentions a friend of his whom he described as that great rarity, a true Canadian eccentric. Coming from a country where everybody is slightly odd, he is certainly in a position to know. But as must be increasingly apparent, the breed was not always rare in Canada. Until the Great Depression, the most damaging aspect of which was its effect on the national self-confidence, a great many Canadians appear to have been individuals of intensity.

Murrough O'Brien was one of them.

23

Two Prairie Surgeons

O NE OF WILFRED Bigelow's earliest cases reveals the directness of the
man, his self-certainty, decisiveness, and a certain arrogance ameliorated by an awareness of the absurdity of human beings, himself
among them. After graduating from the Medical College in Winnipeg in
1903, he practiced for a while in Hartney, Manitoba. His acquaintances
there were young bachelors in the trades and professions, and they were
in the habit of gathering for lunch at a large, oval table in the dining room
of the Hartney Hotel to exchange gossip and slander. Sometimes other
diners, such as commercial travelers, would try to join them at table, but
these outsiders soon gave up, discouraged by the deliberately crude
manners of the Hartney Hotel gang, who among other unseemly demonstrations were in the habit of passing the butter balls to each other by
firing them across the table with a quick flick of the knife. The recipient
would catch the butter balls by holding up their plates vertically, facing
the server.

The hotel had recently hired a redheaded, cross-eyed waitress, a large,
muscular lady by the name of Maude. One day Dr. Bigelow was called
into the kitchen. There he found Maude lying face down on the floor,
shrieking every time anyone tried to touch her. The entire hotel staff were
huddled nearby, terrorized by the nerve-shredding spectacle. Bigelow
studied her for a moment, reached for a large wooden paddle, walked
over to Maude, pulled up her skirts and whacked her on the behind with
"a good solid blow."

The treatment confirmed his diagnosis of hysteria, for it was instantly
effective; except that it placed the doctor in some jeopardy. The crack of

the butter paddle against her ample buttocks had hardly died away before Maude jumped up and made for him with blood in her eyes. Bigelow lurched from the kitchen on his bad leg and across the dining room, with Maude in hot pursuit. She was still chasing him far up the street when the rest of the staff and his fellow diners all rushed out to see the denouement; which looked dangerously close—hindered by his gammy leg, Bigelow was rapidly being gained upon.

In his later years as a successful surgeon, as a pioneer user of the X-ray in Western Canada, and as the founder of what is believed to be the first private medical clinic in the country, Dr. Bigelow turned rude, forceful, and bombastic, but there was always an inner sense of proportion that raised these qualities, which in a humourless man might have seemed intolerable, to the sum total of the colourful personality.

He used to puzzle his family by standing in front of a mirror each morning, engaging in a one-man wrestling match, until he was polished with sweat, compensating for a semi-crippled condition through iso-metrics, long before the value of such muscle-opposing exercises was generally understood.

He was convinced that the welfare of the autonomic nervous system depended on frequent hunting and fishing trips. During the fishing trips he employed eccentric trolling methods, somewhere between the tech-niques of West Coast salmon fishing and Bay of Fundy high-tide cod fishing.

Wilfred once attempted to drum up some cardiac arrest business among a storeful of men in Kentville, Nova Scotia, by reproducing the call of a mallard at full volume.

He was rigidly Victorian at home, lustily humorous in the operating theatre. To combat post-operative pulmonary collapse, he insisted that his hospital patients sleep in their long-handle underwear, and prescribed *spiritus fermenti* for them, in the form of rye whisky.

He used his armpit as an incubator, sleeping at night with test-tubes of virulent bacteria under his arm.

Wilfred Bigelow arrived in Winnipeg during the year following O'Brien's graduation from the Manitoba Medical College, after a long train journey from his native Kingsport in Nova Scotia. That town had been founded by an ancestor of his, Isaac Bigelow. In the early part of the century, Kingsport was a vigorous shipbuilding centre specializing in three- and four-masted sailing ships, but the coming of the steamship had ruined the industry, and left the town with no reason for being except as a shipping port for apples and potatoes.

Like most of his friends, Wilfred looked forward to a seaman's life, and to this end had taken up the study of trigonometry and navigation. "This ambition of mine was suddenly cut short by an accident when I was sixteen," he wrote in his memoirs. " I injured my leg and this resulted in infection of a leg bone as well as the infection and complete destruction of an ankle joint and a hipjoint." He was out of action for a year, and stiff-hipped for life.

Two years after the accident, having painfully adjusted his ambition, he accepted an offer to teach public school at Delhaven, "because nobody else would take it." By then he saw college as the only gateway to a reasonable career for a cripple, and the school job seemed to be the only one that would enable him to save enough money to accomplish this. He was just starting his second year at Delhaven when he received a telegram from his sister in Winnipeg, telling him about a job "as an office boy and assistant in surgery to Dr. J. O. Todd," his brother-in-law.

Wilfred accepted immediately, for he had discovered that despite a handsome salary of one hundred and sixty dollars a year, he had not been able to save a bean. "I left Nova Scotia on a Saturday and arrived in Winnipeg on Labour Day, nine days later. It was a long and, I might say, romantic trip on a harvest train, which was comparable to a cattle train. This was one of the early excursion harvest trains that at that time went west from Nova Scotia. The fare to Moose Jaw, Saskatchewan, was ten dollars."

The train consisted of seven coaches of the Colonist type, with wooden seats and no upholstery, and a caboose filled with trainmen. After one look at the rough crowd from Nova Scotia, the trainmen had retreated to the caboose, and from then on were rarely seen.

The train hands had good reason to keep out of the way. At one stop on the single track C.P.R. line, the locomotive crew made the mistake of stopping opposite a shack with a sign on it reading "Bar Room." Immediately, half a dozen of the Nova Scotian harvesters ran forward to the engine and ordered the fireman and engineer, with suitable threats, to hold up the train until they were told to move on. "In the meantime about two hundred men started loading bottles, kegs, and anything that contained liquor from the bar and cellar. This performance did not take very long. The liquor was all put aboard the train. It took us two days to get to Fort William and those days were really something that cannot be properly decribed. The men were singing, yelling, fighting and vomiting." Wilfred, who had teamed up with another young fellow named Armstrong, spent most of the time in an upper bunk. The two boys watched the alcoholic frenzy in wide-eyed amazement, though they enjoyed it once they had adjusted to the smell and noise. It was a new experience. "When we got into Fort William on Sunday morning," Bigelow continued, "we had been seven days on the train. We were all herded out of the cars and the water hose was turned on and every car washed down. The only drying it got was from some big mops that the men pushed along the floor. We left Fort William just before dark and the cars were still wet."

The day after his arrival in Winnipeg, the wide-eyed nineteen-year-old went to work for Dr. Todd, assisting his brother-in-law at St. Boniface Hospital. The job lasted five mornings a week for five years, four of them as an official medical student. "My first job at assisting, the first few months, was learning the names of the various instruments and passing them when called for, and holding a retractor at the proper tension," Bigelow said. "By keeping my eyes open and following the surgical procedures carefully, I was able, in a few months, to anticipate the procedures and have my hand on the proper instrument before it was called for. One common bit of disciplining that I got almost daily for some time was, when I appeared to have become interested in something else and allowed my gaze to wander round the operating room. I was immediately brought into line by, 'Wake up, where are your eyes?' Also in these early days of surgery there was an occasional rap over the bare knuckles with an artery forcep."

A year after the start of this apprenticeship with Dr. Todd, Wilfred formally entered the profession, and graduated four years later from the Manitoba Medical College. The year 1906 found the frozen-hipped Nova Scotian with the heavy-lidded eyes and the firmly intolerant mouth practicing in Brandon, Manitoba. The seven G.P.s already established there were not exactly overjoyed at the arrival of yet another doctor, especially one who looked as if he might become a formidable competitor. As a student Wilfred had had unusual experience in surgery through his association with Dr. Todd. Extensive post-graduate work in the United States had followed. It had included a sojourn at the Mayo Clinic in Minnesota. As a result he was familiar with the latest surgical techniques. Worse, he was dismayingly up-to-date in many other fields of medical science, including the new-fangled X-Ray, long-wave treatment in physiotherapy, and the suspicious development known as local anesthesia. He was also knowledgeable in bacteriology, already doing his own smears and microscopic examinations.

Some of the established G.P.'s in Brandon were quite cool to the newcomer. Two of them greeted Wilfred with the suggestion that he go back where he had come from. Another mistook him for a patient when he came limping into the office, and was all warmth and sympathy, until Bigelow told him that he had come not to complain but to compete.

At least none of the new colleagues were violent, like the crazed doctor who helped Wilfred to pay for his honeymoon.

The lady he was to marry was a rosy-cheeked blonde from Scotland by the name of Grace Ann Carnegie Gordon. She was not only a lovely-looking girl, but, a highly qualified nurse, with a gold medal from her training days in Sunderland and a licentiate in obstetrical surgery from London. Wilfred met her when she came out to join her parents in Manitoba.

Actually he had already heard about Grace Gordon from a fortune teller. A traveling palmist had visited Hartney while he was practicing there. The palmist had hired a room for a week over Dr. Woodhull's drug store, but nobody would go near her, for fear of what the neighbours would say. Wilfred, already an independent cuss, lurched upstairs on his rigid leg to see what his palm and her crystal ball had to say about his future.

The moment he walked in, she said, "'You are a doctor aren't you?' Later she remarked, 'You have not a wife, you are not married?' and I said, 'No. I do not expect to be, as women do not marry cripples.' She said, 'No, you are wrong. Your wife-to-be is now on the Atlantic Ocean coming over from the Old Country.'"

Wilfred treated the session with the old girl as a joke. But the woman with whom he had fallen in love while she was assisting him in an obstetrics case, proved to have been crossing the Atlantic exactly according to the palmist's prognostication.

Even so, Wilfred did not really believe that Grace would "ever see anything in me, a cripple." Besides, she had five other suitors in town including the manager of the grain elevator, who were all far more successful than he was, and fine-looking men into the bargain.

Still, "with more courage than sense I proposed to her in a horse-drawn cutter while driving her home one night. I nearly fell off the seat when she said, 'Yes.'"

She agreed to marry him even though they would be starting out with a stake of only ninety dollars; all he had left after his expensive post-graduate training. Theirs would obviously have to be a very thrifty honeymoon. But three days before he was due to join her at her sister's place in Minneapolis, he got an urgent midnight call to go to the Imperial Hotel in Brandon, Manitoba, where a doctor from a nearby village was running amuck with a loaded pistol. "The doctor had been a college mate of mine and he was drunkenly crazy, having the delusion that some man was trying to get him, so he set out with a pistol to get his imaginary man.

"When I got down to the Imperial Hotel, Mr. Hannah, the owner, and his clerk, Mr. Evans, had locked themselves in the bar room on the first floor and all the guests had locked themselves in their bedrooms. The crazed man, at that time, was walking through the hallways of the second and third floor, searching for his 'victim' with a pistol in hand. Since I had known this man for four years, Mr. Hannah thought I could handle him. He was afraid to call the police in case he might shoot a policeman coming up the stairs."

Wilfred limped cautiously upward, and found the doctor prowling the second floor. He decided that the best way to calm the man was to offer to help him hunt for his imaginary victim. While he was doing so, he managed to maneuver the mad doctor into a spare room, and got him to lie down. After the doctor had quietened somewhat, Wilfred said that he would go out and "find this fellow and drive him out from wherever he is hiding and when he walks by the door, you shoot him."

Naturally, nobody in the hotel was foolish enough to walk past the door until the drunken doctor had fallen asleep. He was then entirely disarmed. Whereupon a vastly relieved Mr. Hannah presented Wilfred with a hundred dollars, which made all the difference to the honeymoon trip. It enabled the happy couple to travel to Rochester to watch surgical operations at the Mayo Clinic.

It was significant that Wilfred Bigelow's postgraduate studies were confined almost entirely to his own continent. The days when ambitious North American graduates went as a matter of course to Europe to complete their education were drawing to a close. Increasingly, because of enlightened people like the Rockefeller staff member who had persuaded his boss to invest in the sciences, the United States was replacing Europe as the centre of medical research and development, and specialist training.

The formation of the American College of Surgeons in 1912 was another indication that the profession at home was keeping up with international standards. The college was formed principally to identify properly trained surgeons in the United States and Canada. (Herbert Bruce of Toronto, featured in a later chapter, was one of the founding members.) It was a proof of Dr. Bigelow's standing in the profession that he was invited to become a fellow of the college prior to its first convocation in 1913—though when he arrived at the convocation in Chicago in a rented tuxedo, one of the surgeons present mistook him for a flunkey, handed over his coat, and pressed a silver dollar into his palm.

"Thank you, sir," said the distinguished Canadian surgeon, vastly enjoying his own far from characteristic obsequiousness.

Another result of Dr. Bigelow's orientation towards United States developments in medicine was his receptivity to the idea of the medical clinic, where a group of specialists could work together professionally and with a common financial arrangement. In 1913, he started his own clinic in Brandon. The partners included himself and another surgeon; a bacteriologist; a girl to do the blood counts, stains, differentials, cultures, vaccines, blood ureas, and blood sugars; and an eye, ear, nose, and throat specialist. A few years later, a pathologist joined them. "The concept of a clinic," Bigelow said, "where a complete examination and treatment could be provided by specialists working together and submitting one common account proved to be successful. It functioned for nearly half a century, providing services to patients who came from all over the prairies."

During his postgraduate studies in the United States, Bigelow became particularly interested in the development work being done there on Rontgen's "accidental" discovery.

Many scientific discoveries have been termed accidental, from the sight of a swinging lamp in a Pisa cathedral that led to the theory of the pendulum and the boiling kettle that inspired the idea of the steam engine, to Newton's apple and Fleming's penicillin mould. The discovery of X-rays was similarly described as accidental, though, as in the other great scientific breakthroughs, the phenomenon would not have been developed had it not been observed by the right man at the right time. In the case of Rontgen, the "accident" was that he had been working on barium platinocyanide-treated surfaces in connection with his work as a physicist in Wurzburg. One dark November afternoon in 1895, while experimenting with electrical discharges in a highly evacuated glass tube, he noticed that the sensitized surface, which was some distance away across the room, glowed brightly whenever the power was switched on in the tube. The surface continued to glow even when opaque paper was interposed between the tube and the surface; though the fluorescence died when much denser material was placed in the way. Thus the unknown ray seemed to be capable of penetrating certain material.

Naturally Rontgen was curious, as the phenomenon had not previously been observed. He investigated, and found that the "X" ray was capable of penetrating many kinds of solid objects. One of the objects was his hand. To his astonishment he saw the outline of his own bones, surrounded by the softer outlines of the flesh. The bones could not only be seen when the hand was placed in the way of the unknown or X-ray, but could be captured on a photographic plate.

As had happened so often in the past, the medical profession was slow to grasp the revolutionary advances in diagnosis that the X-ray made possible. The public, though, were quick enough to seize on what they thought were certain other possibilities. They had read in the newspapers that X-rays could penetrate clothing. Thinking that the invisible ray would reveal the human form in all its naked inglory, that the device was a kind of electrical peeping tom, they raised an outcry against this invasion of Victorian decency. According to Harvey Graham, "A London firm rose to the occasion, and made a small fortune from the sale of X-ray proof underwear," and in New York there was an attempt to legislate against the use of X-rays in opera glasses.

Gradually the public realized, with considerable disappointment, that the X-ray picture was of purely scientific value. A few months later, royalty completed the process of making X-rays respectable. Just as Queen Victoria had popularized anesthesia when she accepted chloro-

form to ease the birth of one of her children, and Edward VII had made
the appendix fashionable when his own was removed at the turn of the
century, so now other members of royalty showed the way, when Kaiser
Wilhelm permitted a radiograph to be taken of his crippled left arm, and
Queen Amelia of Portugal had her ladies-in-waiting X-rayed, to show
them the awful constricting effects on their livers of their sixteen-inch
corsets.

Intensive research into more efficient methods of producing X-rays
followed. It was an indication of Bigelow's spirit that, despite the opinion
of many doctors that X-ray treatment was a sort of quackery, he went
ahead and bought one of the earliest machines, a Kelly-Koit, and used it
in treatment as well as in diagnosis.

"This X-ray work was of such interest that the following spring after
my period of post-graduate work in New York, I attended a meeting of
the New York Academy of Medicine, and listened to a Dr. Musser. He
brought with him a large number of glass X-ray plates since X-ray films
did not come in for years afterwards. These X-ray plates which I saw that
evening were the first demonstration or outline of the stomach. With this
technique you were able to watch a meal go through the intestinal tract
with periodic pictures and to time the emptying of the stomach.

"The X-Ray opaque meal used in this demonstration was bismuth
subnitrate ½ ounce, which was given in a tumbler of buttermilk. Before
the plate was taken, a coin was fastened over the navel to mark as a
boundary to the upper gastric area. The plates were usually taken every
six hours. It was interesting to see a case of obstruction in which the
stomach was still partly outlined with bismuth the next day."

Bigelow used this method for one of his first X-ray exposures, to
examine a possible obstruction in the stomach of a female patient. As per
the New York method, he taped a twenty-five-cent piece over her navel,
but forgot to remove it. When he saw her again four months later he
found her still sporting the quarter. Not one to waste money, he snatched
it off her stomach and popped it into his pocket.

Ever alert to new methods and techniques, Dr. Bigelow became, in
partnership with a druggist friend, a dental pioneer, shortly after purchasing his Kelly-Koit. One of his patients, a Mr. Armstrong, had been
kicked by a horse and his jaw had been fractured. The fracture could not
be properly reduced. It kept slipping out of place. When Bigelow examined the man in the hospital his druggist friend, Jerry Hughes, was with
him. Bigelow mentioned that he could not get a clear picture of the side of
the jaw on his X-ray glass plates, and said, "If only I had a small X-ray
plate which would go inside the mouth, I could put it against the side of
the fracture and expose it from outside." Hughes replied, "Do you think
that an ordinary Eastman Kodak would work?"

Bigelow decided to try. Jerry Hughes went back to the drug store and cut off a couple of inches of camera film, wrapped it up in black paper in the darkroom and returned with it to the patient. He held the film inside Armstrong's mouth with his fingers against the fractured area, then developed three films. Each one, according to Bigelow, was perfect. "It showed part of one molar tooth lying between the fractured ends of the bone. It was exposed for about one-half minute and besides showing the fracture, there was a lovely outline of the bones of Jerry's fingers.

"Monday morning I did an open operation upon the jaw, removing the tooth without going into the mouth, and wired it. The operation was successful and I think this gentleman is still living.

"I believe this is one of the earliest films used in X-ray work in Western Canada, as I had never heard of film being used before."

In this case, the doctor did not mention whether or not he used local anesthesia, but he was just as alert to the advantages of that development, though many of his colleagues ridiculed the idea. As with X-rays, Bigelow first saw it demonstrated in New York, on a patient who was being operated on for hemorrhoids. "It was such a striking demonstration, I felt there was a real field for local anesthesia. I saw no one doing such work with local anesthesia until 1907 when Novocaine was used." As he had difficulty in getting satisfactory general anesthesia, he devised a technique of his own, and from then on did a good deal of his major surgery with local anesthetics.

Bigelow was just as up-to-date in the matter of transportation. Other medical men might swear by—as well as at—the horse and buggy in summer and the horse and cutter in winter, but Bigelow was not at all locked-off to the equine quadruped, especially when, in the winter of 1908, a pair that he had hired took a wrong turning in thirty-below-zero weather. So much for the assertion that horses always knew their way home. To make matters worse, the dumb beasts were quite content to stay where they were because they were nicely protected behind a nine-foot wall of snow, whereas the doctor was on the cold ground, under the overturned cutter.

Soon after this experience Bigelow bought his first car. It was a wooden-bodied, three-seater Ford with coal oil tail lights and no doors. Drafty or not, he was thrilled with it, and if the worst drawback was that he had to stop the engine when meeting horse-drawn vehicles, that was the fault of the highway system rather than the vehicle. The roads were so narrow that it took quite a while for another rig to get by. However, Bigelow used the delay to advantage. While he was waiting for the other vehicle to pass, he cleaned his spark plugs.

"You could drive for a week in these districts, out to Deloraine, Boissevain, Killarney and then west, and never meet a car. The drawback in the city was the taillight. As the taillight was coal oil, the darn thing would jiggle out, or go out very frequently." This was serious, as there was a two-dollar fine if the Brandon police caught you with your taillight out.

The carbide headlamps could also be balky. From about the first of November, the water in them would freeze. However, after a year Bigelow had a magneto installed, and from then on jounced contentedly along with electric lighting. Which left one major problem. Every time he filled up, the gasoline had to be strained or filtered. Bigelow solved that problem by carrying a funnel with him, and using his hat to strain the gasoline. His hat, he said, gave wonderful service, and the sodden haberdashery, replaced on his head, did not appear to do much harm to his scalp. In fact he had an idea that it made his hair grow all the more luxuriantly.

Both Murrough O'Brien and Wilfred Bigelow had received their degrees after a four-year course at the medical school in Winnipeg. In 1906 the course was increased to five years, following premedical requirements. Given the increasing complexity of medicine, this was a necessary change, but not a very welcome one to the students, whose graduating years suddenly seemed to have receded far into the distance.

The reaction of one of the students, Gordon Fahrni from Gladstone, Manitoba, was typical. At first he was furious at missing the four-year course by a matter of months, but the feeling gradually faded when he discovered how much there was to absorb, especially in surgery in which he was particularly interested.

Four years later he discovered another advantage to the lengthened course. With no graduating class in 1910, the hospitals found themselves short of interns, with the result that Fahrni and his friends were able to spend most of their final year on intern duty at the Winnipeg General. Thus they were being given an earlier-than-usual opportunity to grasp the clinical situation of the sick.

Fahrni became one of the new breed of unofficial specialists, led into his field by a spontaneous concern rather than by a formal course in the specialty. As an intern he had been shocked at the high mortality rate following operations for goitre (enlargement of the thyroid gland), especially after thyroidectomies on those suffering with toxic goitre. The patient, usually young, would come into the hospital in a nervous, jumpy, and apprehensive state, with staring eyes, hot skin, heart racing, and manner agitated. During the next day or two, the thyroidectomy would be performed with the usual heavy blood loss because of the duration of the operation. (There was no blood transfusion service available.)

"To see this patient twenty-four hours later, thrashing about in bed, pulse racing and temperature ascending, the orgy to end in death forty-eight to seventy-two hours following operation," Dr. Fahrni wrote in his memoirs, "was an emotional experience for nurses and all others in attendance and a shock to the family. To many of us it appeared vital to learn more about the thyroid gland and its diseases and if a surgical approach in treating some of them was needed."

As Fahrni became more involved in the thyroid problem, the Manitoba minister of health asked him to look into the incidence of goitre among school children of Winnipeg. He discovered that 48 percent of those surveyed had thyroid enlargement. With the advent of iodine prophylaxis (as defined in the *Penguin Medical Encyclopedia*: prophylaxis, the prevention of disease, means "anything from vaccination to a daily walk."), the disorder largely disappeared, but there were forms of goitre that were not susceptible to medical treatment, particularly hyperthyroidism. These had to be dealt with by the surgeon.

"This was the situation when I began to practice medicine," Fahrni continued, "and from what I had seen during my intern training, the surgical results were somewhat appalling. The alternative seemed to be more knowledge in depth of what constituted hyperthyroidism, a recognition of how susceptible its subjects were to trauma of any kind and the importance of a surgical program to successfully meet the need of these fragile sick patients.

"With this mental attitude, I began to take a keen interest in diseases of the thyroid gland from the time I was an intern in the Winnipeg General Hospital. It was obvious that with the lack of medical help, surgery must be applied in a manner consistent with a lower mortality rate and fewer serious complications." Accordingly, Fahrni applied it in that manner, and in time began to cut down the death and complication rate, and to rehabilitate patients who would otherwise have been invalids for life.

The new local anesthesia was not the least of his revised techniques. "Early in my career, I learned the advantage of local anesthesia in the operating room," he wrote in his book *Prairie Surgeon*. "In those early days Ether inhalation was just taking over from chloroform. Next, Ethyl Chloride was introduced and had the advantage of a quick recovery of consciousness when the face mask was removed. All of these general anesthetics, however, took something out of the patient, particularly when nausea and vomiting were common sequelae. By using local anesthesia this extra burden was removed from the operative dose and this was an added asset to the recovery of borderline cases. The results were so satisfactory that I was soon using this method in all my goitre operations."

Gordon Fahrni found himself becoming a specialist in the subject whether he wanted to or not. As his skills increased, other doctors began to refer patients to him from greater and greater distances, until his thyroid work threatened to crowd out the general surgical work in which he was still deeply interested. Within a short time he was doing three hundred thyroidectomies a year.

Not all of Fahrni's colleagues approved of his work. One of them exemplified the age-old rift between the physician and the surgeon.

"Dr. Charles Hunter, who came to Winnipeg from Scotland, was an internist on the Medical Faculty and prominent as such in the community. He had an idea that surgeons were too ready to operate when perhaps a medical regime was indicated. He had a great propensity to challenge, in a sarcastic manner, the statements of senior surgeons at clinics or medical meetings. I had been working hard to lower the surgical risk in operations on toxic goitres and as usual, as my following grew, there were some of my confreres who were skeptical.

"At a regular meeing of the Winnipeg Medical Society I presented a report on fifty consecutive thyroidectomies without a death. I was proud of this accomplishment, because it was in the very early days before iodine was in use as a pre-operative measure. In the discussion that followed, Dr. Hunter, with his broad Scottish accent, said that in that day and age it was quite a feat, but he felt that goitres were not surgical cases and that if operated upon they often died and he felt that 'Gaarden' as he called me in his Scottish brogue, should not as such a young man, be operating on goitres."

Dr. Fahrni was rocked by this attack from such a prominent quarter, but a month later, after a careful investigation, reported back with a long list of toxic goitre cases where surgery was not involved. All of the patients had died. Fahrni had already proved that he had reduced the surgical mortality rate from twenty percent to as little as one percent; now he was showing that Hunter was talking through his hat when he asserted that goitre cases "if left alone never died."

Fortunately, Hunter had enough humility to apologize for his lack of knowledge on the subject, and for impugning Dr. Fahrni's motives and integrity; and thereafter further burdened "Gaarden" by referring many additional goitre cases to him for operation.

By 1929, Dr. Fahrni was working at St. Boniface Hospital. Among the patients in his teaching ward was a boy suffering from an incurable disease, ostetitis fibrosa cystica, that Fahrni had first heard about when he was a student. Clinically the picture was of a loss of calcium leading to the softening and eventual collapse of the bones. Fahrni also observed a nodule in the left lobe of the boy's thyroid gland, but was unable to account for it. The disease was incurable.

The boy was still in the ward when the doctor went to Europe on a study trip. While he was in Vienna, he was excited to learn of recent work on the parathyroid bodies which showed that ostetitis fibrosa cystica was caused by a tumour in the parathyroid body; and that removal of the tumour allowed the bone system to recalcify itself. My God, he thought to himself, that nodule in the boy's thyroid must have been a parathyroid adenoma!

As soon as he reached home, Fahrni hurried to the hospital to learn that the boy had been discharged and sent to the Home of the Friendless. When he went there he found that the boy had died three weeks previously.

Two years went by, but not a single case of parathyroid adenoma was reported anywhere in the country. Then one day, Fahrni was golfing with a friend, Dr. A.C. Scott, who had a practice at Indian Head, Saskatchewan. While they were propelling balls and divots down the fairway, Scott happened to mention a patient he had left behind in his hospital while he was making a trip to the East. He was wondering if she would still be alive when he got back. His description of the case so excited Fahrni that he instantly abandoned the game, walked to the clubhouse and telephoned the hospital at Indian Head to find out if the girl was still alive. He learned that she was, though in great distress.

This was an understatement, as he found when he took the night train to Indian Head. "I was amazed," he wrote, "to see on the bed an emaciated girl [eighteen years of age] gasping for breath with her mobile chest wall collapsing and expanding with each respiratory cycle. Her thighs were crossed and her legs drawn up to her body. The slightest movement of any part of her body caused her to cry out with pain."

Unfortunately, on examining her neck, Fahrni could not feel a tumour. Still, X-rays and other tests suggested it might be a case of hyperparathyroidism. "Her present poor condition was the end result of four years of illness and it seemed the only thing to do was to explore her neck. She was given some sedative premedication and with one person holding each corner of the bed sheet, she was carried to the operating room table. Fortunately, I had brought with me equipment for local anaesthesia, as I hardly think any one would dare give a general anaesthetic to this gasping dyspnoeix girl. I was so happy to find the missing upper left parathyroid body (there are four and I had demonstrated three normal in size and position) globular in shape and enlarged to an inch in diameter in the mediastinal area behind the upper breastbone. No difficulty was encountered in removing it. I brought it home where our pathologist in the General Hospital confirmed it as a parathyroid adenoma."

Gordon Fahrni added the case to his growing list of articles on thyroid diseases. The girl later had to have an operation in her thigh bones to correct the deformity that the disease had caused, otherwise her recovery seemed almost magical. She was relieved of her agonizing pain, her bones recalcified and grew strong again and soon she was not only able to walk but to work. The last Gordon Fahrni heard of her was as a stenographer in a western prairie city.

24

And Four Psychiatrists

I T IS FASHIONABLE to present contemporary man as a debased creature, with his frightful inventions, ferocities, and deformed desires. Yet even the most superficial reading of history suggests that ours is an increasingly enlightened, sensitive, and compassionate society in which, to a remarkable extent, pain has been banished, intolerance subdued, and inhumanity effectively condemned. Though highly imperfect, the normal human being of the 1980s is a more sensitive and civilized person than his counterpart even of a mere fifty or sixty years ago.

Consider the treatment of the mentally sick. There have been periods in history when they were treated humanely, but, for the most part, superstitious fear or crude insensitivity prevailed. The problem with the madman was that his condition could not be explained in physical terms. Even five thousand years ago, a patient could be treated with a measure of success if he had a wart, a wound, or whooping cough, but how was he to be helped when the cause of his frantic excitement or depression, his gibberings or unnatural silences, his compulsions or delusions, could not be determined by the methods of science or even satisfactorily localized in the body? Worse, there was a reluctance to put as much effort into understanding his mental state as went into investigating his physical functions. A madman was frightening, sometimes because of his dangerous behaviour, but also because he reminded people that his elemental emotional forces were their forces, with only the slight difference that his had been unchained. How easily one's own primitive impulses might similarly be let out of their subconscious dungeon.

Paradoxically, while we might look upon the sufferer of an obviously

318

physical misfortune—a sword-thrust, a stroke of bad luck—in terms of There But For the Grace of God Go I, this empathy was denied the madman, out of fear; the fear of the self. Better that the madman should be out of sight, out of mind. "We incarcerate these miserable creatures," wrote Johann Reil at the beginning of the nineteenth century, as if they were criminals in abandoned jails, near to the lairs of owls in barren canyons beyond the city gates, or in damp dungeons of prisons, where never a pitying look of a humanitarian penetrates; and we let them, in chains, rot in their own excrement. Their fetters have eaten off the flesh of their bones, and their emaciated pale faces look expectantly toward the graves which will end their misery and cover up our shamefulness."

It took a long time for psychiatry to be accepted as a significant part of medical science. The shamans probably ascribed mental illness to supernatural forces and treated it through magic. Hippocrates swept aside some of mystical clutter through his insistence on rational knowledge: "I assert that the brain is the interpreter of consciousness." That bawdy Greek, Aristophanes, in his play *The Clouds* even anticipated the Freudian psychoanalytical technique:

> SOCRATES: Come! On to the couch!
> STREPSIADES: What cruel fate! What a torture the bugs will this day put me too!
> SOCRATES: Ponder and examine closely, gather your thoughts together, let your mind turn to every side of things; if you meet with a difficulty, spring quickly to some other idea, above all, keep your eyes away from gentle sleep.
> STREPSIADES: Oh, Woe, woe! Oh, woe, woe!

(But when Socrates, thinking that Strepsiades is now deep in psychoanalysis, enquires about the reason for his anguish, Strepsiades confides that the problem is the couch; the bugs are nibbling at his gonads.)

In Roman times, Soranus treated the mentally ill by psychological methods and managed them humanely and as comfortably as he could. The collapse of the empire brought anarchy, and with it a return to supernatural explanations for life's mad mysteries. Briefly, in the early Middle Ages, the insane were again treated with sympathy—the influence of the Greeks had revived. "One of the earliest asylums for the mentally ill, the Bethlehem Hospital in London, was originally far different from the snake pit that later became known as Bedlam. In those early days patients were treated with concern. When they were able to leave the hospital in the care of their relatives, they were given arm badges to wear so that they could be returned to the hospital if their symptons should recur. These patients received so much attention and sympathy from the community that vagrants often counterfeited badges so they would be taken for former patients of Bethlehem. In the thirteenth century, in Gheel, Belgium, an institution was established to take care of the retarded and psychotic children, who were often boarded out to and adopted by sympathetic families in the neighbourhood."

In the fourteenth century the mentally ill came to be considered as witches or demons, and were persecuted accordingly. The process by which this came about was a complex one, but stemmed basically from a series of fires, famines, and epidemics that caused Europeans to suspect that God had turned against them. The church, custodian of the public soul, searched for diabolical scapegoats. They found them at work not only among the flock but in their own fold. "Centuries of imposed celibacy had not inhibited the erotic drives of monks or nuns," wrote Alexander and Selesnick in their *History of Psychiatry*, "and underground passageways were known to connect some monasteries and nunneries. Townspeople often had to send prostitutes to the monasteries in order to protect the maidens of the village. It became increasingly imperative to the Church to start an anti-erotic movement, which meant that women, the stimulants of men's licentiousness, were made suspect. Men's unsavory impulses could no longer be tolerated, so they were projected upon women under a misogynic banner whose motto was: 'Woman is a temple built over a sewer.' Women stirred men's passions, therefore they must be the carriers of the devil. Psychotic women with little control over voicing their sexual fantasies and sacrilegious feelings were the clearest examples of demoniacal possession; and in turning against them the Church increased an already mounting fear of the mentally deranged."

Mass psychotic movements, such as that of the flagellants who whipped themselves across the continent in the hope of placating God, further panicked the church into extremism. Its worst excess was a book written by a pair of Dominican monks: *Malleus Maleficarum*, a sort of textbook of psychopatholgy.

It was also a text for the Inquisition. After proving conclusively that demons and witches existed—conclusively because, if the reader were not convinced, he was *ipso facto*, a witch, demon, or a heretic himself—the book went on to show how witchcraft worked, complete with explicit descriptions of sexual orgies. It described how witches were to be tried and punished. The text was followed faithfully enough over the next three hundred years, hundreds of thousands of women and girls being burned at the stake.

The judicial process was not without its kicks. The Inquisitors were given an opportunity to grope the comlier witches under the pretext that they were searching their private parts for hidden charms or tokens; and the judges' voyeuristic tendencies were indulged by the requirement that the witch was to be paraded naked before them, complete with shaved pubis. The excuse for this later touch was to deny the devil the opportunity to hide in her pubic hair.

Unfortunately for other members of their sex, some emotionally disturbed women co-operated with their tormentors. It was not until such Renaissance men as Johann Weyer began to investigate cases of witchcraft objectively that the ecclesiastical malevolence began to subside. One of Weyer's cases involved a sixteen-year-old girl who asserted that the devil had put foreign objects, including pieces of cloth, into her stomach. Weyer showed that she had taken the cloth orally; it was damp only from saliva, not from gastric juice.

In the seventeenth century, Thomas Sydenham made notable contributions in recognizing that psychological factors had much to do with disease, or even that disease could be simulated by such factors, for example hysteria. Generally the Age of Reason produced a great advance in the realistic approach to psychiatry. The first person to employ the term "neurosis" was William Cullen, though his methods of combating anxieties and depressions were primitive: purging, bloodletting, use of emetics, and so forth. Another pioneer, Philippe Pinel, wrote systematic descriptions of psychotic illnesses. At the same time, the treatment of the mentally sick as a whole grew steadily worse. Bethlehem Hospital had now become Bedlam, a tourist attraction for Londoners, who could spend an enjoyable afternoon laughing at and taunting the mad people. There were a few rather more enlightened institutions such as the Narrenthurm in Vienna and the Pennsylvania Hospital, which had been founded in Philadelphia in 1751, but for the most part conditions were frightful, with atrocious treatment from brutal attendants. Symptomatic of the fear that insanity inspired was the professional reaction to Pinel when he took over the administration of the Bicêtre in Paris, unchained the inmates, and gave them fresh air, fed them palatable food, and treated them humanely. His colleagues thought that he himself had gone mad.

The most important figure in the study of psychology, personality, and psychiatry and its disorders, Sigmund Freud, "succeeded for the first time in explaining human behaviour in psychological terms and in demonstrating that behaviour can be changed under the proper circumstances." As one of the greatest of pioneers, his path was also perhaps the most difficult because his research, however scientifically conducted, lay in the quicksands of personality rather than the solid grounds of measurable fact. In later life he would say of Einstein that, "The lucky fellow has had a much easier time than I have. He had the support of a long series of predecessors from Newton onward, while I have had to hack every step of my way through a tangled jungle alone. No wonder that my path is not a very broad one, and that I have not got far on it."

Nevertheless, many of the observations could be repeated, his conclusions checked. For the first time he made the psychological approach to psychiatry work. He postulated that mental illness is the outcome of an individual life experience. His chief accomplishment was his study of unconcious phenomena and the psychoanalytic method of treatment. As J. A. C. Brown described it, "Patients were asked to relax on a couch and say whatever came into their minds, however absurd, unpleasant, or obscene it might appear by everyday standards. When this was done it appeared that powerful emotional drives swept the uncontrolled thoughts in the direction of the psychic conflict as logs floating on the surface of a great river are whirled about by the currents beneath the surface of the water." The resulting painful memories were frequently found to relate to traumatic sexual experiences in childhood.

Freud later modified these findings, especially in the light of the terrifying dreams of battle-shocked soldiers in the First World War, which could hardly be interpreted in terms of sexual symbolism. In fact, psychiatry as it is known today, began with the thousands of First World War shell-shock victims. For the first time it was clearly recognized that everyone, however emotionally stable, was vulnerable to psychological, physical, and social stress, and had a breaking point.

On the other side of the Atlantic, Benjamin Rush, one of the signatories of the Declaration of Independence, anticipated in a minor way Freud's theory of the subconscious. He encouraged his Pennsylvania patients to write down their psychobiologies in the belief that the script would shock the patient out of his morbid ideas. Rush, described by the historical geneologists as the Father of American Psychiatry, had been influenced in his restricted humanitarianism by Pinel; restricted because, though he believed in considerate treatment for the mentally disturbed—occupational therapy, good food, and comfortable lodgings—he remained committed to eighteenth-century methods: dosing with emetics and purges, bloodletting, restraint, punishment, and shock. Tricking the patient out of his delusion was one of his methods. For example, if a patient was convinced that he could not empty his bladder, Rush might tell him that the world was on fire and that only his urine would put out the conflagration. If that failed to work, Rush recommended dropping the patient into icy water, or some similar jolt designed to scare the delusive piss out of the poor fellow.

Rush's *Medical Inquiries and Observations upon the Diseases of the Mind* was the first American textbook on psychiatry. It was based on his thirty years experience at the Pennsylvania Hospital.

A successor at the same hospital, Thomas Kirkbridge, and a non-medical crusader, Dorothea Lynde Dix, also advanced the cause of the mentally ill in the United States. Dr. Kirkbridge's greatest achievements were in mental hospital administration, design, and planning. Dorothea Dix's impact was on the consciences of the politicians. She shocked state legislatures into doing something about the appalling plight of the insane under their jurisdiction. The career that made her famous began when she visited the East Cambrige jail in Massachusets, and found that the mental patients were being confined indiscriminately with criminals and degenerates. Appalled by their plight, she became a reformer in their cause, in Canada as well as in her own country. It was through her efforts, money, and concern, that a mental hospital was built at St. John's, Newfoundland in 1855. She also lobbied the Nova Scotia Legislative Assembly on behalf of the mentally sick of their province, for whom there was then no treatement centre. She prevailed on the assembly to pass the necessary legislation, and personally supervised the building of an institution for such patients.

Writing about Dorothea, a Canadian psychiatrist, Joseph Workman, wrote to one of his friends, "Have you seen Tiffany's book, the biography of Miss Dorothy L. Dix? If you have not, just wait until somebody lends it to you. It is truly (?) a florid production—very captivating to those who can appreciate spread eagle-ism. I, however, read between the lines. I see that her father was a real *paranoiac*—a religious propagandist who spent all his money (or that of other people) in the publication of pamphlets which Dorothy was condemned to stitch and address, until she ran away from Worcester to Boston when she was eleven years of age. That was in 1813, when travelling was not easy—on foot. The history of her achievements is nothing short of miraculous. It shows how much a good crank can accomplish when fortune puts him (or her) on the right track."

Workman was one of the Canadian pioneers who made notable contributions in the humanitarian and scientific treatment of mental illness.

The situation that Dr. Workman experienced in the mid-nineteenth century was similar to that obtaining in most western countries, a basic insensitivity to the needs of the mentally ill. During the French regime in Canada, an early start had been made in treating mental patients in a hospital environment. In 1714, the General Hospital in Quebec provided a special ward for mentally sick women, and later, accommodation was found for about a dozen men. Otherwise, harmless lunatics were allowed to drift about the countryside, finding what food and comfort they could from those who did not share the superstitious fear of madness. By the early nineteenth century, most of the insane were being segregated in the usual way, in jails or asylums, or, at best, hidden away in shameful attics.

The first Canadian asylum for the insane was opened in Saint John, New Brunswick in 1835, the year of Joseph Workman's graduation from the McGill medical school. The asylum in Toronto, which was opened six years later, exemplified the prevailing attitude to the insane. It was an abandoned jail.

William Canniff had high praise and unbounded admiration and affection for Joseph Workman. He wrote of Workman that, "He stands equally high as a physican, as a teacher, as a writer to the medical and secular press, as a critic, as a linguist, and especially high in that branch of medical science to which he gave the riper years of his active, practical life." By the end of Workman's life he was, according to Canniff, internationally admired, "particularly by advance psychologists of Italy." Yet at one point in his life, Workman actually gave up the practice of medicine to become a shopkeeper.

After obtaining his M.D. at McGill, Workman hurriedly married his girl friend, Miss Wasinge, daughter of an English manufacturer of cutlery. The reason for the haste was not the usual one. He was afraid of losing her. The Wasinge family had threatened to cart her off to Toronto, where they owned a hardware business.

Workman practiced in Montreal for a year, until his brother-in-law in Toronto, who was running the hardware store, died in an accident. Workman was persuaded to take over the business. Accordingly, with his wife and baby, he moved to Toronto in 1836, and gave up medicine; though to be on the safe side he procured his licence to practice in Upper Canada, just in case he failed as an ironmonger.

Instead, to his dismay, the business thrived. He seemed to be stuck with it. At one point, escape from seeders and adzes, Japanned ware and blue-flamed stoves, Labradors, mangles, Manilla rope, and shovels, seemed possible when his friend, Dr. John Rolph, invited him to teach at his new medical school. (Dr. Rolph had been persuaded that Workman was a good doctor because his sympathies were with the reformers against the tin-pot Establishment). "But Dr. Workman deemed it to be incongruous to deal in hardware and teach medical science at the same time, and therefore declined Dr. Rolph's invitation."

After ten years of shopkeeping, however, Workman had had enough, and when Rolph again invited him to lecture at his school of medicine, he accepted. His first course was in midwifery and diseases of women and children. Fortunately he had kept up with developments in the medical arts by extensive reading of medical journals, to which he also contributed, so that his lack of practical experience in midwifery was partly offset by an up-to-date knowledge of the theory.

Meanwhile, on the asylum front, those responsible for the Provincial Lunatic Asylum were busy maintaining the Toronto tradition of vicious controversy in matters medical (in the stimulation of which Dr. Rolph was particularly adept). The asylum, which had started out in an abandoned jail, had subsequently transferred to a wing of the Parliament Building which was then on Front Street, Toronto, and finally to ominous-looking quarters at 999 Queen Street.

By the 1850s the asylum had already used up several superintendents.

They had displeased the board of directors and as a result had been forced to resign. "The natural result," as one superintendent said, "was anarchy and neglect of the patients."

The insane were neglected enough to begin with. Describing the asylum in its original prison quarters, a contemporary observer, J. Henry Toke, said that, "It was dark, and the faces of the seventy patients showed misery, starvation and suffering. The doctor in charge pursued a system of constant cupping, bleeding, blistering, and purging the patients, giving them the smallest quantity and poorest quality of food. No meat was allowed." William Canniff, who always knew the juiciest details of any local medical intrigue but who was too gentlemanly to impart them to his scandal-loving readers, merely informs us in reserved language that some verbal pushing and shoving went on in the highest quarters to fill the superintendent's position after the "retirement" of the last incumbent.

Naturally, John Rolph was one of the pushers and shovers, undeterred by the fact that one of his rivals was backed by the governor-general, Lord Elgin. Elgin had a candidate, Dr. John Hunter Robinson, who happened to be from Lord Elgin's home town in Scotland. But Rolph's chirurgical clout had been augmented by his appointment as a cabinet minister. His protégé was Dr. Workman. Dr. Workman got the job.

Administratively, Workman's task was made easier by the replacement of the squabbling board of directors by a government committee. This resulted in increased powers for the superintendent that enabled him to actually superintend. Hygienically, though, he ran into trouble with an outbreak of cholera that carried off several of the patients. After a lengthy and malodorous investigation, he discovered that the builders had failed to connect the drains to the main sewers, thus converting the entire basement into a seething cesspool. (To his chagrin, Dorothea Dix would have to pick this of all times to visit the Toronto asylum.) After the drains problem was rectified, "perforating Dysenteries, intractable Diarrhoeas, and the whole Typhoid family of deadly complications ceased to perplex the Medical staff."

Workman remained as superintendent for over twenty years, during which period the conditions at the asylum improved enormously. For the first time the staff had a director whom they could admire and respect. One of his clinical assistants who was later put in charge of the Verdun Protestant Hospital in Montreal, said of Workman that "I can scarcely recall an evening on which this gifted man did not pass an hour or more in one or another of his wards, the centre of a circle of patients, for whom he never failed to find some topic of interest by which to divert them from their morbid thoughts."

Workman soon confirmed what Pinel in France, Chiarugi in Italy, and others had demonstrated: "that to a remarkable degree the mentally ill would respond to what was expected of them. Treated like dangerous beasts, they behaved as such. Treated with dignity, humanity and understanding, they responded in a more socially acceptable manner. Conversation, reading aloud, games and useful and interesting activities of all kinds were shown to have beneficial effects. This type of program was called 'moral treatment.'" (The authors of *A Study of Psychiatric Services in Canada* point out that this program resembled in many ways the programs now used in most modern mental hospitals—milieu therapy, remotivation therapy, and activity programs.)

In his extensive writings, Workman was much exercised over the contemporary theory of moral insanity—behaviour ascribed to immorality rather than to pathology. In one of his papers, published in the *American Journal of Insanity*, he argued against the momentarily fashionable concept of moral insanity, backing up his argument with such cases as that of the lady, who, "by a series of the most extraordinary misrepresentations and cleverly carried out impostures, raised large sums of money on no security whatever, and spent them as recklessly; imposed on jewelers, so that they trusted her with goods worth hundreds of pounds; furnished grand houses at the expense of trusting upholsterers; introduced herself by sheer impudence to one great nobleman after another, and then introduced her dupes, who, on the faith of these distinguished social connections, at once disgorged more money. To one person she was a great literary character; to another, of royal descent; to another, she had immense expectations; to another, she was a stern religionist."

It was only when she developed marked insanity and brain disease from which she soon died, that the people she had lied to, conned, and cheated, realized that they had been duped by a lunatic. But, "had this poor woman's insanity not culminated speedily, but progressed slowly and insidiously, as it does in thousands of cases, she would, beyond all question, have been consigned to a penal prison,... the judge would have frowned, the prosecuting counsel would have sneered, the jury would have been astounded, and the press would have applauded their verdict of guilty."

In the same article, rather more tenuously, Workman discussed the case of a girl of fifteen, Kate, whose behaviour had convinced her mother that she was destined for a life of shame. Three physicians had certified her as being morally insane. After she had spent several months in the asylum, Workman found nothing wrong with Kate, and sent her home. Two days later the mother brought her back, "and presented to me a large bagful of various articles of dress, on which Kate had been practising dissections. I looked over them considerably, and on closing my inspection, I said to the mother, 'There is too much method in this madness to convince me of its genuineness. We have had the girl here over four months, during which she had never spoken one word indicative of insanity, nor has she done one act pointing in that direction. I can not re-admit her, for I believe she is not insane." But the mother became distracted, terrified that the girl would end up as a prostitute. Workman took the girl back for another thirteen months, "during all which she was just as good, as gentle, obedient and obliging, as she had been throughout her former residence. I now talked to her in a very serious and paternal manner, showing her the impropriety and irrationality of her conduct at home, and pressing on her the consideration of her own best interests, which must be ruined by her continuance in a lunatic asylum. She listened to all I said with much deference, but finally told me she would like to leave the asylum, but not to go home to live with her mother. Now, her mother was neither harsh nor capricious, but, on the contrary, she had been both kind and forbearing; and her father and brothers had been equally so. I must say that this ultimate enunciation of my gentle patient let in a little light; for I well knew that the likings and dislikings of the insane are almost always unaccountable, and that both fall upon objects or persons apparently the most foreign to the rational incidence of either."

Workman finally arranged for the girl to live elsewhere. Three years later he saw her again, during which time she had shown "no more symptoms of insanity, either moral or intellectural."

The story is interesting in its explication of pre-Freudian thinking. Workman argued that if he had believed that Kate was morally wrong-headed rather than having a "constitutional strain of insanity in her frame," and had treated her accordingly, as a felon, she would have ended up as a hardened criminal. In light of Freudian theory, the girl would surely be considered neither morally nor constitutionally insane, but rather the victim of some subconscious trauma connected with her family.

Workman wrote enlightenedly on witchcraft in his book *Demonamania and Witchcraft*.

Throughout his sympathetic administration and decades of scientific study, Dr. Workman kept a diary. A researcher's perusal of the manuscript, at the University of Toronto, inspires affection for the man as revealed through his private thoughts and comments; on his children (Son Fred, Son Will), and his acquaintances, and on other topics, such as books, birds, politics, and the weather. He gets mad at the post office, particularly over an increase in its postal rates. He cries over his wife's death, and writes a poem about it. On a visit to Montreal he is tickled to find his mother reading away, as bright and alert as ever, even though she is a hundred years old; he gets very annoyed over his daughter's honeymoon on "A boat to Montreal, on one of those stupid modern excursions, called Marriage Tours," and offers her fifty pounds sterling if she will give up this expensive nonsense. He is told to keep his fifty quid, and scrawls peevishly in his diary, "I *shall* keep it. My disbursements for a dress and other marriage fooleries, including $40 to Annie have been over $350." Then follows a diatribe on modern children, but he adds that, "She has been a good and dutiful child. I never raised a finger in correction of her. May God bless her." He trips fifteen hundred miles through several American states, and is pleased with everything he sees except Chicago, which he describes as "a huge den of scoundrels, sharks, pickpockets, and other human cattle." And he writes with Canadian resignation on the prospects for the future of the country: "1867, Monday, July 1st. Today is celebrated the Confederation of the British American Provinces. May our new state of political existence realize all the benefits promised by the promoters of the measure. My fear, however, over-weighs my hopes."

He was nearly as pessimistic about the prospects for another association, the Canadian Medical Association, to which he was elected president. Commenting on it in the 1880s, he said that, "The discussions were spiritless and vapid. Those who spoke merely showed that they could not be silent, but had they held their tongues, they might have passed for wiser men. The meetings were full, but a few more of such will bring the Association to a natural death."

The C.M.A. Members at the time were mentally so rigid that they regarded even Dr. Richard Bucke with suspicion. Soon after taking over the London, Ontario lunatic asylum in 1877, Dr. Bucke had abandoned the usual mechanical and chemical restraints on the inmates. His critics called him impractical. When excellent results were obtained, they called him a visionary.

"There is something very curious about this non-restraint movement," Bucke replied. "To those who practise it, it seems very simple, but those who do not practise it do not, and apparently will not, believe in it."

Bucke's approach to psychiatry was partly organic. What particularly upset his colleagues were his surgical interventions, his operations on the female patients to correct uterine and ovarian disease. According to Dr. Cyril Greenland in his paper on Richard Bucke, the bushy-bearded medico claimed that the increase in the discharge rates of female patients fully justified these procedures. He quotes Bucke as saying that, "It comes to this, that the treatment of the mind resolves itself into an endeavour to place the whole physical system on the best possible basis of health and efficiency." Greenland comments to Dr. Bucke that, "mental illness was not simply an accidental aberration necessitating skilled and humane treatment, but evidence of a failure of the biological process by which mankind adapts to change."

Recent developments have shown that the organic approach in some areas of psychiatry is entirely valid. Many of the new medical theories of disease apply to the problems of mental illness. For instance, vitamin deficiency can cause psychotic symptoms. Chromosome disarray and biochemical mistiming are other causes of mental malfunctioning. A whole new direction in such scientific exploration had been plotted in the twentieth century. "Oxygen consumption in the brain, how muscles convert chemical energy into work activity, the metabolism of nervous tissue, and the action of hormones were under investigation. It was discovered that the efficiency of certain organs can be measured electrically, since there are variations in the electric potential within their tissues. In 1929, Hans Berger showed that variations in the electrical activity of the brain could be recorded on graphs, and he invented the electroencephalogram, an invaluable tool in diagnosing brain abnormality."

Richard Maurice Bucke was yet another of the wide-ranging, intensely individualistic doctors who have made the Canadian medical scene so distinctive; one of a host of great men and women whose lives expound the early history of the country, its crudeness and simplicity, its pains and morality, and its burgeoning sensitivity to the human plight. Like so many pioneer doctors, Bucke was the son of a clergyman, imbued with the spirit of service to others, but also a self-interested spirit that allowed him a stake in fortune and fame. With the rest of the family of Horatio Bucke, a Church of England curate, and his wife Clarissa, Richard was brought to Canada when he was one year old. The family of nine settled at Creek Farm, three miles east of London. There the curate gradually transformed a valley of elms and its trout stream into an English country estate, complete with a gabled house of great chimneys and drafty fireplaces. As in so many pioneer families, it was the wife who held the family together. When Clarissa died fifteen years later, the fortunes of the family started to decline. There was the inevitable conflict between Richard and his father, and soon after his mother's death, Richard decided to "live elsewhere." He had not yet come to appreciate the great benefit he had derived from his father. He left home in 1853, when he was sixteen years old. Over the next three years he worked as a gardener in Columbus and on railroad construction in the same state, Ohio; as a fireman on a Mississippi steamer; then later as a maker of barrel staves in the Louisiana swamps. In 1856 he went west, as a driver in a wagon train traveling from Fort Leavenworth, Kansas, to Salt Lake City.

He wrote about this and subsequent adventures long afterward, in a pamphlet entitled *Twenty-Five Years Ago*. Richard's experiences were so colourful and dramatic that certain fictional accounts of the opening of the American West were based on them. When he arrived at Salt Lake

City, Utah, after a journey of twelve hundred miles lasting five months, he heard about a gold strike in California, and decided with several other drivers to continue onward and obtain a share of the rumoured riches. Four parties of drivers were formed, each with its "prairie schooner" for carrying supplies, and a team of horses to draw a large water cask. Richard was a member of the second party to set off toward what he called the Great American Desert.

Fortunately he and his nine companions possessed a few weapons, including a shotgun, five rifles, and two revolvers; for at dawn one morning they were attacked by a large band of Soshone Indians. A series of skirmishes ensued. The Indians wounded two of the invaders, one with an arrow in the shoulder, the other, a man named Butler, with a bullet in the intestines. Richard shot at least one of the Indians. After several others had been wounded they withdrew; just in time, for by then the white men were almost out of ammunition.

The Indian attack was only part of the ordeal, for the water cask was now empty, and their provisions almost exhausted. Their thirst, at least, was relieved when they managed to veer back to the Humboldt River, but it took them another six days to reach their immediate destination, Sam Black's trading post at the edge of the great American desert.

There they were joined by other wagon drivers, some of whom had also been wounded in skirmishes with the Soshone. One of the drivers had asked to be left behind with a pistol so that before dying he would be able to take at least one of the Indians with him.

Richard's party continued onward, carrying Butler in one of the wagons. Butler eventually recovered from his intestinal wound. Being deprived of food and water had saved his life. By the time the party reached the Sierra Nevada Mountains, winter was approaching, so they did not dare to cross. Richard, now twenty years old, remained there until the following spring. He bought tools and staked a claim in a mountain cleft named Gold Canyon. There he made friends with two boys who were about his own age, Hosea and Allen Grosh. They too, were sons of a clergyman. They had been prospecting since they were about fourteen years old.

The previous year, Hosea and Allen had found not gold but silver in Gold Canyon, and when Richard met them they had just returned to exploit the find. Richard joined up with the brothers, and the trio determined to hack it on their own. But their luck seemed to have run out. That fall, Hosea struck his foot with a pick, and died of an infection.

In November 1857, Allen and Richard decided to push on to San Francisco. Loading as much food and rock samples as they dared onto Allen's donkey, they set off to cross the mountains, and by nightfall had reached Washoe Lake. The donkey, however, objected to an unfair share of the load. When the boys woke up the next morning they found that it had scarpered. Richard had to trudge a total of sixty miles before he could locate the beast and bring it back.

In Squaw Valley they were held up by a heavy snowfall that blocked the pass. As the donkey could not negotiate the deep snow, they killed it, and parceled it up—and thus ended up carrying the donkey.

Seven days later they were still in Squaw Valley, hemmed in by snow. Desperately they pressed onward, wearing improvised snowshoes, traveling along thousand-foot-deep ravines and across ice-fields. By December they were hopelessly lost. They had been forced to throw away their weapons, their geological specimens and most of their tools and personal possessions, and had eaten the last piece of donkey meat. They kept on, for there was no alternative, sometimes covering only six or eight miles a day through the snow, along the American River, up cliffs, down tangled slopes. Allen grew weak from hunger and exposure, and Richard despaired, and at one point proposed that they lie down in the snow and end it all. Allen insisted on going on, though his condition was even worse than Richard's. Bucke later admitted that Allen was much the braver of the two.

By December 6 they were reduced to traveling on hands and knees, and were almost dead with exhaustion when they reached a mountain cabin occupied by two prospectors, an Italian and a Chilean. The boys' feet were frozen, but the two men still hoped to save them by wrapping them in blankets and washing them in brine. Unfortunately Allen was too far gone. One morning he appeared to rally, and talked enthusiastically about the fortune they would make when they reached the gold field at Sugar Loaf. Twelve days after their arrival at the cabin, he died.

Richard's feet were not in much better shape and finally the miners sent for a surgeon, who announced that one foot and part of the other would have to be amputated. The surgeon, unfortunately, had little skill and the operation was so crudely performed that forty years later Bucke would still be suffering such pain as to incapacitate him for days on end.

Only once during those forty years did he complain. This was in Paris when, engaged in postgraduate study, he suddenly gave way to loneliness and despair, seeing himself as a wreck, hobbling through life with the aid of a cane. But at the time, during and after the amputation in the mountains, he was exultant, crying that though it had cost him his feet, yet it was worth the price. For, "I was born again."

The "rebirth" was Richard's new perspective on life, his determination to do something useful for the sake of himself and others. Perhaps it was inspired by the realization that if he had known something about medicine his friend Allen Grosh might have been saved. He determined to return home and apply to the best school of medicine in the country.

McGill University accepted Richard, though he had no formal education. In London, neither he nor his brothers and sisters had been sent to school, but had been taught instead by their father. That Horatio's tuition had been effective was now revealed when Richard proved to be a well-rounded student. In the year of his graduation, 1862, he carried off two of the nine prizes awarded that year. (Altogether, three of Horatio's sons became doctors, and another became a distinguished civil servant.)

After graduation, Dr. Bucke continued his medical education in Britain and France. In the following year he set up practice in Sarnia, Ontario. Three months later he received a letter from the Gould and Curry Silver Mining Company, which had taken over the mine established by the Grosh brothers. The company's claim to the title was being contested in the courts, and they needed Dr. Bucke's testimony to support it. Richard jumped at the chance to view again the wild grandeur of the western wilderness that he had come to know so painfully and well, not least because the company offered to pay his expenses to the tune of $250 a week, with a retainer of ten times that amount.

Just as Dr. Workman had nearly abandoned medicine for hardware, now Dr. Bucke almost abandoned it under the influence of nostalgia. He was sorely tempted to make Lake Tahoe his home. In California, according to Edwin Seaborn in his sketch of Bucke's life, while waiting for many weeks for the case to come to court, "he spent some of the happiest moments of his life driving here and there with 'Billy', his horse, catching trout in the streams, sailing to Cascade Lake, Emerald Bay, Sugar Pine Point, Falling Leaf Lake and Cave Rock. He rode over the Sierras by the trail he and Allen had followed, found the barrel of their gun near Squaw Valley, rusted and not worth taking away with him." And renewed acquaintances with his rough oxen-driving and mining friends. One of them was a fourty-four-year-old Trenton, Ontario man named Henry Comstock, who had staked claims at what is now Virginia City, Nevada, and discovered the fabulous Comstock Lode. "He talks as wild as ever," Richard recorded, and "says he has lost one hundred million since he saw me—thinks he is worth twenty-five million now." In fact, Comstock sold his holdings for minor sums; otherwise he never profited from the incredibly rich mining property to which he gave his name.

In time the court case was settled, and Bucke, throwing off his somewhat premature nostalgia, returned to Sarnia. To make sure he was not tempted to roam again, he married, and proceeded to build up a family of eight children, and an extensive practice that still gave him time to write and to translate foreign literary works into English. One of his translations was Renan's *Job*.

Eleven years after his return to Canada Bucke became the superintendent of the new asylum at Hamilton. A year later he moved to

London, where as superintendent of the asylum there, he found himself living hardly more than a few yards from the home that he had abandoned twenty-four years previously.

At the time of his appointment, the work of Pinel and others for the mentally ill was hardly known in Canada, and during his first year in office, Bucke accepted without protest the degrading methods of restraining the "lunatics." A year later, though, he began the improvements that caused consternation among his colleagues. His reforms started with alcohol, which at a few pennies a gallon, was lavishly used in the lunatic asylums to pacify the inmates. Bucke slashed the institution's annual expenditure on raw, pioneer spirits by 66 percent. If that wasn't bad enough, over the next five years, he was converted to the practice of non-restraint. The medical profession felt that this was madness.

There was even worse to come. According to Dr. Seaborn, "Bucke sought for and corrected whenever possible the physical ills of the inmates, adopting surgical methods when these were indicated. The infirmary installed in a small room adapted to the purpose, he saw grow to the proportions of a hospital. Concerts for which many of the most talented of London's artists appeared were given for the benefit of patients. Dances for them were given, the music being provided by members of the staff. It was common knowledge that the ability to play some musical instrument was the key to position on the staff. Sports among patients and between them and their attendants were encouraged. A field day of sports for patients was inaugurated to which the elite of the city appeared in a fashionable promenade. Lastly a chapel was erected at which the priests and ministers of all the denominations performed their respective rites."

Dr. Bucke had objected to the former practice of conducting services in an amusement hall. "The sight of a stage," he wrote, "is not favourable to the state of mind which ought to accompany the worship of God."

By 1884, Bucke could report that, "During the year just closed and for three months before that,...we have not used at this Asylum any mechanical restraint or seclusion of any kind whatever; neither have we during that time used any morphia, chloral, or other sedative drug for the purpose of quieting or calming any noisy or violent patient. Two years ago we began in earnest this non-restraint movement, and I must confess I have been as much surprised as any one else can be at the success we have had in carrying it out. It is not simply that we have disused mechanical restraints and seclusion, but we have revolutionized at the same time the whole morale of the institutuion, the disuse of restraint and seclusion being only a small part of the revolution."

To Bucke, Dr. Greenland writes, "mental illness was not simply an accidental aberration necessitating skilled and humane treatment, but evidence of a failure of the biological process by which mankind adapts to change." Bucke explored this theme in his two most important books, *Man's Moral Nature* and *Cosmic Consciousness*.

Bucke's main contribution to Canadian medicine was to introduce modern medical and surgical procedures not previously available to asylum inmates, thus bringing Canadian psychiatry, previously considered an outcas, into closer relationship with the rest of the medical family. Later his work was greatly extended by the third of our psychiatric pioneers, a man dedicated to the cause of psychiatry almost in spite of himself.

Dr. Charles K. Clarke first experienced the uneasy world of the insane at the age of seventeen, when he became an assistant to Dr. Workman, at the Toronto asylum. It was this experience rather than any real interest in the management of the insane that got him the position of assistant superintendent at the Hamilton asylum, following his graduation from the University of Toronto in 1878. He had hoped to set up in private practice, but medical school costs and the illness of his wife temporarily scrubbed that ambition.

The job in the Hamilton asylum did not exactly increase Charles Clarke's enthusiasm for psychiatry. "This experience was like a horrible dream," he wrote. "The staff were impossible, and in many instances an immoral and uncontrolled rabble."

The lonely ordeal lasted for a year, until William Metcalf took over the superintendency. Dr. Metcalf was a close friend as well as a relative — he had married one of Clarke's sisters. Between them, Metcalf and Clarke did what they could to make life easier for the mental patients. Three years later when Dr. Metcalf moved to the asylum at Kingston, he asked Clarke to go with him as his assistant. Clarke agreed, out of friendship and admiration for the older man rather than through any real commitment to psychiatry. He was as determined as ever to establish a private practice as soon as he could afford to do so.

This decision was, if anything, reinforced at Kingston, when he observed the extent to which the politicians were perpetuating the system of brutal restraint and seclusion through their interference in the running of the asylum. Finally he had had enough. Not even his friendship with Metcalf was proof against his frustrations. He sent in his resignation.

Usually it is the winds of circumstance that drive people off the course they had hoped to follow, mocking the poetic assertion that one is the captain of one's ship, the master of one's soul. In Clarke's case, the winds seemed to be holding him to a course he had no real desire to follow. The latest circumstance was the killing of Dr. Metcalf.

The danger from patients who were liable at any time to give way to homicidal impulse was not one that particularly alarmed Dr. Clarke, though the danger was always present. Richard Bucke also had a narrow escape from death when a patient named Joyce suddenly seized him by the throat and jumped with him into Lake Ontario, shouting "We will sink together, Doctor." On that occasion the doctor survived, though he was nearly dead by the time a passing blacksmith hauled them both out of the water. Dr. Metcalf was not so fortunate. While making his rounds one day, he was attacked by a patient and stabbed in the stomach. He died shortly afterwards.

As a result, Clarke was asked by the government to withdraw his resignation and take up the post of superintendent. Thus, once again his ambitions were thwarted by chance. He agreed, his motives in staying on purely humanitarian. He accepted, he said, in order "to protect several hundred defenseless creatures from a political hireling who might be pitchforked into the job."

As the years went by, however, his own energy and independent spirit created the career that he had attempted to resist. Circumstances had forced him into psychiatry, but he would become its foremost Canadian pioneer by his own efforts.

Clarke began by turning the asylum from a jail into a hospital. "Brutal and feckless" attendants were replaced by nurses. By 1887 he was providing the nurses and attendants with formal training in the care of the mentally ill. He removed the chafing linen, the leather harnesses, the iron chains, and other restraints that had worsened the condition of so many of the patients. But as others had shown he found that non-restraint was not enough; also required was the companionship of active therapy. Searching for some therapeutic occupation, he chose brush-making, because one of his patients had been a brush-maker. The therapy proved to be not only good for the patients but for the institution, his brush factory started to make a fair profit, until he could hardly keep up with the demand for its products.

The competition, though, was too much for other brush manufacturers, and for organized labour. Their protests brought a visit from the inspector of asylums. He ordered Clarke to close the workshop.

Bitterly disappointed, Clarke turned to music to soothe the savage breast. Learning that one of his patients was an old military bandsman "whose only fault," Clarke put in, "was that of looking upon the wine that is red," he persuaded the old fellow to form a band from among the dementia praecox patients. "Though in the end the band became quite proficient it was not easy to listen to, at first." The superintendent reported that initially, "they could only play a few selections, not too intricate, not too difficult, and I'm afraid not too harmonious."

The noise must have been particularly painful to the superintendent's ears for he was quite a skilled musician himself. His instruments were the violin and cello, and he would later become one of the three non-professional players in the Toronto Symphony Orchestra. But according to his son Eric (who later became a psychiatrist himself) Dr. Clarke was not quite as proficient with the cornet. Father must have been aware of this," Eric said, for "I noticed that he only played on it when I was in the house, so that the neighbours, particularly the family next door, thought I was responsible for the noise."

By 1893, Clarke was calling for the abandonment of the word *asylum*. "It is a difficult matter," he said in that year's annual report, "to get the non-professional and sometimes the professional men to realize that an insane person is one suffering from bodily disease just as much as the patient with typhoid fever.... We have hospitals for patients suffering from fever, etc. Why not hospitals for persons suffering from insanity?"

In time, the Kingston asylum became such an important centre in mental hospital administration that it attracted visitors from Europe and the United States. By the turn of the century, Dr. Clarke had become the country's most renowned psychiatrist, not least through his appearances as a forensic psychiatrist in many sensational murder trials. During the next quarter-century he was appointed dean of the Faculty of Medicine at Toronto and professor of psychiatry, superintendent of the Toronto General Hospital, and director of the Mental Deficiency Clinic and of the psychological laboratory. During these years he also developed the ambition to establish a psychiatry institute. It was finally realized after the First World War, with the building of the Toronto Psychiatric Hospital.

The lives of these three pioneers tell much of the story of psychiatry in Canada. "Dr. Workman brought decency and order into the asylum. With great courage and vision Bucke treated his patients as individuals. Synthesizing these elements Dr. Clarke laid the foundation for the development of psychiatry in Canada as a medical specialty. By emphasizing the need for research and enlightened public interest and participation, he also gave meaning to the idea that the scourge of mental illness would one day be prevented as well as cured."

Prevention was particularly the watchword of Clarence Hincks, founder of the National Committee for Mental Hygiene, which later became the Canadian Mental Health Association.

Hincks's predecessors had largely been concerned with the treatment of people already psychotic, neurotic, or otherwise mentally disturbed. He was one of the first to recognize the value of dealing with mental trouble before it incapacitated the sufferers, especially children. A super salesman in the cause of mental health, he obtained the funds for the project that later became the renowned Institute of Child Study, at the University of Toronto (headed by William Blatz); and he inspired the creation of many other psychiatric clinics, including the Crease Clinic in

Burnaby, B.C., one of the most modern treatment centres in the country, where at one time as many as 89 percent of patients were being returned to the community in a matter of months. During his lifetime, through his personal appeals, it was estimated that Hincks contributed half a billion dollars to projects related to psychological treatment, prevention, and research. He made sure that he himself never earned more than nine thousand dollars in any one year.

Dr. Hinck's crusade in the cause of mental health was inspired to some extent by his own neurosis. Periodically he lapsed into such profound depression that the best he could do was wait for the storm to pass. Thus, "My knowledge of psychiatry," he said, "comes from the inside, from my own personal suffering. Physical pain is like a pinprick compared to mental anguish." In a conversation with Sydney Katz, he once recalled the circumstances of his first attack. I was sixteen years old, he said, "A University of Toronto undergraduate, and I was spending a social evening at a friend's house on St. George Street. As I was playing cards, I suddenly became aware that there was something wrong with me. I had become self-conscious; I had lost all spontaneity of thought of action, and my world seemed to change in some queer way. When I spoke it was as though someone else was speaking and that I was more of a listener. My usually buoyant mood left me. I was not depressed but I lost the joy of living. I had become conscious of what had been previously automatic actions, such as using my handkerchief, shuffling my cards, moving about on my chair, etc. All these things became uncomfortable to me.

"I found it difficult to carry on a conversation, even small talk among intimate friends. There was a paralysis of my thinking; the free association of ideas was blocked. Thus, I was suddenly struck by a condition that affected me intellectually and emotionally. This was the attack that was to repeat itself each year up til the present. It usually comes in late winter or early spring and has lasted as long as four or five months.

"One of the things that has constantly amazed me is the way in which outsiders are unaware of what I am going through. Here I am with my entire inner life changed—anxious, wanting to be alone, thinking process slowed down, no zest for living—yet no one aware of it except two or three people who are closest to me. This led me to conclude that human beings are so wrapped up in themselves that we don't observe anything obvious like a bad limp or a blackened eye. . . . I have known people to visit mental hospitals and be unable to distinguish between staff and patients, unless staff wore their uniforms.

"My former chief, Dr. C. K. Clarke, noted this on many occasions and once conducted an experiment. At the time he was professor of psychiatry at Queen's University and superintendent of Rockwood Mental Hospital, in Kingston, Ontario. One evening, he invited to his home six leading

Queen's University professors, and without an introduction included one
of his patients from the mental hospital.

"Everybody had a good time. The conversation was animated and
ranged from music, history, world politics, to philosophy and science.
One of the most active participants was the mental-hospital patient.
After two hours of chatting, Clarke arranged for the patient to sit in
another room with his own family. Clarke took advantage of this absence
to ask the professors what they thought of his guest. They agreed that he
was a man of culture, widely read and an interesting conversationalist.
They wondered if it was Clarke's intention to propose this stranger for a
Queen's post. Clarke said, 'No, not at present because he happens to be a
patient of mine at the mental hospital.' The guests were astonished and
outraged and said that he had no right to be in a hospital; he was as sane
as anybody. Clarke then brought the patient back in and asked him this
direct question: 'Jim, please tell these gentlemen who you really are?'
Jim, slightly displeased by their ignorance, replied, 'Why, I thought they
knew. I am, of course, the strongest man in the world. I am Atlas. I
balance the world on my shoulders.'"

Jim was perhaps an exceptional subject for Dr. Clarke's experiment.
Edmund Brasset, who studied mental disease while acting as assistant
physician in the Nova Scotia Hospital in Halifax in the 1930s, noted that
most of his patients were people without much education. By and large,
Brasset wrote, "it seems that the person who is least likely to become
insane is the person of more than average intelligence, who has a broad
formal or informal education, who reads books, and who is 'nervous.'"

"This is my own observation at least, and I have my own theory about
the matter. The intelligent person is, I believe, better able to cope with
what Shakespeare calls 'the slings and arrows of outrageous fortune.'
Most nervous people are intelligent. Their nervousness is often a price
they have to pay for their superior mental equipment. Confronted with
too great and prolonged adversity, they may go into a state of temporary
exhaustion—exactly the same thing as the so-called combat fatigue
experienced by fighting men who have been exposed too long to the stress
of battle. It never of itself leads to insanity. The nervous person, the
chronic worrier, may develop ulcers of the stomach but his mind is likely
to remain intact."

Brasset's exception was an unusually intelligent clergyman and scholar
who often tried to explain to Dr. Brasset what it felt like to be insane.

"'It's like this. My mind seems to go around and work so fast and I
can't stop it. Let me give you an example. You say to me, "How are you
today, Mr. Smith?" Now, I answer you right away without hesitation. I
don't hesitate even a split second, but in that split second, this is what I
think: What does he mean by saying, "How are you today?" Does he

want to know how I am mentally or physically or does he really want to know anything at all? That is a mechanical phrase, "How are you today?" It really does not deserve an answer at all. Wasted words, wasted words, wasted words. Words should not be wasted. Should I answer him or not? If I don't answer him, he'll think I'm crazy, which of course I am after all. Maybe I had better answer him. So here goes with the answer, "I'm all right, thanks." Only the answers don't all come out right like that.'"

Clare Hincks' reaction to the same kind of question was similar, though of course his problem, albeit personally hellish, was insignificant compared with the clergyman's psychosis. (The basic difference between neurosis, suffered by millions who are still able to function well enough in everyday life, and psychosis, is that the neurotic is aware of his illness, while the psychotic has little or no insight into it, and does not attribute his troubles to his own mental health—if anybody is sick it is those around him, not himself.) "The best way friends and colleagues can act," Dr. Hincks said, "is not to ask me how I feel because the answer has to be "Like hell!'"

The neurosis that periodically incapacitated Clare Hincks through his life possibly had its origins in his family history. He was the only child of a Hamilton schoolteacher, a cultivated and capable woman to whom he was strongly attached. At the age of forty, Maud had married one of her former students, William Hincks. Hincks was twenty-six at the time. She put him through college. Their son, Clarence was born in 1885 at St. Mary's, near Stratford, Ontario. As he grew up he became increasingly aware that between himself and his father there was a rivalry for Maud's attention so marked that "it was as though mother had two sons."

When Clare was nine years old, his father, a Methodist minister, was transferred to Toronto, where, through the continued support of his wife, Clare's mother, he won wide recognition as a hellfire preacher. As Sydney Katz put it, "Every Sunday morning he staged spirited attacks on sin in all its guises, drinking, smoking, gambling, sex and Sunday streetcars."

The estrangement between father and son lasted right up to the day in 1936, when Clare, now fifty years old, invited his widower father on a trip to England. On the first night out on board ship the Reverend Mr. Hincks walked into the lounge to find his son not only drinking and smoking, but playing cards with total strangers. It was the first time he realized just what kind of a son he had. He was shocked, and as soon as he could talk to Clare in private, he lit into him, saying, "'I didn't know that I had a son who is a wastrel, a drunkard, a gambler and who keeps evil companions.'"

An unrepentent Hincks struck a bargain with his father. He would give up cards for the duration of the trip if his father joined him in a few drinks.

His father agreed. In the privacy of their cabin, the Reverend Mr. Hincks sipped a glass of crème de menthe and reported his sensations in detail. "'Now it's warm in my mouth...have a hot sensation in my throat...it's going through me like electricity...now I feel pleasant, good.'" A few minutes later he embarked on another experiment, this time using whiskey and soda. His findings were again positive. By the time the ship docked in Southampton, Clare and his father were close friends, a friendship, concluded Katz, "that lasted until his death."

The great turning point in Hinck's career came during a professional visit to New York when he met Clifford Beers, the founder of the mental health movement in North America. An engineer, Beers had been incarcerated in several asylums following a suicide attempt, and had been so shaken by the treatment he saw being meted out to the inmates and which he also experienced personally—that after his discharge he wrote a book, *A Mind That Found Itself.* It caused a sensation, and stimulated many wealthy citizens into supporting Beers' National Committee for Mental Hygiene.

Hincks returned home to establish a similar institution in Canada. Part of his objective was to improve the lot of mental patients throughout the country. Accordingly, over the years following the First World War he visited almost every asylum in Canada. The situation was even worse than he had expected. Along with an associate, Marjorie Keyes, he visited a "hospital" in Manitoba, where he came upon what appeared to be a coffin standing on end. When it was unlocked a woman fell out. She had been imprisoned in the coffin for three years. In the attic of a New Brunswick institution he found ten cages with straw on the floor where patients were kept. In Prince Edward Island he met inmates who were sequestered for no good reason, including a child who had merely been rebellious in school. Throughout the country he found cages, shackes, muffs, camisoles, and other forms of restraint in common use—this sixty years after Joseph Workman had unchained his first "lunatic."

It was quite possible that at least one of the inmates whom Hincks encountered was normal but had been incarcerated by unscrupulous relatives. R. J. Manion, practicing about this time at Fort William, suspected a number of such attempts on his patients. One of them was "a pretty little woman whose husband apparently tired of her and had decided that he would get rid of her by putting her into an asylum. She was an excitable little thing, but quite as sane as any excitable woman is. I knew her husband very well, and had known him for many years (though he was not Canadian-born), and warned him that, if he endeavoured to go any further with this case, it would be brought to the attention of the law officers, with whom he had had dealings in the past."

Another of Manion's clients had already been certified as insane by two Port Arthur physicians when Manion and a colleague were called in by a suspicious lawyer. The doctor found no hint of insanity; instead he found a passel of scheming relatives intent on confining the man in order to get possession of his substantial savings. "The physicians who had certified him were quite outstanding and reputable," Manion wrote, "the elder one being particularly able and intelligent. Probably they had been carried away by the stories of the patient's actions given them by these interested relatives, and had perfunctorily signed the certificate." Fortunately Manion managed to persuade the elder physician to rescind his signature.

Clare Hincks was so shocked by what he had seen during the tour of the country's asylums that he set about raising prodigious sums of money through the Canadian Mental Health Association. Subsequently he introduced widespread reforms: occupational therapy to mental institutions, hygiene courses to schools and among social workers, hygiene clinics and training for psychiatrists, and inspired research into mental deficiency. When he died in 1964, he had become one of the honoured figures in North American psychiatry, through his vision, his drive, and his selfless concern for the anguish of his fellow human beings.

25

The Most Famous Woman Doctor
of Her Time

WILLIAM OSLER INFLUENCED the lives of an extraordinary number of
people in the profession, and none more than Maude Abbott,
another great Canadian institution. In 1898 this plump, husky-voiced
work-demon had just been appointed curator of the McGill Medical
Museum when she attracted the renowned physician's attention under
distinctly painful circumstances. Following a professional tour of several
museums in the United States she arrived in Baltimore and sought out
Dr. Osler with a letter of introduction. She was invited to join his retinue
while he made his ward rounds. "The visit over, the procession had just
left the wards when an unpleasant, but certainly fortunate, accident
befell me, which threw me suddenly into personal contact with him to an
extent which even my connection with McGill was not likely to have
done. Standing for a moment with my hand on the lintel of the half-closed
door, someone swung the other heavy half-door to, crushing my finger
and neatly extracting the nail. Dr. Osler's concern took the form, after
the finger had been dressed by an intern, and a profitable morning given
to me in the pathological department on his introduction, of an invitation
to dinner that evening....

"Dinner over, the great experience of the evening came, for this was
one of Dr. Osler's student nights, in which I had been invited to participate. Seated at the head of the long dinner-table, now covered with a
dark cloth, with nine young men and three women ranged around it, and
me beside him at the end, and with a little pile of books before him, he
began by introducing four rare editions from the classics of medicine to
his hearers, with a few wise words of appreciation on each.

"Then followed a delightful talk upon points of interest or difficulty in the week's work, for these were all his clinical clerks, the reporters of his cases in his hospital service.

"And then, as I sat there with heart beating at the wonderful new world that had opened so unexpectedly before me, he turned suddenly upon me.

"'I wonder now, if you realize what an opportunity *you* have? That McGill museum is a great place. As soon as you go home, look up the *British Medical Journal* for 1893, and read the article by Mr. Jonathan Hutchinson on "A Clinical Museum." That is what he calls his museum in London, and it is the greatest place I know for teaching students in. Pictures of life and death together. Wonderful. You read it and see what you can do.'

"And so he gently dropped a seed that dominated all my future work. This is but an illustration of how his influence worked in many lives."

Dr. Abbott's primary responsibility at the McGill museum was to bring order to a large collection of specimens that had never been properly described and classified. At first the museum work seemed "a dreary and unpromising drudgery; but as Dr. Osler had prophesied, it blossomed into wonderful things." By the time Osler visited her six years later, the prodigious undertaking was almost complete. Among the remaining specimens that still required labeling were eighty-three that Osler himself had contributed while he was working in Montreal. Maude arranged the bottles on a table and waited, among the crowd that invariably assembled whenever Osler was expected, her heart fluttering as if awaiting a lover of exceptional tangency.

"I shall never forget him," she said in her autobiography, "as I saw him walking down the old museum towards me, with his great dark, burning eyes fixed full upon me." For the rest of the morning she listened to him and regarded him with the purest intellectual adoration, as he sat there talking about his beloved specimens. "'That fellow, now, I remember well,'" he said as he studied a large aneurism of the aorta that was innocent of any trace of laminated clot, and that had ruptured into the right pleura. "It took a long while before the diagnosis was made, but he came back into the hospital with a pulsation in the second and third interspaces. So we put him to bed and tried to cure him with Pot. Iodid. He got 120 grains a day, and the pulsation disappeared. We were talking of discharging him in triumph, when one day he died suddenly, and we found—that.

"'And this,' seizing suddenly upon a small unlabelled specimen which had completely mystified me, for it represented a small piece of apparently quite healthy thoracic aorta, with a round hole in its wall leading into a sac the size of a tangerine orange, which lay between it and the oesophagus, and opened into this by a small jagged tear. 'This is that extraordinary case of mycotic aneurism of the aorta rupturing into the oesophagus. She died without any warning at all. It is reported by me in the *International Clinics*. There is a beautiful coloured frontispiece of it done by old Mr. Raphael.'" And, as Maude shyly handed over a pickled heart, like a child who had been delegated to proffer a posey to a distinguished visitor, Osler remarked in his mysterious, dramatic way, "If that heart had not petered out when it did, in all probability I would not be where I am now." The heart had belonged to Osler's predecessor at McGill, whose professorship Osler had succeeded to.

Maude listened, entranced by the poet of pathology, and for the rest of her life would adore Dr. Osler with a love in which there was no trace of sexual sublimation. For her, passion was of the intellect, and her love was for those who aroused her mind. There is no hint in her life of any standard relationship with men, of desire and exploitation, duplicity, neglect, affection. She remained, it seemed, contentedly *virgo intacta*. It was the yearning for knowledge that possessed her, as it had been since she was eleven years old, in her birthplace, St. Andrews East, Quebec, on the north shore of the Ottawa River. Her childhood was affectionate and stable, even though she was the product of a failed marriage. Her father, the Reverend Jeremiah Babin, of French-Canadian extraction, had married the daughter of another clergyman named Abbott, but had abandoned his wife even before Maude was born in 1869. When Mrs. Babin died a few months later of tuberculosis, the grandmother, Mrs. William Abbott, adopted Maude and her sister Alice, and had their names changed by an act of parliament, to Abbott. Mrs. Abbott proved to be a perfect maternal substitute, being as intelligent as she was kind. She was remarkably cheerful, despite the loss of her husband and every one of her nine children.

Maude's motivation would earn sighs of envy from today's parents. She was educated at home by a governess, but the governess could not satisfy her desire for knowledge. "March 1884, one of my day-dreams, which I feel to be selfish, is that of going to school. I know Alice would like it herself so much, but I do so *long* to go. And here I go again; once begin dreaming of the possibilities and I become half daft over what I know will never come to pass. Oh, to *think* of studying with other girls! Think of learning German, Latin and other languages in general. Think of the loveliness of thinking that it entirely depended on myself whether I got on, and that I had the advantages I have always longed for."

Maude could hardly believe that other girls did not appreciate their incredibly good fortune in being allowed to go to school. "What geese some girls are. Why, there are hundreds of them going to school and longing to get away from it, and lots who would envy us a governess."

She was ecstatic when, at the age of fifteen, she was allowed to attend a private school in Montreal. But, "We are never satisfied. My next wish is to go to college, and now I am wishing for that almost as ardently as I did last winter for my present good fortune." A scholarship to McGill enabled her to realize this ambition, though not without difficulty. Men did not approve of higher education for women, not least because women were thought to be incapable of bearing the mental strain. The chancellor of McGill certainly thought so. When Grace Ritchie, one of the first women to graduate from McGill, had finished delivering the valedictory speech, he was quite solicitous. "And are you not tired?" he asked her.

It had been difficult enough getting into the arts course at McGill. When Maude's thoughts drifted towards a career in medicine she found that the medical barricades were much better manned than those thrown up by the arts people. She was refused admission. Members of the medical faculty were thoroughly alarmed at the prospect of teaching mixed classes. Besides, women, it was believed, did not have the stamina, mental or physical. And they would distract the men, with their undulating forms and promising eyes. Worst of all, the professors would have to cut the risqué sallies from their lectures.

She was finally admitted to the medical faculty of Bishop's College, but for Maude, this was very much a second best. "I was literally in love with McGill," she wrote, "and I have never really fallen out of love with her ever since." Later: "Those were dark days. No longer within the walls of my beloved McGill, among rough students, many of whom seemed to have lower standards than those among whom we had worked together for the pure love of working, and struggling, as only a first year student in medicine does struggle."

There were further difficulties when the time came to enter the teaching wards of the Montreal General Hospital. Grace Ritchie had managed to obtain her ticket of admission, but when a number of her friends from Queen's University also applied for admission, the hospital committee took fright at the prospect of an onslaught from a monstrous regiment of women students, and ruled that no further tickets should be issued to females. Fortunately, on Ritchie's advice, Maude had applied for a ticket while she was still in her first year, and the Hospital had given her a receipt for her twenty dollars, though they had not yet issued the ticket. When the hospital refused to hand it over, a number of men took up her cause in the newspapers. The ensuing typographical uproar caused the committee to hand over the ticket in a hurry.

On the whole, her three sessions in full attendance at the Montreal General were not too much of an ordeal, though there were moments of genteel embarrassment. As the only girl in the class, should she or shouldn't she stay and watch operations involving the private parts of the patients? To withdraw in confusion was sometimes as embarrassing as to remain.

The professors also made the occasional snide comment about their lady student. Francis Shepherd made one, and "The stamping and applause that greeted such a remark as this was the only unchivalrous act on the part of the men which I remember. A number of them had been my fellow-graduates in Arts, and I used to look longingly across at them, but I was now in an alien school, and I think over-sensitive, and somehow we did not grow intimate; and I was very lonely."

Part of the trouble was that she was personally unpopular. She was a glutton for work, and as her biographer, H. E. MacDermot, remarked, "such over-zealousness is never popular among students. She had no special charm of manner and with strangers was apt to be shy and awkward." To many she seemed uncouth. She was too free with her elbows, shoving her way through the crowd to obtain the best view. Even the superintendent of nurses, Miss Livingston, found her aggressive.

But then, a meek and mild Maude might not have graduated as brilliantly as she did, with the Chancellor's Prize, and the Senior Anatomy Prize.

Certainly, as Maude grew older and more confident about her place in a male profession, the warmth and simplicity of her nature was allowed its proper expression. Years later, Osler even described her as a "saint."

She was hardly that. She could be quite selfish, though she would have been astounded and upset if anybody had said so to her face. One of her characteristics, according to a friend, "was her power to make others conform to her time and plans. If, at times, one resented this," the friend quickly adds, "one realized that only in that way could she have accomplished her contributions to medical science." Another friend characterized her as "a most dynamic, amusing, lovable and sometimes maddening person. Always in such a fever of activity, with more paper, talks, and reports than anyone could possibly do; working all night, catnapping during the day."

Nowhere is Maude's concern for others better illustrated than in her relations with her sister. Her devotion to Alice was perhaps especially intense because Alice was the only close family she had. Even so, her concern for her elder sister's welfare was exceptional, especially after Alice, at the age of thirty, suffered complications following an attack of diphtheria, and became an incurable mental invalid. Formerly a placid and attractive person, Alice's nature changed completely. Maude refused to give up hope; she consulted one specialist after another, and steadfastly refused to place her sister in an institution, though Alice was sometimes quite violent. Much of what little money she earned from a small private practice and her museum work went to supporting and caring for Alice.

Maude particularly enjoyed picnics with her colleagues and friends. She took Alice with her whenever the young woman was enjoying one of her periods of serenity.

The museum work, meanwhile, though poorly paid, was going well, and was beginning to establish Maude's international reputation in the field. By the time of Osler's visit, she had transformed the place from a repository of shriveled kidneys and disregarded hearts, into a living force in the life of the university. She had communicated her enthusiasm for her pickled charges to the students. "The museum teaching was quite a spontaneous development," she wrote in her autobiography. "As I came to know the specimens intimately, the students began dropping in and asking questions about them. Professor Adami put up a notice saying that the students of the final year who wished the specimens demonstrated to them might arrange with me for this at hours mutually suitable." In time, these sessions became so popular that some of the best students returned again and again for demonstrations of the same material. The faculty, which until then had not taken Dr. Abbott too seriously, were so impressed by her work that they placed the museum demonstrations on the curriculum as a compulsory part of the course.

Members of the faculty had not taken Maude too seriously at first because she had not yet learned to associate freely enough with her male colleagues. She wanted to be accepted by the men as if only her shape differentiated her from them. But what they saw as her womanly disorganization got in the way. "She has her own peculiar methods of work," wrote H. E. MacDermot, who knew her in the days when she was working with her usual haste and energy in a small, screened-off portion of the museum, "in which system and orderliness were conspicuously absent, but everything she did was quite clear in her own mind, and no one ever found her at a loss for details. Her desk usually looked as if the papers had been deposited on it by a passing gust of wind, which might just as easily blow them all off again. But she would pass her hands through and over them and find what she wanted quite readily."

Maude was also touchy if she thought that the others were not giving her the respect that would have been accorded her had she been a man. She was furious if Dr. Roddick or Dr. Shepherd addressed her as Miss rather than Dr. Abbott. Naturally, Shepherd persisted in so addressing her, purely to rile her. She had not yet learned to take a joke against herself.

Maude took her work just as seriously, plunging into it so exclusively that the leisure of others was in constant danger. "In one afternoon she could suggest enough research to occupy a man for a hundred years," said a student. Her conversations also tended to be exceedingly time-consuming, so that at least one member of the faculty would hide when he saw her approaching. Those who failed to dodge out of the way in time might find themselves not only frustrated over her blithe disregard for their schedules, but increasingly confused over her dissertations. She modulated from one topic to another without making it entirely clear where one subject ended and the next began.

Her museum assistants could not, of course, escape, and were consequently loaded down with work, though admittedly the moment she realized that she had, for instance, kept her private secretary frantically at work for twelve hours at a stretch, she would be most contrite, and insist on the secretary going home at once. Maude herself was likely to forget all about minutes or meals.

Maude's simple, demanding nature did not affect the spirit of loyalty among her staff, though their admiration for her was sometimes tinged with irritation over her disorganized ways.

"It was not long," said one of them, "before we discovered Dr. Abbott's special trait in her work. She had about a dozen irons in the fire at the same time and all seemed in confusion. Moreover, she took on any new thing that came up with the greatest of enthusiasm, indeed as if she had nothing else to do. In her demonstrations to the students she would speak rapidly, showing specimen after specimen, with an enthusiasm which never faltered.

"At the time of which I speak she was working on the catalogue of the war museum; she was collecting material for the Osler Memorial number of the *Canadian Medical Association Journal*, she was engaged in a tremendous correspondence related to the Association of Medical Museums, of which she was treasurer as well as editor of its *Journal*, she was working on literature relating to several interesting specimens of congenital heart disease, and of course, she had her teaching.

"Her private affairs seemed to be no less complicated; she was superintending the transformation of an old church which stood on the grounds of her property in St. Andrews, into a duplex dwelling. The rent from this property was to provide income for the maintenance of the old home which was occupied by her sister, who had been an invalid for many years.

"She had far too many things for one person to do. But she had the talent of getting others to help her, either willingly or otherwise, but the protests, if there were any, were always silent. It was said by some that no one could have a five-minute interview with Dr. Abbott without getting something to do. She was like an economical housewife who never wastes anything! She never missed the opportunity of using a friend's time and energy, and if the individual was not a friend, she assumed that he very soon would be. It must be added that her manifestations of appreciation were warm and generous, taking the form of appropriate gifts or flattering references in the presence of others, or in print."

Maude was busy on numerous other tasks during the period to which this student was referring; so many tasks that frequently she ran out of hours and was forced to borrow from eating and sleeping time, and take out loans on the patience of others. Referring to a long-delayed manuscript of hers, and its even longer-delayed illustrations, one of Maude's correspondents wrote, "When I started editing this work, I had a beautiful suit of chestnut hair. Now it is completely white and almost gone. I hate to say who is responsible for this, but as you are a woman I know that I can leave it to your intuition." To which she apologized for the tenth time, replying that, "I am dreadfully distressed about your hair. I am sure when you get my illustrations it will begin to grow again."

Months later he was still trying to get the work completed.

In the 1920s, Maude was appointed professor of pathology at the University of Pennsylvania for a period of two years. By then she had learned to relax and to chuckle at herself as heartily as others did. Whereas formerly she had been disliked for her perfections, she was now loved for her faults. "She was always surrounded by a cortège of eager, happy admirers," wrote a Philadelphia colleague, "to whom she gave herself unreservedly and who in turn helped her with the details of life that we ordinary mortals fuss over but on which her mind did not dwell. We gathered up her belongings which she usually dropped at intervals, tried to remember where she had put the various papers she was going to need, and sorted out her kaleidoscopic plans.

"Journeys in her company never had a dull moment. Someone usually managed to pack her things in order, although there was nearly always something which had to be pulled out of the bottom of the trunk at the last moment. At the station there was always a crowd of her friends to see her off. She greeted each one warmly and invariably remembered some special thing that she wished to show to one or other of them, or some gift she wanted them to have. And the suitcases would be opened on the platform and the contents scattered while she hunted for the treasured articles. All aboard! Friends frantically pushed everything back again and she and her belongings would somehow scramble in just as the train started....

"Her amazing ability and persevering energy might not always be apparent behind this camouflage of scattered belongings, but one has only to turn to her writings and to consider what she accomplished in an age when a woman was anything but welcome in the field of medicine to realize her greatness."

By middle age, Maude had become quite eccentric, in the time-honoured tradition of the absent-minded professor. "She displayed," wrote Dr. MacDermot, "a curious mixture of fondness for clothes and conventional dress, together with carelessness about them. Her assistants say that she would come into the museum with a new dress on, which she would proudly display and would then proceed immediately to ruin it with the drippings from the specimens she handled."

At the age of sixty-four, Maude was still lighting the way for others with the midnight oil. Dr. William Gibson: "When I was a student in first-year medicine at McGill in 1933, I began a study of a set of little memo. books in the Osler Library which were used by Sir William Osler for jotting down all manner of quotations and case histories. One day a heavy gray-haired woman came into the library where I was working, and recognizing the Osler notebooks, asked if I was an out-of-town reasearcher in medical history. I replied that I was a first-year student at McGill and was interested in Osler. That was my fatal mistake! I was at once whisked downstairs by this bustling human dynamo who seemed only to cling to the stair rail, letting her feet find the step if they could. Within a few minutes I was in the midst of a sea of charts, books and pictures. A new edition of the Osler bibliography was about to be born — but first, 'some medical student with spare time' must be found to help with a few simple details."

Dr. Gibson was the simple medical student. Five years later he was still desperately thrashing through a sea of Oslerian publications on everything from tapeworms to nurses' education. Even when he departed for Oxford he could not escape, for "Dr. Abbott was sure that the Oslerian atmosphere of Oxford would contribute enormously to the success of the work." At one point he had accumulated so many bits and pieces of text for her that he had to paste them onto a roll of wallpaper, and post the enormous bundle off to Montreal where "Maudie" received it with rejoicing.

Maude Abbott's major accomplishment was her work on congenital heart disease. Once again it was Osler who aroused her intellect to its most passionate endeavour when he asked her to contribute on the subject to his *System of Medicine*, in 1905. When Maude asked him how she should go about it, he answered with typical loaded brevity: "Statistically."

"So," she said, " I began on the *Transactions of the Pathological Society of London*, and summarized all the cardiac anomalies there, and from this passed to other articles until I had records of 412 cases, with autopsies. I analysed all the individual cases in large charts spwn from our museum specimens."

It took her two years to complete the work. Fortunately it was not affected by the 1907 calamity, when fire destroyed the medical building, along with most of the Osler and Shepherd Pathological Society of London, and summarized all the cardiac anomalies there, and from this passed to other articles until I had records of 412 cases, with autopsies. I analysed all the individual cases in large charts spcollections of pathological and anatomical specimens. Maude's chief, Dr. Adami, lost his library and the manuscript of a new textbook on pathology. It happened that Maude's notes were all at home, where she did most of her writing, but even so, she was acutely distressed. An onlooker described her that morning as standing in the snow "with her hair all dishevelled, and her skirt on back to front, looking the picture of misery as she surveyed damaged museum specimens."

Later, Maude expanded her work and ultimately became, in the words of an American colleague, "the world's authority on congenital heart disease." This despite the fact that her work was not original. But it was a vital contribution, for until her extensive analysis, congenital heart disease was an obscure and ill-mapped area of medicine. Her monograph brilliantly illuminated the subject for the first time — and a clear definition of a subject is often as valuable as an original contribution to it.

"When we review Maude Abbott's influence in the field of cardiovascular disease," Dr. Paul White concludes, "we find that far more important than any of her written works was her vital stimulus to other workers. Her spirit was indefatigable. She inspired innumerable other workers throughout the world and was always very willing, in fact eager, to place at the disposal of anyone who sought it, her own vast experience and the details of pathological and clinical findings in the cases she had studied herself or analysed in the literature.

"Thus it may be said that many of the contributions, sometimes very important, to our knowledge of congenital heart disease made by others are due directly to Maude Abbott's influence."

It was that same spirit of informed enthusiasm that she had put into her museum work which made her a major figure in the international museum field and in Canadian social and medical history. Her life was not an easy one. "She had to contend with a combination of indifference and condescension in the attitude of many of the Faculty regarding her work. Maude had many good friends at McGill, but even the best of them were inclined to be merely tolerant of her activities. It was several years before she received from her Faculty colleagues the full and deserved recognition which was accorded her outside Canada."

Osler was Maude Abbott's one consistent guiding light. "He gave direction to her intensity of purpose, and took her work as seriously as it deserved. His encouragement was naturally of immeasurable solace and support. Little wonder that he was her hero."

26

Establishment Figures

WHILE TORONTO WAS still sixty years distant from the handsome, cosmopolitan city it is today, the life of a successful doctor in a then-complacent bastion of Anglo-Saxon respectability could nonetheless be stimulating. The city was on the international cultural trail, so that surgeons like Herbert Bruce had the opportunity to meet many a renowned colleague, among them William Osler, who was a frequent visitor until his departure for Oxford, and Joseph Lister, whom Dr. Bruce met at a dinner given in the visitor's honour at the Toronto Club in 1897. Governors-general, portrait painters, dukes and countesses, and even authors, dined at his table. His friends included Lord Tweedsmuir (John Buchan), Nancy Astor, R. S. McLaughlin, the automotive pioneer, Hamar Greenwood, who climbed high in British politics, Lewellys Barker, Lord Beaverbrook, Chief Justice William Mulock, Poet Laureate John Masefield, and Sir Victor Horsley and Lord Moynihan, who were internationally distinguished surgeons. At one time or another, Dr. Bruce met W. B. Yeats, poet, John McCormack, singer, Sir Ernest Shackleton, explorer, Sir John Martin Harvey, actor, and Generals Evangeline Booth and Sam Hughes of the Salvation and Canadian Armies, respectively. Frederick Banting and Vincent Massey, Dr. Charles Mayo and Queen Marie of Roumania, and Sir Richard Paget were also acquaintances, the last encountered at a Toronto meeting of the British Association for the Advancement of Science, when he demonstrated a machine, powered by a bellows, that was designed to aid people who could not speak. ("At any hour of the day we would hear the machine emitting its only sentence, 'Hello Lila! Hello Lila!'")

In contrast to the zigzag course of the Mathesons and the O'Briens, Herbert Bruce's medical career ran in a perfect straight line; the measurements of his achievements neatly marked off at the right intervals: B.A., M.D., F.A.C.S., L.R.C.P., F.R.C.S. (the second Canadian to receive this highest of all degrees in surgery by examination), and, toward the end of his distinguished career, the inevitable Ll.D. Not that Herbert Bruce was born with a silver tongue depressor in his mouth. His privilege lay in his mental ability and the sensitivity of his small, precise hands. The son of a self-educated farmer, he was born in 1868 at Port Perry on Lake Scugog, and matriculated at the age of fifteen. Being too young to enter medical school—his ambition to become a doctor had not wavered from his earliest years when he used to dose his family with prescriptions of cold tea—he did the next best thing and went to work in Allison's drugstore.

"Allison's drugstore gave me plenty of experience and responsibility," he wrote in his autobiography. "Of course, I was only an apprentice, not a qualified pharmacist such as Mr. Allison, and he would be responsible for any mistakes that I might make. But my responsibility was not lessened by the fact that the proprietor was addicted to laudanum. This meant that I was left in charge of the store when Mr. Allison took his dose and disappeared upstairs to sleep it off. The work was, however, not uninteresting, and the knowledge I gained in the composition and mixing of drugs was to prove of great value to me in my professional career. Then, unlike today, the doctors usually mixed their own prescriptions and no doubt in this way augmented their income. The store could sell many drugs without a prescription and it amazed me to find the confidence men and women placed in me, a boy of sixteen and only an apprentice, to provide them with a suitable remedy for their various complaints. They would tell me their symptoms and I was expected to sell them a cure."

Bruce's own addiction was to a new invention, the telephone, over which he held long conversations with Lewellys Barker, who was also working in a drugstore, a few miles away in Whitby.

"After about two years of apprenticeship in Port Perry, I saw an advertisement for a clerk with a knowledge of drugs to work in a drugstore in Toronto operated by Dr. Jehu Ogden. I applied for the job and was accepted. With two years of experience behind me I was now able to command a salary of five dollars a week and —what was more—was also provided with food and lodging. The store was situated on Queen Street at the corner of Bathurst. It had a little room over it in which I slept and I was given my meals at Dr. Ogden's house which was around the corner on Bathurst Street. He was a man of many parts for he not only practised medicine and owned a drug store, but also ran a milk route. Occasionally he took a few days' holiday and left me in charge of his patients. I remember once I had to look after a case of typhoid in a boy of eighteen (my age). He was very ill and delirious, and when a distended bladder developed I had to pass a catheter although I had never done this before. The patient lived, but I was very relieved when Dr. Ogden returned and assumed his responsibilities."

As soon as he was old enough, Bruce enroled in the school that John Rolph had established on his return from exile, the Toronto School of Medicine. "A two storey building with no pretence at architecture," it was located almost opposite the old Toronto General Hospital at Gerrard and Sumach Streets, where Bruce served as a house surgeon after receiving his B.A. degree in the spring of 1892.

It was typical of the irregular scene among the city's rival medical colleges that one should award the M.B., bachelor of medicine, another the M.D., doctor of medicine, and a third the M.D., C.M., doctor of medicine, master of surgery. To earn his M.D., Bruce had to submit a thesis. His subject was intestinal anastomosis. He did most of the work on the thesis at home in Port Perry. "During my last holiday after graduation, I was allowed to use the cool summer kitchen for my experiment. Catching a stray dog, I removed a portion of the small intestine under ether anesthesia. I then brought the ends together, keeping the channel open with two small plates fashioned out of turnip. Up to that time, such joining had been kept open until healing had taken place by a 'Murphy button.' This button was made first of steel and later of bone and was devised by Dr. J. B. Murphy of Chicago, surgeon and teacher. Later these methods were discarded and clamps were used which enabled the ends to be held together during suturing, after which the clamps were removed.

"My idea was that, after healing, the vegetable would disintegrate and avoid difficulties in the form of possible stoppage or ulceration as might be caused by the Murphy method. At all events, my operation was a success and the report, which I submitted to the Faculty describing it gave me both my M.D. degree in 1893 and also the Ferguson medal awarded for the best original paper."

After three years' study in London, with the F.R.C.S. after his name, Bruce was offered the position of associate professor of clinical surgery in his alma mater, which was now part of the University of Toronto. But on his return to Canada Bruce found that, true to the controversial tradition of the medical school scene in Toronto, the appointment had aroused more than a smidgin of spite and jealousy. It had been forced through by the vice-chancellor, the Hon. William Mulock, over the objections of the professor of surgery, Irving Cameron, who had been pushing a favourite of his own. Mulock wanted the best man for the job and had concluded that this man Bruce, gold medalist for his graduating year and Fellow of the Royal College of Surgeons, was the man for the job, despite his youth and the fact that he had not even started up in practice.

So when Dr. Bruce, unaware of the controversy, went along to Professor Cameron's place to thank him for the support, it was rather an awkward meeting. About the best Cameron could manage in the way of congratulations was a comment on the blueness of Herbert's eyes.

It was only then that Bruce recollected a couple of incidents involving Cameron when he, Bruce, was a house surgeon at the Toronto General Hospital. A patient had been admitted late one night with a dislocated hip joint, and without thinking, young Dr. Bruce had reduced the dislocation on the spot. The following morning, Cameron had reprimanded him, saying that Bruce's prompt treatment had deprived Cameron of the opportunity to demonstrate the problem and its solution to his class of students.

On another occasion, Cameron was giving a clinical lecture on a lump in the upper arm of a patient, and had diagnosed it as a fatty tumour. Bruce piped up with a request to be allowed to puncture the swelling. He said that he thought it might be an abscess rather than a tumour. Cameron reluctantly gave his permission, and was considerably put out when, following the puncture, a quantity of pus emerged.

Bruce wondered if Cameron's antagonism would sustain itself into their new professional relationship. He soon found out. For three years, Cameron gave him no chance to operate at the General Hospital, and would allow him into the out-patients department only once a week. As for teaching, he was assigned only a small class. The subject: bandaging.

Fortunately, Bruce managed to keep up his skills in the operating theatre at St. Michael's Hospital, where, "The kindly treatment I always received from the Mother Superior and Sisters... has remained a happy memory throughout my life." He was hoping to specialize in brain surgery. At St. Michael's he performed the first operation of its kind in Canada on a patient suffering from *tic douloureux*, a severe spasmodic pain affecting the distribution of the fifth sensory nerve; but given too few other opportunities to operate on the brain, he was forced to return to general surgery.

As the university appointment was unpaid—the prestige was considered to be remuneration enough—Bruce diverted much of his energy into building up a general practice. His second office was in a house, purchased in 1900, at 64 Bloor Street East. (Dr. Bruce would be as secure inside his property lines as within his social and professional circles. Every house and acre he purchased was in a perfect position to soar in value. The Bloor Street East property would later be bought by the Crown Life

Insurance Company, while his first farm would similarly make a huge profit, as it was located on Bayview Avenue — 120 acres of some of the choicest land around the city.)

At first Bruce visited his patients on a bicycle, or by the new electric streetcars. As the practice rapidly expanded he invested in a horse and buggy, the horse being a dual-purpose vehicle: he rode behind it on his way to hospital in the mornings, and on top of it in the afternoons, for exercise — liver-shaking gallops along Bloor Street, or up through the Rosedale ravines and through Moore Park. In his first year as a general practitioner he earned nine hundred dollars, in the second, two thousand dollars. Three years later he had paid back all the money he had borrowed to support himself through his postgraduate studies abroad.

By 1910, Bruce had a very large practice indeed, some of it out of town. In one such case, he received an urgent call on a Sunday, and he had to pay for a special train to take him to a village some hundred miles away, where a female patient was reported to be in great distress from a centrally placed abdominal tumour. When he got there, he found that the problem was quite a simple one; the patient was suffering merely from an over-distended bladder.

It was a ticklish situation. Bruce did not wish to embarrass the local physician by telling him that he had made an expensive mistake, especially as a rival doctor was present, who would be thrilled to witness a colleague's discomfiture. The two doctors did not get on at all well together. So, while he was placing the patient in the gynecological position, Bruce did some quick thinking. He decided to keep the rival doctor occupied and out of sight of the surgical work by appointing him as anesthesiologist. The doctor who had called him in would act as assistant. That left him the nurse. She would certainly be in a position to see that Dr. Bruce was merely emptying the bladder with a catheter. So just as he was about to start, he purposely dropped an instrument on the floor, and sent her out of the room to boil it for ten minutes. Immediately, while pretending to operate through the vagina, he hurriedly passed the catheter into the bladder and emptied it, and when the nurse returned, fussed around with various instruments to convince her that something important was going on.

The doctor who had called him in could see what Bruce was really up to, and must by then have been sweating with embarrassment over his faulty diagnosis. Afterwards, he was suitably grateful that the consultant had protected his professional standing in the community — but not so grateful as to call upon Bruce ever again for assistance.

As was usual in such cases, the work was done on a kitchen table under the light of kerosene lamps. Later, Bruce made a collapsible steel table that would fit into his car. The car also supplied the illumination. His chauffeur, whom he had imported from England along with the car, a Fiat, would detach an acetylene headlight and direct it on the patient. Bruce's only remaining problem when visiting out-of-town patients was the condition of the roads, which were sometimes surfaced with gravel, and usually with mud; but there was nothing he could do about that.

This was not the only occasion when Herbert Bruce protected a colleague. He was once called in to finish an operation that had been begun by a family doctor. The G.P. had been working on the patient for two hours, trying to remove a kidney. "On arrival," Bruce wrote, "I found him running between a textbook and the patient, hoping that the book would tell him what to do next."

By 1910, Dr. Bruce's practice was so extensive that he needed hospital space for at least fifty patients at any one time. As the General could not supply it, he solved the problem by creating a hospital of his own. For $65,000, he obtained a house in four and a half acres of land at the head of Homewood Avenue, and had it converted to provide for a hundred patients, with three operating rooms on the top floor. "The bedrooms were furnished by the well-known firm of Thomas Jenkins with the aim of providing a home-like atmosphere. The beds, of course, were of hospital construction. The china imported from Limoges, France, and the silver from England. Both china and silver bore the hospital crest."

The crest was that of the Duke of Wellington, who also supplied the name for the hospital: the Wellesley.

Dr. Bruce's thirty-five-years of experience in surgery ranged from an elbow operation, at which he assisted while still a student, to his extensive head-wound surgery as a medical officer during the First World War. In the process he was involved in many developments in surgery, from the imperfect first years of antisepsis, through X-ray and radium treatment, to plastic surgery.

The elbow operation took place in the 1890s. Bruce and a fellow student were chosen to assist the professor of surgery at an operation in a private house, on a young woman with an immovable elbow joint. He saw his professor begin the operation by removing his coat, turning up the cuffs of his shirt, washing his hands and dipping them in a solution of bichloride, putting his instruments in a solution of carbolic acid and after a few minutes, transferring them to a dish of boiling water. Meanwhile, the other student administered the anesthetic, pouring ether onto the gauze that was stretched over a metal frame and held over the patient's nose and mouth.

When the girl's struggles subsided, the professor proceeded to operate—sticking the knife between his teeth whenever he needed somewhere to park it.

The operation was at a private home on Gerrard Street and began at nine o'clock in the morning. The professor being a rather slow and deliberate worker, it had still not been completed by one o'clock, so the anesthesiologist remained behind to keep the girl quiet with occasional drips of ether, while the surgeon and his two student assistants repaired to their hostess' dining room, and partook of a hearty lunch. They then resumed work on the still-unconscious girl at two o'clock, and the operation was successfully completed at four. The girl had spent seven hours under ether.

As a true professional (and also because as a teacher he had to face medical students who seemed to become more alert and critical with every passing year), Dr. Bruce kept pace with new methods and developments in his subject, clinical surgery, by subscribing to British, German, and French medical journals, and by periodic visits to European clinics. His admiration for the European leaders in medical science was not always unreserved. When he went to see Ernst Wertheim of Vienna perform a radically new operation for cancer of the uterus in the early 1900s, he was shocked by the insensitivity toward the feelings of the patient. He found the procedure grotesque. "The patient was brought into a room stark naked and placed on a slab-like table," he recounted. "They then lifted and spread her legs. When this was done, her cervix was cauterized with a red-hot iron and without any anesthetic. Of course, certain precautions such as the washing of the body and shaving had been taken. She was then removed to the next room which was the operating room where an anesthetic was administered and the hysterectomy was performed with certain technicalities I need not describe. The Listerian emphasis on antisepsis was, however, recognized by the surgeon and his assistants, all of whom wore high rubber boots; and the floor was being constantly washed with buckets of water!"

But at least the operation needed to be done. Unlike the case back home, where a general practitioner who fancied himself as a surgeon performed an abortion on a woman under the impression that he was removing a fibroid tumour. The doctor made the further mistake of demonstrating the result only a few hours later at a meeting of the Pathological Society in Toronto. He showed his colleagues the uterus that he had removed, with, he said, the tumour enclosed. One of the members asked him to open it. He did so, and exposed a small infant.

Dr. Bruce appeared to have encountered his fair share of incompetents in the profession. Also the jealous and vindictive. Noting that the medical calling is second only to the church in professional jealousies, he described an early case of his, also involving the removal of a uterus for cancer. He took the uterus from a patient at the Toronto General, and sent it to the Pathological Laboratory, which was under Dr. J. J. MacKenzie.

Unfortunately, MacKenzie not only lacked experience in pathological work—he had previously been professor of botany—but was lacking in common courtesy. Without giving young Herbert Bruce a chance to speak, he ran to the hospital board of trustees, claiming that the uterus showed the remains of decidual cells—indicating that Bruce had removed not cancerous tissue but a recently pregnant uterus.

When he was informed that he would be called before the board for disciplinary action, Bruce demanded that three outside authorties be consulted. Accordingly, sections were submitted to three well-known pathologists, including William Welch of Johns Hopkins. Their reports were unanimous: there were no decidua. It was cancer.

Furious at the attempt to injure him in this manner at the outset of his career, Bruce announced that he would bring the case before the next meeting of the medical faculty. Cornered, MacKenzie turned to a friend, the professor of pathology at McGill, hoping for a report that would repair his reputation; but the best his friend could do was to say that the specimen resembled decidual cells but was in fact early cancer.

When the circumstances were reported to the president of the university, he told Bruce that he would ask for Dr. MacKenzie's resignation if Bruce requested it. Bruce, satisfied that he had been vindicated, refused, not wishing to ruin MacKenzie's career.

As well as incompetents, officious and otherwise, Bruce also encountered quite a few eccentrics. "Surgeons usually operate in the morning hours," he said, "but one surgeon who was on the staff of St. Michael's Hospital before the turn of the century, Dr. L. M. Sweatnam, had in this respect some idiosyncrasies which were not always appreciated by the authorities and nurses. He had studied surgery under Dr. Kelly of Baltimore. For several years he had made a practise of operating at night. On one occasion, he had finished an operation of a female patient at about 10 p.m. for some abdominal condition and went home. He returned to the hospital about 2 a.m. and decided to operate again, this time on the patient's gall-bladder."

Dr. Sweatnam also liked to take care of himself. He would often go into a room adjoining the operating theatre, insert a tube and wash out his own stomach.

"Another of my Toronto colleagues in the early days was Dr. Robert J. Dwyer. He was a very fine old physician. Once, he reported a patient to a young house surgeon as having died and instructed him to perform the necessary duties on such occasions. The houseman started on what he thought was a dead man and had the scare of his life when the patient awoke and asked what he was doing. 'Lie down—you're dead,' said the house surgeon. 'Indeed, I'm not,' came the reply 'Yes you are,' the house surgeon insisted. 'Dr. Dwyer said you were and he knows better than you.'"

Occasionally, doctors have found that nature knows better than they. Dr. Bruce once examined a young woman who had a large mass almost circling her neck and restricting head movements. He diagnosed the condition as sarcoma, a form of cancer, and a pathological examination of the tissue confirmed this. But, "The growth was so extensive and so fixed to the vessels and other structures of the neck that operation was out of the question and I had to tell her so. It was before treatment by X-ray and radium for malignant disease. A few weeks later she had a fall, hitting her head on the ground, and in a matter of weeks the mass spontaneously disappeared. It is impossible to understand the reason for this unless the body possesses some natural defence of which we know nothing."

During his career, Dr. Bruce performed thousands of appendectomies, though as a medical student he had seen only one such operation. It was first performed in 1887, by George Morton, the son of the dentist who had first used ether anesthesia in the operating theatre. This was shortly after it was recognized, again in the United States, that the seat of this type of inflammation was the vermiform appendix. Until then it had been described as perityphilitis.

Bruce was to encounter some mighty strange treatments by the public to combat appendicitis, or "inflamation of the bowels." "I remember in the early days of my practise," he recalled, "being called in to see a boy, eighteen years of age, who had developed such an inflammation. A cat had been killed by his parents, and while still hot, its warm body, split down the middle, had been put on his abdomen!"

Among Herbert Bruce's contributions to surgery was his advocacy of a two-stage method of removing the prostate gland. During a meeting of the British Medical Association in Toronto in 1906, he described a case where a man of over eighty was suffering from urinary obstruction owing to an enlarged prostate. "To give him immediate relief I opened the bladder above the pubis and drained it through a tube for a couple of weeks; and then I operated and went through this suprapubic opening and removed the prostate. This aroused considerable interest and...surgeons generally adopted this two-stage method."

Many of his operations were highly unusual. One was on a woman in her late twenties, who appeared to have a tumour. "When I was called in to see her in consultation with two other doctors, none of us was able to make a correct diagnosis. The mass was easily felt—apparently in the stomach—but we were by no means certain of its nature. It might have been an inflammatory mass or an unusually placed cyst. Operation was decided upon and when I opened the abdomen I found it to be within the stomach itself. I made a vertical incision from the lesser of the greater curvature to open the stomach, as in this way I would encounter fewer blood vessels, and there I found the tumour to consist of an accumulation of hair which had been woven together into a firm mass. It was about nine inches in length and two and a half inches in diameter. At one end it was bent and tapered to the extent of another two and half inches." Apparently the woman had been swallowing her hair combings for years, a habit that Dr. Bruce found disgusting and almost unbelievable, considering that the woman (he believed) was quite sane.

If any further proof were needed, beyond his highly successful practice, his golden touch in investment in land and property, and his acceptance by Toronto and international society, that Dr. Bruce was at the summit of the establishment, it came in 1932 when he was cajoled by Prime Minister Bennett into taking up the regal posture of lieutenant-governor of the province. He thus became host, in the glorious French chateau-style Government House in Chorley Park, overlooking the Rosedale ravine, to still further hordes of international celebrities in the arts, science, royalty, and diplomacy. But then, Herbert Bruce had always been a right-thinking member of the conservative, hard-working and honourable class that was then considered the only proper foundation for a stable, creative society.

A remarkable number of Canadian doctors, notably Herbert Dunscombe, Rolph, Tolmie, Helmcken, and Sir Charles Tupper, went into politics. They were drawn into legislative chambers partly out of vanity, perhaps, but mostly because they were needed, being among the better-educated pioneers, and because their profession made them more sensitive to social conditions. One who rose almost to the top in national politics was a student of Herbert Bruce's, R. J. Manion.

Manion considered his instructors at the University of Toronto to be among the ablest in the profession, and none more so than Dr. Bruce, who was then, at the turn of the century, teaching surgery. "I venture to assert," Manion intoned many years later in good parliamentary style, "that no one of the old school aristocracy of England could fill the position with more grace, courtesy and distinction than does this brilliant Canadian, Herbert A. Bruce. He is one of the few teachers of that time who still remains with us, and it is the wish of every student who ever saw his graceful and skilful surgical technique, or who ever listened to his splendid lectures, that he continues long as an inspiration to other Canadian youngsters in our hinterlands."

Dr. Bruce would no doubt have approved of Robert Manion, too, had he noticed him. Robert was a positive Frank Merrivale of a lad, honest, straightforward and true, stalwart, brave and virtuous, manly as a boy, boyish as a man. His father was an Ottawa Valley farmer who had given up tilling and stump-pulling and headed west, to become a general merchant to the railroad construction crews of the Canadian Pacific. His wife and four children joined him in 1886, and the following year they settled in Fort William.

For years the family lived in hotels, of the rude jerrybuilt sort heated by box stoves, illuminated by oil lamps, and subsidized by the bar-room take. Though young Robert admitted that the proprietors of these establishments were quite worthy fellows—they must have been, he thought, because at least two of them later became members of Parliament—he found the hotel life repellant, with its omnipresent stink of booze, its kitchen percussion, bellowed altercations, squealing fiddles and wall-shaking hoedowns. He would slip away whenever he could, to soothe his soul in the silence of the little wooden church nearby. Not that he was a coward or snob. Far from it. He was a sturdy, God-fearing lad, brimming with moral certitude. He was quite ready to intervene in the sordid affairs of the bushmen, railroad workers, or Indians, if there was a principle at stake. His reaction to the rotten behaviour of a hotel regular named Harvey was not untypical. Harvey was a cardsharp, and one day he made the mistake of showing the boy a few of his dirty tricks. The next day when Robert saw him cheating a newcomer out of his hard-earned pay, the fifteen-year-old quietly laid a note in front of the gambler, informing him that if he did not cease and desist, Robert would expose him. "What a damn fool I was," Harvey said later, "to tell a boy like you my tricks."

At the same age, Robert repelled, with anger and disgust, an attempt at bribery. He was working for the Canadian Pacific at the time, at a wage of thirty dollars a month. A grain merchant offered to double Robert's earnings if he would supply confidential information from the railway records. He was properly shamed (blushing all over his face, according to Robert), when the boy stoutly replied that the merchant had made a mistake—he was not that sort of fellow.

Priggish was the sort of fellow R. J. Manion appears to have been in his youth; though his righteousness was redeemed by qualities of courage that would win him a Military Cross in the First World War. He took considerable risks with his life as a youth, as in dangerous swimming contests in Lake Superior. These contests developed in Robert a moral as well as physical courage, and a better understanding of his limits as well as his potential. As a student, first at Queen's University, then at Trinity in Toronto, he recognized that he was not a brilliant student but that he had the ability to see what was important, the ability to pick out the salient points from any subject, and throw out the irrelevant. At college he worked four nights a week, summarizing the subjects so that long before the examinations were due he could abandon the textbooks and concentrate on his synopses. "One recalls very well indeed (with perhaps a little pardonable pride)," he wrote, "that many of the nurses whom one met, and even sometimes flirted with, were greatly worried about my results in the final examinations.

"Consequently toward the time of examinations a number of them pleaded with me to give at least enough attention to my work to get my degree. Knowing that I was really, in my working hours, giving intense application to my studies, and feeling quite sure of getting into the honours class in my final examination, I derived a good deal of fun in letting them conclude that I was likely to have great difficulty. When the final results were published in the morning papers, showing—very much to my own surprise and much more to theirs—that I had carried off the gold medal, fifteen or twenty letters were delivered to me at my rooming place by special delivery early in the morning, letters of congratulations and apology from these kind, good women who had offered me such sisterly advice in the hope that I would forswear my wayward ways long enough to get my examinations. I experienced a great boyish thrill out of these letters—boyish for I was the youngest member of my year."

Forty years later, a book of instruction, *Doctor in the Making*, by A. W. Ham and M. D. Salter, was written on the subject of getting the most out of medical school, a book designed to overcome a host of blocks and hang-ups in the medical student's progress, and to clarify his mind on everything from proper motivation to the do's and don'ts of the profession. Don't pay any attention to the curious tradition of loutish behaviour in which some students indulge to compensate for an inferiority complex about the value of medicine; don't neglect personal cleanliness; don't try to practice before you graduate; do develop a sensitive personality to understand the patient more fully. The authors of the book heartily agreed with Manion about the importance of organizing knowledge in preparation for examinations. They gave an example, first of a poorly organized student and then a well-organized student in their answers to a hypothetical exam question, "Discuss the cells of the blood."

"The first student reads this question. In looking into his mind we should see something like the following:

"Cells of the blood, polymorphonuclear leukocytes, phagocytes, infection, boils, pus, leukocytosis, fever, lymphocytes are blood cells also then there are eosinophils and basophils and monocytes, there are more polymorphs than the others, let's see if I can remember the percentages, eosinophils are more numerous in allergic conditions, what about macrophages, they aren't in the blood, they're in the tissues, now what do lymphocytes do? Well, I'd better describe all these cells, monocytes can turn into macrophages. I've hardly ever seen a good basophil—are platelets cells? No, they're just parts of cells, guess I can leave them out, not much time left, my gosh! I forgot about red blood cells—I was thinking about cells with nuclei, how did that question read anyway?"

When the second student reads the same question, he is enabled to write an orderly answer because a kind of synopsis something like the following flashes into his mind:

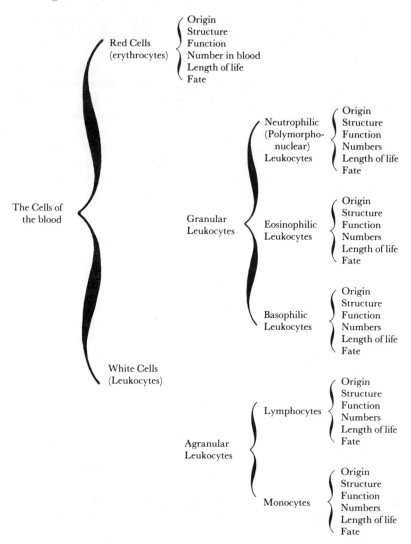

The above would be Manion's method.

As for the undergraduate behaviour analysed by Ham and Salter as being a compensation for feelings of inferiority and manifested in lurid descriptions of medical details to non-professional friends, and in loutish acts, Manion provides one example, in the behaviour of a group of his fellow students, who stole a cadaver from the dissection room and hung it from hooks in front of a butcher shop. Naturally Manion disapproved of this, especially two years later when he and a friend were invited into the butcher's house for a friendly glass of beer, and were promptly thrown out again when the butcher learned that they were medical students.

In his autobiography, Manion noted that in the first years of the twentieth century, studying medicine took up much less of a student's time than it does today. Moreover, the course ran a mere four years, without any requirement for internship. What with a relatively undemanding course and his own efficient methods, it left the fine-looking, clean-cut young man with plenty of opportunity to enjoy the night life of the city, particularly its five theatres: The princess (high-class drama and opera), the Grand (popular plays rather than Shakespeare), the Toronto (melodrama), Shea's (vaudeville) and the Star (shapely girls indecently exposed). He would line up for hours to see Sir Henry Irving in *The Bells,* Edward Smith Willard in *The Cardinal,* Otis Skinner in *Francesca da Rimini,* Johnston Forbes-Robertson in *The Light That Failed,* Sir John Martin-Harvey in *The Only Way,* Richard Mansfield in *Cyrano de Bergerac,* and Lulu Glaser in *Dolly Varden,* and other musical comedies such as *Floradora* and *The Prince of Pilsen,* and to hear Paderewski at Massey Hall.

Manion also dated girls and pranked in Mrs. Gee's boarding house on Parliament Street. But what he appreciated most from his student days was the mental discipline of the medical schools, enabling him to think out any problem from cause to effect in a systematic and logical way.

When he returned to Fort William to practice, Manion was only twenty-three years old, yet had four medical degrees after his name, two of them obtained during postgraduate study in Scotland. During those two years he had become more the tolerant man of the world. He had also become somewhat garrulous and unorthodox in his views, and outspoken. "I never succeeded in curbing my sometimes too outspoken habits to any great extent," he wrote. He had also learned a little humility. "For all doctors," he said, "nature is the real physician, and we are merely the aides-de-camp, for most patients if left alone get better, this being true of probably ninety-five percent of ill people. Consequently the intelligent physician merely tries to assist nature through diet, fresh air, and exercise or rest, to bring about the return of health more quickly."

His father, unfortunately, proved to be among the remaining five percent. Diagnosing cancer of the bladder in his parent, Robert called in a specialist from Chicago, Dr. B., from whom he received his first lesson in the manipulation of the medical fee. Dr. B. offered to make the trip for fifteen hundred dollars, but, "having made the trip, he submitted a bill for two thousand. My father had no objection to the fee as stipulated, but did object quite justly to the increase. He paid it *after having received a very optimistic prognosis,* though the specialist changed his prognosis as soon as he had arrived back in Chicago with his fee in his pocket; and the cancer carried my father off four months later."

Dr. B. also collected a few other fees while he was in Fort William. For local residents, a visit from a Chicago specialist was too good an opportunity to miss, whether their problems were genito-urinary or not. One of them was a man who had been informed by Manion that his daughter had a tumour of the leg. The father called in the Chicago specialist, who confirmed the diagnosis. For this the father was quite happy to fork out fifty dollars, but to Manion who did the actual operation he paid not a cent. Another patient, an Irishman, was happy to pay the visitor two hundred dollars, though his advice was "indefinite and useless." When Manion pointed out that the Irishman had grumbled terribly when he, Manion, had spent half the night treating him, the Irishman replied that after all, the Chicago man was a specialist, while Manion was merely a local man.

Such incidents taught R. J. Manion the psychology of fee-charging. "Medical men are often accused of... putting heavy fees upon those who can pay for the same treatment which they give to someone else for nothing," he said. "This is quite a proper policy. Doctors necessarily cannot refuse to attend the poorest of people, and since perhaps a third of their work is done for nothing, they must get good fees from those able to pay. Even the fairest-minded physician or surgeon usually works on this theory, for medical men doing general practice lead a very difficult life. They are called out at irregular hours; a good deal of their work is of a repulsive character; and they are subjected at all times to the charge of ignorant patients that they were maltreated. Consequently, when they get good results with wealthy patients, it is only fair that these rich should pay in proportion to their wealth. It is the same principle as in taxation."

Another example of patient ingratitude was a comfortably-off contractor who broke his leg while at work. After Manion had set the leg, the fracture healed and the limb functioned as well as before; "but as this case occurred before the X-ray was used to any great extent, and we were without one in my small city, I had set the fracture by manipulation. The *tibia* (that is, the shinbone) healed in such a manner that there was a slight unevenness as one ran his fingers down over the sharp edge of the shin, which in no way interfered with a perfect functional result." But the contractor refused to pay because of the slight unevenness around the shinbone. When Manion angrily informed him that he was expected to pay his account, the man replied slyly that, "If I showed that to a jury, they would think it was a pretty bad result." Which ended the argument right there. The contractor knew, and Manion knew he knew, that his leg was as sound as ever. "But no doctor can afford to take a chance of being drawn into suits for malpractice, no matter how unjust those suits may be, since human nature is prone to think the worst of anybody anyway, and besides, malpractice suits do not help a doctor's reputation."

(One of Manion's friends risked such a suit when he advised a mother that her baby boy required a minor tongue-tie operation. But he forgot his own advice, and circumcised the child instead. Fortunately the mother agreed that circumcision was a good thing anyway.)

Another lesson that Dr. Manion soon learned was that, "Generally speaking, women are more courageous in illness than men, though this is not always the rule, as some men who are impatient, bad-tempered and irritable in little things, when seriously ill and suffering severe pain from one cause or another bear it with the utmost fortitude. And sometimes men who are very courageous in every other way are very great cowards in pain or sickness."

Two years before the First World War, Manion became an alderman in Fort William. It so stimulated his interest in politics that when, upon returning from the war—serving part of the time with the French army—he entered national politics, representing Fort William. Four years later, he was a cabinet minister; in 1926, postmaster-general; and from 1930 to 1935 was minister of railways and canals under Prime Minister Bennett. By 1938 he was leader of the Conservative opposition, as staunch and upright in old age as he had been as a cardsharp-foiling, bribe-spurning lad of fifteen.

27

War Heroes

HERBERT BRUCE DID not in the least conform to the characterization of the surgeon as a prima donna of the operating theatre, so he was all the more upset at being cast as the villain in a First World War skit that was still being reviewed a quarter century later when, as a member of Parliament, he uttered some comment on the conduct of the prime minister, MacKenzie King, and a fellow member riposted with a snide reference to the 1916 affair.

Soon after the First World War exploded in Europe, Dr. Bruce, despite his lucrative practice, his duties as professor of clinical medicine at the University of Toronto, and his responsibility for the Wellesley Hospital, crossed the Atlantic to offer his services to the Canadian surgeon-general, G. Carleton Jones. Or tried to, but when he got to England, he learned that Jones was in France. To catch up with him, Bruce, who was a lieutenant-colonel in the Medical Reserve Corps, had himself posted to the Canadian hospital at Le Tréport, where, as a skilled surgeon with a fine reputation, he was most respectfully welcomed.

The welcome from the surgeon-general was not nearly as cordial. Bruce had some difficulty in obtaining an interview with Jones. The trouble started from the moment they met. They took an instant dislike to each other.

G. Carleton Jones was an old army man. He had joined the Canadian militia the previous century, and had first seen active service in the Boer War. He had been appointed director of the medical services as long ago as 1906, and by 1914 appears to have adopted the inflexible posture that distinguishes so many of the First World War brass hats. Within minutes he was dismissing Bruce with the information, curtly delivered, that he had no need of a surgeon.

As the first task that Bruce had been given upon arrival at Le Tréport was the removal of a piece of shrapnel adjacent to the spinal column of one of an already large number of surgical casualties, an operation that the hospital staff had not themselves dared to perform, this response astounded him. His reply was decidedly disrespectful. He informed the director of medical services that in that case, he would return to Canada where a great many people *did* have need of a surgeon.

Whereupon Carleton Jones barked that Colonel Bruce would stay where he was until ordered to do otherwise.

In a fury, Bruce determined to go home, whether Jones liked it or not. There was just one difficulty. He was now under Jones's jurisdiction, and could not get onto the cross-channel steamer to England without order papers. He solved the problem by waiting on the pier at Boulogne until the rest of the passengers had had their papers examined and had been issued with embarkation cards. Seconds before the boat was due to sail, he rushed up to the transport officer, being careful to flash his pips and crowns, and asked for an embarkation card, hoping that his rank and his air of urgency would get him through without having to show his papers. The ruse worked, and he was back in Canada before the surgeon-general was even aware that he had left France.

The reaction of G. Carleton Jones can be gathered from the action he took when he heard that Bruce had not only removed himself from army jurisdiction but he had also removed a number of X-ray plates. Bruce wanted to show the profession back home the kind of fractures that were being received in action, but the surgeon-general saw it as plain theft. He accused Bruce of stealing government property.

Jones's attitude toward Bruce was not in the least softened when he heard that Sam Hughes, the minister of militia and national defence, had not only dismissed the accusation but had done so with a laugh.

Worse was to follow. A few months later, when Jones's organization came under criticism from soldiers abroad and civilians at home, the minister appointed Bruce to the post of special inspector-general, with orders to investigate the medical service, and prepare a report. When he heard about this, Jones might have been excused a slight feeling of paranoia.

The secret report was completed in 1916, and contained fourteen recommendations, the first of which must have given Jones still further cause for chagrin. It proposed that the Canadian medical service be reorganized "from top to bottom." As Carleton Jones represented the top, the significance of the proposal was humiliatingly clear.

But then things began to go wrong for Herbert Bruce as well. The report upset many others as well as Jones, including certain officials who had been receiving a kick back from merchants who were supplying food to military hospitals, and from several medical officers whose wisdom or efficiency had been questioned. Bruce, mistakenly assuming that the government and the military wanted the whole truth and nothing but it, had named names.

It would not have been so bad if the report had remained confidential, but shortly after Bruce handed it over to the minister, the contents were leaked to the press. One of the surgeons, criticized by name, threatened Bruce with a suit for libel. Bruce had to apologize for using the name, though he did not retract the criticism. Nevertheless, the surgeon publicized the apology in a way that made it look as if the criticism had been unfounded.

This and other enmities roused by the report so distorted the truth that after the war, Bruce felt obliged to publish a book, *Politics and the Canadian Army Medical Corps,* in order to establish the facts, not least those that had been suppressed by the government at the height of the controversy.

Even then the attacks continued. A few years later, in his *Official History of the Medical Services,* Sir Andrew Macphail, commenting on Sam Hughes's choice of Bruce as his medical trouble-shooter, wrote, "It would be interesting to inquire into the mental process by which the Minister arrived at the conclusion that he selected the proper person for so exacting a task; but that would be a problem in psychology." To which Herbert Bruce, in his official history of himself, snarled back, "Possibly so, but knowing something of the services which Sir Andrew Macphail performed in England during the war, and of his political activities, one is inclined to add that it would be equally a problem in psychology and also in politics to inquire into the question why these particular services secured for Sir Andrew his knighthood!"

(Bruce was probably all the more miffed at Sir Andrew because the controversy had put paid to his own knighthood.)

As special inspector-general, Bruce had not only prepared the report but had been given the job of implementing it; but before he could do much about it, Sam Hughes was forced to resign. His successors wasted little time in discrediting the report, apparently being more concerned to prove it false and thus vindicate the medical establishment than to discover what was useful in it. In Bruce's opinion, his enemies were engaged in "an effort to protect the Government and provide an extensive and thick coat of whitewash to a situation which was in danger of becoming intolerable." But in the meantime, the discrediting of his report and the attacks on him damaged Bruce's reputation, and ultimately ended his services with the Canadian Army Medical Corps. The irony, according to Bruce, was that his proposals, which contributed to his and Sam Hughes's downfall, were nearly all implemented by the end of the war.

One of Bruce's criticisms had been leveled at the inadequate inspection of recruits in Canada. Many volunteers were arriving in Europe unfit for military service. Murrough O'Brien, our Dominion City saddle-bag surgeon, was partly responsible for at least one of them.

The outbreak of war found O'Brien in Winnipeg, attired in a 1907 cavalry uniform with the rank of major. "There was no lack of volunteers for the Canadian Expeditionary Force," Major O'Brien recounted. "Indeed, one of my big problems as medical officer was catching and weeding out the unfit. They tried all sorts of tricks to get by me with their bum hearts and bad lungs and all for the privilege of serving at a dollar and ten cents a day and dying, lots of them, in the rat and lice infested trenches of France.

"One case that I remember well was that of a Boer War Veteran. He diddled me nicely. He was in good shape physically but his teeth were in a hell of a mess. I couldn't pass him on that account. He said he couldn't afford to pay for extractions and a plate. He pleaded and argued but I was adamant. The Army of 1914 had no free dental service for its recruits. 'Come back with a dental plate and I'll pass you.' I told him. He was thoughtful for a second or two and then he said softly, 'Will you put that in writing, Major?' I was surprised at the request but I gave him the agreement in writing."

Two weeks later, Murrough saw him in uniform. Apparently the man had gone straight to the medical college and persuaded a student to extract his rotten teeth free of charge. He had then borrowed his sister's dental plate, presented himself before another medical examiner and shown him: 1. his bare gums; 2. Murrough's statement; and 3. his sister's false teeth, explaining that he wasn't wearing the teeth at the moment because his gums were too sore to tolerate the plates after the extractions. The examiner had then passed him for active service and the old veteran had then returned the teeth to his sister and gone off to war, toothlessly triumphant.

Murrough's overseas contribution to the war was as a medical officer to a railway unit in arctic Russia. His orders were to establish a chain of hospitals along a railway line that the unit was supposed to build between the Murmansk coast of northwest Russia and Petrograd, eighteen hundred miles away. As millions of men would find out on the Western Front, there was a considerable gap between the military theory and the geographical reality. The weather was so severe in northwest Russia that not one foot of track could be laid. As for hospital construction, the only hospital he was able to establish was the one he stole from the Russians.

Murrough had been told before he left Canada that there were hospital facilities at Simeniova. In fact there were none whatsoever. He solved that problem by raiding a railway siding and stealing two boxcars. His men lifted the boxes from their bogies by sheer muscle power, and hauled them to the camp site under cover of darkness. By daylight the two boxcars were in business. Murrough used part of the end space in one for office and sleeping quarters, and the balance as a hospital.

The first disease Murrough encountered in northwest Russia was the one that had afflicted the first white settlers in Canada: scurvy. But O'Brien had anticipated the problem. While he was in Winnipeg, the government had charged him with the task of purchasing the unit's supply of drugs and medical and surgical equipment. With considerable foresight Murrough had included a supply of lime juice. But somebody had dumped it onto the shores of Kola Bay, and it had frozen and spoiled. "I was in a bit of a pickle until I recalled something I had read to the effect that scrapings from the skins of potatoes were effective in treating scurvy. This seemed worth a try, but unfortunately at this time we had run out of potatoes. In spite of the fact that my scurvy patients were Russians, I saw little hope of persuading that suspicious fellow Popoloff [the local commander] to give me some spuds, and anyway even if he had been generously inclined it would have meant some very involved negotiations and delay. I took the easiest way out. I called in three of four of my best filchers and sent them after the tubers. I got my potatoes, fed the patients skin scrapings, and the scurvy cleared up like magic."

The railway project was finally abandoned in May 1916, and the unit returned to Canada. There O'Brien, like Bruce, offended his superiors with his criticisms, in Murrough's case some typically forthright remarks on the totally useless and costly expedition to Russia. Which may have been the reason he ended up as a sanitary officer in Winnipeg, with little to do except draw his pay.

Military and political leaders in the First World War were not noted for their hospitality to the facts.

Shortly afterwards, Murrough O'Brien resigned his commission, and disappeared thankfully back into civilian life.

The contribution of another sanitary officer, Colonel George Nasmith, was rather more heroic. A consulting engineer as well as a doctor of public health, Nasmith saved a great many lives through his prompt identification of the poison gas that was used for the first time by the Germans against the Canadians at Vimy Ridge.

At the outbreak of war, George Nasmith was in charge of a sanitary section in Toronto. Upon his arrival in France in 1915, he was given the job of establishing a medical laboratory in a small town in the Amiens sector. He picked out a splendid quarters in the town hall, comprising the banquet hall and band room, which was well-lit and had a fine view of the village square. "Our laboratory," he wrote, "had charge of both the bacteriological and hygiene work of a given area; it was the only laboratory that did both types of work. When our apparatus had been unpacked and set up in the old ball room of the Hôtel de Ville, it made quite an imposing show, and after we saw what equipment the other laboratories had we were decidedly proud of ours.

"Our first bit of work proved to be the examination of a number of soldiers who had been in contact with a case of cerebro-spinal meningitis, to detect 'carriers' of the specific germ. Then material of all sorts began to come in for examination from the casualty clearing stations, field ambulances, sanitary and medical officers, rest stations and other places. Most of the routine bacteriological work proved to be of much the same nature as that done in a health laboratory at home, and consisted of examinations to detect some of the ordinary communicable diseases such as diphtheria, cerebro-spinal meningitis, typhoid fever, malaria, dysentery, tuberculosis, and venereal diseases."

Along with a well-equipped lab, Nasmith had two highly qualified men on his staff, Major Rankin, an Alberta Government pathologist and bacteriologist who had been engaged in tropical medicine in Siam for five years before the war, and Captain Ellis, a research worker with the Rockefeller hospital laboratories in New York. Ellis was thoroughly up-to-date on the latest developments in vaccine and serum therapy. Between the three of them there was no problem in bacteriology, pathology, sanitation, or the treatment of disease that they could not handle.

One of the worst problems they had to face was the Flanders soil. It had been liberally manured for centuries, and every cubic yard was rich in virulent germs, particularly those that produced gas gangrene and tetanus. Nasmith's laboratory was kept exceedingly busy, identifying matter from wounds sent in by hospital surgeons.

The hygiene work of the laboratory included the examining of milk and foods, the evolving of methods to purify effluents discharged into streams, and particularly the analysis of the water in the water carts that supplied the various units. "Well, springs, creeks, and ponds used as sources of supply were also examined, and not infrequently samples from 'springs' encountered while digging new trenches, were sent in to be tested. The tremendous number of bacteria found in some of the 'spring' samples were on several occasions reported as indicating the presence of buried animal matter in the immediate vicinity of the springs, and resulted in finding this to be correct. In one case in which a badly polluted water was so reported upon, the burial place of some fifty Germans was found only a few feet away."

It was while he was checking on the purity of the water supply to the Canadians who were holding the Ypres salient, one spring day in April

1915, that Nasmith saw a yellowish-green cloud rolling over the front line trenches. He guessed instantly that this was a gas attack. The attack was accompanied by a ferocious bombardment.

Straddled by bursting shells, and well aware that an infantry attack would soon follow, Nasmith waited out in the open to confirm that it was gas, and to test it on himself. When the first thin swirls reached him, he stood there, calmly noting the irritating effects on his throat and lungs, and the way it was making his eyes run and turn bloodshot. He decided that the gas was chiefly chlorine, with perhaps an admixture of bromine, but that there was probably something else present, to account for the irritating effect on the eyes.

While Nasmith was thus acting in the time-honoured medical tradition of experimenting on himself, a Canadian Highlander came trudging up the road. He confirmed that his platoon had been gassed, and that the Germans had infiltrated behind their sector. With the platoon surrounded, the order, "Every man for himself" had been given. The soldier told Nasmith that he was the only one who had managed to get out.

It was night by the time Nasmith had dodged through the barrage and sniper fire to reach No. 3 Field Ambulance at Vlamertinghe. There he saw the effects of the gas for the first time. "Lying on the floors were scores of soldiers with faces blue or ghastly green in colour, choking, vomiting, and gasping for air, in their struggle with death, while a faint odour of chlorine hung about the place.

"These were some of our own Canadians who had been gassed, and I felt, as I stood and watched them, that the nation who had planned in cold blood, the use of such a foul method of warfare, should not be allowed to exist as a nation but should be taken and choked until it, too, cried for mercy."

(Such sentiments were common when they were intended, as in this account in Nasmith's memoirs, for public consumption in wartime, but among the fighting men, expressions of hatred for the enemy were rare. As the war blundered onward, if there was any hatred it was usually directed toward their own staff officers.)

Though he had inhaled only a few whiffs of the gas, Nasmith had to take to his bed, suffering from bronchitis. In the afternoon he dragged himself along to corps headquarters to give his opinion on the constituents of the gas and to suggest the type of mask that could be used to counter its effects.

The effects had already proved devastating. Within three days of the attack, 2,600 Canadian casualties had passed through the No. 3 Canadian Field Ambulance alone. One of them was a friend of Nasmith's, a medical officer who had been lying out in no man's land for two days. "This," said Nasmith, "was one of those personal experiences which bring the war home to us with startling reality.... You hear of the loss of a thousand men and it affects you very little, but if you know personally a single one of the thousand, the news of his death may give you the blues for days."

In this, the second battle of Ypres, the Canadian division stemmed the onslaught that followed the gas attack, though they lost nearly half their infantry. In the meantime, Nasmith's laboratory became an important centre, visited by hosts of generals and distinguished medical men, who were anxious to find out about the gas and methods of combating it. General headquarters called him in as an advisor, and he was given the authority to carry out large-scale experiments in counter-measures. "We also did a good deal of experimental laboratory work with other gases which might possibly be used, with the object of discovering their antidotes." For his part in the emergency, Nasmith was made a Companion of the Order of St. Michael and St. George.

The emotional impact of the war, as described by another medical officer, Captain Boyd, was typical. Like George Nasmith and a million other men, he entered the war in a spirit of adventure. He came out of it rent with anguish.

William Boyd spent only five months at the front, but it was enough to change his life. The University of Manitoba's professor of pathology, William Boyd's war service included a brief spell in charge of an infectious diseases hospital at Bailleul. The rest of his time was spent at Ypres with a field ambulance.

A field ambulance was a self-contained unit with its own transport. "A wonderfully interesting day," he wrote on March 12, 1915, near the headquarters of the Canadian division. Filled with anticipation of adventures to come and with patriotic ardour, he rejoiced when he saw a column of drab, dejected prisoners-of-war being marched rearward. They had been captured that morning at Neuve Chapelle. They were a symbol, as he saw it, of a defeated enemy. The column was followed, as if the contrast had been deliberately arranged by a propagandist, by "a magnificent procession of British lancers."

The reality was not far behind the lancers. "The whole training of a medical man tends to inure him to unpleasant sights and smells," wrote the pathologist a day later, "but I must confess that we needed all our training this morning. The dressing-station was formerly a school, and every room was so packed with wounded, lying on stretchers on the floor, that it was with the greatest difficulty that we could move about. It was literally almost impossible to put your foot down without treading on a wounded man. The condition of the wounds was indescribable, for many of them were two days old, and during that time the wounded men had simply lain out on the battlefield, the furious fighting rendering the evacuation of casualties an impossibility. In this country of heavily-manured soil, every wound becomes septic at once, and unless treated thoroughly soon swarms with the microbes of putrefaction. You can imagine what the condition of these great gaping cavities was at the end of forty-eight hours. There were all sorts and conditions of wounded, from a Colonel of the Guards, who died shortly after admission, to English, Scotch, Indian and even German privates. One poor Scotch laddie, whose bowels were hanging outside his abdomen, told me that he came from Fife. It was quite like a message from home to hear the broad, kindly Scot's tongue again. 'I've an awfu' sair belly, doctor,' was the only complaint the poor boy made.... In some instances the men appeared to be partly anesthetized by the extreme fatigue from which they suffered — a merciful dispensation. The head injuries were the most frightful, for in some cases the greater part of the face was smashed in by shrapnel."

Five months later, as Boyd prepared to return home to Winnipeg, he was suffused with dread melancholy, wishing simultaneously that he had "never set foot in this stricken land, where death stalks beside you by day, and takes you by the arm as you walk the roads at night," and torn with regret at giving up the emotional intensity of the front line experience. These were feelings shared by so very many others in the war, by those who, in spite of the awful conditions, were always glad to return from leave, to get away from the selfish home front, back to an intense, elemental comradeship. "If, as Aristotle says, tragedy purifies the mind through terror and pity," Boyd concluded, "how much more does war thoroughly purge it of all dross. For war is the great tester; it brings out the best that is in a man, even as also it brings out the worst that is in him. 'The beauty and the terror of the world,' have never held so much meaning for me as during these past months. And tomorrow I am going to leave it behind, perhaps for ever."

First World War military leaders were remarkable for their ignorance of the dreadful conditions at the front, an ignorance that sometimes seemed almost deliberate, as if an understanding of the reality would expose their bankrupt strategy. This was the reason that staff officers were regarded by the fighting men with such venomous hatred. One of the few generals to set a clear view of the facts was Launcelot Kiggell. Paying his first visit to the fighting zone in 1917, general Kiggell grew more and more agitated when he saw the tortured terrain, the mud, and the overlapping shell holes, and finally burst into tears, saying, "Good God, did we really send men to fight in that?"

Army chaplains, too, would rouse the scorn of the fighting men. With the notable exception of the Roman Catholics, army chaplains rarely appeared in the front lines, where they were most needed. There was no such dereliction on the part of the medical personnel of the regimental aid posts, field ambulances, and dressing and casualty-clearing stations. They worked so close to the fighting that their casualties were often as severe, proportionally, as those among the infantry. John MacCrae, the Canadian doctor who wrote one of the most famous of all poems, *In Flanders Fields,* and about whom Wilder Penfield would muse during a crisis twenty years later, was at one time working so close to the trenches that the soldiers became his patients by falling wounded at his feet.

Torn with the anguish over the pain and suffering and wholesale slaughter, the medical officers regarded their working conditions with far more concern than the danger to themselves. The conditions under which they had to repair the human damage, in dirty, verminous barns, dugouts, tents, cellars, would have appalled even their pioneer forerunners in kitchen-table surgery. But whereas doctors like Murrough O'Brien had steadily increased their surgical skills through domestic improvisation and constant practice, the work of front line surgeons was often so rushed, so desperate, so urgent, that even the most sympathetic and conscientious medical officer had to abandon surgical subtly to avoid becoming totally overwhelmed by the fleshly carnage. The Western Front was no great training ground for surgeons, except in terms of desperate haste, as in pre-anesthesia days.

One effect of the war experience was a devotion to duty carried to irrational lengths, a half-demented drive beyond the point of shock or exhaustion, until death or incapacity gave out the final orders. Captain F. G. Banting's behaviour in this respect was typical. A twenty-seven-year-old native of Alliston, Ontario, Banting appeared to be average in his abilities, not as experienced as most of his fellow officers, for he was just out of medical school, a product of the University of Toronto's war-accelerated course where the final two years had been compressed into a single fifteen-month stretch.

Otherwise he was competent enough, braver than some—he won the Military Cross, an award that had to be well-earned—and more studious than most—his commanding officer was startled one day to see him sitting in a trench during a bombardment, engrossed in a pocket manual of anatomy. He was also mature and considerate enough to have earned the devotion of his batman, Private Kels from British Columbia, one of those army impresarios who could fix, arrange or supply anything at short notice, conjure luxury out of spartanism, plenitude out of scarcity.

In September 1918, the studious captain was at Lilac Farm in the Cambrai sector with the 13th Field Ambulance. He had been working for many hours without a break, treating hundreds of wounded and helping to evacuate them to the rear by motor ambulance and horse and stretcher. As the fighting blazed around the farm, his unit suffered so many casualties that by early evening there were only two officers left, himself and Major L. C. Palmer, and a few sergeants acting as dressers.

The field ambulance was also sharing the farm with a field gun, which was firing eighteen-pounder shells at the enemy. The Germans appreciated its efforts as little as the Canadians, and after a while they began to return its fire with whizz-bangs, a particularly deadly kind of missile that arrived without the usual warning whistle, moan or howl, to the alarm of the Canadians and several German prisoners who were being held in a farm building close by. One of the Germans, a major, was the first casualty; he was decapitated by a piece of shrapnel. The same shell also wounded Captain Banting in the arm.

During a lull in the bombardment, Major Palmer examined his friend's arm and found that a shell fragment had stuck the right forearm, severing the interoseous artery. Palmer applied a tourniquet, then removed the fragment, tied a field dressing in place, then told the captain that the ambulance would take him to the rear. As the major removed the tourniquet, Banting protested the orders, insisting that it was just a superficial wound. He couldn't possibly run out on the boys just for a scratch like this.

Palmer, noting signs of shock from loss of blood as well as extreme fatigue, was equally insistent that Banting would have to go. At that moment, Palmer was ordered to Cambrai, which had just been captured, to set up an advanced dressing station.

Over the next few hours Palmer had no time to think about his friend, for, soon after he arrived at Cambrai, the Germans counterattacked and he was forced to hide in a cellar.

A see-saw battle continued for hours, and it was after midnight before the British retook the town. At four in the morning, Palmer returned to Lilac Farm. There he found Captain Banting, still attending to the wounded, though he was reeling with fatigue and gray with shock.

Angrily, Palmer ordered him out, and this time Banting obeyed, and made his way to a waiting ambulance.

His wound was bleeding again by the time he arrived at the casualty-clearing station, necessitating a hurried transfusion. Later, still weak from loss of blood, and also from lack of food, for he had eaten nothing since the beginning of the action, save for a piece of angel cake given to him by one of the men, he was taken to an operating room to have his wound cleaned, and drying tissue excised. A few days afterwards, he was shipped to the No. 1 General Hospital in Manchester.

It was for his fortitude during the Cambrai action that he was awarded the Military Cross.

Banting needed almost as much fortitude on the home front. He arrived in Manchester on a Wednesday, but his wound was not examined until the Sunday, by which time it was infected. The captain had further cause for complaint about the roughness of the treatment at the No. 1 General, in the unfeeling way that the packing in the wound was ripped out, and later over the careless procedure during an operation to extend the wound and improve drainage. "When there is too much hurry and flurry, treatment sometimes becomes sloppy, especially when men are overworked," he observed. And decided that if this was the best that the hospital could do, he would take over and thenceforth supervise his own treatment.

That captain was fortunate. The war ended before he could be recycled into the horror of the Western Front. The world was equally fortunate, for the captain was to become one of the supreme benefactors of mankind, through his discovery of insulin.

28

A Most Unlikely Genius

FREDERICK BANTING HAD no grea confidence in his abilities, so the anti-climax of peace and the uncertainties of the future abraded him, as they did many another returning veteran. He had long had a fear of failure, and his accomplishments thus far had not reassured his ego. At university he had manifested no special talent, except as a glee club singer. He was slow, solemn, and painstaking, dun characteristics that did little to vivify his personality. In the slanguage of his day he would have been described as a poler or grind.

In appearance he was just as ordinary. Though tall and husky, he looked nondescript in his civilian suit. With his long face and large nose and the studious crease between his brow, he was neither good-looking nor interestingly ugly. In personality he had no quirks or eccentricities, and nobody remembered him saying anything particularly amusing, perceptive, or unexpected. At the university, his instructors had taken no particular interest in him, and if his fellow students even remembered him, they were likely to assume that he was well on his way to obscurity, doing neither much good nor much harm to a list of patients who were never likely to be enraptured by his bedside manner.

Though he claimed that as a youth, "it was my greatest ambition to be a doctor," the ambition did not appear to have greatly energized him. When he enroled at the University of Toronto in 1911, it was as a divinity student. This was to please his father, who was a farmer and a devout trustee of the Methodist Church. Months jittered by before Fred summoned up the courage to tell the old man that he was not really suited to

380

the ministry. He put off the painful—and pained—interview for so long that another year was lost before he could transfer to medical school.

Accordingly he was forced to spend much of 1912 working on the farm at Alliston, though he did devote a few evenings a week to the study of an anatomy textbook that he had borrowed from the local G.P.

He also found time to plod attendance on a local girl named Mary. She was the daughter of a local minister. Their courtship was as conventional as their respective characters. He had known Mary since childhood. Everybody assumed that they would marry as soon as Fred could afford to do so.

At medical school, Fred's attitude remained dutiful, his progress undistinguished, his outlook priggish. "Fred considered the study of medicine very seriously," said his cousin, Dr. Hipwell. "The hours of work were hard and long. Often he took those of us, seemingly more frivolous, to task for our shortcomings. But it was done invariably in that kindly and sincere way of his own, and without rancour." Struggling to recollect one memorable thing about Banting, Dr. Hipwell added that, "I recall his pride in the possession of a three-volume Sabotta McMurrich."

Fred certainly did not have the self-certainty of the prig. After his discharge from the army, anxiety and self-doubt once again began to erode his confidence. Here he was, nearly twenty-eight years old and he had not even served an internship, let alone established a career. He was not even sure what kind of a career it would be. While in England he had developed an interest in orthopedic surgery—the mechanical correction of human deformity—but the interest was not intense enough to give his life unalterable purpose. And his conscience still nagged him. In striving for his medical degree, he had received more than his share of the family resources. He tried to make up for the filial imbalance by renouncing any future share of his father's estate, but his conscience was not fooled. He knew that he would have to call on the family for further help when it came time to establish a practice. Nor did the voluntary sacrifice reduce his feelings of inferiority. He could not help comparing himself unfavourably with his four elder brothers, who, at his age, had been self-supporting for ten years.

Luckily there was still another year to go before he would have to lean again on the family. His self-confidence revived somewhat when he was accepted as an intern at the Hospital for Sick Children. He was particularly pleased to be an intern there, for he was fond of children. This sympathy was partly derived from a childhood experience, when his best friend in Alliston had died of infantile diabetes.

That friend must have flicked across his memory more than once when he saw so many of the children in the hospital suffering from, and, inevitably dying of, that incurable disease.

The children are said to have responded to Fred with a matching affection. Perhaps his conduct with the children, his joshings, his jokes, and his amusing nicknames for them, were a compensation for his often unsatisfactory relations with adults. He had developed no deep or rewarding friendship with his contemporaries, not even with his childhood sweetheart, Mary.

Mary, who was now, in 1919, teaching in a rural school near London, Ontario, was a blonde and pretty girl with a conventional soul, though no doubt she had the usual romantic conceptions of what a love affair should be. If so, they must have been sadly eroded by Fred's conduct, which suggested that he regarded their friendship, not so much as a love affair as a habit. Nevertheless, until his discharge from the army, she continued to believe that he would make a satisfactory husband, despite a number of disappointments, such as his rejection of a career in the church—she had rather fancied herself as a minister's wife—and his failure to propose before going overseas, not to mention his letters from France, which had been a little too laconic to cause much of a fuss in her bosom.

His only romantic gesture so far had been the impulsive purchase of a diamond ring for her, when he was in England. It had suddenly occurred to him one day that he had been keeping Mary in suspense for an awfully long time, and that he had better do something about it. The gesture had, for a while, refueled her affection. She had written back in a rush of loving terms—suppressing the concomitant disappointment that he had seen fit to mail the ring to her, instead of waiting to deliver it personally, gift-wrapped in Cyrano eloquence.

Almost as soon as he returned from the wars, he cast her down again, with a request for a further postponement of their wedding until he had established himself in a career.

By then, Mary had been waiting for him for over nine years. Even the diamond ring could not allay a suspicion that the reason for his caution and lack of ardour was apathy, rather than concern for their common welfare. And gradually the ring became a symbol of her resentment. She would return it more than once over the next two years.

In the meantime, Banting camouflaged his doubts and uncertainties under the cover of his work for the hospital. He was proud to be working there, for already, in 1919, the Hospital for Sick Children had an international reputation. It had been established forty-four years previously by a group of public-spirited women who had been appalled at the plight of the children of the city. The children had suffered, become crippled, and had died, with little effort having been made to treat or comfort them.

Since 1875, the hospital had grown rapidly, mainly through the money, dynamism, and compassion of John Ross Robertson, the abrasive publisher of the *Evening Telegram*. Robertson had no great respect for doctors. One of them described a job-application interview with Robertson. He recorded the publisher's first words as, "Are you any good?" and his last words, delivered a few glares later, as "Well, tell them I said to give you a try. Now get out of here!" But he had a generous love of children. Determined to create the biggest and best children's hospital in the world, he studied hospitals and their facilities throughout the United States and Europe, and incorporated their best features in a new hospital building on College Street, a boastful edifice of stone carvings, peaked towers, and terra cotta ornamentation.

Another formidable character who would shape the hospital in the mould of his ego was Dr. Alan Brown. He became physician-in-chief within weeks of Fred Banting's appointment as an intern. Nobody found Fred remarkable, but Brown was another matter. Over the next thirty-two years of his captaincy, he would command the staff as if they were the complement of a seventy-gun ship-of-the-line, and become one of the most feared, hated, and respected medical men in the country.

In the new age of specialization, which was essentially a post-World War I phenomenon, Dr. Brown's field was pediatrics. He subordinated every other consideration to the welfare of his babies. "Brown supervised the treatment of every medical patient and many of the surgical ones," wrote Max Braithwaite in his history of the hospital, "and heaven help the intern or nurse or resident or even staff doctor who wasn't doing his job at peak efficiency. He once told a doctor concerning the 'history' prepared on a patient that, 'The idiot elevator boy could have prepared a better history!'

"Hurrying through the corridors, he'd pause long enough to take the lid off a cart of food being wheeled to a ward. If he didn't like it, back it went. He inspected every corner for dirt that might harbour germs." For Dr. Brown was ruthless with anybody who did not put a baby's health far above any other consideration. If he found a nurse being slovenly or careless, she would be fired on the spot. The little man's bullying ways earned him considerable hatred in some quarters, but others revered him for his accomplishments in protecting his charges from infection, and for his support for any development that would increase their chances of survival, such as Bruce Robertson's work in blood transfusions for children.

Blood transfusion is a comparatively recent development, and Bruce Robertson was one of its pioneers. He had worked on transfusion techniques as a major in the Canadian Medical Corps. Upon his return to Canada, he "became convinced that a change of blood (exsanguination-transfusion) could greatly benefit children suffering from infection in the blood." According to Braithwaite, after careful experimentation in the hospital's research lab, Robertson worked out a technique for treating children suffering from severe burns, erysipelas, blood poisoning, malignant scarlet fever or that old devil, acute intestinal intoxication.

"He reasoned that the best means of tapping an infant's blood supply was through the top of his head. On all babies there is a soft spot or fontanelle where the bones of the cranium haven't yet grown together and where mothers can watch their baby's pulse beating. A needle with a lead stopper on it was inserted into this soft spot and the required amount of blood drained off.

"At the same time new blood, uninfected blood from a donor, mixed with a 3.5 percent solium citrate solution and placed in a basin, was introduced into a vein of the tiny patient. As the bad blood went out and the good blood went in the baby showed a dramatic improvement." The procedure reduced the mortality rate by twenty-five to fifty percent.

Fred Banting does not appear to have earned Dr. Brown's displeasure, not least because shyness and reserve tended to make him inconspicuous. Besides, he was pretty much out of Brown's line-of-sight, being on the surgical side, in orthopedics.

Even by the turn of the century, the hospital had become a renowned centre for orthopedic surgery. John Ross Robertson had been particularly proud of the orthopedic workshop "which looked like a blacksmith shop with forge, workbenches, pulleys and belts turning and grinding wheels, hammers, tongs, files and a great variety of other tools, many of which were invented and made right in the shop." Ross had promoted the workshop in the hospital's 1901 annual report. "Aids for Every Form of Bodily Deformity," read the advertisement, "for deformities of the feet; for flat feet—a special boot; for bow legs; for knock knees; for short legs, for wry neck; for round shoulders; for diseases of the joints, hip joint; ankle joints; for club feet— splints and special boots; for paralytic deformities; for weak ankles; for spinal disease—special braces and jackets; for lateral curvature; for Potts disease; for knee joints. Crutches made of maple or hickory."

By the time that Banting joined the hospital, the department was pre-eminent in the field, mainly through the work of C. L. Starr, an international authority in orthopedics. Banting idolized Dr. Starr. According to Dr. Seale Harris, who knew Banting, "The younger man developed into the older one's devoted disciple, tireless in his effort to emulate his master's marvelous operative technique and his independent, sometimes radical methods of curing chronic diseases of bones and joints. From [his earliest] days, Fred Banting had had a tendency to hero worship. Some deep inner need in his rather undemonstrative nature apparently was satisfied by someone who embodied the qualities which he himself was striving to attain. During that year of internship, his ideas centered around Dr. Starr, and for many years afterwards Starr remained his valued preceptor.''

On his part, Starr thought well enough of Banting to recommend him to Western University (soon to be renamed the University of Western Ontario) as instructor in orthopedic surgery. Accordingly, as soon as his intern year was up, in July 1920, Banting moved to London, then a pleasant little tree-camouflaged town of sixty thousand.

Given Fred's cautious nature, one would have expected him merely to rent accommodation in London until he had placated his bank manager. Instead, in a surge of optimism he splurged on a house on Adelaide Street North. Admittedly it was not in the best part of town, and the purchase put him another two thousand dollars in debt to his family back in Alliston. All the same, he felt sure that he was finally on the road to success—complete with a second-hand Ford Tourer, for traveling along it.

For a whole month he was sure that he would do well in London. After all, there were no others specializing in orthopedic surgery in that city, or indeed anywhere else in western Ontario. So there would be little competition, except for local men doing minor orthopedic work. Also, the prestige of his connection with the university was bound to help him build up a private practice.

There was a further advantage to living in London. It put him within easy reach of his fiancée. Mary had finished the school term by the time he arrived, and would not be returning to her rural school until September. But that was all right. It would give him time to build up his bank account with a steadily increasing income from private practice, and with the few dollars he would earn from his six hours a week at the university.

Even the unsatisfactory arrangement over the Adelaide Street property could not douse his glowing anticipation of success. The former owner of the gray brick home had asked to be allowed to occupy part of it for another year. Fred agreed. Thus, for the time being, his share of the house amounted to only two rooms, a combination office/living room, and a bedroom.

He remained optimistic as he set about furnishing the rooms and purchasing orthopedic apparatus and surgical instruments. After which he sat down in his office to wait for the expected rush—or at least shuffle—of patients, meanwhile reading up on anatomy, to while away the time.

Twenty-eight days later he was still whiling away the time. Not a single patient had appeared, and his income had reached, in his words, ''the grand total of nothing.''

By the time Mary returned to London, his confidence had begun to drain away again, to be replaced by the old fear of failure. His spirits failed to soar even when Mary came to see him. She was not at all impressed either by the restricted accommodation or by the neighbourhood.

Even so, had Fred welcomed her warmly and eagerly, it is quite likely that she would have responded with matching enthusiasm. Instead, Fred's dejection infected her as well. Their first day together in months ended dismally. It is not hard to imagine Banting going back to his sparse office at the end of the day in an even greater state of depression, and Mary returning to her boarding house to seethe or weep in bitter frustration over what seemed to be an emotional impotence on his part, over what increasingly seemed to her to be a decade of wasted years.

During the next few months he made the situation even worse by repeatedly offering to release her from the engagement. He kept saying that it wasn't fair to her to keep her waiting any longer.

How she must have hated him sometimes.

Gradually their weekend meetings became fewer, their correspondence more distant. She began to make excuses why she could not visit him on the weekends. Fred grew more withdrawn than ever. And so the frustrating affair coasted slowly downhill throughout Banting's year in London, with many breaks in their relationship, symbolized by the repeated return of the diamond ring. Admittedly the ring did not entirely go to waste. According to Lloyd Stevenson in his biography of Banting, "During the intervals of estrangement Banting wore the ring on his watch chain and occasionally used the diamond to scratch a slide in the laboratory; his associates could thus keep themselves more or less informed of his current status."

The ring was finally rejected about a year later, and the affair dribbled to its miserable conclusion.

The failure of his love life was bad enough, but far worse, as Fred saw it, was the humiliating state of his professional life. He was proving totally unsuccessful, not just in general practice, but in the field in which he had thought himself to be reasonably well qualified.

The trouble was that the other doctors could not see that he was anything special as an orthopedist. Accordingly, they handled the simpler problems themselves, or if they could not, passed them on to George Ramsay, who was on his way to becoming the city's most prominent orthopedist, or else referred them to Starr or Robertson in Toronto — certainly not to this morose fellow Banting, about whom nothing was known, except that he was suspicipusly late to be starting up in practice, and who, with his increasingly round-shouldered posture and furrowed brow, was aging like a refugee from Shangri-la.

It was not surprising that poor Fred was looking old and careworn. He had worked hard all his life, and the enforced idleness left him aching with bewilderment, guilt, and frustration. He could not even begin to fill in his time. At the university he was showing himself to be a competent teacher, clear and precise in his anatomical and physiological demonstrations, but the demonstrations took up only six hours a week. In his private practice, the gaps between patients yawned so wide that in an attempt to span them he had taken up painting again. As a youth he had been quite interested in art. All the same, he would have preferred to illuminate his account book with figures rather than canvases with paint, and the amateurish daublings still left him with too little to do, except to study half-heartedly, pace up and down, smoke too many cigarettes, drive about listlessly in his Ford Tourer, and reminisce almost with nostalgia about his days as an army medical officer, when his life had some meaning and purpose.

Not that Fred's talent for painstaking hard work lay entirely fallow. In late summer he undertook a research project for Professor F. R. Miller, chief of the physiology department. The work temporarily lifted the weight of depression from his stooped shoulders. Miller, a neurophysiologist at the university, had invited Banting to assist him in a research problem concerning the cerebellar cortex.

Given Fred's sense of failure and his feelings of humiliation over his showing so far in London, he must have felt an enormous gratitude for this token of confidence in his ability that far outweighed the importance of the research. But the project, to investigate the excitability of the cerebellar cortex, was more significant than Banting realized. It initiated him into the techniques of medical research.

Unfortunately the investigation was all too soon concluded, and once again he found himself reduced to semi-idleness, to the frustrating routine of a class or two at Western, a patient or two in his office, hours and hours of nervous puffing at cigarettes, while he waited, waited, waited; painting the occasional uninspired landscape, playing the occasional game of bridge, studying three days a week with an old college friend, Dr. Tew, who had also decided to try his luck in London, and, when the remaining hours in his two rooms became unbearable, walking or driving up to the reading room of the medical school library, to read the latest batch of technical journals — though what with the tedium, the debts, the loneliness, and Mary's withdrawn letters, and the awful feeling that life and love were slipping past unconsummated, it was sometimes hard to concentrate on the dense, esoteric texts. Until one day, October 30, 1920, he read an article that would transform not just his life but the lives of millions.

The journal was the latest copy of *Surgery, Gynecology and Obstretrics*. The lead article was a long, detailed account on *The Relation of the Islets of Langerhans to Diabetes, with Special Reference to cases of Pancreatic Lithiasis.* It was by Dr. Moses Barron of Minneapolis.

Banting borrowed the copy because, as it happened, he was to discuss the pancreas next day with his students. His recent readings in physiology and some dissection and histological work had made him reasonably familiar with the pancreas, the small organ seated behind the stomach and across the spinal column that secreted the three enzymes: trypsin, amylopsin, and lipase; that helped the body to digest protein, starch, and fat, and that also appeared to control the amount of sugar in the blood.

Thus, among its other virtues, the pancreas prevented diabetes, a disease caused by the body's inability to burn sugar as a fuel.

Everybody knew that, of course. What wasn't known was exactly how the pancreas helped the body to assimilate sugar. It was probable that the metabolism was aided by a hormone secreted by tiny spots in the pancreas known as the islets of Langerhans. Although Osler had surmised many years earlier that if someone could isolate this secretion he would be able to control diabetes, physiologists had failed to do so. The pancreas was still an enigma. No matter how many extracts had been made from the pancreas of animals, the product was unable to control the lethal disease of diabetes mellitus.

As Fred reread the article that evening, he underlined one particular paragraph in which certain experiments were recalled, wherein the pancreatic ducts of rabbits had been tied off, and the experimenters had found "that within twenty-four hours the ducts became dilated, the epithelial cells were desquamated, and there were protoplasmic changes in the acinic cells... at the fourteenth day a great deal of the parenchyma had been replaced by connective tissue.... Ssobolew ligated the ducts in rabbits, cats, and dogs. He found a gradual atrophy and sclerosis of the organ with relatively intact islets and no glycosuria."

With relatively intact islets. As Fred looked at these words again, an idea occurred to him. It was such a simple idea that he would probably have lost confidence in it instantly, feeling sure that the thought must have occured to others in the field long ago—had the article not been the latest word on the subject.

"We do not know whence ideas come," he said much later, during a speech in Chicago—a speech that showed just how desperately unhappy he had been in London, "but the importance of the idea in medical research cannot be overestimated. From the nature of things ideas do not come from prosperity, affluence and contentment, but rather from the blackness of despair." Whether his recipe for inspiration—a weight of despair, an over-flowing cup of loneliness—was universally applicable or not, the ingredients certainly did not distract Fred from the revelation he now obtained from that underlined passage in the article by Dr. Barron: that *if* the tying of the pancreatic ducts caused atrophy of the pancreas except for the islets of Langerhans — and *if* the islets were the source of the diabetes-preventing hormone — then there *must* be a way to extract the hormone, no matter how many times great physiologists had failed to do so — perhaps because of interference from other ferments, such as trypsin. It was simply (he thought) a matter of eliminating that interference.

The more he thought about it, the more excited he became. He telephoned his friend William Tew and asked him to come over. He had something important he wanted to talk about. When Billy arrived, Fred showed him the article, drawing his attention particularly to the part where Moses Barron, in his study of the formation of gallstones, "had noticed that the glands of the pancreas secreting vital digestive ferments were likely to atrophy if gallstones obstructed the passageways from the pancreas to the small intestines. Experiments on animals.... had shown that these glands would also shrivel when the pancreatic ducts were tied."

After Tew had read the article Banting outlined his idea. He said he wished he could get hold of a pancreas of the type that Barron had described, because it seemed to him that if the glands which secrete trypsin, the most powerful of the digestive ferments, were not functioning, it might be possible to make a pancreatic extract containing that mysterious substance secreted by the islets of Langerhans — the still-unidentified hormone that apparently controlled the metabolism of blood sugar. And if they could only get hold of that, they might find a way of treating diabetes.

That night, Banting could not sleep for thinking about Barron's experiments in tying off the pancreatic ducts. He could not understand why Barron had not considered the next step, which seemed so logical. That step, as Banting put it in his notebook at two o'clock in the morning, was to "Ligate the pancreatic ducts of dogs. Wait six to eight weeks for degeneration. Remove the residue and extract."

Next day, heartened by Billy Tew's lively response, he discussed the idea with F. R. Miller. But the professor was not quite so encouraging. His field was the physiology of the nervous system, and he had no particular interest in endocrinology. He told Banting regretfully that he could not help him. His facilities were limited. He suggested that the man to consult was MacLeod of Toronto, who was an authority on carbohydrate metabolism, and would be better able to judge whether Banting's idea was worth pursuing.

Accordingly, Banting made an appointment with J. J. R. MacLeod and a few days later drove to Toronto in the Ford Tourer and stated his case.

MacLeod was not the least impressed. How on earth, he asked with lofty amusement, could Banting, with his lack of training in research, expect to isolate the internal secretion of the pancreas when so many world-renowned physiologists had failed—quite apart from the uncertainty as to whether such a secretion existed in the first place. No, there was not the slightest chance that MacLeod could see his way to allocating either subjects or space for experiments by someone who was barely qualified to be considered even an amateur researcher. No, the idea was absurd.

The germ of Banting's later enmity toward Professor MacLeod must have insinuated itself at that first meeting in the medical building of the university. Not everybody had the warmth, sympathy, and perception of an Osler. When he brushed aside Banting's idea, MacLeod's contempt for the younger man's qualifications and experience must have shown through a little too clearly.

Unfortunately his verdict could not be challenged. He was the supreme authority on the subject. Though he was, at forty-four, not that much older than Banting, J. J. R. MacLeod was far above him in achievement. He was a Scotsman with degrees from Aberdeen and Cambridge, and with years spent in the study of physiology at Leipzig and Berlin, and in imparting that knowledge to hosts of students in England, the United States, and Canada. He was a superb teacher. He was renowned for his physiology textbooks and scientific papers and for his original research, especially in carbohydrate metabolism. He knew more about diabetes than any other man, and had written about it extensively. So he knew what he was talking about.

In character he was said to be an honourable man, but one who was perhaps overinfluenced by the honours that had been heaped upon him, and by his training as a graduate student in Germany. There he had perforce been a nonentity to his Teutonic masters. He had resented their high-handed manner. But he had apparently not learned from that experience to treat others, like Banting—admittedly a rather drab and unpolished person, whose suasions did not come trippingly off the tongue—with the tact or consideration that he himself would have appreciated from his German professors.

Fred was crushed by the encounter. He needed no reminder that he was unworthy. He was quite capable of regarding himself realistically. After twenty-nine years of struggle, he knew he had little to show and tell. He had no experience in physiology. He had produced not a single paper. He had no background to speak of in research. All he had to show, really, were two years in rough-and-ready martial surgery, and a few hours as a demonstrator, and a few months as a failed G.P. He knew all that, and could understand the celebrated professor's reluctance to provide him with research facilities. All the same, surely the idea he had brought with him should have been evaluated more thoughtfully on its own merits, and not ignored on account of its bearer's accomplishments.

Nevertheless, such was the growing force of Banting's belief in the idea that, despite the blow to his self-confidence by MacLeod's "thinly veiled scorn," he persisted in his efforts to convince the professor. He journeyed to Toronto a second time, and a second time failed. Once again, Banting returned to his drab routine in London, teaching, reading, painting uninspired snowscapes, waiting for patients. There were no women in his life now that he had let Mary slip out of communication range, no close friends at all, except for Billy Tew.

The routine also included his old, compulsive studying. But at least it now had a direction: diabetic research. And his drab, passive nature was transformed. That winter, the idea ceased to be a midnight intuition, and became an obsession, powerful enough that even the prospect of another humiliation from Professor MacLeod could not deter him from trying again.

On this third attempt, in the spring of 1921, he penetrated the professorial defences. Wearied by Banting's persistence, and perhaps impressed in spite of himself by the man's conviction which seemed to be generating its own energy, MacLeod compromised. He was going to be away in Britain for two months that summer. Reluctantly he agreed to let Banting use the physiology lab for those eight weeks—which MacLeod, well aware of the time-consuming difficulties of physiological research, knew to be hopelessly few.

At this reluctant and probably exasperated concession, Banting must have had great difficulty in supressing his excitement. The opportunity to put his hypothesis to the test was high. Except that, Oh God, he would have to wring a further concession from the professor. At the risk of upsetting the arrangement, he reminded the older man of his total ignorance of most of the techniques of research. He would need, Banting faltered, an assistant to do the blood chemistry work, and certain other calculations. And he would also need a free supply of experimental animals, for he had no money to pay for them himself.

He waited tensely for the response. But perhaps because MacLeod had gone this far and realized that he would either have to take the next essential step or cancel the arrangement and risk having this fellow badgering him again in another few weeks, or perhaps because Banting's confession of his deficiencies showed that he was not entirely a fool rushing in where angels had fallen flat on their faces—that he was prepared to undertake the task in the proper (and all too appropriate) spirit of humility—MacLeod agreed. He would supply Banting with ten dogs and a research assistant.

Thus reluctantly committed, MacLeod followed through by mentioning to his senior class in physiology that a Dr. Banting would be investigating the function of the pancreatic islets in the hope of isolating the antidiabetic hormone—if there was such a hormone. (Some authorities believed that the function of the islets of Langerhans was to detoxify, to defend the body against organic poisons.) Would anybody be interested in this line of enquiry? Two of them were: Mr. Noble and Mr. Best.

Charles Best, a twenty-one-year-old who had just passed his B.A. exams in physiology and biochemistry, and who had been doing experimental research in diabetes, was interested enough to come to MacLeod's office to hear what Banting had to say.

Best, a muscular young man with fair hair and a ready smile, liked the sound of the project, but was dismayed by the financial aspect. Professor MacLeod was prepared to provide a maximum of ten dogs for vivisection, but no funds whatsoever. Banting could not afford to pay a salary. He had barely enough to support himself, let alone an assistant.

That summer, Best had planned on earning money as a demonstrator in physiology. It is to his eternal credit that he agreed, with very little hesitation, to start work with Banting as soon as the spring term ended—a tribute to his integrity as a scientist.

They started work together as soon as MacLeod had left on vacation, the careworn older man and the carefree youth. Banting had already established a methodology in consultation with his young assistant. He began by ligating the pancreatic ducts of several of the experimental animals, and Charlie soon discovered that in his modest demeanour and humble approach to the task ahead of them, Banting had not done himself justice. He was both knowledgeable and organized in his approach. He had been working in the lab for only a brief period before he showed that there were depths of knowledge and originality beneath his drab exterior. He devised a new technique for removing the pancreas in a single operation. Until then it had always been done in two stages. Again, while they were waiting for seven anxious weeks for the results of the operations, Charlie discovered that though Banting had played down his competence as a linguist, his French and German were quite up to the task of translating and reviewing the latest work by the European authorities on the dreaded disease of diabetes mellitus.

When the hypothesis first occurred to Banting, he had, in his ignorance, no idea of just how formidable was the task that he was undertaking. Now, in this waiting period of reading and reviewing between operations on the dogs and the next stage, he began to realize just how brash he had been in hoping to do in a few weeks what others had failed to accomplish in years of work in well-equipped labs. He would confess later that if he had been fully conversant with the work of others in the field he would never had had the nerve to start.

Diabetes was a terrible affliction. The ancient Greek had given it its name, which meant "to pass through," so named after its most conspicuous symptom, the quick passage of water through the body. "The patients never stop making water," wrote Aretaeus in the second century, "for the melting is rapid, the death speedy. Moreover, life is disgusting and painful, thirst unquenchable, drinking excessive."

As Seale Harris wrote in his book, *Banting's Miracle*, 'From that far-away time until 1921, when Banting and Best came tilting their lances at the foe, there had been comparatively little advance in the treatment of diabetes mellitus. Physicians did learn, to be sure, that the illness might be controlled to some extent by extremely rigid diet, excluding many of the foods that the average person craves....Patients might continue to exist for five or six years under such a regimen, but only at the cost of a continual morbid preoccupation with the thought of food, an incessant hunger that was likely to make of life a savorless ordeal, with temptation to forbidden indulgence a constant threat."

In addition, the danger of complications was omnipresent. "Some diabetic patients developed gangrene and had to have their feet amputated. Others suffered agonies from neuritis and were never free from pain except by addiction to morphine. Still others were victims of pneumonia, tuberculosis, or acidosis. Boils and carbuncles were frequent and often resulted in blood poisoning and death. A wound which in an ordinary patient might have been trivial usually led to serious infection in a diabetic, while a surgical operation meant almost certain death."

By the twentieth century it was generally agreed that the immediate cause of the disease was the failure of the pancreas to secrete a substance that helped the normal body to burn carbohydrates, to assimilate sugar. Professor MacLeod's reaction to Banting can be more fully appreciated when the vast literature on the subject and the abortive efforts of over more than a quarter century of a host of brilliant physiologists is considered. None had tracked down the mysterious hormone, extracted it, and injected it into the diabetic body on the assumption that the injected material would compensate for the lack of the natural substance. In the circumstances, it was hardly suspicious that J. J. R. MacLeod would regard Banting as a scientific parvenu and could be excused his failure to perceive that this incomplete, uncertain fellow, Frederick Banting, had been granted an insight into the problem and that his comparative ignorance of the work of prior researchers would help him to validate it by protecting him from his own intellectual insecurity.

By the twenty-seventh of July that momentous summer, Banting had two dogs prepared for the crucial stage of the experiment. One of them had its pancreas removed, the other its duct tied. "From this point onward," wrote Lloyd Stevenson, "the pace of the work was accelerated. The changes to be studied required not weeks but hours, even minutes, to become apparent. If an internal secretion of the pancreas existed, it must now be proved. Banting was about to take the final step in the program which he had outlined for himself in London.

"A duct-tied dog was chloroformed, Banting and Best, clad in their customary white cotton gowns, stood over it. With decisive strokes of his practised scalpel, Banting opened the abdominal cavity and displaced the stomach to reveal the shrivelled remnant of the pancreas. This he removed. The degenerated gland was chopped into small pieces in a chilled mortar and frozen in brine. The mass was ground up and about 100 c.c. (a little more than three ounces) of saline were added. Of this extract 5 c.c. were administered intravenously to the depancreatized dog. Samples of blood were taken at half-hour intervals and analyzed for sugar content. It was shown that the blood sugar had fallen from 0.200 to 0.11 percent, in two hours, and at the same time the clinical condition of the dog was much improved."

The excitement of the researchers, as they calculated the reduction of the blood sugar under the action of the extract "isletin" must have been intense. But it was a disciplined excitement, perhaps hardly more than a flush of pleasure, a smile exchanged, a brief hand clasp. For though this result suggested that Banting's idea might not be leading into yet another physiological cul de sac, that it might just possibly not be another of his failures, it was equally possible that some other factor was present to account for the fall in blood sugar. They would have to check the result over and over again to be certain. They might, for instance, have obtained the result because of conditions that could not be duplicated.

All the same, there was no doubt about *this* experiment. Without a pancreas, the canine subject should have lapsed into a coma and died. After the extract had been injected into its veins, its blood sugar had gone back to normal, its urine was free of sugar. In fact it was soon running around the lab like a normal animal.

Unfortunately, there was only a limited quantity of "isletin." When it ran out, eight days later, the dog died. The researchers were both saddened. They were also perturbed at the thought of the number of dogs that would have to be sacrificed to produce a sufficient quantity of "isletin."

The search for an alternative source for the extract led Banting to the slaughterhouse. As a farmboy he had seen that his father had prepared cows for slaughter by having them impregnated, to cause them to eat more heartily. He also remembered that there were more and larger islets of Langerhans in the pancreas of a fetus than in the offspring after birth. Drawing again on his bank account of ideas that in the paradoxical way of the creative imagination seemed to be increasing with every withdrawal, it occurred to him that the fetus of a steer during its first four months of growth might be a prime source for "isletin." There would be no digestion in the fetus, and therefore the pancreas would surely be free of trypsin, the digestive ferment that made the job of isolating "isletin" so difficult.

The hypothesis was proved: such fetuses, obtained from a local slaughterhouse, were found to be free from trypsin, and their expanded islets a rich source of "isletin"—or as it was soon to be renamed "insulin." Further, by late August, Banting and Best had developed a method of using the whole pancreas of adult cattle, the method that is still essentially in use today.

Then, Professor MacLeod returned.

It would surely have been a rich moment for an outside observer when MacLeod strode into his laboratory that September, ruddy and refreshed after his Scottish vacation, confident and ready to sweep the amateurs out of his laboratory so that he could get on with the *real* work—his researches into anoxemia—to be told that Banting with a twenty-one-year-old assistant had not only proved his hypothesis, but had developed it in technique and production to an astounding degree in only two months.

It was perhaps to be expected that the professor, who himself had researched frustratedly for so many years into the problem of diabetes, refused to believe it. Banting's account of the confrontation with MacLeod was coolly objective. "In view of the great importance of the fundamental observation that the active principle of the extract exerted a definite influence upon the blood sugar and sugar secretion of diabetic animals," he wrote, "Professor MacLeod advised us to secure even more results along this line." This note, as objective as if he were merely recording some mechanical day-night ratios of urine, was, in fact, the residue of a seething conflict that, unsoothed, would have had disastrous consequences for insulin research.

The professor, as contemptuous as ever of Banting's ability, questioned the accuracy of his notes. "Banting, interpreting this as a reflection on his integrity, allowed his native tendency to pugnacity to overcome the restraint with which he previously had bridled his resentment at MacLeod's attitude toward him," Harris writes. "His temper flared, a bitter argument followed, and MacLeod practically requested Banting to cease work in his laboratory."

When Banting threatened to take his discovery to the United States, his supporters on the faculty intervened and applied the field dressing of their appeasement. But the wound underneath continued to fester in an animosity on Banting's part that would intensify during the crisis still to come, and on MacLeod's part, an aloof scorn. To which he added a stubborn insistence, not just that the experimenters give him further proof of the efficacy of insulin but that they tackle other problems in metabolism "having no immediate connection with the treatment of diabetes."

Thus, as Banting saw it, while diabetics were suffering and dying, weeks were squandered in unnecessary experimentation. He resented it with a fury that caused concern among his acquaintances. The emotion was all the more harmful to him because he was too unaggressive to express it in the presence of its cause, the professor. Naturally the emaciated condition of his finances did not ameliorate his ire. It was all very well for the lab chief to insist on these further weeks of work. *He* was receiving a good salary as professor of physiology, while Fred had liquidated his every asset in an effort to keep going that summer, even to the extent of selling his beloved jalopy. He was deeply in debt, so that even the sixty dollars a month that the physiology department now started to pay him did little to ease his plight.

It took a professor from another department to accomplish that. During the summer, Banting had consulted Dr. Velyien Henderson on certain chemical problems. Henderson had become steadily more impressed with Banting's work. Sensitive to Banting's predicament, he obtained for Banting a sinecure in the department of pharmacology, with a salary of $2,200.

It was the largest sum that Banting had ever earned. For the first time in almost thirty years he would be able to look forward to a few months of financial security.

But Banting was probably even more grateful for the facilities that the position afforded him: a lab of his own. In this space at least, MacLeod would have no jurisdiction over him.

Professor MacLeod may not have cared a jot about Dr. Banting's financial situation, but when the results were verified beyond the boundary of his skepticism he was quick enough to accord the discovery his unqualified support. He reoriented most of the resources of his lab to the insulin experiments and transferred every available man to the work, including himself, E. C. Noble and Dr. J. B. Collip.

Noble was Charlie Best's fellow student, who had not been able to join the team until later on in the summer. Collip was the most notable addition to the group, although not according to his own over-modest account. "I recall quite vividly," he wrote, "how impressed I was with Banting and his problem, which was nothing less than a frontal attack on the pancreas to obtain its elusive internal secretion. My own problem, the effect of PH upon the blood sugar, seemed insignificant by comparison, but I had come to work with a man, whereas Banting had a problem which even at that time superceded such things as personalities and graduate training. I feel that I was very fortunate to have been a worker in MacLeod's laboratory at the time that Banting started his first investigations and to have known of the progress of this work at first hand. He was most anxious that I should become a co-worker with him. I assured him that I would be delighted to do this, but that I would have to wait until my revered Chief, Professor MacLeod, said the word. Some weeks later, at a time when Banting's early experiments, in which he had been assisted by C. H. Best (now Professor Best), had in my opinion established completely the existence of insulin, Dr. MacLeod asked me to join in the work. The part which I was able to contribute subsequently to the work of the team was only that which any well-trained biochemist could be expected to contribute, and was indeed very trivial by comparison with Banting's contribution."

In fact, James Collip did a great deal to develop the process for the preparation of insulin on the scale necessary to make it available to the millions of diabetics. He worked principally at the Connaught Laboratories of the University of Toronto, which, together with the Lilly Company of Indianapolis, would be initially responsible for the production of insulin. His career indicates the quality of the man. A native of Belleville, he had graduated from Trinity College at the head of his class in the honour course in physiology and biochemistry, and had gone on to a Ph.D. in biochemistry. During the First World War he organized the University of Alberta's department of biochemistry. When Banting met him in MacLeod's department, he was on a sabbatical leave. After his return to Alberta he isolated the active principle, parathormone, from the parathyroid gland. In 1928 he went to McGill to do major work on the pituitary hormones. "Here he isolated the sex hormones and tropic hormones from the anterior pituitary and extracted oestrogens from the placenta." He also was the first to isolate the adrenocorticoltrophic hormone (ACTH), making him one of Canada's major contributors to medical science.

Collip's contribution to the insulin story was far from trivial, either in technical or human terms. He did not in the least share Banting's antipathy to the professor. Where Banting saw the chief as a hostile martinet, Collip saw him as a dignified friend, fair-minded, genial, and human. Though Drs. Banting and Collip later became close friends, this difference of opinion actually led to one of the most scandalous things that can happen in academic circles, beside which anything short of sodomy appears inconsequential. They had a fist fight. One day when they were both working in the physiology laboratory, Banting's expressions of hostility toward MacLeod became so excessive that in a fit of exasperation, Collip threatened to walk out and carry on his share of the work independently. At which Banting lost his temper completely. He threw a punch at the biochemist, knocking him to the floor, where he lay, in Seale Harris' words, "dazed and amazed."

Though the clashing emanations from the hopelessly incompatible professor and his pugnacious protégé created considerable tension in the lab, it did not hinder the team from making rapid progress. Fred and Charlie had worked out the proper doses and their frequency for a variety of conditions and complications in dogs, and by the end of the year they were ready to test the findings on people. The first test on a human diabetic came on January 11, 1922, at the Toronto General. The patient was a fourteen-year-old boy who had at best only a few more weeks to live.

In a room crowded with observers, including Banting, Best, the physicians in charge who were from the university faculty, and several extra nurses and interns, the boy was injected with a weak solution of insulin.

It was not a particularly dramatic inauguration of a clinical trial, an instantaneous marvel like the first official anesthetization of the surgical patient in the Boston General. Hours passed before it was determined that the boy's blood sugar level had dropped by a quarter, and the urine sugar had slightly decreased. In fact, the treatment continued for two weeks, the dosage being gradually increased. But at the end of that period the physicians were as impressed as if the change had occurred in the first hour. The boy had improved so greatly in appearance and in vigour that the physicians, Walter Campbell and A. A. Fletcher, were astounded.

To be quite sure that no other factor was involved in the improvement of his condition, the course of injections was discontinued. Sugar again appeared in the urine in large amounts, with traces of acetone. Administration of the extract was resumed ten days later, on February 16, with a gradual lowering of sugar excretion and the disappearance of acetone from the urine. Again "the boy became brighter, more active, looked better and said he felt stronger."

When the boy, "L. T.," had entered the hospital at the beginning of December, he had received what hitherto had been a death sentence: a diagnosis of juvenile diabetes. "On admission he was poorly nourished," ran the hospital report, "pale, weight 65 pounds, hair falling out, odour of acetone on the breath....abdomen large and tympanic...dull, talked rather slowly, quite willing to lie about all day." Except when, on the essential starvation diet, the boy dragged himself to the beds of the other patients to steal leftovers from their food trays. By January 11, he was approaching the end of his life.

Now, a few weeks later, he had been transformed from a wasted wreck to a healthy child, distinguishable from normal boys only by his dependence on insulin; the first of uncountable millions to be saved, thanks to the experiments that had begun a mere eight months previously.

It was one of the supreme moments in medical history. To the observers, the change in young L.T. was astonishing. Even more incredible was what followed, the Lazarus-like raising of children from the diabetic coma. To the doctors and nurses who had spent a professional lifetime watching helplessly while death staked its inexorable claim on such victims, the transformation in the patients injected with insulin was awesome. Until now, those who had gone into coma had never returned. Yet even though the extract was still lacking in potency and worryingly impure, out of ten patients in complete coma treated with the extract, six were revived. They were still alive and in sound health by the end of the Second World War.

Others, too, in that series of clinical tests, might have survived had the problem of adequate production of insulin been solved. But it had not, and in one case the staff were forced to watch in anguish while the patient, a child, whom they had restored to consciousness with insulin, and who was on the way to recovery, died because they had no more extract to give him.

It was at this worst of all possible moments that the press caught on to the significance of the objective communications between the physiologists about the miracle that was taking place in Toronto. Just as the experimenters were facing the fact that they must not treat any more patients until they could produce insulin in suitable quantities, the news of its miraculous powers was flashed around the world. Diabetic millions from Chudleigh to Chungking were informed that they were about to be reprieved from their sentence of thirst, hunger, and sickness unto death. The disease had been conquered by a Dr. Frederick G. Banting, working at the University of Toronto. All it took, to release them instantly from their torment, were injections of his specific.

Naturally the afflicted responded with some urgency. Banting was inundated with letters from diabetics, imploring him to help them. Those who could afford it struggled to the new medical Mecca from the Americas, Europe, the most distant parts of Asia. He achieved worldwide fame almost overnight, from the profession as well as the public; for there had been a remarkably short interval between the announcement of the discovery and its acceptance by the usually ultra-cautious scientific community. The evidence had been too strong; it had been presented with a speed, clarity, and precision that left no room for skepticism. As we have seen, it was not uncommon for the profession to scorn and neglect great discoveries until long after their work was proved. In Banting's case, the world's scientists lavished him with praise almost from the start. It was not so much a matter of a modern speed of communication as of overwhelming irrefutable evidence. As for the public, he became an instant hero of science, from whom further miracles were expected almost hourly.

The abrupt, spectacular fame caught Fred entirely unprepared. One moment he had been a self-doubting recluse, walking, hunched, between the lab and his room on Grenville Street where he had lived since his return from London, Ontario. A room so crowded with books, journals and papers that his landlady would hardly have been able to enter even had she been allowed to do so; a room where he would sit until the early hours of the morning, reading and scanning and making notes until his eyes grew too raw from fatigue and cigarette smoke to take in any further detail on carbohydrate metabolism. And so to bed, until it was time to shamble anonymously back to the lab.

Now, suddenly, he was being pointed out on the street and worse, hunted by reporters. He was not prepared for their aggressive ways, nor was his the kind of tolerance or sophistication that could handle their uniformed importunities. No doubt, like everybody else, he had youthfully daydreamed of eminence, but when it came he found it almost as intolerable as his former neglect by the profession in London. Fame moved into his life like a squatter into an abandoned tenement. He had no time to adjust to the ways of the news media. From the start, he took its stories far too seriously, pshawing and snorting over the journalistic simplifications, seething over the premature assurances that insulin was an instantly available "cure" for diabetes when in fact it was a control, not a cure, and as for its being a finished product, ready for mass consumption, like corn flakes, *Rubbish!!* Couldn't they understand how premature all this fuss was, that the extract was still in the experimental stage? His contemptuous attitude to the press—not unlike MacLeod's behaviour toward him—made him a good many enemies.

The reaction of one roughly handled newspaperman was typical. After Fred Banting had given him the verbal bum's-rush, the reporter revenged himself under a headline reading, "Banting Pearls Not for Swine." He accused Banting of using bad language, and quoted his description of other newspaper stories about him as rot. In general the reporter presented a picture of a peevish and violent churl. He also referred to Banting's "alleged" discovery.

A reporter in London, Ontario, was slightly more objective when Banting dismissed him with a rude word that was rendered in the newspaper as "Bah!" The reporter merely described Fred as being "Refreshingly Rude."

The reaction of some former acquaintances was rather more satisfying. Until now they had avoided him as a mediocrity. Now they started to cultivate him assiduously, hanging onto his every halting word with a respect not unmixed with amazement at the wizardry of fate that had transmuted a leaden swot into a golden boy of science.

On the whole, Banting did not adapt gracefully to world fame. He gives the impression of being oppressed by a sense of his own unworthiness. He seemed to be negatively charged, despite outbursts of self-interested pugnacity. The first time he was publicly honoured by a huge audience at the King Edward Hotel in March 1923, he received a standing ovation, a tribute that has now become grossly devalued by the synthetic enthusiasms of the trendy, but was then accorded only to superlative achievement. But then, as later, he gave little of himself in terms of personality or self-expression. Wrote one reporter, "He reminds one of a little of a small boy asked to recite something in front of the class when he wants to go fishing." And though the world continued to heap accolades on him, his reaction seemed to be one almost of anger, as if from a deep-seated feeling that his renown had not been properly earned.

Certainly, nobody could say he was suffering from inflammation of the ego. His ineptness as a speaker—his speeches were usually as badly presented as they were ill written—appears to have been a manifestation of a profound heart-sinking self-doubt, of which an immutable modesty was only a superficial symptom. When invited to Buckingham Palace for an interview with the King, he went not to the main entrance but to a side door. Sweating with trepidation in his brand-new morning coat, he was escorted to "a Chinese room" and asked to wait. However, his fears subsided somewhat when presently, "in came a sloppy individual with the sort of trousers that have pockets on the front. He was some sort of official. He had bad teeth, very bad teeth, and he lounged against the fireplace with his arms on the mantelpiece while he talked to me." Fred was greatly reassured by the sight. "'Lord' I thought to myself, 'if the King can stand you around him, he'll be able to stand me for a while. I won't be thrown out inside the first few minutes.'"

By the summer of 1923, Banting had earned the absolute and unqualified respect of the entire scientific community. In Europe the attitude of many of the most respected medical men and scientists verged on reverence. Yet his performance at, for instance, the London Congress of the International Society of Surgeons suggested that his presence there was a case of mistaken identity. "Four hundred of the greatest surgeons from every nation awaited Dr. Banting's address with breathless interest," reported the *Daily Express*, "but Dr. Banting occupied a back seat and refused to speak until later. The learned surgeons who preceded mounted the rostrum and delivered deliberate and eloquent addresses.

"Then came Dr. Banting's turn. There was an expectant hush as a short man, clean shaven, with large, round, gold-rimmed spectacles, rushed breathlessly on the stage. He would not use the rostrum erected for the Congress. He had to overcome shyness. He clasped his notes behind his back, fixed his eyes on the ceiling, and began in a rapid colourless monotone an address that was technical and unintelligible to the layman. There was no hint of triumph in the even enthusiasm of his tone.

"He stopped as abruptly as an interrupted gramophone record, and scuttled from the hall before the audience had brought their hands together in the first clap of eager applause. He rushed straight into the street and lit a cigarette with intense agitation."

Presumably it was poor Fred's hunched, self-conscious posture that convinced the reporter that he was "a short man." Actually Banting was just short of six feet tall.

He failed to turn up for the second day of the Congress, and thus thankfully missed many speeches in his honour—except for one speech that would have given him great pleasure. A distinguished member rose to describe Banting as a benefactor of mankind whose discovery ranked in importance with those of Louis Pasteur.

It was a breathtaking comparison, rendered all the more thrilling because Pasteur happened to be Banting's greatest hero.

The one consequence of Banting's work that gave him the profoundest satisfaction was the feedback from the increasing numbers of patients whose lives he had saved. By 1924, the Connaught Laboratories of the university and the Eli Lilly Company of Indianapolis were producing insulin in sufficient quantities to keep large numbers of diabetics alive. The gratitude of patients and their relatives, expressed in letters and in person, touched Banting deeply. One woman, describing her son's recovery, said, "His weight was 65 pounds, his teeth were all decaying; his hair thin and lifeless, his skin drawn and sallow; and nothing was left but a skeleton. Today his weight is 145 pounds, his teeth are in perfect condition, hair thick and glossy, and the most glorious color in his cheeks I have ever seen in anyone. He is a frolicking, joyous happy boy.... He has no *craving* for food, swims, plays tennis, anything else without the slightest fatigue.... I owe his life to you."

The gratitude of the physicians of the formerly doomed victims of the disease was almost as intense. At first a few of them had tested the new product with a doubt born of long experience with faulty new remedies. They hardly dared to believe that the suffering they had witnessed since first clinical experience of diabetes had really come to an end. For a while their reservations had seemed justified when, using dosages not precisely calculated, some of their patients went into insulin shock; the symptoms ranging from nervousness to convulsions. A few physicians became frightened or disillusioned. Most of them, however, realized that there must be ways of avoiding unfavourable reactions, and a great many of them visited Banting in Toronto to accompany him on his daily rounds in the diabetic wards of the General Hospital and to observe his methods. These, in fact, included the giving of deliberate overdoses to the patients, so that the patients would learn to recognize and counteract the symptoms of the resulting hypoglycemia when they went home and became responsible for their own treatment. "The visiting physicians learned also to teach their patients how to give themselves the necessary injections of insulin two or three times a day just under the skin of the upper arm or thigh or in the rump, taking care to vary the location of the spots for inserting the needle from one injection to the next so as to avoid all danger of injuring the tissue by repeated puncture in one spot." Thus the uncertainties of those attending Banting's clinics in Toronto, or in seminars conducted throughout the continent were quickly dispelled, and they realized that insulin really was one of the truly great miracles of modern medicine.

Among the host of visitors, those who were most impressed, and who were most grateful for the discovery, were the diabetic specialists, who had spent a lifetime trying, and invariably failing, to keep their adult patients alive for more than one year. Their awe and gratitude when they saw the effect of insulin was profound. Some of them were so moved that their expressions of gratitude to Banting were almost incoherent. When they returned home and began to apply the methods with results that, no matter how hard they resisted the word, seemed miraculous, they wrote back in almost loving terms, like the southern American doctor who, practically within minutes of his return from Toronto, was called to the bedside of a fifteen-year-old boy who was in such distress that he was groaning, though unconscious. He had already passed through stages of thirst, hunger, emaciation, nausea, vomiting, and excessive urination. Another physician had diagnosed appendicits, but the returning pilgrim decided to try insulin. At first he went about it timidly, but soon his confidence was soaring. The boy came out of the coma within six hours. In less than a day he had lost every one of his adverse symptoms. Within ten days he was in perfect health.

Though deep down, Banting felt himself to be little more than an obscure country boy from Alliston, and had difficulty in adjusting to the idea that he was now an important man, he bristled fiercely enough when a certain other person agreed with his low opinion of himself. And when that person appeared to be taking the credit for the discovery of insulin, Banting's attitude darkened into outright hatred.

Inevitably, the somebody was J. J. R. MacLeod. The original announcement of the discovery came from him, rather from Banting. Even Banting's biographer, Lloyd Stevenson, who seemed to be a MacLeod supporter and disapproved of his subject's thin-lipped attitude to the Chief ("the spectacle of the young man turning away in anger from the old one, refusing for years to speak to him, cannot be said to add to our admiration for Banting") had to admit that the professor worded the original announcement in such a way as to make it appear that most of the credit was due to him rather than to his junior. He was lauded accordingly.

404 *Rogues, Rebels, and Geniuses*

Both Stevenson and Seale Harris maintain that MacLeod was not being willfully dishonest in snatching at the largest possible share of the honours. "He was profoundly inbued with the ideas of the German *geheimeraths*. He believed that heads of departments should receive the principal credit for researches which had been carried out in their laboratories, even if they themselves had not initiated, directed, or actively participated in the experiments. He was convinced that reports of his subordinates' achievements should be made by him, not by the subordinates. Acting on this belief, he made a number of reports, both spoken and written, which (perhaps unintentionally) gave his hearers and readers the impression that J. J. R. MacLeod was the principal discoverer of insulin and that Frederick G. Banting and Charles H. Best were merely two among a number of assistants who had happened to work under his direction."

To a modern reader, MacLeod's behaviour appears presumptuous, especially as he was working in North America where it is customary to give the credit to the person who had earned it. This view is sharpened by the article that MacLeod wrote for the *Encyclopaedia Britannica*. The 1929 edition was supposed to contain the definitive word on the subject of diabetes, yet there was not a hint in the article that Banting was the discoverer of insulin, or that Best played any part in the discovery. As early as May 1922, at a meeting in Atlantic City attended by some of the continent's most eminent clinicians and teachers of medicine, MacLeod made only a passing reference to the experiments, and referred to their principal researcher only as "F.G.B." The result was that, following the address, the speakers reserved their praise exclusively for Dr. MacLeod.

That any praise at all should go to the lab chief was almost more than Banting could bear. Apart from the fact that MacLeod had consistently demeaned him, just what had the Scots *geheimerath* contributed? He had provided facilities and collaborators. He had insisted on painstaking verification of the work done in his absence, and the repetition of certain control experiments. And he had given his undoubtedly valuable advice. But to the creative work, as distinct from the back-up support, he had contributed not one jot. And here he was, hogging the honours, and worse still, getting away with it, not least because of his skill in persuading the audiences that he was already a scientist from whom such achievements were only to be expected. Banting's rage was such that on one occasion it even overwhelmed his inborn fear of his own emotions. When MacLeod followed up the Atlantic City meeting with an article in the *British Medical Journal*, which similarly gave the impression "that MacLeod was the father of Banting's baby," the pressure of Banting's resentment grew so unbearable that it actually propelled him along to the professor's office. Then he proceeded to spatter MacLeod with accusations. It only made the situation worse. Banting was self-conscious and inhibited even when he was in a tranquil mood. In a state of seething fury he was well-nigh incoherent; whereas MacLeod had a fine command of the language, supported by a dignity that rose to the challenge of his authority by becoming cutting and contemptuous. Banting was finally forced to retire in disorder, realizing, when he calmed down, that he had probably confirmed MacLeod's opinion of him as a thoroughgoing boor and country bumpkin.

The chief's behaviour had the further effect on Banting of intensifying his loyalty to Charlie Best. From now on, on every possible occasion, he insisted on giving Best rather more of the credit than was his due. (Best admitted that in assigning equal credit to him, Banting had been "generous.") When Banting received a substantial international award in 1923, he dispatched a telegram reading, "I ASCRIBE TO BEST EQUAL SHARE IN THE DISCOVERY," adding that he was hurt that Best's contribution had not been properly acknowledged.

It was as if Banting hoped that by adding Charlie's weight to his end of the teeter-totter of fame, he would catapult the professor off the other end.

Admittedly, Banting viewed Best's contribution from a calmer perspective on another occasion that same year. In recognition of his achievement, the provincial government offered to establish a special post for him at the University of Toronto, to be known as the Banting Chair of Medical Research. When Dr. George Ross told Banting about it, he replied that he wished it to be known as the Banting and Best Chair of Medical Research. "I wanted to know why," Ross recounted, "since the plan was devised to honour him as the discoverer of insulin. The only answer I received was, 'Well, Best stood by me at a time of difficulty.'"

Ontario's gesture toward science was not the only government accolade that year. The federal government acknowledged Banting's contribution to the country's prestige by granting him a lifetime annuity of $7,500. In Europe, the award of state pensions to great scientists and artists was not uncommon, but it was unprecedented in North America. What was even more remarkable, not a single Parliamentarian objected.

With this generous annuity, Banting's money troubles were finally resolved, after five years of being "worse off than a beggar." He was able to pay back his father a loan of four thousand dollars. "I have never known anything like the relief I felt when that was all paid back, with interest," he confided to a friend; though he remained as concerned as ever with Best's credit. "Dear Charlie," he wrote, "I have just had a marconigram telling me about the Dominion Government. I wish they would give you an equal amount. Surely blessings are falling on us fast enough now. We must keep our heads. Fred."

Fred certainly kept his scientific head as far as money was concerned. When a patent was secured for insulin in the names of himself, Best, and Collip, he assigned it to the university. To accommodate the diabetics who insisted on the attentions of the great man himself, he opened an office at 160 Bloor Street West, and though he could have made a fortune as a specialist, he soon abandoned the practice, and returned to research work. He might have adjusted with difficulty to the publicity his fame had brought, but he had no difficulty in resisting the temptation to capitalize on it. "He might easily have asked, as easily received, fantastic fees," wrote one of his biographers, "but his charges were exceptionally modest. Some of his colleagues, unfortunately, were not so fastidiously restrained, and a few were frankly opportunists and quite ready to 'scalp' the more well-to-do-visitors. An Atlantic City millionaire came to Toronto with his wife and daughter because the latter was a diabetic. During their stay in the city the millionaire's wife had an attack of acute abdominal pain and her case was diagnosed by a leading Toronto surgeon as appendicitis. He accordingly proceeded to remove her appendix—at a cost to the unprotesting millionaire of five thousand dollars. To this was added a bill for two thousand five hundred dollars, submitted by the physician who had first been called to see the case and had referred it to the eminent surgeon. Banting was furiously angry. He felt that the visitors from Atlantic City had come to Toronto on his account, as indeed they had, and that two of his colleagues had taken advantage of them in a manner which he considered shameful."

Meanwhile, though the "Insulin Rush" of diabetics to Toronto subsided as the extract became more generally available, the publicity continued unabated, and in fact would alternate between the raucous and the muted for the rest of Banting's life. In October 1923, he was still being hounded by reporters, and he was having difficulty in convincing them that he was not about to trot out another epoch-making discovery; that though his discovery had been made in only a few weeks, normally it took years of research to accomplish even a minor breakthrough.

He was now making more of an effort to treat the press with tact. But his new appeasement policy soon broke down. That month, several international news services announced that Dr. Banting was working on a cure for pernicious anemia. Fred immediately issued a furious denial, calling the story a lie and asking them to, for God's sake, leave him alone to get on with his work.

(In a way, Banting did make possible a cure for pernicious anemia. Two years previously, a Harvard doctor, George R. Minot, had developed diabetes, and a strict diet was only partially successful in controlling it. Then came insulin. It enabled Minot to carry on his researches with a vigour that was essential for the work. In 1926, he discovered that liver could make up for the failure of the red blood cells to reach maturity. He had thus found a working cure for pernicious anemia. Without Banting's contribution, it is quite possible that Minot would have died, or at least would not have had the energy to complete the work.)

Banting's irate response to the news stories once again caused the press to castigate him. They soon felt as frustrated as he was; for just as their diatribes were reaching fortissimo level, they were forced to sing his praises all over again, when it was announced that Banting was to receive the supreme tribute to medical achievement: the Nobel Prize for Medicine.

Yet Banting must have been in danger of bursting several minor blood vessels when the announcement came from Stockholm. For who should be named as co-discoverer of insulin but Dr. J. J. R. MacLeod. Unfortunately there was nothing he could do about it without damaging his own reputation. The best he could do to rectify the injustice was to share his half of the $40,000 prize with Charles Best.

Even then, not to be outdone, MacLeod offered to share his portion with Dr. Collip—thus thinning out the award still further.

Frederick Banting's public life gave him little personal satisfaction. His private life brought him even less.

The fault lay in his own lonely, stilted nature. He had many virtues: he was honest with himself, and usually considerate of the feelings of others. But at the same time there were elements in his character that made it difficult for others, particularly women, to match their esteem for his achievement with an affection for the man. He behaved churlishly at times. He bore grudges and he made them last. He was often gauche and unresponsive in his relations with women, partly out of shyness and inhibition, but also out of the kind of insensitivity that can arise from an acutely sensitive nature. He considered himself to have been ill-done-to by their sex, as represented by Mary, who, he believed, had cruelly jilted him. Even by 1924, when fame and fortune encouraged him to modify his bitter attitude and he started to cultivate the company of several nurses at the General Hospital, he soon earned their "enduring dislike," by courting first one, then another; trifling, as they saw it, with their affections. They resented it, especially after he unceremoniously ditched one of their number, who had considered herself engaged, as insouciantly as he had used Mary's ring to etch laboratory slides. For a man who was easily hurt, he could be quite deficient in insight into the sensibilities of others.

He paid the price of this impassivity when, at the age of thirty-two he rushed into marriage with an X-ray technician.

Marion Robertson was a doctor's daughter from Elora, and she seemed almost too promising a mate to be true. She was not only pretty, charming, exceedingly feminine, and as lively as a flapper, but her job in the radiology department seemed to indicate that she was interested in science. Fred approved of women who had serious intellectual interests. No doubt Marion, flattered by the attentions of a great man, did her best to emphasize that interest. Fred quickly convinced himself that he was in love with her.

Had he given himself time to know her better, he might have drawn back in time. Or possibly not. Perhaps he feared that another long engagement would lead to another humiliation, or perhaps his yearning for a warm and stable home life was urgent enough to blind him to an incompatibility, and deafen him to the cautious warnings of his friends.

In any event Fred felt he had to decide quickly, for in the spring of 1924, he and several other prominent British and American scientists were invited by the United Fruit Company to study health problems in tropical America. As the trip was to be made by steamer, it seemed too good an opportunity to miss, to combine the study of yellow fever, pellagra, malaria, and dysentery, with an all-expenses-paid honeymoon. Accordingly, he shortened an already short engagement, and in June 1924, married Marion at the home of her uncle in Toronto. He had known her for one month.

As a newspaper account had it, "The pretty bride and her distinguished groom received the full and frank benediction of a summer sun. Even between the closely drawn curtains of the upstairs sunroom, where the ceremony took place, its warm rays filtered."

They departed on their honeymoon in Banting's shiny new roadster immediately after the ceremony, and, after he had collected an honorary degree from Yale University en route, they sailed from New York on the S.S. *Calamaris*.

Fred had been looking forward tremendously to the trip, not least to the opportunity to meet a number of his heroes among the scientists and medical men, and at the chance to escape the glare of publicity that had frazzled him over the past three years. But there was no escape, even among men whom he had thought, in his overweening modesty, to be superior in scientific endeavour. The enduring value of his discovery and the prestige of the Nobel Prize was too great. Even these celebrities sought him out, and deferred to him almost as if they believed that he belonged in their august company. That he did not truly believe it himself was immediately obvious to the others, and many of them were quite touched by his lack of side, his honesty and humility. One of them was Colonel B. K. Ashford, an American pioneer in tropical medicine whose discovery of uncinariasis, the hookworm disease, had brought him international renown. He wrote that, "Of all the friends I made on that trip, none became closer than Banting. We sat together at a table all the way to

Kingston; and timidly—it was his honeymoon—he made friends with me."

In Jamaica, the night before he was to deliver a paper on the causes of diabetes and the use of insulin, Banting hesitantly asked if he could rehearse the paper with Ashford, to get the benefit of his advice. Ashford agreed, and together they sneaked away from the ball that was being given to honour the delegates, and sat together on the seashore. "And there," wrote Colonel Ashford, "under a swaying electric light beneath the palms he read me the wonderful story of his work, the light that has flooded the dark corners of a hitherto incurable disease, a genuine conquest of Medical Science. He read it just like a boy who had been told to write a composition and is afraid it isn't good enough. I interjected a few phrases simply for clarity of expression. He was so grateful that I felt guilty, and exclaimed:

"'Good God, man!—it's the substance, not the words!'

"He told me that he knew now what had drawn the two of us together. It was that opportunity which we both had had of directly applying our own remedy, curing our patient, and getting immediately therefrom the powerful stimulus to ambition in research which a successful case brings. 'But,' said he with charming naïveté—'after all, you know, I am only a laboratory man. I know next to nothing of the art of medicine. I'm the greenest man here. All this is new to me.'"

The friendship with Ashford was the kind of empathy that Banting had hoped to develop with his wife. But even by that night on the seashore he had begun to realize that he would never achieve a meaningful closeness with Marion. He was already giving up. When he sneaked away from the ballroom, he left Marion behind to dance with other men.

In Marion's correspondence, there is not a hint of the sundering relationship between the newlyweds. Her letters home suggest no real involvement with her husband. Monday: "We have just finished playing games on deck." Tuesday: "Last night the moon was full, and we danced on deck and had such a good time." Thursday: "It's very hot— unquestionably hot—and we are not allowed to bathe at all here (Havana) because the water in the harbour is not pure. One has to be so careful in the tropics it seems. One indiscreet move and you get something awful the matter with you. The gentlemen had a meeting in the morning to visit hospitals, so we decided to stay home and try to keep cool. I was sorry though that I hadn't gone because some one had sent word that I was interested in X-rays and they had the X-ray department all ready for inspection and asked for me specially. However, the rest was no doubt better for us—it was so hot."

A week later they were in Jamaica for the International Conference on Health Problems in Tropical America, with Marion reporting that

"Tuesday afternoon we had a bathing party...then at night the formal opening by the Governor-General, and a dance. Fred sent me a huge armful of American beauty shaded roses and I wore my white dress and had a beautiful time. Wonderful floor—good music—everything." The next day she is thinking of aiding a New York *Times* reporter in delivering a spoof, a take-off on a medical report, entitled *Feminensis Amorita.* By the end of the conference she is begging off an official trip so that she and a friend, Laura Carter, can get a rest and write a letter or two. "We just haven't a minute left to us—they have entertained us so lavishly." By late July, they are entertaining the officers of the world's largest warship, H.M.S. *Hood.* "The officers were all here for a dinner and a dance on Saturday night and we met them—some of them, for there seems to be so many—and we had a splendid time." On July 29, "Fred made his speech today at three, so that hurried up the end of the luncheon and as soon as that was finished we all went over to an At Home on the H.M.S. *Hood.* Fred's speech was just splendid. Sir Thos. Oliver spoke so nicely after—about his directness and his simple modest manner and his sincerity and his genius....All the others too spoke of it and what a splendid paper it was.

"The At Home today was very fine....Tonight there's a meeting and Fred is there and there's a dance later on—and then a swimming party."

A few days later, from Honduras: "We saw over the place all day and at night they had a dance on board and all the people came down and we had a great old time. You'd be surprised at the people here. All young married people—charming girls who dress so well and live so nicely in spite of their isolation. There are a great number of young college men here too who are so glad to see people again from home. In the afternoon there was a big reception here. After supper, when we sat opposite Lady Newsholme and His Excellency, we danced on the roof to the 'Marimba Band'—the national music of Guatemala and my beau the Minister (I can't even say his name) and I led off the dance, as Lady Newsholme didn't dance. More excitement. Fred thinks this is a fool of a country. They separate us at all the functions."

In fact, Fred and Marion were already separated by their totally different characters, and Seale Harris, who was there as an American delegate to the conference, saw it with sad clarity.

"It would have been pleasant," he wrote on Fred's behalf, "to have a wife with whom he could laugh wryly at the penalties of fame and in whose company he could have escaped occasionally to the quiet anonymity he enjoyed. But all too soon he found that this was not the kind of wife he had. She enjoyed the recognition she got as the wife of a famous man, but even more she enjoyed her recognition as a beautiful and charming young woman in her own right. The music, the dancing, the luxury, the tropical verdure and tropical languor—it was all so romantic, or it would have been romantic if she had not found herself tied to a husband who seemed to be more interested in all kinds of nauseating disease problems than in moonlight and dancing and having a good time while you were young. Well, at least she didn't have to be tied to him all the time; if he didn't care to dance at least she could dance while he watched, and she could let him see that other men seemed to enjoy her company."

Fred did not care to dance because he could not dance. So he was forced to watch her being whirled around in the arms of others for hour after hour, until exhaustion drove him to bed in the small hours of the morning, where lack of sleep and growing anxiety about the future fogged his concentration at the next day's conference sessions.

Even with such a sympathetic friend as Harris he tried to hide his feelings. When Harris asked him why he did not join his wife on the dance floor, "he passed the whole thing off as a joke, saying that dancing was strenuous business on a hot night and that he preferred to let his be done by proxy. But those who knew him best were not deceived by his professed unconcern; they guessed rightly that he was suffering. Never since he was a little boy enduring the agonies and embarrassment of his first party had he felt as miserable as this, for this was not the sort of social life for which he had a gift, and yet as each day passed he saw more and more clearly that it was the breath of life to Marion." Outside he was sweating with humiliation; inside, chilled with shock at the discovery that he had known nothing at all about Marion when he married her. By the end of the three-month cruise, he was dreading the return home. "The newspapers would be panting for belated reports of his sudden marriage; all his friends would be anxious to greet the happy bride and groom; everyone would be wanting to felicitate him. But by now he knew too well—and Marion knew too—that no felicitations were in order; there was no happy bride, no happy groom; there was no lasting love, no mutual understanding."

The rest of the story is just as unhappy. The estrangement of their first weeks together was never mended, though the dishonest conventions of the day dictated the pretence of a happily married life.

They did not separate officially for some years, and were not finally divorced until 1932.

It was not until 1939, with his marriage to a woman of warmth and intellect, Henrietta Ball of New Brunswick, that Banting achieved the kind of communication he had yearned for all his life. The marriage lasted eighteen months. On a wartime flight to England, the bomber in which he was flying crashed. Twenty hours later he died in the shattered fuselage, as unreachable in the wastes of Newfoundland as he had been throughout the early part of a lonely, painful life.

29

Perspective: The Inside Story

BANTING'S DISCOVERY OF the hormone, insulin, was one of the peaks in the endocrine range that had been hazily viewed by a Paris physician, de Bordeu, as early as 1775. De Bordeu was intrigued by the changes that took place in a man's body after his testicles had been snipped off. Castration was not uncommon in bygone centuries as treatment for disease or injury to the organs, and also for security and esthetic reasons. Male slaves, destined for Eastern harems, had the operation performed on them to ensure that they would stand only on guard duty. The lord of the harem naturally preferred to minimize competition, to deny his ladies a standard of comparison with his own prowess, or lack of it. In seventeenth-century Rome, Sistine Chapel choirmasters, running short of Spanish "falsettists," substituted *castrati*. For nearly two hundred years, the artificial male soprano, created by an operation on the sexual organs in boyhood, contributed his pure tones to church music, notably in Italy, but also in England, which has a long, alto-voice tradition that has continued into twentieth-century pop music, as perpetuated by The Beatles. The operation was barbaric but it produced a fine choral effect — unlike the effect on the castrated rooster which loses heart as well as testis, and abandons its dawn tantara.

In eighteenth-century France, de Bordeu, noting such physical changes in the castrated male as an exuberance of fat and an austerity of hair, speculated that there might be some substance formed by the testicles that affected such growth, and that other organs might similarly contribute to the bodily economy.

It was late in the following century, though, before advances in

412

chemistry enabled the endocrine glands to be properly studied, an endocrine gland being one that releases its product, a hormone, into the blood stream to act on other parts of the body. Endocrinology became one of the important new studies in world medicine. Its modern development stems from Claude Bernard's concept of the glands as producers of secretions that feed directly into the bloodstream rather than into ducts such as the sweat glands; and which act as bodily environmental protection agencies.

We have already encountered Claude Bernard—the scientist who contributed to an understanding of curare, the use of which, in anesthesia, was climaxed by the work of Harold Griffith in Montreal. Bernard was a dome-foreheaded man with the small, sensuous lips formed by the lip-pursing French language (the other extreme being the mouth-widening American pronunciation of English). He was born in St. Julien in 1813 and, like Herbert Bruce and Lewellys Barker, first found work as a pharmacist's assistant. Unlike the Lake Scugog apprentices, the experience did not lead him directly into medicine. He had little interest in mortar and pestle work, but dreamed of stage success, and spent much of his spare time writing five-act dramas and other entertainments.

The pharmacist, however, was not entertained, and finally fired him. Bernard journeyed to Paris and showed a couple of his plays, entitled *The Rose of Rhone* and *Arthur of Brittany*, to a well-known critic, who was also a Sorbonne professor. The critic read the dramas, and was greatly impressed—by how bad they were. He recommended that Bernard abandon all thoughts of a writing career. On the other hand, it would be a pity to waste the pharmacy experience. Perhaps Monsieur Bernard should worship sombre Minerva, goddess of medicine, rather than continue to pluck at the gaudy skirts of the theatrical muse?

The footlight-dazzled are rarely receptive to the truth about their abilities, but Bernard appears to have recognized his Melpomenean or Dionysian deficiencies, and, to the world's subsequent advantage, promptly enroled in the faculty of medicine. By the time he graduated he had shown enough promise to be taken on as an assistant by the noted physiologist, Magendie. He continued and greatly extended Magendie's work, and by the climactic year of his life at the age of sixty-five, had established endocrinology on firm, scientific foundations. Bernard was also the discoverer of the vasomotor system, the nerves of which regulate the calibre of blood vessels.

The line of research between Bernard and Banting was straight and direct, for Bernard was the first to observe scientifically that the liver of a dog had a sugar-forming function. Similarly he found that the human liver releases glucose into the blood. The blood then carries this form of sugar to the tissues. Bernard called this an internal secretion, the term "hormone" not being used until 1902 (or 1905, according to some sources) by E. H. Starling, a British physiologist. While others had maintained that digestion took place only in the stomach, Bernard demonstrated the pancreatic connection: the job of the pancreatic juice in breaking down fats, starch, and protein.

Bernard's attitude during his life of experimentation and direct observation amply justified the critic-professor's assessment of him as being well suited to science. He soon came to realize that while imagination was a good thing in the theatre, it was a downright drawback in the laboratory. Upon entering the lab, he said, one had to remove not just one's hat and coat but one's imagination, leaving the totally objective observer. Moreover, "One must break the bonds of philosophical and scientific systems as one would break the chains of scientific slavery," he added in his 1865 *Study of Experimental Medicine.* "Systems tend to enslave the human spirit." Particularly the human medical spirit, which has always tended to be enslaved by past systems or doctrines.

Endocrinology advanced rapidly after Bernard's pioneering work. E. H. Starling was one of the stoutest builders on the Frenchman's foundations. He discovered that the pancreatic digestive enzymes and hydrochloric acid were incited into production by substances secreted by the stomach, thus completing Bernard's pancreatic equation. After Starling, hormones, "the blood-borne secretions of the endocrine glands," became a favourite subject for scientists. The thyroid hormone was next to be investigated, then the two hormones adrenaline and noradrenaline, the first constricting the skin and digestive blood vessels and relaxing the visceral muscles, and the second affecting nerve impulses.

Researchers like Bernard and Starling greatly accelerated progress in pharmacology, immunology, chemotherapy, and radiology, as well as endocrinology, because they were traveling along roads paved by social and technological forces. The industrial revolution was one of the forces, encouraging the development of new instruments. The one that most profoundly affected progress in research, especially in microbiology, was the microscope.

Though its origins lay in the Middle Ages, the first major advance in microscopy took place in he mid-seventeenth century, through the lens-grinding genius of a Dutch haberdasher, Leeuwenhoek. A pure amateur, Leeuwenhoek managed to overcome some of the distortion that had plagued scientists since Malpighi first saw the capillaries in a frog's lung. With his three-inch microscope, the Dutchman was the first to watch the contortions of "animalcules" — bacteria. Examining every substance he could find, from pond water to his own semen, Leeuwenhoek described what he saw in jaunty Dutch. When some ladies looked through Leeuwenhoek's microscope at a drop of vinegar and saw some little wiggly things swimming about in it, he wrote that "some of 'em were so disgusted at the spectacle that they vowed they'd never use vinegar again. But what if one should tell such people in future that there are more animals living on the scum on the teeth in a man's mouth, than there are men in a whole kingdom? Especially in those who don't even clean their teeth?"

About eighty years later, another amateur, Lister's father, Joseph, designed a two-lens-in-one microscope that made high-power instruments possible, and greatly eased Pasteur's investigations. But the most significant advance came through the German physicist, Ernst Abe, who, working for the industrialist, Carl Zeiss, completely redesigned the microscope, working out the optics from mathematical formulae to allow the most perfect possible view of micro-organisms.

Another instrument, basic to the practice of medicine, was the one invented by René Laennec in 1819. Laennec was the first to create a complete diagnostic system for pulmonary and cardiac sufferers. For years he had urgently desired to hear the heart beat clearly enough to help him achieve a more informed diagnosis. Placing his head on the patient's chest was simply not good enough. It was particularly embarrassing, having to rest his ear on a woman's left breast. One day, while crossing the courtyard of the Louvre, he stopped to watch a small boy who had his head pressed to a wooden beam. At the other end of the beam a friend was tapping messages with a nail.

Laennec wandered off, thinking about it, and the next time he examined a patient he thought he would employ the same principle. Rolling up a sheet of paper, he applied one end to the heart region and listened at the other end. He was amazed at the clarity of the heartbeat. A more permanent aid followed, a wooden cylinder. The telltale heart spoke more eloquently still. Laennec called this aid a stethoscope—from the Greek word *stethos*: chest.

A rather more sophisticated instrument was Helmholtz's ophthalmoscope, used for inspecting the inside of the eye, partly for diagnosing eye diseases but also for obtaining valuable evidence on the whole body as varied as signs of high blood pressure or diabetes. The ophthalmoscope also allowed an observer to see the body's only visible nerve, the optic nerve. Then, in 1853 a new means of administering drugs came along: the hypodermic syringe, invented by Charles Pravaz of France and Alexander Wood of Scotland.

Among the discoveries that progress in other fields, specifically the electrical, made possible, none was more portentous than the X-ray apparatus. Until it came into use, physicians could press, probe and palpate only from the outside, comparing overt symptoms against check lists of clinical knowledge; but the delicate covering of the body might as well have been as thick as Hadrian's Wall when it came to inspecting the inner sanctum of living man. William Röntgen's discovery enabled, for the first time, the tissues and internal anatomy to be seen, and pathological changes noted. X-rays would have the most profound influence on medical practice since Hippocrates brought his unprejudiced eye and reasoning brain to the art of diagnosis.

When Röntgen made his announcement in the final week of 1895, the significance of his discovery was almost immediately appreciated throughout the world by laymen, and even by the medical profession; though, as already noted, a few Victorian souls considered purchasing X-ray-proof drawers, fearful that the see-through rays might turn them into involuntary exhibitionists. (Lead-lined loin cloths did come into use eventually, though for protection against genetic damage rather than the lascivious eye.) Radiography joined that tiny, privileged company of medical developments that would be exploited immediately. Like Banting's discovery, the need for it was very great. It was quickly put to use in hospitals throughout the world, to diagnose fractures, locate foreign objects, and confirm bone diseases. Its value even outweighed the dangers. The exposure-time of the first X-ray machines could be as long as half an hour, resulting in troublesome skin burns and, ultimately, cancers. The need to reduce the exposure-time was quickly realized, and by 1913 improvements in the cathode tube had reduced it to only a few seconds—just in time for the First World War, when tens of thousands of men became human junkyards of shell fragments.

Nowadays the film that replaced the early X-ray plates requires exposures of mere fractions of a second.

Other developments in radiography include the ingestion of materials (contrast media) to help expose parts of the body that would not otherwise show up on the X-ray, such as radio-opaque barium sulphate which, when swallowed, outlines the gastro-intestinal tract, and iodine-containing agents injected into veins and arteries which show kidneys and blood circulation.

A view of the heart, however, was denied to radiologists until 1929, when a young German doctor, Werner Forssmann, in an astounding experiment, showed that an iodine-containing contrast agent could be introduced directly into the heart, to make it opaque. He did this by experimenting on his own body—introducing a catheter into a vein in his elbow and insinuating it all the way to his heart—while watching the process through a fluoroscopic screen, and taking X-ray pictures. His chief came into the laboratory while he was doing so, and almost had a heart attack, screaming at Forssmann, "What the hell are you doing?" Horrified, the chief tried to intervene and was only prevented from doing so by several well-aimed kicks to the shin.

When the astounding X-ray shots were published, they caused a sensation, and Forssmann, who had graduated from medical school only a few weeks previously, was smothered with newspapermen. He was also fired from the university department—German *geheimeraths* were not noted for their admiration of private enterprise in underlings.

Unfazed, Forssmann later repeated the experiment on himself, and completed it by injecting a contrast agent through the catheter and into his heart, experiencing only "a slight haziness, a disturbance of consciousness and vision which lasted only a second or two, presumably as the concentrated fluid first flowed through the brain." In the thirties, two Americans, André Cournand and D. W. Richards, Jr., perfected the technique of making damaged hearts visible. Thus they inaugurated the era of the heart operation, a once spectacular and dramatic event, now quite routine. The work of all three men was recognized some years later when they were jointly awarded the Nobel Prize in Medicine.

While excessive exposure to the new man-made radiation could cause cancer, natural radiation was found to be useful in combating it. The most powerful radioactive element in nature was radium, discoverd in 1902 by Pierre and Marie Curie.

The Curies were a fascinating couple who exemplify the mysterious intensity of the research worker, as well as the transference of devotion in the post-Darwinian age from religion to science. Marie came to maturity caring a good deal more about learning and the fate of her country than about spiritual matters. Poland was under the hated tsarist bureaucracy when she was born in Warsaw in 1867, and she was well into middle age before her beloved country was freed from an oppression that had not even allowed her to learn her native language. She was forced to recite her school lessons in Russian, and study Polish in secret.

France was her cultural Valhalla and Marie was twenty-four in 1891 when she finally reached Paris, to enroll in the faculty of sciences of the Sorbonne. With few friends, except those among the expatriate Polish community, including the pianist Paderewski (who would be the first prime minister of the Polish Republic in 1919), she settled into a life of relentless study and grinding poverty in the Latin Quarter (though as George Orwell noted, being poor in Paris was preferable to being in reduced circumstances anywhere else; in Paris, nobody cared whether you lived or died, whereas in other places, particularly London, conditions were just appalling—you were at the mercy of charitable organizations). In 1893 Marie obtained her master's in physics, and the following year in mathematics, having survived the entire period on three francs a day, a sum which, if offered as a tip for coffee and croissants in a superior French restaurant, would have brought a glaucous glare from the waiter.

Thin, blonde, and severe, Marie had apparently had no love affairs by the time she met Pierre Curie. Her ambitions were intellectual, her passion, which in an earlier generation might have been directed into religion, was for science, her loyalty, to Poland. Which were precisely the qualtities that brought her the love of Pierre Curie, then thirty-five, who was already well known for his research into magnetism and piezo-electricity—electricity due to pressure, especially in crystals. It was her knowledgeable mind that attracted him when she called on him one day at the School of Physics and Chemistry. Better still, there was not a hint of coquetry in her gray eyes. In his experience, women like Marie were rare. He was intrigued, and over the next few weeks, before her return to Poland, he made excuses to see her whenever he could. He asked permission to visit her in the Rue des Feuillantines, and in the words of her daughter and biographer, Eve Curie, "she received him in her little room, and Pierre, his heart constricted by so much poverty, nevertheless appreciated, in the depths of his spirit, the subtle agreement between the character and the setting. In an almost empty attic, with her threadbare dress and her ardent, stubborn features, Marie had never seemed more beautiful to him. Her young face, thin and worn from the effort of an ascetic life, could not have found a more perfect frame than this denuded garret."

After repeated attempts to persuade Marie to become his mistress, Pierre finally gave up, and proposed marriage. By which time, according to Eve, he had "gradually made a human being out of the young hermit." She accepted. It was typical of Marie that when a friend offered to spring for a wedding dress, she replied, "If you are going to be kind enough to give me one, please let it be practical and dark, so that I can put it on afterwards to go to the laboratory." Two years later she was working in that laboratory on the thesis she had chosen for her doctor's degree: the nature of natural radiation.

Following Röntgen's discovery, Henri Becquerel had started to investigate X-rays himself, to confirm his theory that such rays were emitted under the action of light. He began to experiment with uranium, but to his surprise he found that that rare metal emitted its rays spontaneously, with or without exposure to light. The discovery was made when he left some uranium salt crystals on top of a photographic plate. Even though the plate had been thoroughly protected by stout black paper, the salts had darkened the plate through the wrapping. An English physician, Sylvanus Thompson, noted the same phenomenon—radioactivity, as Marie Currie later named it—almost simultaneously, but Becquerel got his findings into print first. He showed that the uranium continued to emit rays even after it had been kept in darkness for months.

The Curies seized on this discovery as a promising field for investigation into the nature and origin of radiation. Working in the School of Physics and Chemistry, using the electrometer that her husband had invented, Marie became certain after a few weeks that the radiation from the uranium was proportional to the quantity of uranium, and was unaffected by any external factors—such as the freezing cold of the studio she was using. Further experiments indicated that uranium might not be the only element that emitted radiation. Accordingly, she put uranium aside and began to examine all known chemical elements, and discovered that thorium also emitted spontaneous rays. The discovery propelled her still deeper into unknown territory. One of the first revelations was that the radioactivity in some minerals was far stronger than it should have been, given the amount of uranium or thorium they contained. Her detailed and prolonged researches ultimately convinced her that a much more powerful radioactive substance must exist—an entirely new element, hitherto unsuspected by physicists. And in April 1898, she and Pierre announced that it must surely be present in pitchblende, the ore from which uranium was mined, because pitchblende produced a radioactivity hundreds of times more powerful than that from uranium.

In December of that year the Curies gave the new element a name: radium. But to characterize it properly they needed a larger amount. As she and her husband earned barely enough money to live on, there was no way they could afford to buy the necessary quantity of pitchblende, which was mined in Bohemia, then part of the Austrian Empire. Until it occurred to them that the radium would not be in the ore from which uranium was extracted, but in the waste material. And surely the Austrians would be willing to part with material that they had no use for.

Through the intercession of the Vienna Academy of Science, the Bohemian mine agreed to sell their rubbish for a small fee, and early the following year, sacks of it arrived at the School of Physics and Chemistry. Joyfully, the Curies pounced on the heavy brown dust, and quietly established that even though all the uranium had been extracted, the residue was even more radioactive than it had been before the miners had gone to work on the parent pitchblende. This was certainly confirmation that the by-product might prove to be far more valuable that the product.

Marie Curie's findings were increasingly at variance with fundamental theories on the composition of matter. In the fifteenth-century days of the reactionary Galen-fixed Paris establishment, such an upsetting of hallowed ideas would have earned Marie scorn and contumely; but scientists were at last becoming cautious about condeming heretics, whose explorations had all too often opened up and settled splendid new scientific territory. Which was fortunate for Marie, for she had a particularly sensitive and vulnerable personality.

For two years she continued to slave over the hot laboratory stove, working in a leaky shed formerly used by the faculty of medicine as a dissecting room until it was found unfit even to house corpses. She and Pierre worked patiently and undramatically, absorbed in their weights and measures, in the slow elimination of their chemical analysis, watching for the telltale flicker of the electrometer. "In spite of the difficulties of our working conditions, we felt very happy," Marie wrote. "Our days were spent at the laboratory. In our poor shed there reigned a great tranquillity: sometimes, as we watched over some operation, we would walk up and down, talking about work in the present and in the future; when we were cold a cup of hot tea taken near the stove comforted us. We lived in our single preoccupation as if in a dream."

They had few visitors, mostly physicists or chemists, anxious to bounce their ideas off the tall, rough-bearded, peaceful-eyed Pierre, or to converse with both — "the sort of conversation one remembers well," Marie wrote, "because it acts as a stimulant for scientific interest and the ardor for work without interrupting the course of reflection and without troubling that atmosphere of peace and meditation which is the true atmosphere of the laboratory."

The other half of the realm was their flat in the Rue de la Glacière, now shared by their first-born, Irene. Their domestic life was as orderly as any bourgeois couple. Pierre had come a long way from his free-thinking, convention-spurning days. He noted, not at all detachedly, the cutting of Irene's teeth — though he was jealous enough when he thought that Marie was spending too much time with the baby, even when she was merely recording its first words: "Gogli, gogli, go." Even at home, scientific precision did not entirely desert Marie. Describing her jam-making: "I took eight pounds of fruit and the same weight in crystallized sugar. After an ebullition of ten minutes, I passed the mixture through a rather fine seive, I obtained fourteen pots of very good jelly, not transparent, which 'took' perfectly."

It was March 1902 before Marie succeeded in isolating radium: one-tenth of a gram of a beautiful blue light. She left it in the lab, but in the evening she could not resist returning with her husband to look at it again. For a long time they sat in the dark, wondering at the power of such a minute quantity of salt — which was so radioactive that Pierre's electrometer could not begin to handle it. They continued to sit side by side, admiring the deadly glow worm. Like the X-ray workers, they had no idea of the hazards they would face — and had already faced. Their notebooks were soon so contaminated that they would be considered too dangerous to handle three-quarters of a century later.

Ultimately, radium proved to be two million times more powerful than uranium — and uranium was dangerous enough as it was. Yet to the end of her life, Marie, so utterly objective in all things scientific, refused to believe that her beloved element could be hazardous, even though she had already observed its effects on herself and her husband: scarred skin, rheumatic pains, and dragging fatigue. It would have been characteristic of her to ignore radiation sickness herself, but it could not have been easy to shut her eyes to Pierre's condition. In him the radiation sickness grew steadily worse, until he was killed in a traffic accident four years later. His head was smashed into more than a dozen pieces by a horse and cart.

Maire Curie shared with her husband and Henri Becquerel the Nobel Prize for Physics in 1903. Later she became the first person of either sex to win the Nobel Prize twice, when she received the chemistry award in 1911; but before the second award she had undergone an ordeal that brought her to the brink of suicide and madness.

After her husband's dreadful death, Marie's life for a time had gone into a numbing decline. Slowly recovering from her grief she threw herself back into research, into her duties as director of the physical laboratory at the Sorbonne, and as mother of two precocious daughters. But the girl who had originally seen herself as a bride only of science, was now a woman with a whetted sensual appetite. She took up with a young physicist, Paul Langevin. In time-honoured Parisian style, Langevin, who had a wife and children, took a *pied-à-terre*, and there the physicists delighted in the chemistry of love. Unfortunately a newspaperman learned of the liaison in 1911, and published the story in *Le Journal*.

In Paris, a fellow, whether painter or postal clerk, was expected to have a mistress. The arrangement was looked on with tolerance and no particular interest—unless the partners were so immoral as to flaunt the affair, or unless they were of the elite. In this case, of course, the woman was a world-famous scientist and Nobel laureate. The story, in typically flowery French journalese ("the fire of radium has lit a flame in the heart of a scientist, and the scientist's wife and children were now in tears"), quickly spread to the world's sensational press and created a scandal.

The public reaction appears to have contained a good deal of spite and jealousy. There was even a suggestion that Pierre Curie had not been accidentally killed but had been driven to suicide upon learning of his wife's liaison with a former pupil. Marie was hounded by newsmen, and reviled in anonymous letters, and her life was threatened. The French xenophobia, having been aroused, the public reminded itself that she was a foreigner of the worst sort—Russian, German or Polish—and probably Jewish into the bargain. (The anti-Semitic Dreyfus Affair had been resolved only five years previously.)

The journalist who had first broken the story was challenged to a duel by an enraged Langevin, but did nothing to diminish the libel and slander—especially as the duel took place in a bicycle stadium and neither of the duelists could bring himself to fire. As for Marie, her health broke down completely, and she was taken to hospital on a stretcher, close to death. She was still a sick woman two years later when she went to Warsaw for the inauguration of a new radioactivity institute.

Marie lived to see radium adopted throughout the world in the treatment of cancer, refusing to the end to believe that the element was inherently dangerous, despite the radiation burns to her hands, and despite the nature of the sickness that finally killed her in 1934: leukemia.

The practical result of the Röntgen and Curie discoveries was a new treatment for disease through radiotherapy, which used X-rays and radium, the same unit of dosage, the Röntgen, being applied to both. It was mainly the slow cancers, such as those of the face, breast, bladder, cervix, and uterus, that proved to be most susceptible to radiotherapy. For deep-seated cancers, surgery, sometimes in combination with radio-therapy, is now thought to be the best form of treatment; though, considering the progress of medicine since Pasteur, it is quite likely that doctors in the future, having gained a better understanding of the human system in all its incredible physical, mental, and perceptual complexity, will shake their heads indulgently at the barbaric twentieth-century custom of cutting into people with knives. (But at the present time, surgeons are busier than ever, repairing the ravages of degenerative disorders in an increasingly elderly population.)

By 1930 it had become evident that X-ray and radium treatment was destroying healthy as well as diseased tissue. There followed a lull in such therapy until the mid-1940s when radioisotopes came into use, these being forms of chemical elements used in medicine for tracing the movements of chemical substances in the body. Radioisotopes were the products of nuclear fission. (Incidentally it was at McGill University between the years 1898 and 1907 that Ernest Rutherford and his associate Frederick Soddy established the theory that led to the nuclear reactor: that the atom consisted of a positively charged nucleus orbited by negatively charged electrons.) By the 1960s, radioisotopes, in partnership with their scanners, enabled the liver, thyroid, lung, spleen, kidney, heart, or pancreas to be seen with amazing clarity, and, better still, allowed them to be seen at work. Brain tumours, too, could be revealed, using isotopes from such substances as iodine, gold, or arsenic.

Thus nuclear medicine had arrived, to which the University of Saskatchewan contributed in the late fifties with its "Cobalt Bomb," a machine used for bombarding cancerous tissue with pinpoint accuracy. And this development completes the story of Frederick Banting, for it was his heirs in endocrinology who were the first to take advantage of nuclear technology. Nuclear medicine was only later taken up by hematologists for the study of blood and its disorders, next by radiologists, then by clinical pathologists, until now it spans the entire field of medicine.

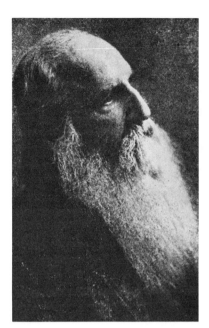 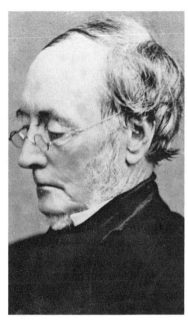

ABOVE: Richard Bucke (*left*) and Joseph Workman (*right*), two fathers of Canadian psychiatry. (Public Archives Canada/C9596; PAC/C52307) BELOW: Dr. Jean-Martin Charcot, one of the pioneers of neurology in France, demonstrating a patient with "hysteria." (Museum, Academy of Medicine, Toronto)

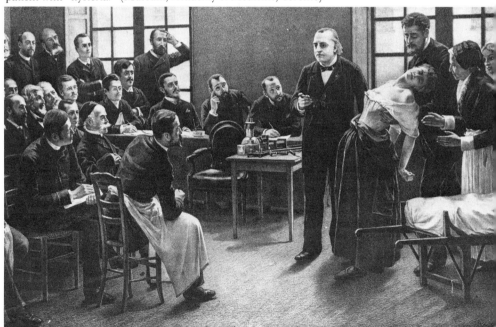

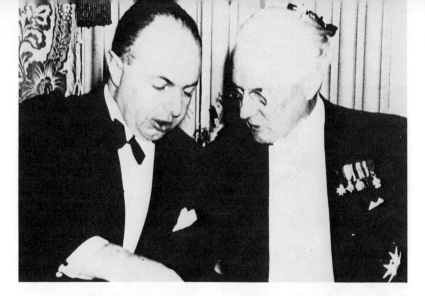

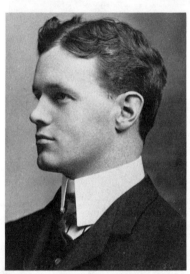

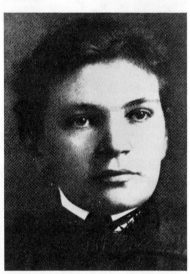

TOP LEFT: Herbert Bruce (*left*) with Premier Mitchell Hepburn. (PAC/C19531) ABOVE LEFT: Robert J. Manion—from private practice to cabinet rank. (PAC/C52055) ABOVE: Maude Abbott of McGill—museums and the human heart. (PAC/9479) TOP RIGHT: World War I battlefield. (PAC/PA2367) CENTRE RIGHT: Bringing out the wounded. (PAC/PA160) LOWER RIGHT: Operating room in France. (PAC/C59837)

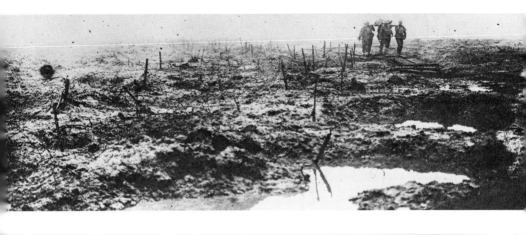

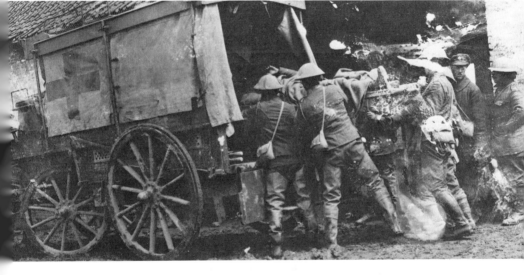

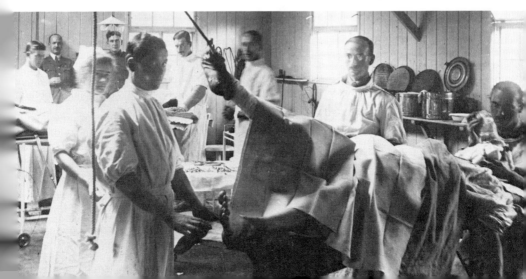

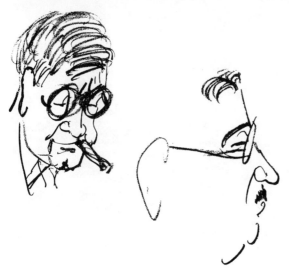

LEFT: Frederick Banting as caricaturist — sketches of colleagues at a convention. (Museum, A of M) BELOW: Banting (*right*) with Charles Best and Banting's dog Marjorie. (Museum, A of M)

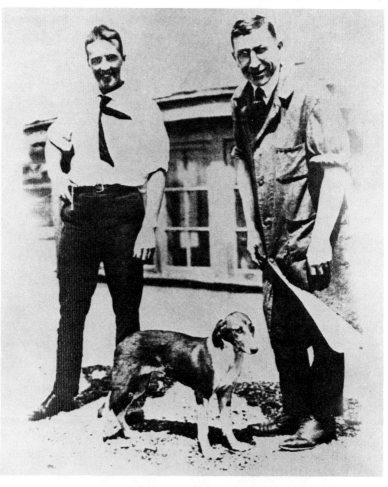

30

The Specialist

PEDIATRICS IS CONCERNED with the care and development of children and their diseases, from the day of birth to sexual maturity, but as Alton Goldbloom found out after his return to Montreal in 1920, a pediatrician also has to be something of a psychologist, a surrogate father, and a detective. The third of these qualifications was called upon at five o'clock one morning, when Goldbloom received an urgent call from the Montreal Maternity Hospital to examine a newborn baby. The infant had suddenly become ill, and had turned a deep indigo blue.

As the baby was being undressed for the examination, Goldbloom noticed that it was wearing what appeared to be new clothes. He asked about that, and one of the flutter of nurses around him confirmed this, and said that all the new babies had been dressed in a new issue. Goldbloom looked over the tiny shirt, nightgown, and diaper, and saw that they had been stamped, as usual, with the hospital name. The ink was fresh. And the little garments had obviously not been to the laundry. He turned to the nurses and asked them to check all the babies in the hospital as fast as they could, to see if any other infants had turned blue. They sped off, and some minutes later came rushing back to say that they had found thirteen other blue babies.

Goldbloom had once come across a case of shoe dye poisoning. He reasoned that the cause might be the same: the absorption of analin-dye from the stamp ink. There was a considerable commotion in the hospital when he ordered that every baby wearing new clothes should be stripped as quickly as possible, and dressed in garments that had been laundered at least once. There were a hundred babies to attend to. The ones who were affected soon recovered, and Dr. Goldbloom's reputation as a diagnostician went up another notch.

Further along the pediatric scale was four-year-old Susie, a bright little chatterbox who had been vomiting every morning for six weeks. Goldbloom examined her but could find nothing wrong. He thought for a moment, then asked the mother if by any chance she was pregnant. She confirmed that she was, about two months. Goldbloom promptly sat Susie on his knee and asked her if her mother was also vomiting. On receiving a cheerful affirmative he then asked Susie if she knew why her mother was being sick every morning. The child said it was because her mother had a baby in her tummy.

"And why do you vomit, Susie?"

"Because I want a baby in my tummy too, and I want it all the time."

Goldbloom convinced her that only grown-up ladies could have babies, and she would have to wait a few years before she could have one. The vomiting ceased.

Benny, a few years older than Susie, was also vomiting, but his trouble was quite plainly physical. His symptoms, including a drunken walk, had suggested a brain tumour to at least one specialist. The anxious parents, hoping for a less serious diagnosis, called in Alton Goldbloom.

Right away he suspected lead poisoning. He had seen many such cases in children, usually from lead toys or from house paint. Except that Benny did not have such toys, he was too old for them. He did chew his lead pencils, but of course, as everyone knew, there was no lead in the lead of a lead pencil. All the same, the symptoms, including the telltale line in the gums, suggested that lead poisoning was the cause.

On the day that Goldbloom examined him, Benny had his worst attack. He had severe convulsions, and was rushed to the Children's Hospital, in Montreal, and lay there unconscious for several days. Quite often, death or permanent brain damage followed such severe symptoms, but happily Benny recovered.

However, the source of the poisoning had still not been established. If it were not determined soon, next time Benny was likely to die. The only possible source of the trouble was his pencils. Goldbloom asked the mother to bring one of them to the hospital. The "lead" of course was harmless, but what about the paint on the foreign-made pencil? He scraped some of the paint onto filter paper, soaked it in potassium iodide solution, waited a few moments, then added drops of acetic acid. The filter paper turned deep yellow. So there was lead in the pencil after all, in the paint.

At the far end of the pediatric scale was a fourteen-year-old boy who had become so thin and weak that his frail mother had to carry him to and from the bathroom, and up and down the stairs. There were no physical signs of disease, and a psychiatrist had been called in. He found that the youth was reverting to infantile behaviour, and could not be shaken out of it. Goldbloom went to visit the patient, but he refused to go up to the boy's bedroom. He insisted that the patient must come down to him. The boy did so, making a production number out of it—slithering down the stairs and collapsing on a couch in the living room.

Goldbloom regarded him coldly. The boy's hair was revoltingly long, and he was wearing a fuzzy moustache and beard. Goldbloom feigned anger, and stormed at him to shave immediately. The boy said that his father wouldn't let him have an electric razor. Goldbloom, who had once been an actor, further sharpened his characterization of a man of authority who was not to be trifled with, and turned to the mother. He ordered her to phone her husband and tell him to bring back an electric razor. At the same time he was noting the response from the boy. He was beginning to revive. "Do you want to keep him a baby all his life?" Goldbloom shouted at the mother, but really addressing the boy. "and what about a haircut?"

On being told that the boy wanted a crew cut but his mother wouldn't let him, Goldbloom glared at her. "Let him have any kind of haircut he wants," he ordered; then rounded on the son, and told him to get dressed and then go out and get a haircut this minute. Whereupon the boy, beaming, went back upstairs, two at a time, and was dressed and running from the house within minutes, a dollar bill clutched in his hand.

The doctor did not say what the psychiatrist thought of this summary treatment.

When Alton Goldbloom, a Montreal-born descendant of Lithuanian parents, and a McGill graduate, returned to that city in 1920, pediatrics was starting to stride rapidly from the cozy darkness of folklore and superstition into the light of medical science. The United States was the leader in the new study of calcium metabolism, vitamins, nutrition, and immunity; appropriately enough since the United States was a land where children were worshipped to excess. Consequently it was in that country that the shy, rather formal young man obtained his training as a pediatrician, under one of the American pioneers, Emmett Holt. In the process, his name became known throughout the medical world as the inventor of the Goldbloom Needle, and for his research into pyloric stenosis, a disorder common in first-born children.

Despite his reputation, Alton had two strikes against him when he started up in practice in the city of Montreal, which had a population of 640,000 at the time. The first was that as one of these newfangled pediatricians, he was muscling in on obstetrical territory. In conservative Montreal, obstetricians were still considered to be the experts in child care. The second strike was his race. The atmosphere in Montreal, as in the rest of the country, was often unpleasant for a Jewish physician. There was both outright and covert anti-Semitism. The medical establishment did not think of Jews as members of the club. Years went by before the Protestant hospitals would admit either a Jew or a Catholic to a staff position, and even when a few Jews finally attained such positions, there were implied or unofficially expressed limitations. And the English hospitals were the only ones that the Jewish doctor could approach for his training, for the French hospitals were worse. In 1920, "No Protestant or Jew had ever been appointed to the attending staff of these hospitals." When one French hospital took on a Jewish graduate, the French interns went on strike, and despite worldwide condemnation, they had their way, and the student had to leave.

"The French hospitals," Dr. Goldbloom wrote in his autobiography *Small Patients*, "suffered from a stifling chauvinism and from an exclusive devotion to the medicine of France. A young man who had trained in the United States or in England could not hope for the recognition that he would get if he could put *des hôpitaux de Paris* on his shingle or his letterhead. There were no internships in France as we know them, nothing more than hospital walks as members of large coteries, but six months of this and a man would return to Canada as a specialist. The English hospitals were broader in their outlook and sent future Canadian leaders abroad for long periods of intensive training. Today the French hospitals are doing the same and their quality and professional attainments in many respects rival the English. What I came to in 1920, was a situation in which there were two rival camps, superficially friendly and correct and actually hostile, each with its own medical society and its own publication and with a minimum of contacts. There were two schools, McGill, smug with its world reputation, well-equipped laboratories, a famous library and some renowned teachers; and Laval (later the University of Montreal) essentially provincial, with poor facilities and little reputation and also a bit smug; a far cry from the present medical school of the University of Montreal with its massive pile, its beautiful laboratories, its excellent hospital facilities and some men on its staff with world reputations."

Alton desperately wanted a teaching appointment at his alma mater, McGill, but to do so he would have to establish himself in one of the two teaching hospitals. The first, the Royal Victoria, was not even worth trying. The man who ran the inconsequential pediatrics department there was ignorant of the latest advances in pediatrics, and was determined to keep newcomers out, so that his own deficiencies would not be exposed. When Goldbloom asked the powerful professor of gynecology to intercede on his behalf, he was reminded that he was a Jew.

The situation was not much better at the Montreal General. The man in charge of child care was not even a proper pediatrician. He was a dermatologist. When Alton interviewed him, the first question the dermatologist asked was whether Alton had volunteered for military service. A warm testimonial from the great Emmet Holt elicited only criticism of Holt and his methods.

The chief kept Alton waiting for a month before announcing his decision: he would give Alton a provisional six months appointment, but with no duties. The dermatologist said that there was no room for him in the outpatient department. However, Dr. Goldbloom could accompany the dermatologist on his rounds if he wished; but there would be no advancement or any teaching appointment.

These were humiliating conditions for a man as well trained as Alton. Still, he suppressed his pride and accepted, in the hope that the situation would improve. Which it did, very rapidly, when the dermatologist began to appreciate the depth of Alton's knowledge. After only a few days, the chief, uncomfortably aware of his own ignorance of the new science, began to make excuses why he could not make the rounds today, or teach his group. Within a week or so Dr. Goldbloom found himself in unofficial command. He had run of the children's ward in one of the country's top hospitals. Further, he had taken over the chief's students, doing what he most wanted, teaching. He could hardly believe that he had attained within days what he had hoped to achieve within years.

Moreover, the students appreciated him, and told him so; that he was the best teacher in pediatrics they had ever had. Until then he had had little confidence in his lecturing ability, even though he was used to addressing audiences. Before taking up medicine he had been an actor. Through his friendship with S. N. Berman (the future playwright) he had received a massive transfusion of theatrical blood, and had played in American stock companies before his father, who traveled across Canada peddling diamonds to merchants, railwaymen, and lumberjacks, asked him to abandon his misspent youth on the boards and take up a respectable profession.

Fat and foppish in appearance, brazenly confident on the stage but shy and stilted in real life, Alton went to Manitoba College, which gave a matriculation course for older students; and from thence to McGill, where he discovered in medicine a new and lasting love.

Now his audience was no longer one of rowdy ankle-fanciers, henna-haired doxies and tired businessmen, but senior medical students, who appreciated his theatrics more than the theatre-goers had ever done; and he found a new confidence in himself.

The confidence was needed. It was almost unprecedented for a young man to be placed even unofficially in charge of a ward without having served a long apprenticeship in the outpatient department. In a ploy that should have ended his rising influence, his jealous colleagues invited him into outpatients', thinking that this would lose him his ward privileges and teaching duties. Instead, he managed to keep the other jobs as well. Within eighteen months he was confirmed as an instructor with the rank of assistant demonstrator.

At the same time, he was establishing a private practice in pediatrics, working out of an office in the mansion of his in-laws. (He had married the petite and vivacious daughter of a prominent Montreal family, the Ballons.) The practice was an instant success. The idea of a specially trained physician for children caught on quickly with the general public, long before McGill University understood the need for a pediatrics department.

It was the general practitioners, the obstetricians and other specialists who resisted the idea. Alton had to be extremely tactful to avoid giving offence to his colleagues. He couldn't help showing them how little they knew of the latest child care developments in everything from nutrition to the latest equipment, such as the electric otoscope. This was an instrument that could bring the tiny ear canal of a child clearly into focus. It made the incising of a child's eardrum seem like child's play. Which was precisely why ear specialists, for instance, resented the pediatrician. The use of the otoscope took the mumbo-jumbo out of the operation for piercing abscessed ears, made it look ridiculously simple.

One such resentful specialist was a pompous little man who, along with Dr. Goldbloom, was called in to examine a small boy named Malcolm, who had an earache. In this decade before antibiotics, earaches often developed into abscesses and from abscesses to mastoids, and Malcolm's earache was well on the way. But when Alton suggested that the eardrum, which was bulging with pus, should be opened, the ear specialist disdainfully disagreed that the time and the eardrum were ripe. Because the child was being looked after by two impressionable grandmothers, he had his way. The specialist was not going to be advised or have the authority of his old age and experience challenged by a young whippersnapper in a totally superfluous field like pediatrics.

The child suffered agonies for three days before the ear man condescended to operate; by which time Alton could see that Malcolm was headed for an acute mastoid. But, "my consultant," he wrote, "was constantly demonstrating the superiority of his knowledge by assuring the grandmothers that things were progressing satisfactorily. After ten days of wavering, Malcolm developed swelling of the face and bloody urine. To me this meant that unless the mastoid was drained without delay the situation could soon become hopeless. I tried to make this clear to my stubborn consultant. He countered that it was up to me to clear up the kidney condition first before he would consent to operate on the mastoid."

Though it was almost heresy for a young physician to differ with the opinion of an established big-wig, Alton grew so desperate that he went to see the dean of the faculty of medicine, Charles Martin. When he heard the story and saw the child for himself, the dean's language might have created two more patients out of the grandmothers by giving them heart attacks, had they heard the dean's explosion. He called the ear specialist on the telephone and told him that unless he opened up the mastoid immediately the kidneys would never recover and the boy would die. After which, "Martin hung up the receiver, put his arm about me as if to comfort me and assured me that all would be well. This was at noon and the operation was peformed at four. Malcolm improved rapidly."

By no means all of Dr. Goldbloom's "rivals" resisted the new science. A notable exception was the obstetrician, James Duncan, who had the humility to admit his ignorance when faced with a problem in a child that was outside his field of expertise. He consulted Goldbloom soon after he arrived in Montreal, and after the newcomer had saved several two- or three-pound premature babies—before pediatrics they would probably not have survived—Duncan's faith in pediatrics slowly began to influence other obstetricians.

One of James Duncan's cases got Goldbloom into a spot of trouble with a haughty, lorgnetted dowager. Dr. Duncan called on him one day and said he wanted Goldbloom to replace an attending doctor who was getting nowhere with the first and only child of a middle-aged socialite couple. The baby was not thriving and was crying constantly. Goldbloom found that the replaced doctor had been giving the baby an unsatisfactory folklore formula: whey, cream, and milk sugar. Like many a child that was being fed the old, time-honoured formulas, it was simply not getting enough to eat. The baby was literally starving. As soon as Alton put it on to milk, water, and cane sugar, and a side order of cod-liver oil, the baby began to thrive. He also prescribed orange juice, but the baby refused to accept it. "But already at that stage in our pediatric knowledge," Goldbloom wrote, "it was becoming known that canned tomato juice had about half the content of Vitamin C that orange juice had. What we had done in New York and what I suggested in this case was that they drain the juice from a tin of canned tomatoes (the now widely used canned tomato juice was not yet commercially available) and feed it to the baby. The mother was horrified at the thought of giving her baby something out of a can. She would do it, she said, but only because I said so. She certainly would not think of doing it if anyone else had advised it, but I had done so well with her baby, surely I must be right. The baby thrived, enjoyed the tomato juice, and that was that."

All the same, it was not accepted practice, and shocked many in the lady's social circle, including the dowager who upbraided him at a hospital meeting. She demanded to know what the devil he thought he was doing, giving babies things out of cans. It was typical of the restricted radius of her prominent social circle that, "The story was constantly coming back to me in newer and stranger forms. Sometimes as the rash and foolhardy act of an unscrupulous upstart, sometimes as a daring and miraculous feat: I was now hero, now demon. The final metamorphosis went as follows: a baby was dying and all the Montreal doctors had given up. They said to the parents, apparently in chorus, 'There is nothing more that we can do; there is, however, a young man who recently came from New York, from Dr. Holt, who might be able to help you; why not try him?' I was then sent for, came in, took the traditional 'one look' at the baby and cried, 'For heaven's sake, open a can of tomatoes, quick!'"

Despite the depth of his training and a gathering renown as a pediatrician, Alton Goldbloom had to haul himself up a ladder of success whose rungs were widely spaced. Confirmed as a lecturer by 1926, it took him another thirteen years to reach the dizzy heights of assistant professor, when McGill finally formed a department of pediatrics (partly because the University of Toronto had established such a department, and McGill "dared not stay behind Toronto"). In the meantime his practice expanded still further, even into French territory.

His first French patients came to him in a roundabout way through the money-grubbing of a devious charlatan. This was a Montreal doctor who, despite a poor reputation in the profession, earned a considerable income which he was careful not to share with the young physicians whom he frequently called into consultation. Put another way, he cheated his colleagues. He would ask his consultants not to charge a fee this time because the patient had been under great expense. He would, he said, compensate the young physician later by calling him in again on some future occasion. But from the patient he would extract a hefty fee, saying it was for the consultant's services. He would then pocket the money himself. Goldbloom was caught twice before he realized what was going on.

Still, maybe the old charlatan wasn't so bad after all, for on the third occasion he actually offered to refer a patient to Goldbloom. It was a child with scarlet fever, he said, but he couldn't handle it because he might carry the infection to his surgical patients. So Goldbloom could have the case free.

It turned out that it was, indeed, free. The father of the patient was a doctor—and doctors and their families were traditionally treated free of charge. Which of course was why the old devil had handed over the case.

However, Goldbloom's success with the scarlet fever patient earned the gratitude of the child's father, and he recommended the pediatrician to a prominent French family living in the same apartment house. After them "came their cousins and their friends, in great profusion, and after that it was a geometric progression."

Alton hurriedly learned the language, including its patois—*Il feel pas bien, Elle est bien smart*—and his French practice soon outstripped his English practice. Even doctors in Paris began referring patients to him. As for the French hospitals, "I found myself welcomed and respected beyond my worth and I was being used extensively as a consultant by French physicians. The phenomenon was unique. I was able to prove to my own satisfaction that the barriers were not as impassable as I had been led to believe."

One of Goldbloom's French-Canadian patients was a five-year-old girl, Ginette, who was admitted to the Children's Hospital suffering from malnutrition. But she had been puzzling the doctors there with symptoms that could not be explained by her emaciation. She had little appetite but a lot of diarrhea, a beefy red tongue, rough, scaly and cracked skin, and was ferociously irritable, suggesting a disturbance in the nervous system. The chief, Harold Cushing, and the house staff were quite startled when Goldbloom suggested—though he had never seen a case—that it was pellagra.

Pellagra in Montreal? That was a disease associated with the southern states, where people ate maize because there was nothing much else to eat in the way of vegetables. It was a vitamin-deficiency disease. Because of a certain toxic effect of maize, the people who ate it needed more niacin than others, but frequently got less because the rest of their diet was so poor. "Yet here it was in a native Montreal child, typical and unmistakable in all its details. Its cause—Ginette was one of eight children, the father was only occasionally employed, food at home was always meager, only one pint of milk a day was brought the eight children, meat and green vegetables were rarities." Ginette's rapid recovery following proper treatment showed that it was pellagra. Subsequently, Goldbloom discovered many other cases, including a variation of pellagra where adequate food was being given but not being physiologically utilized.

One of his English patients, the son of Stephen Leacock, was the one to whom he felt the most gratitude, as it led to a lifelong friendship with the father. One day Goldbloom brought his friend Sam Berman—who was having his first success on Broadway—specially to Montreal to meet Leacock, and their dinner together at Leacock's house led to one of the most exhilarating occasions in Goldbloom's life, for their host, normally not a funny man but a serious economist and historian, was inspired that evening; telling many good stories and improvising a series of criticisms of famous books and plays as they might have been reviewed had they appeared in the 1920s, such as the first performance of *Hamlet*: *It is hard to see what possible relevance this play can have for a present-day audience*, Leacock's review might have begun. *Why Mr. Shakespeare seems to think that the sanguinary ditherings of a Danish aristocrat can have the least appeal to an audience attuned to the pertinent profundities of* Up in Mabel's Room *we simply cannot....*

Otherwise, most of Dr. Goldbloom's exhilarating moments, and the ones that made his life complete, came through teaching. "As part of the dramatizing of my undergraduate teaching, I gave each beginning group a demonstration on the unlearned behaviour of the newborn infant. I would demonstrate the postural patters, the behaviour, the various reflexes and responses with which the brand-new baby is endowed as forerunners to his behaviour as a human being. Students are always fascinated by such a demonstration, the newborn infant grasping my fingers so tightly that he may be lifted into the air without any danger of his letting go; the almost perfect walking movements, when held up by his thorax, his feet touching a hard table, the turning of his head in the direction of a stroke on the cheek, followed by a wide opening of the mouth. In this last, I could not resist a bit of showmanship and a bit of misdirection. I would stroke the infant's cheek and at the same time say, 'Now open your mouth wide.' The infant would open his mouth and the students would applaud as in a theatre. To them, there was no connection between the stroking of the cheek (which they never noticed) and the result. The only heard the command, and, amazed, saw the immediate response, and the impression was a lasting one."

As for the academic realization of his ambitions, Goldbloom achieved this when he was finally put in charge of the Children's Memorial Hospital toward the end of the Second World War, and was made professor of pediatrics at McGill University — the first Jew to hold a chair in any Canadian university.

31

Jews Were Not Gentlemen

ABRAHAM WILLINSKY overate, which did nothing for his already somewhat ungainly figure. By middle age the celebrated genitourinary specialist tended, as he admitted himself, to waddle like a duck. Otherwise he was a lovely man, kind, tolerant, sympathetic, unaffected by the frictions of pride that fray the simple strands of friendship. One of his first patients was a jolly fellow in the fur trade, who called on the doctor one day to treat a severe attack of asthma. After relieving the man's distress with an injection, Willinsky sat down for a chat, to see if he could determine the cause of the asthma. There was little he could do if it was the result of a childhood anxiety. After a while he began to suspect a physical cause, the furs that the man periodically delivered to the wholesalers. He suggested that the man should avoid contact with the furs for a while, and see what happened. The patient was delighted by such a simple therapy. By then he was feeling well enough to go to work, so Willinsky gave him a lift uptown to his warehouse. The fur trader called the doctor again a week later, but when Willinsky arrived, he found that the man, having kept away from the furs, was in perfect health and spirits. It turned out that he merely wanted another lift uptown. He had been about to call a cab when it occurred to him that the doctor's fee for a house call was less than the cost of a cab.

Willinsky understood the true priorities of pride. He was proud of his profession, his race, and his family, but not of a stiff neck or a spurious dignity. He merely laughed, and obligingly dropped the patient off at the warehouse; though he raised his fee subsequently, to ensure that he was not re-employed as a chauffeur.

Otherwise, if there had been any real doubt about the patient's ability
to pay, Willinsky would have made no effort to collect. At one point in his
career there was such a discrepancy between his declared income and his
heavy case-load that the internal revenue department sent an inspector
to audit his books. The inspector found an astonishing number of accounts
open, going back for years, or even ones that had simply been written off.
He advised Willinsky to send out a collector if he wanted to avoid trouble.

One of the debts was paid, after a fashion, thirty-five years after it was
incurred. One day, during his bicycle-riding period, he was called to
Grange Avenue to deliver the baby of a poor pedlar's wife. His usual
charge was ten dollars, but when he saw the discomfort with which the
woman counted out the first five dollars, as if giving birth to quintuplets,
"'You don't need to pay me,' I said. 'Anyway, it is a very small baby. It's
premature, and I can't be sure it will live. Keep that five dollars for
yourself, for food, what the baby needs.'" Thirty-five years later, in the
1950s, Willinsky was in Los Angeles to read a paper at a meeting of the
International College of Surgeons. During one of the meetings he was
called to the telephone. The call was from a woman who had seen his
name in the papers. She identified herself as the child that had been born
that night.

"You want to pay the five dollars now?" Willinsky asked.

"She laughed. 'I want you to meet my husband. I want to entertain
you. And Mother would like to see you when you are back in Toronto.
She has heard that you have become a well-known doctor. Can I pick
you up at your hotel there?'

"'Yes, I am free at five o'clock.'

"It was a big Cadillac that came, and they made a fuss over me. But
that wasn't the worst of it. She gave the whole story to the papers, the old
Grange address, her name, my name—all of it, telephoned in to *The Los
Angeles Times*. It came out all garbled and of course it caught the press
dispatches. Even in England they had the story, or some version of it, for
it went through all sorts of changes in its course: 'DOCTOR COLLECTS OLD
DEBT...', CANADIAN PROFESSOR...', her picture, my picture, 'CAST YOUR BREAD
UPON THE WATERS...'—all the variations. By the time I came home every-
body had seen it. How they kidded me back in the hospital."

Even when his patient was a multi-millionaire, Willinsky showed the
same material non-attachment. In late middle age, now one of the
country's foremost specialists, he allowed the Baron de Rothschild to
cheat him out of three-fifths of his fee. The baron's reasoning went as
follows: "If I paid you $5,000," he told Willinsky, referring to the
prearranged fee for a bladder operation, "the Canadian Government
could get $3,000 of it. Maybe even more. Why should I make payment to
the Canadian Government? I am a citizen of France, only in town for a
short time. So I've decided to make the fee the net amount and simply

give you the $2,000 outright," declared the great banker, ignoring the fact that the government would also get a chunk of the $2,000. Then, to prove to Dr. Willinsky how well he was being treated, Rothschild added, "I *could* leave without paying you a cent. You forgot to put anything in writing."

Willinsky merely shrugged, and made out a receipt for two thousand dollars.

Abraham I. Willinsky, or A. I. as he was called by his friends, was not entirely without faults. He was not above telling lies. One evening his wife Sadie ushered a peculiar trio into his consulting room; a small, sturdy immigrant woman, her attractive daughter, and a weedy-looking young man. Abraham soon discovered that he was being approached as an arbiter rather than as a practitioner. The girl, a bright and lively sort, worked in the office of a large firm, and her fiancé, the weedy young man, had heard rumours that she was fooling around with her boss. He had told the girl's mother that before he would marry the daughter she must be examined, to establish her virginity. The mother, though infuriated by his suggestion, had agreed nonetheless. Hence their presence in Willinsky's office.

"When I went into the surgery at the girl's signal," Willinsky related, "I was surprised to see her still fully dressed, perched on the corner of a table.

"'You don't need to examine me, doc,' she said in a friendly matter-of-fact voice. 'I'm no virgin. You saw that puny morsel of a man out there. I couldn't marry him if he was the last fellow on earth. Do me a favour. Just tell my mother I'm all right.'

"'That wouldn't be straight.'

"'Let's be practical,' she said. 'Any fee you're paid comes from us, not him.'

Willinsky pointed out that she could get rid of him simply by telling the truth.

"'Look,' she said. 'I promise you nobody is going to force me to marry him anyway. Especially after this. But why give him a victory first?' She drew a full breath: 'If I tell the truth, my mother will die of shame. Can't you see that?'"

Willinsky did see that, and to avoid such a disaster informed the mother that her daughter was, as far as he could tell, still a virgin. The boy jumped up to congratulate the girl; whereupon she announced coldly that she never wanted to see him again. Smug in his certainty that she could not possibly mean this, he started toward her with approving arms akimbo. Her arms were somewhat less welcoming. She swung at him with her fist. He went flailing back and hit his head on the desk. So the doctor had a little medical work to do after all.

One of the most marked characteristics of so many of the meritorious men and women in this medical gallery is their intense awareness of others, the result of an apperception in human relationships that in our time has been dissipated by the desensitizing effect of mass communication. Abraham Willinsky shared that sensibility, not least because he was yet another doctor to come under the spell of William Osler. It was Osler who turned Willinsky to medicine in the first place. Willinsky heard a lecture by the great physician in Toronto in 1903, the occasion being the opening of a new medical building. The theme was one of Oslers' favourites: Work, the Master Word. Listening from the back row among the arts students, Willinsky felt elated. It was as if Osler were addressing him personally.

Not that the boy needed the Oslerian exhortation to fulfil his life through love and industry. He had always worked hard in school, immeasurably helped by that great gift, a photographic memory, and by a protection from other distractions—an undesired protection—imposed by his character, his race, and his dress. He was quiet and manageable, Jewish, and dressed by his mother in clothes that made him look like Little Lord Fauntleroy, a combination that made him an outcast among the rowdy lads of Queen Street where his family owned a dry goods store. His family was from Russian Poland, where it was bad enough being a Pole, but even worse being a Jew. Not least among the ordeals his antecedents were subjected to in Poland were the Russian press-gangs that raided Jewish homes in the middle of the night to carry off likely recruits for labour projects in Siberia. His mother's uncle had been kidnapped in this fashion when he was thirteen years old, and was never heard from again. Which was a good enough reason in itself for the family move to the New World. There Abraham's opportunities, and his marvellous exploitation of them, filled his parents with wonder, and also with apprehension. Oppression was in their souls and it seemed to them that it was dangerous for a Jew to become too prominent. "You have to learn not to make yourself conspicuous," his mother told the boy.

Abraham's marked difference from the other boys, from the Queen Street cliques and the Jarvis Collegiate conventionalists, deepened his sensitivity to others by orienting him more intensely toward his own family, to a keener perception of their quirks and passions, hopes and fears; so that when he heard Osler say, that day in the new medical building, that "More than any other the practitioner of medicine may illustrate...that we are here not to get all we can out of life for ourselves, but to try to make the lives of others happier," he was already halfway there, to attaining the Oslerian generosity of spirit. It flowered in Willinsky, despite the prejudice he had to face. He was the third Jewish doctor to graduate in Toronto, and anti-Jewish sentiment was as strong in that city as it was in the rest of the Western world. When he tried to sign on in

1914 as a medical corps man he was told that it would create problems to have a Jew in the officers' mess. Officers were supposed to be gentlemen. Though he yearned for it, he could not get hospital experience at the Toronto General. Eddie Robertson (a doctor who was trapped for days in the Moose River gold mine cave-in in Nova Scotia many years later, in the mid-thirties), put it quite plainly. "To be honest with you," he told Dr. Willinsky, "they say you would be a good man for the staff here. You may as well know that I'd hate to see any Jew get on in this hospital. Once you opened the door, they'd be running the place in no time." At least Robertson was forthright about it. Abraham appreciated the medium if not the message. What was harder to stand was the silent acceptance of such attitudes by the rest of the profession. According to Willinsky, it was ten years after this conversation before one Jewish intern a year was accepted in the teaching hospitals in Toronto, and thirty years before a Jewish doctor was given a clinical appointment on the indoor staff of a hospital affiliated with the university; though he conceded that many leaders in the profession fought for the principle that a doctor should be judged by professional standards alone.

Willinsky's generosity of spirit ("Above all, in the hard years, Osler helped to keep me steady"), did not allow him to become embittered. Sometimes when the anti-Semitism was flagrant he fought back, as during a court case when he was racially slandered by a chief inspector. Willinsky lit into the policeman, greatly relieving the boredom of the newspapermen present. The outburst was duly reported in the papers next day. Otherwise, Willinsky detoured around the domestic roadblock by completing his education at various European and American medical centres, and when he returned to Canada, concentrated his energies in private practice, rather than in bruising onslaughts against the ramparts of bigotry.

Even his first practical experience as a doctor had a somewhat prejudicial preface. Upon answering an ad for a medical assistant at Carp, Ontario, he received a reply form the doctor, Charles Franklin Magee, to the effect that the name Abraham Isaac Willinsky might cause wholesale riots in the district, or at least retail resistance. So, Dr. Magee wrote back, "I have a proposition. There is a Grand Trunk line that gets you to Carp at 12:25 p.m. Get off that train next Thursday, and go into the station waiting-room. Stay there. If you'll do, a messenger will tell you. There is a train back to Toronto at 3:52 p.m. If no messenger has come along for you by that time, take the train home again."

Intrigued, A. I. turned up at Carp as instructed, and walked into the station waiting room. He set his overnight bag on a varnished bench, then drifted around, studying the cuspidors, listening to a dog barking in the distance, and peering with bright, humorous eyes through the empty wicket. After a while he settled down with a book, glancing occasionally at the station clock. "An hour passed. Nobody appeared. Once I heard wheels on the road, the jingle of a horse being tethered, and crunching footsteps.... But it was only the ticket agent arriving. He disappeared into his cubicle. Occasionally he scraped a chair back, rustled papers. Once a stranger passed through the room on his way out to the pump for a drink. I went outside too and paced the platform, but the sun was too dazzling. I returned to my book. The stranger apparently went his way—I never saw him again. The clock stared off over my head and a fly buzzed up and down a sealed window above me."

Finally Willinsky gave up and went to the wicket.

"'May I have a single to Toronto?'

"'No, not today.'

"'But I understood that there was a train at 3:50 or so,' I protested.

"He shrugged, turned away and came out of the cubicle. Ignoring me, he opened a side door and bellowed: 'Mike! Hey, Mike!' He tossed his uniform cap down on a nearby bench, waved toward my suitcases, and said, 'Come on, we can go now. I'm Magee.'"

Whereupon the real station-master again appeared and, wordlessly morose, replaced Dr. Magee in the cage.

"'I couldn't be dead sure until you spoke,' Magee explained as he led the way to his buggy. 'Your looks were all right. But I had to make sure you had no accent.'"

Upon his return from postgraduate study in Vienna, Willinsky set up in a practice of his own, traveling to his patients in an absurd contraption that inspired a good deal of merriment on the street, a tiny horse and an outsized buggy. A. I. didn't mind. "A doctor might as well shed cheerfulness when he makes his rounds." Later he exchanged the horse and buggy for an Everitt-Metzger-Flanders auto.

By the end of the First World War, Willinsky found that he had become a specialist—still a rarity in Canada—almost by accident. Since graduating from the University of Toronto in 1908, he had taken special courses in venereal diseases. His knowledge of the subject led him to one of the city's first VD clinics, at the Toronto Western Hospital. It was the increasingly close association with this hospital that focused his interest on genito-urinary disease in general. In 1918, he was listed as head of the department of urology. This did not bring him any closer to the longed-for university teaching, but at least it gave him a reputation in the city, and a prestige that was not lightly dismissed, for the Western, after a bad start as the "Bathurst Street Butcher Shop," was on its way to becoming, according to a distinguished British medical visitor, a hospital unrivaled for its efficiency in either Europe or America.

"Initially it was primarily my course in venereal diseases with Stokes that brought me into close contact with the hospital," Willinsky wrote. "Exact methods of diagnosis and promising treatment had just been worked out: the Wassermann reaction was introduced in 1907 and salvarsan, or 606 because of the number of preliminary experiments, was discovered in 1912. Neo-salvarsan, or 914, came much later. Our treatment of gonorrhea in the twenties was irrigation with potassium permanganate, a mild antiseptic. Diagnosis was stressed in the Stokes course, a great benefit when I began work in the Western's VD clinic." The clinic was set up quite apart from the outpatients' clinics, as if its problems were too sordid to permit intimate contact with more moral afflictions, and this separate status led to some awkward situations. "One man who had been tested and found syphilitic had gone on to the regular Out-Patients' Clinic, and there the sore of his leg had been diagnosed as a traumatic ulcer. By the time I looked into his failure to turn up for treatment, he was already booked for an amputation. There was no choice for me but to hunt up the surgeon: 'I'm Buttinsky Willinsky, I know. But that leg will respond to treatment, I believe,'" he told the surgeon, and showed him the clinical notes. Since the hospital pathologist would have identified the syphilis and exposed an exceedingly faulty diagnosis when it was too late—after the leg was amputated—the surgeon must have experienced a mixture of chagrin and gratitude.

Another error in diagnosis involved a woman who was overwhelmed with shame when the outpatients' clinic insisted over her scarlet-faced protestations, that she had venereal disease. Fortunately Willinsky was one of the two men in the city who owned a cystoscope—an optical instrument for examining the inside of the urinary bladder—and when she was passed on to him, the instrument showed that the woman's discharge was being caused by a stone in the bladder that had formed around a hairpin. It was cases such as this, and Willinsky's generosity in contributing the latest sophisticated equipment to the clinic, that got him his staff appointment.

Among his instruments were those that had been developed for regional anesthesia. Willinsky was a Canadian pioneer in this field, as well as, and often in combination with, his urological work. It was quite an occasion in the hospital when he performed an appendectomy without general anesthesia. The regional anesthesia technique was quite novel in Canada, so a large crowd came to witness the demonstration.

Not that all of his patients appreciated the efficiency with which he could operate in fairly informal circumstances and without the discomforts of general anesthesia. "One man, a big Polish fellow, came back three weeks after his operation, highly indignant. 'I pay you $35 to take my tonsils out' (it sounded like *consuls* as he pronounced it). 'I come here for operation, remember? You prick me and leave me alone. Then you come back, prick my throat and show me two bits of meat, "These are your consuls"—remember?' I nodded. 'Well,' with a scornful rush, 'now my friends have the *real* consul operation. He must go to hospital. There they put over his nose'—he cupped his hand to show me—'and he have sleep, a long time. Then coughing, sick much blood. Again they make him have the long sleep. He stay sick for many days. That is how they make the real consul operation—and I pay you for this operation, but have none of it. Give me back my money.'"

Willinsky promised to return the fee and also to pay for such a bloody operation if the Polish chap could find a doctor to operate; which helped to convince the man that the two bits of meat really had been his 'consuls.'

Regional, or conduction, anesthesia stressed that pain is conducted by the nerves. August Bier of Germany had been able to anesthetize the lower half of the body by spinal injection as early as 1899, using a weak solution of cocaine, and there had been a flurry of improvements in the first two decades of the twentieth century which were particularly effective in reducing surgical shock. The nerve-blocking technique, that Willinsky had learned initially from George Pitkin of New Jersey, was of enormous help to him in his rapidly expanding surgical work. One of his most notable achievements occurred in the early Depression years, when as a noted diagnostician, he was called upon to examine the young wife of a university staff member. She was having fits, but a series of tests at the Toronto General had found nothing organically wrong. The hospital people concluded that she was mentally ill, but her husband was convinced the cause was physical and refused to send her to an institution.

When Willinsky saw the patient she was drawn with pain. There would be very little warning of the attacks. She would suddenly clutch her side and fall writhing to the floor.

"The location of the pain indicated that a kidney was affected," Willinsky wrote. "Under partial nerve-block I inserted a catheter—and touched off an attack exactly as she had described it. The suffering seemed intense. "It suggests the acute pain of *tic douloureux*,' I told her husband. 'This is usually a disease of the trigeminal nerve in the face, but I remember a case described by a French doctor, E. Papin, where a nerve on the kidney was so affected.' What I suggested was a denervation of the ureter, i.e., removing the sympathetic nerve supply to cut its connection with the nervous system. Once again I gave spinal anesthetic so that, with the patient's co-operation, the sensitive spot could be located. I made an incision over the kidney and stripped back the nerves until I touched the one that started up that pain. This nerve was then severed."

During the woman's convalescence there were no further attacks, even when she was again probed by the catheter.

Straightfaced, Willinsky told the lady that he could not guarantee that the pain would not return. He said that she had better come and see him again—in twenty-five years.

"I reported the case," he added, "at a local medical meeting, for this operation was a relatively unknown procedure in Toronto although not in France; but the group was not convinced that there had been an organic lesion. 'She felt better because the operation had a temporary effect,' they said. 'The attacks will recur when it wears off.'"

The lady did in fact report to A. I. twenty-five years later, to confirm that she had had no further trouble.

32

The Missionary Position

IN THE DAYS when Protestant and Roman Catholic clergymen were still sure of the superiority of their moral values, they assumed the duty of putting less-well-organized societies, from Mampoko to Manchuria, on an evangelical paying basis. Acting on the assumption that the way to a heathen's heart was through his stomach ache, the missionaries recruited medical people in the cause. They had no great difficulty in doing so. Even though doctors tended to be skeptics in matters of religion, they were also noted for what Dr. Hans Selye calls altruistic egoism; that is, doing good to others without sacrificing one's own interests.

This is not to say that all missionary doctors lacked true religious conviction. A few of them were genuine believers, and heard "the call" quite as clearly as their clerical friends. Dr. William E. Smith was one. He was the ninth child of a family living on a rented farm in Durham County, Ontario. William loved his widowed mother, as much for her cheerful and uncomplaining nature as for her sayings, such as "Early to bed, early to rise, makes a man healthy, wealthy, and wise," and "Speech is silver, but silence is golden," and for her delicious gravy. In his early years, he was unusually pious. At the age of twelve he took three days off work in the fields to attend a religious convention in Kendall, four miles from home. "I had a glorious time studying the Bible and those spiritually-minded leaders of our Church. It exhilarated me to testify that I was conscious of Jesus Christ in my life, giving me strength to do the work on the farm." Otherwise he was a normal, healthy boy, enjoying sports, books, and fist fights. One of his favourite adventures was to ride the wagon wheel. He would cling to the rim and spokes, with his head thrust through the wheel for better purchase. The faster the wheel revolved the more exciting it became. Until one day, a wagon driver, fearful that the boy would be thrown off, pushed his head further through the wheel, in which position it was struck by the iron end of the wagon bolster. William bore the resulting scar for the rest of his life.

The only other scar of childhood was religious doubt. He read books on agnosticism, and his piety was sorely affected. He convinced himself that there was no God and that religion was superstition, and he came to hate old Mr. Patterson, the revivalist, who kept asking his congregations to pray for William, to save a young infidel who had once loved Jesus.

William's doubts gnawed at him for three years, until "I realized that my study of agnosticism was unsatisfactory, and I became anxious to find God. I had recently been listening to the Salvation Army in Kendall, and learned that drunkards' lives had been completely changed, which seemed positive evidence that God reigned in their lives. I called upon God to save me from my sins, through Jesus Christ, and to restore unto me the years in my spiritual life which the locusts had destroyed." On his knees that night in his bedroom he pleaded to God to be forgiven. His prayers were answered. "His spirit flooded my soul. Once again I received the witness of being born again, with my name written in the Book of Life, an experience that has remained and been renewed many times on my journey through life. I kept humming the words of the hymn — 'What a friend we have in Jesus,' and, 'Oh the good we all may do, while the days are going by.'"

By then the family owned a store; although William enjoyed serving people in it, "yet I had a deep longing for more education, but not for the purpose of learning how to make a living, but for already I was successful along that line. The real urge was spiritual; to be of greater service to Him, and help to bring in the Brotherhood of Man. Through the reading of mission books on Africa I wanted to witness for Jesus Christ in that field, and tell the people of His love and power to change lives and hopes."

After talking it over with his mother and older brother, Jim, William went to college in Toronto to take the arts course in preparation for the Methodist ministry. After some preaching experience on the Methodist circuit, he was persuaded by the general secretary of the foreign mission, Dr. Sutherland, to take the medical course as well as the theological, and become an ordained medical missionary.

He married shortly after graduation in 1895, still intent on missionary work in Aftica, until he heard of riots in West China; whereupon he informed Dr. Sutherland that, "The Chinese people evidently need the Gospel message just as much as the Africans, so you may send us to China." Sutherland obliged, and Dr. Smith worked there in a missionary hospital for forty years under three unruly Chinese regimes. "It was His Spirit that sent us to West China," he wrote, "to bear witness to the love of Christ to a people who wanted neither us nor our Christianity." Adding that by the time he retured in 1939 "the Chinese attitude had entirely changed and that they now wanted missionaries to be brothers with them in the fight for righteousness."

Florence Murray, M.D., also came from an earnest Christian household, in her case in Pictou Landing, Nova Scotia. "I wanted," said the blonde with the plump, gentle face, "to use my life where it could count most. I wanted to serve others and share my knowledge of God as our loving heavenly Father with people living in fear of evil spirits." The evil spirits resided in Manchuria and Korea, where she spent most of the next half century, following her graduation in 1918 from Dalhousie University Medical College in Halifax.

At first Florence wished to emulate her father and become a Presbyterian minister. Later, she decided to become a doctor. Her years of medical college were uneventful, until December 6, 1917; the day of a great explosion when a French munitions ship collided with a Belgian vessel in Halifax harbour and blew up, devastating half the city. One thousand five hundred people were killed. All senior medical students were called in to tend to the uncountable thousands of wounded. When Florence reported for duty at a military hospital she was told to give the anesthetics. As it happened, through no fault of her own, she had missed that part of her training, but she felt that this was no time for excuses. Her first patient was six years old. Florence was terrified, not knowing how large or small a dose of ether to give. "I knew I should watch the eye reflexes to help judge the depth of anesthesia, but this unfortunate child had lost both eyes." She did so well that next day she was appointed official anesthesiologist to the hospital.

A few weeks later another emergency arose when the Spanish influenza, that was to kill twenty to thirty million people during and after the First World War, struck the Maritimes in full force. She was sent to minister to the survivors of a small fishing port, where she organized an emergency hospital, and learned to handle such citizens as one who swore that if he contracted the disease he would have no petticoat doctor fiddling with him. However, he soon changed his mind when he caught the flu.

After interning experience in an American hospital Florence was offered a position as assistant to one of the most prominent surgeons in Nova Scotia. She was also made demonstrator of anatomy in the medical college. It seems likely that in time she would have become a prominent member of the medical profession in Nova Scotia, had she not long since taken a vow that she would volunteer for missionary work in teaching, preaching, and healing. As soon as she paid back most of the money she had borrowed from the family to see her through college, she reported to the Mission Board of the Canadian Presbyterian Church that she was now ready to go overseas.

Her first posting was to Yongjung in Manchuria, to a Presbyterian mission hospital which had been designed and built by a Newfoundland doctor, Stanley Martin. Florence learned of the work-load she would have to face when she was told that Dr. Martin had been seeing 22,000 patients a year.

Manchuria was then mostly populated by Koreans. When Japan annexed Korea in 1910, many Koreans had been forced off their land and had moved to Manchuria and Siberia where the land was as plentiful as the snow. The descendents of these Siberian Koreans ultimately became the North Korean communist leaders of today. Japan had also taken over Manchuria as part of their planned conquest of China. As the Japanese tended to isolate themselves in compounds, the missionaries had little contact with them.

There was plenty of contact with the Korean-speaking population, and though Florence was, at the age of twenty-eight, a sensible and well-balanced person, she was shaken at the primitive life of the inhabitants, particularly that of the women. Many of the women did not even have names. Girl children were valued so little that they might simply be addressed as "Hi, you," or as "Back Room," if they happened to have been born in a back room. Boys were not much better off. They were likely to be given such names as "Dog Dung" — in order to fool the evil spirits that the boy was not really worth malevolent attention.

Domestically the Korean women were not allowed to eat with the men. As for the Chinese women among the population, they were crippled physically as well as socially. Florence was appalled when she first saw their traditionally bound feet — the toes bent under the sole and the heels forced forward by bandaging, until the feet of the grown women might be only four inches long. Florence was uncertain as to whether the practice was aesthetic — that the Chinese really believed such deformities to be beautiful — or whether it was done originally in order to make it difficult for wives to flee from cruel husbands. In any event the practice, though beginning to die out in China, was still carried out in Manchuria, causing great pain when the process was first begun on a little girl.

The appearance and culture of the Western woman doctor was just as intriguing to the Koreans. As Florence learned the language and was able to communicate directly with the people, they would usually ask her how old she was. Her blonde hair was so unfamiliar a sight that they thought it was dark hair that had faded with advancing years. They were surprised to learn that she was twenty-eight, and absolutely amazed that at that age she had neither husband nor sons. (One of her male patients was a married man of twelve years old.) They felt really sorry for Florence, that nobody had been able to arrange a marriage of convenience for her. They also thought she smelled like a cow. "Don't you drink milk and eat butter and cheese?' they pointed out, 'Why wouldn't you smell like cows?'"

Medically the scene was as disturbing as some of the customs. The diseases that were by then under control in the West were rampant in Manchuria and Korea: typhoid, typhus, diphtheria, leprosy, malaria, sprue, and various parasitic conditions, and especially tuberculosis. In Yongjung, Dr. Murray saw her first case of sleeping sickness. There was also no appreciation for the dangers of infection.

Popular treatment, such as *chim* and *doom* further complicated her task as a surgeon. *Chim* was a crude acupuncture method, where "needles might be wiped off on a dirty sleeve and inserted cold, or else heated and used red hot in which case they were at least sterile.... Another treatment favoured by patient and practitioner alike was known as the *doom*, an ironically appropriate name. In *doom* treatment, the healer placed little piles of powdered leaves of certain plants on the skin over the affected area and then ignited them. He usually did this many times on the same spot and might treat several such spots at once. The burned tissue sloughed away leaving a deep ulcer through the whole thickness of the skin or even deeper. I asked one woman," Florence said, "whose loss of tissue from the *doom* treatment had penetrated the muscular layer, how many times she had had the *doom* in that spot. One hundred times, she told me. I believed her." The treatments often caused serious complications for the surgeon, owing to the creation of adhesions and the added danger of post-operative infection.

Even hospitality could be a problem for a Western doctor. Florence once made a house call on a Chinese who was ill with tuberculosis. She happened to know that the patient's brother was also ill in the same house. He had syphilis, in an infective stage. "At the house, instead of going at once to see the sick man, we [she and an interpreter, Kim] were invited to sit down in an outer room where the hospitable master of the house lighted the family pipe and handed it to me. I didn't know what Chinese etiquette decreed in such cases and feared it might be taken as a slight if I refused. Even had I been a smoker, the family pipe in that house would have had no attraction for me. I declined as politely as I could. The man then lighted a cigarette, took a puff to get it going well, and passed it to me. Again, at the risk of giving offense, I had to decline.

"He then emptied the used teacups onto the floor, poured fresh hot tea, and gave cups to us. Kim accepted his. Fearing to decline a third time, in spite of unhappy thoughts about the infectious diseases in the household, I forced myself to swallow a few drops. The hardships that friends of overseas missionaries sometimes deplore are often more subtle than they imagine."

Faced with unsanitary conditions and with many patients whom it was too late to help, Florence tried repeatedly to explain about infection and the necessity of bringing the sick to the hospital while they were still strong enough to recover from surgery; but the older men, living in a world of evil spirits which were obviously responsible for every ailment from clubfoot to clap, failed to understand—mainly because they wouldn't listen. Gradually though, she began to get through to the younger people and those with a little education. One of them was a man who had been blind for eighteen months from cataracts. He believed that he had been victimized by evil spirits. After Florence had operated on him to remove the cataracts and restore his sight, he was finally convinced that what the Christian missionaries said was true, that the Great Spirit, God, was more powerful than any of his evil spirits.

Part of the process through which the religious missionaries got through to the inhabitants was to accompany the doctors or nurses on their house calls. The medical people were thus a kind of advance guard, establishing lines of communication for the hospital evangelists. The evangelists then made follow-up calls of their own, bringing supplies and sympathy, "as well as preaching the Gospel of the love and mercy of God. The church people often helped out in cases where home care was needed for the children during the illness of the mother, or provided food or clothing. Many people," Florence Murray wrote, "experiencing this kindly concern and help from strangers became interested in their motives for doing it, and often they, too, decided to become Christians."

Abraham Willinsky was the sort of person who was interested in everybody he met, whether they were dull or bright, pitted or polished, and the young man, Bob McClure, who turned up at his clinic one day in 1922 was worthy of special interest. Not just because he was an M.D. at the age of twenty-one, or because he was destined for missionary work in China where he was to take the place of a Presbyterian mission doctor who had been killed by bandits, but because of his unusual background. The boy had spent his early years amidst the chaos that was twentieth-century China, where serenity and barbarism could be manifested in a single incident, such as the one that the young McClure had witnessed in Weihwei: the serene decapitation of several malefactors in bustling, sunlit Horse Market Street.

McClure was still so oriented to the Far East that though he and his family had been living in Toronto now for several years, he still considered China rather than Canada to be his natural environment.

Robert McClure was visually notable, too; a big, red-haired fellow, emanating the restless energy of the kind that has fueled so many men of distinction. He had the power, too, of transmitting the energy. His muscular frame could be accounted for, Willinsky thought, by the fact that he had worked on the Toronto docks as a part-time stevedore, to put himself through medical school.

There was still another reason for taking particular note of Bob McClure. His father, Dr. William McClure, had been a student at McGill under William Osler. Anyone who had the slightest connection with the Great Physician was likely to earn Willinsky's special interest. So when McClure explained that to prepare himself for missionary work he would need some experience in genito-urinary work, Willinsky was quick to respond. He invited McClure to join him at the clinic every Friday evening, and assured him that he would teach him all he knew in the time available.

Like Willinsky, McClure had not been able to obtain an internship following his graduation that year. He had been about to join the British Colonial Service when the Presbyterian Church had offered him the post of medical missionary in Honan province, China. It was through this same connection that he had been taken on as an assistant by one of the best surgeons in the city, Kenneth Perfect. It was on Dr. Perfect's recommendation that he had gone to see Abe Willinsky. So now McClure would have specialized instruction in urology, as well as in Perfect's unofficial specialty, thyroid and goitre operations. Not to mention the training he would also receive in X-ray techniques at the Western Hospital, and in pharmacy. As McClure's biographer, Munroe Scott, put it, "McClure was relentlessly going after whatever training and experience he could find that would be of use in Honan."

Altogether, McClure would devote forty-seven years of his life to the people of China: years of civil strife, three revolutions, the Sino-Japanese War, the Second World War, and the Communist takeover. The country was approaching the Second Revolution when the brand-new M.D. arrived in Honan province in North China, in 1924. The political situation was as usual, a mess. "The infant republic had been struggling on," Scott writes, "but it was a political Siamese twin. One head was at Peking, under which was warlord rule. The other head was down south in Canton where Sun Yat-sen and the Kuomintang were still trying to establish a democracy based upon Greek and Roman ideals most of which were foreign to the cultural traditions of China, and as had become more and more apparent, equally foreign to the Western Powers."

The Western powers were in favour of idealism only if it was their own. They had been victimizing the helpless Chinese giant for over a century, enforcing their commercial contracts with quick-firing guns. The resentment caused by the foreign oppression had not exactly eased the way of the numerous Christian missions that dotted the landscape, as McClure would learn. However, not all of the oppressors were outsiders. In the absence of strong central administration, much of the country was governed by warlords: self-appointed generals with private armies, who levied taxes on the vulnerable towns and villages without fear, favour or risk of retaliation. Which is why, as McClure marched into medical battle as a Christian soldier, it seemed appropriate to him that he should carry a Webley automatic pistol.

The mission station in the city of Hwaiking comprised living quarters for the nurses and doctors, and the Menzies Memorial Hospital. There were two other doctors besides McClure, a Chinese, Dr. Chang, and a Canadian, Dr. Reeds, who was a positive Genghis Khan in the operating room—he spread sawdust on the floor to soak up the gore—but the softest of touches the moment he laid down the scalpel.

Despite McClure's quick temper and a forthright manner that placed medical priorities well ahead of Presbyterian ones, he got on well with his confreres, and they were soon dividing up the work to their common satisfaction. McClure handled most of the abdominal and genito-urinary cases, Dr. Reeds most of the eye work, while Dr. Chang concentrated on the tuberculosis cases.

McClure was soon getting on quite well with the local bandits as well. These were turban-mantled Moslems who were in the habit of darting out of their bamboo groves to rob and kill the unwary traveler. It was such malefactors who had killed McClure's predecessor, Dr. Menzies. As McClure was quite a frequent traveler along the bambooed route to a coal mine near Chinghua, there to attend to injured miners, he found the prospect of imminent ambush somewhat unsettling. As he wasn't in a position to beat the bandits, he decided to, in effect, join them, by making himself so useful that they would grant him immunity.

He found an excuse when he learned that children of the bandits were particulary susceptible to a disease called *kala-azar* which caused the spleen to become hard and swollen. If not treated the victim died. McClure found out where the bandit village was located, and one morning, attired in his khaki shirt and lumberjack boots, he mounted his bicycle and went bandit-hunting. Deep among the high bamboo groves he found a village whose inhabitants, he believed, combined highway robbery with their activities in the bamboo industry.

The appearance of the red-haired, blue-eyed "big nose" caused something of a stir in the village, but there was instant communication. McClure spoke fluent Chinese. He told the villagers that his Jesus people could not only cure their children of *kala-azar*, but also attend to the injuries to which bamboo cutters were susceptible, not excluding the injuries they were likely to suffer following their encounters with the law.

Gunshot wounds, for example. They must not fear that a Christian hospital would turn them away, or give them away. The mission hospital was there for all, regardless of race, creed, colour, or the origin of the bullets in their bodies. But of course, McClure hinted, if this offer, and his skill as a surgeon, were to be fully effective, naturally he must be able to cycle safely through the hundred-foot bamboo trees.

An accommodation was soon arrived at, and from then on Dr. Loa, as he was known to the Chinese, was able to go peacefully about his business everywhere, except in the one place where tranquillity should have reigned most supreme, the Menzies Memorial Hospital.

For there the presence of his wounded bandits created a considerable disturbance, especially when the ward also contained wounded police, their adversaries. The hostility between these forces was bad enough, but during visiting hours the situation was likely to get out of hand. Sometimes the relatives of the bandits and the police arrived simultaneously. As the visitors were unencumbered by splints or bandages, they were able to take much more effective action than the incapacitated inmates.

It was McClure who worked out the formula that would allow bandits and police to coexist while they were being treated. They were placed in separate wards, and to avoid the situation that had obtained in the past in which the law was likely to appear and drag a bandit out of his bed and execute him in the courtyard, McClure ruled that the police were not to be informed about the presence of a bandit until he had been discharged and given a twenty-four-hour head start.

It was a system that did not appeal to the evangelical missionaries. Nor did they approve of the doctor's habit of packing a pistol on his person, even though he insisted that it was merely to keep off rabid dogs. The missionaries were quite disturbed at the idea of a doctor carrying a gun and giving bandits asylum and a head start. They felt that they had a duty to law and order as well as a commitment to non-violence. But, "there was no law and order here in any conventional sense of the term. Even as a student Bob McClure had realized a nurse's duty was to protect the patient from the doctor so there seemed little problem in assuming that a doctor's duty was to protect the patients from each other and from any outside influence, such as broad swords, that would impede recovery."

McClure's sporting attitude toward the bandits brought a far worse problem than the disapproval of the United Church of Canada (which in 1925 inherited the Presbyterian missions in China). Firstly it brought him too many additional clients, in the form of wounded warlord soldiery, and secondly, he caught the eye of the soldiery's warlord, General Li. Li had already made one attempt to recruit a medical officer for his private army. He had sent three invitations to that effect to McClure's colleague,

Dr. Chang. It was a Chinese custom that, while the first two invitations might be politely declined with an excess of thanks, the third was an offer that could not be refused. Having received that final invitation, and having been unwilling to link his destiny with that of a warlord, however powerful, Chang had been forced to flee the Hwaiking mission with his family. Now it was the turn of the doctor who had proved himself a friend of the underdog (except that Li was such a successful general that his enemies were now the underdogs). Li's latest coup was the capture of the city of Hwaiking itself. Soon after his men had entered the city, a troop of his soldiers clattered up to the mission station. There the officer in charge formally invited Dr. Loa to attend an audience with the victorious general. By an amazing coincidence the officer just happened to have a spare mount available for the doctor's conveyance, already bridled and saddled. Would Dr. Loa condescend to accompany the humble officer as an honoured guest of his master? McClure knew better than to decline, even though the officer had asked him only once.

General Li turned out to be a most affable sort, skilled in the Confucian courtesies. After McClure's comfort had been attended to, the general complimented him "on the excellent service the mission hospital was providing in the area in general, and for wounded men in particular. Dr. Loa was affable in return but pointed out that attending to so many wounded soldiers was bankrupting the hospital and that it would proba-bly have to close its doors to combatants. The general felt that would be a regrettable course indeed and would incur the hostility of his men. Dr. Loa felt that if the General would be good enough to pay his back bills, and to attend promptly to current ones, that the hospital might see its way clear to continue to function. The General thought there might be a possibility of suitable financial arragements *if* Dr. Loa would join his army as Chief Medical Officer. Dr. Loa was most touched by the invitation but felt that joining a Chinese army and abandoning his career as a Christian medical missionary was not what he had in mind. General Li was most insistent and showed signs of wanting to extend the invitation at least three times right there and then. Dr. Robert McClure pointed out that he was a Canadian citizen and British subject, and that since Britain still enjoyed extra-territorial rights he still enjoyed His Most Brittanic Majesty's protection.... The General, however, was an accommodating man. He pointed out he was merely trying to solve an administrative problem. It would be much easier for his paymaster to divert funds to the hospital through a Chief Medical Officer. Also, there would be much face for a General of his standing to have a Westerner as Chief M.O. Dr. Loa could sympathize with the General's administrative problem and could understand the implications of face."

McClure finally compromised by agreeing to become an honorary chief medical officer with the rank of colonel; while on his part Li brought his account up to the day by making an immediate payment of five hundred silver dollars to the mission hospital with weekly payments to follow, to cover the cost of repairs to his wounded men. As Scott points out in his two-volume biography of McClure, the appointment of the United Church's twenty-four-year-old medical missionary to a colonelcy in the army of a Chinese warlord was not unduly emphasized in the report to the Church's mission board.

The match between the small, tough warlord and the big, tough Canadian doctor did not end there. By the autumn of 1925, Li was again falling behind in his payments. At the same time he was sending just as many wounded men to the Christian mission, so that the hospital was slowly being forced into bankruptcy. There was one bright patch on the horizon, though. The hospital could survive if it could hold out until the Chinese New Year in February. According to Chinese custom, if General Li was billed before the New Year, he would be honour-bound to pay the bill, or lose so much face that even a plastic surgeon could not save him. Unless, of course, the general could find some way to frustrate the submission of the bill until after the New Year, when the debt would have to be forgiven and forgotten.

It was to ensure such an accommodation that the wily general commissioned a master carver to prepare a *bien-tze*. A *bien-tze* was an elaborately carved plaque, about two by four feet in size, done in brilliant lacquer and gold lettering. It had an almost mystical significance for the Chinese. To be presented with such an honour was to place the recipient at about the same level of prestige as a Knight Commander of the Bath or the winner of a quarter-share in a Nobel Prize. Naturally, the only proper response to such an accumulation of face was for the recipient to forgive the donor any obligation he might otherwise have been forced to fulfill.

McClure did not hear about his magnificent gift until it was almost too late. He was visited one day by a Mr. Li Hung-ch'ang, a member of the Confucian gentry, and principal of a boarding school that the mission had established in Hwaiking.

After the long-drawn-out courtesies had been observed, Mr. Li coyly informed the doctor that there was a master carver at work on a *bien-tze*, and that the name of the recipient, who was being likened on the plaque to the great Hippocrates, was none other than Dr. McClure—a tremendous honour—and that the donor was General Li.

McClure quickly realized the significance of the gift. If it was presented just before the New Year, it would frustrate the hospital from pressing its claim on General Li's treasury. Neither McClure nor the hospital could afford to go against Chinese custom. On the other hand the hospital could not afford to cancel the debt, which now amounted to two thousand dollars.

Despite his agitation, McClure, steeped in Oriental protocol, could not help delighting in the situation, and in the challenge it presented. Accordingly he and Mr. Li put their heads together to find a way around the general's ploy. The main problem was that the master woodcarver, though sympathetic to the mission hospital, was not quite sympathetic enough to stop work on the *bien-tze* and risk being shot. All the same, if he were allowed to continue, the plaque would be finished in time for the presentation before the New Year.

Unless—it suddenly occurred to the mandarin and the medico—there was a way to ensure that it would not be finished in time.

They finally came up with the answer; and the next day the woodcarver turned up at the hospital complaining of a sore right arm. Dr. Loa was so concerned about the possible complications that he immediately immobilized the arm in a plaster cast. It was then put in a sling. So as the carver strolled ostentatiously through the streets of Hwaiking, it was obvious to everybody that he would not be able to work for some time.

Shortly before the end of the year, General Li paid his bill in full, in silver dollars, perhaps almost as pleased by the intrigue as McClure; for when he finally presented the *bien-tze* to the doctor with suitable ceremony outside the mission compound, he also gave McClure a wink.

A year later McClure, who in the meantime had married his sweet-heart, Amy Hislop, was forced to flee China as the nationalist armies under Chiang Kai-shek began to disinfect the country of foreign devils, Communists and warlords. The country was soon aflame with civil war and the only alternative for the various missionaries was flight or conversion of their churches into indigenous, native Chinese. Robert and Amy ended up in Taiwan, seconded to the Presbyterian mission there.

They were back in Hwaiking by late summer of 1931, with their two children. It was the second time that McClure, now superintendent and chief surgeon of the Menzies Hospital, had returned to China in the aftermath of a revolution. By then the Kuomintang under Chiang Kai-shek was more or less in control of the country, though the Communists were still giving Chiang a certain amount of trouble. In the meantime, there had been a few changes at the mission compound. It was not changed physically, but was the same drab, functional complex of two-storey buildings with the same bell tower at the compound entrance. Only now the missionaries were no longer giving the orders, but were guests of the Chinese, invited to participate merely as fraternal delegates. The mission schools were also being run entirely by Chinese, the evangelistic work was under a native pastor, and the hospital, soon to be reorganized as a "Co-operative Society," was also commanded by a Chinese. The United Church, however, was still to pay the expenses of the fraternal delegates.

Otherwise, McClure had to work as hard as ever, so he was relieved to find that his redoubtable head nurse, Janet Brydon, had also returned to Hwaiking. She had even managed to recruit several nurses. One of them was a nineteen-year-old sharpshooter named Loving Lotus. Though Loving Lotus had proved her worth to her landowner father by her horsemanship and her skill at fending off bandits with a rifle, she was only a girl, and had thus not received the benefit of an education. She was quite illiterate. Janet Brydon, though, had spotted her as a potentially useful scrub nurse.

McClure soon discovered that Brydon's instinct was as good as ever. Loving Lotus learned quickly. "Once she had been rehearsed on an operation she never forgot the procedure. The O.R. team practised intestinal repair and stomach re-sections on dogs. By the time a dog had been reassembled, sewn up, and was in recovery, Loving Lotus would have memorized all the detail. She would know what instruments were to be sterilized for that operation and the order in which they were to be used. The O.R. group developed into a smoothly functioning team and Loving Lotus became Dr. Loa's number one scrub nurse. She was with him for the vast majority of operations performed during the next six years and during that time the surgeon never asked for a clamp, a suture, scissors, a needle, or any other instrument. When he extended his hand the correct instrument was always slapped firmly into it. For a surgeon whose major outbursts of temper were always reserved for the slow, the slovenly, or the incompetent, it was an exhilarating experience."

In the operating room and in the wards, including the bandit ward— for the hospital was still treating bandits and giving them a twenty-four-hour head start on the police after they were discharged—Loving Lotus was the very model of an efficient nurse. Even her ferocity was efficient. One evening while she was riding her pony back to the mission after a weekend leave, she was waylaid by bandits and robbed of a ring and a wrist watch. The watch was particularly treasured—it was a present from the chief surgeon himself. She galloped back to the hospital in a very bad temper indeed, not least because she had been caught unarmed—she usually carried a .38 Walther automatic. McClure tried to calm her down, and even promised to replace the watch, but she was not to be placated. She was incensed that the bandits should have done such a thing, after all she had done for them in the operating room, helping to lay open their wounds and remove splinters of metal from home-made bullets, and pick out fragments of bark if they had been sheltering behind trees when they were shot, or flakes of paint if they had been shot through a door, or wads of cotton if they had been shot through their quilted jackets—and repairing femurs shattered by grenades, mines, or shells. Now here they were, rewarding her by stealing two of her most precious possessions. She considered their behaviour to be an example of the grossest ingratitude, and she wished to visit the bandit ward to tell them so.

Knowing his scrub nurse, McClure felt somewhat apprehensive about the confrontation, and insisted that she would have to take along a male orderly for protection—the patients' protection, that is.

When the orderly later reported to McClure what had happened, he still looked a bit stunned. Loving Lotus had marched into the ward and had proceeded to address the bandits and their visitors in terms that ensured their closest attention. She described the robbery, then informed bandits and visitors alike that unless her watch and her ring were returned to her by Thursday morning, she would use certain exceedingly sharp surgical instruments on the reproductive equipment of every bandit she encountered on the operating table from then on.

According to the orderly, she had elaborated so graphically on the surgical techniques to be employed that one of the bandits had been sick and had lost his entire breakfast.

The watch and the ring were returned with commendable promptitude.

Loving Lotus was by no means McClure's only successful medical trainee. As early as 1924 he had been trying to do something about the conflict between the qualified missionary doctors and their highly unqualified competitors, usually former hospital employees who, after some rudimentary experience in the mission hospitals, had hung up their shingles in the neighbourhood claiming to be bona fide practitioners. There was nothing really to stop them from doing so, for there was no uniform licencing system in China.

The situation made for bad blood between the hospital's staff and the former employee and led to unhealthy competition. Many mission doctors were naturally hostile to the medical upstarts, but McClure was not one of them. He was not concerned about the lack of diplomas among the quacks, only about their low standards. He sympathized with those among his former orderlies and male nurses who had genuine aspirations to medical competence. The solution, he felt, lay in co-operation rather than in competition.

Accordingly he began to train young men in laboratory and pharmaceutical work. "Then he would teach them some medicine, and even some surgery," writes Munroe Scott. "He saw ahead to the time when each of his men might be a 'specialist' in a handful of particular ailments and would go out to set up in private practice—with the expertise and the facilities of the hospital to back him up.

"It was an audacious plan and it was destined to grow and to flourish and to become part of China's 'Forgotten' history."

In time, McClure hoped that his best "quacks," as he affectionately

called them, would develop a repertoire of about twenty simple operations, from circumcisions to trachoma operations. (Trachoma was a
common ailment wherein the eyelashes turn inward and cause blindness
by rubbing against the eyeball.)

Before long McClure's Rural Medical System was in full operation.
There were eight counties in the Hwaiking mission's sphere of influence,
and by 1934, eight of McClure's graduates had established clinics, one in
each county. "Each man had served an apprenticeship in the pharmacy
and in the lab. Each had been sent off to Hankow and had earned a
certificate from the inter-mission Institute of Hospital Technology that
had been set up in the Union Hospital in Hankow. Each man had
learned to handle x-ray and to diagnose and treat certain common
diseases. Each man also had acquired a repertoire of minor operations."
And Dr. McClure visited each clinic every fortnight to consult and assist.
It was hardly a system that would have been tolerated at home by the
medical associations, but it was one that worked well in China. The idea
was later adopted by the Communists when they came to power, though
without acknowledging the source of the idea.

"That his system was gaining a considerable reputation was impressed
upon McClure one day when he found one of the practitioners had taken
on an assistant. The assistant was a graduate doctor from one of the
provincial medical schools. He was willing to work with the Hwaiking
practitioner because the practitioner had had a better training under Dr.
Loa than the graduate had had at an accredited institution. This was a
twist. Dr. Loa had always told his quacks they must never compete with a
graduate. If a graduate came to their town they were to co-operate, or,
close the clinic—and now a graduate was joining up as an assistant."

Occasionally, one of McClure's practitioners, affected by his own
prestige, would grow overconfident. Turning up at a clinic run by one of
them, "Dr. Li," McClure was alarmed to find that his protégé had
scheduled an operation for TB glands of the neck for four o'clock that
afternoon. It was one of the situations that McClure had impressed most
strongly on his graduates, that only the simpler operations should be done
at the outlying clinics. The operation for TB glands was definitely not one
of these, and McClure tried to tell the other so. But it was now too late for
Li to draw back without losing face, so McClure reluctantly agreed to
stay and assist.

"'Dr.' Li, assisted by Dr. Loa, began about 4 o'clock. An hour and a
half later they were still at it. The patient was still under anesthetic but
the 'surgeon' was getting deeper and deeper into the neck. Dr. Loa took
over but the light was beginning to fade and the clinic O.R. was not
equipped for efficient night time work. Finally, however, they completed
the operation. Dr. Loa, standing in the midst of a shambles he would
never have tolerated in Hwaiking, was tense and angry. The two men

stood for a moment in the deepening darkness, and then the practitioner bowed a little formal bow.

"'Dr. Loa,' he said, 'I wish to give you strong assurance and fervid hope that this humble doctor will never again attempt to remove TB glands in the clinic.'"

In the summer of 1937, the Sino-Japanese War began. At first McClure thought it was just another of the many conflicts he had worked through, fled from, or compromised with during his years in China. It was not until the Japanese had captured Peking and Tientsin, and had begun a drive toward the key port of Shanghai that he began to take it seriously. In late summer he went to a conference at Hankow called by the Christian Medical Association. At the conference there was ominous talk of extensive bombing by the Japanese on the civilian population. Now filled with foreboding, McClure agreed to serve as the field director for the International Red Cross in North and Central China, to organize and co-ordinate relief work among the civilians. Fortunately he did not have to worry about his wife and children. They had been vacationing on the coast and were already in Japanese-held territory. As neutrals they would be safe enough there.

McClure hurried back to Hwaiking and turned the hospital and the supervision of his now extensive Rural Medical System over to two of his Chinese doctors; and thus ended, temporarily he hoped, his service for the United Church, though the church agreed to continue paying his salary and family allowances.

By Christmas, the Japanese had captured Tsinan, where McClure's father was still teaching medicine at the age of eighty-one. By then the talk of unrestricted bombing of civilians at the Christian Medical Association conference had proved all too prescient. The Japanese had established a clear pattern of attack. Days or weeks ahead of an infantry attack they would make devastating bomber raids on the towns and cities in their path. Dr. McClure would try to guess where the next strike would be made, then hurry to that point, by bicycle and train, to strengthen his relief organizations, hoping to be there when the bombing started, so as to help with the emergency surgery. If there was a train headed in the right direction he would jump aboard with his bicycle. "If the train stopped because of a blown track, or uncoupled to break up the target, he would simply toss out his bike and keep going. He still wore his breeks, leather boots, khaki shirt, and leather jacket. On his back he now carried a pack that contained a blanket, shaving gear, a small typewriter, pictures of Amy and the kids, and a New Testament. He put in almost as much mileage on top of boxcars as inside. He found that driving snow combined with the smoke and sparks from a wood burning engine made for unpleasant travel conditions."

And so McClure scuttled back and forth along the Yellow River, accompanied by Dr. Richard F. Brown, who was in China under the auspices of the Anglican Church of Canada. He traveled into Communist country, to talk to Mao Tse-tung, Chou En-lai, and Chu Teh, about getting Red Cross supplies to their guerrillas, who were dedicatedly fighting the Japanese. The Canadian doctors were courteously received, though Mao and company must have been highly skeptical that Chiang Kai-shek's anti-red nationalists would provide the necessary co-operation.

McClure also ventured on three occasions into Japanese-held territory, until his Chinese friends told him that the enemy had put a price on his head. He would not believe them until he was shown a poster offering a reward of fifty thousand U.S. dollars for "Dr. Lao Tai-fu" dead or alive. Apparently his widespread travels about the front had convinced the Japanese that he was a spy.

McClure's work for the Red Cross brought him into closer contact with other Western missionaries, particularly the American Baptists at Cheng-chow. The experience did nothing to make him more obviously devout. Rather than pay lip-service to God, he let his work for the suffering speak for him. At the height of the conflict in 1938, McClure noted that those who had been most noisily devout had gone to safer pastures. The ones who remained were the true Western representatives of Christianity, people like the American Baptist, Dr. Ayers, the English eccentric Dr. Hankey, and Dr. Brown, who later joined Norman Bethune in exclusive support of the Communists. There were also the Roman Catholic missionaries, who appealed to McClure because they laughed and told jokes and were ready to pour him a beer at the end of a dehydrating day.

If Dr. McClure was impressed by men like Donald Hankey, who was as courageous as he was odd, and Dr. Ayers, who lived in delightful squalor, in a living room heaped with dirty teacups and old clothes, used razor blades, medical books, and instruments, others were even more impressed with him. Two of these were the famous poets, W. H. Auden and Christopher Isherwood. They had been sent to China by their publishers to write a travel book about the East, but they had decided to cover the Sino-Japanese War instead. They met McClure in 1938. They were having breakfast one morning when Dr. McClure, accompanied by Dr. Hankey, burst into the room.

"'Boy,' cried McClure, rubbing his hands, 'I've got a kidney today! Gee, what luck!'

"'Oh, Bob,' said Hankey protestingly. 'You might let me do it.'

"'No, Sir! I want to have a stab at it myself.'"

The poets went on to describe McClure in their *Journey to War* as a "stalwart, sandy bullet-headed Canadian Scot, with the energy of a whirlwind and the high spirtis of a sixteen-year-old boy. He wore a leather blouse, riding breeches and knee-boots with straps. Born in China, educated in Canada, he had earned his college fees by working as a stevedore and a barber. Before the war he had had his own hospital at Wei-hwei, north of the Yellow River. It was now in Japanese hands. At present he was acting as a co-ordinator of Red Cross services, and visiting, in this capacity, all the hospitals and mission-stations up and down the Lung-Hai line.

"After our second breakfast we were taken round the premises. In the compound Dr. Ayres had built a big thatched emergency-hut to accommodate the overflow of wounded. Most of the in-patients were suffering from bomb-injuries: fractured legs and arms. Trunk-wounds, the doctors told us, were mostly fatal; the victims were usually brought in too late, and died of sepsis. The Japanese had been very active in the Cheng-chow region lately, attacking not only the town itself, but many of the surrounding villages. McClure himself had an extremely narrow escape, only a week or two before; the ferry boat in which he was crossing the river had been destroyed a few moments after he had jumped into the water. Two bombs had been dropped here in the mission compound, just beside the enormous outspread American flag."

The poets were obviously fascinated by the tough, extrovert Canadian doctor, and McClure in his turn must have found their company agreeable enough, for he invited them to accompany him while he visited hospitals in the direction of Kai-feng. "After a late supper we started out," said Christopher Isherwood (the author of *Goodbye To Berlin* and other classics). "Chiang was silent this evening, and inclined to be unhelpful; perhaps he was intimidated by McClure's dynamic presence. We were semi-apologetic about the extent of our baggage, uneasily suspecting that McClure considered our possession of beds and a private servant as slightly sissy. He himself carried only a small suitcase. When we reached the station half a dozen coolies sprang out of the darkness, each struggling for a bag. McClure punched one of them hard on the jaw. The man wasn't a bona-fide porter, he explained later, but a railroad thief.

"The train, we were told, would leave at ten minutes to two. We had several hours to wait. The platform, unlighted, crowded with troops, was bitterly cold. But McClure's energy warmed us like a brazier.

"Himself a Presbyterian, he had no use for dogma in mission work; it was silly to bother the Chinese with theological language which they couldn't understand. Phrases like 'washed in the Blood' merely disgust them; 'The King of Heaven' suggests to their minds only a sort of super-tax-collector. If you stand up on a soap-box you only get hold of the loafer who's on the look-out for an easy job. The people we want are the farmers. And they're too busy to come and listen to a lot of talk. This crusader-stuff is the bunk."

The odd quartet—two fine-featured English poets, a hearty, driving Canadian, and an intimidated servant—waited all night on the bone-aching, dust-blown platform, and there was still no sign of a train. "But McClure didn't despair. The station-master had assured him that a troop-train would be passing through Cheng-chow at three. 'That suits me all right. They're apt to be a bit overcrowded. We'll have to sit on the roof. I guess....Only thing—if the Japs come over you've got to jump. Quick. Those trains are loaded full of amunition. You wouldn't have a chance. Not a chance.'"

To Isherwood's relief, the troop train failed to arrive, so they returned to the mission hospital, where McClure went back to the operating room, where he worked, "tinkering away at the casualties with unimpaired vigour.

"At tea-time we came in to find McClure and two bearded Italian missionaries listening with grave faces to the wireless. The Italians had brought news that Kwei-teh had already fallen; even the Chinese news-paper admitted that the Japanese had captured a town only twenty-five miles further north. But the wireless-bulletin told us nothing new; and we agreed that we had better attempt the journey, at any rate as far as Kai-feng. 'Whatever happens,' said McClure joyfully, 'we'll be in the thick of it!'

"Tonight a train was promised for eleven o'clock. At twelve-thirty we were told that it had actually reached the North Station, only a mile away. McClure decided that he and I should walk there, along the track, leaving Auden and Chiang to look after the luggage. In this way we should be more likely to get seats. As we set out it began to rain. Several hundred yards down the line there was a most unpleasant bridge, open to the water beneath. You had to cross it by stepping delicately from girder to girder, hoping that the gaps, invisible in the darkness, would be roughly equidistant. 'What shall we do,' I asked timidly, 'if the train comes now?' 'Jump it,' replied McClure promptly, and proceeded to explain the proper technique of jumping trains, if you didn't want a broken neck.

"But to my surprise and relief, the train was actually waiting. McClure efficiently identified it from a dozen others. We even found a sleeping-compartment with four vacant berths. At first he was inclined to turn up his nose at so much unnecessary comfort; but I cunningly pleaded with him to accept it for the sake of Auden, who, I hinted, was far from well."

At nine in the morning they reached a place whose name, translated, meant "Democracy." It comprised a loop-line, a railroad signal, and a hut, set in the midst of an immense mud plain. Auden, amending Pearl Buck's classic title, called it "The Bad Earth."

They were stuck at Democracy for six hours. After a while, Isherwood couldn't help noticing that McClure's morale seemed to be declining. The doctor explained that it was because his system was short of sugar. "'If I can only get something sweet, I'll be all right. What I need, right now, is a box of candy.'

"Out of the rainy mist, as if in answer to his request, a crowd began to gather. They were neighbouring peasants who had come to sell their wares, scenting from afar the presence of our train. Standing in the drizzle, in their fur hats and straw capes, they offered boiled chicken varnished red with soya beans, sausage-shaped waffles made from bean-flour, gray vermicelli, sugar-cane and hard-boiled eggs. We bought eggs, waffles, and a stick of cane, which McClure sucked contentedly. Its tonic effect upon him was almost immediately apparent. Soon The Bad Earth was forgotten, and we were listening to a further instalment of his lavishly-illustrated autobiography. Our only hope was that it would continue until this journey was over.

"In Cheng-chow he had bought a lorry and run it into quicksand, while disembarking from the Yellow River ferry. Within half an hour the sand had been up to the instrument board, but they had got it out, nevertheless. 'I had to take it apart and clean it, nut by nut. And, boy, when I'd got it apart, I couldn't put the darned thing together again! So I went to Peking, and worked in a Chevrolet garage for a month—learning how.'"

McClure also related the story of General Li and the *bien-tze* tablet, until the train moved off again at three-thirty that afternoon. "Towards five o'clock we arrived at Shang-kui, Kwei-teh's nearest railway station. The distance between Kwei-teh and Shang-kui is about five miles; we covered it in rickshaws, along a flat, rough road, lined with trees. The buildings of the Church of Canada Mission Hospital stand in their own large compound-garden, beyond the air-field, just outside the city. It seems strangely touching, in the midst of the alien plain, to come upon these prim, manse-like walls of gray brick, so isolated, so stubbornly Anglo-Saxon, despite the pointed, upcurving eaves of their corrugated iron roofs. After the drillground barrenness of Cheng-chow, the garden itself seemed wonderfully fruitful and pleasant. The trees were full of birds—crows and beautiful blue-jays, with white throat-collars and long sky-blue tails.

"McClure entered like Father Christmas, with a double postman's knock, and soon, amidst back-slappings and kidney-punching, we were being introduced to his two Canadian colleagues, Dr. Gilbert and Dr. Brown."

On the following afternoon they visited the Roman Catholic bishop and the local American Baptist mission. On the way they admired the massive walls of the town, its gateways plastered with the posters which

seemed to decorate the portals rather than disfigure them; though the
handsome walls enclosed a maze of muddy, stinking streets that made
Auden think of Europe in the Middle Ages. In the Baptist compound
they saw that the American flag had stuck halfway up the pole, and
nobody knew how to free it. "McClure volunteered, of course, to shin up
and get it down. McClure was in his element here. When the centrifugal
pump at the hospital went wrong, he knew why; when the gas-plant
failed, he could put it right; when the engine was making the wrong kind
of noise, McClure detected it at once. Dr. Brown, his friend since college
days, provided a mock-admiring audience for all these feats of energy and
skill."

Later, when Auden offered a cigarette to Dr. Gilbert, he got an insight
into the attitude of some of the missionaries that was not at all to his taste.
Dr. Gilbert accepted the cigarette as if giving way to sheer vice. "Elsewhere in the mission-field," Isherwood wrote, "so we had heard, the
sternest taboos prevailed. Mission-doctors were obliged to smoke in
secret, like schoolboys. If they were discovered there would be a public
prayer-meeting for the salvation of their souls. In some places a doctor
caught drinking a glass of wine by his minister would be liable to lose his
job altogether. (It must be added that, in the course of our Yellow River
Journey, we witnessed few serious signs of this stupid and contemptible
tyranny—no doubt because the tyrants themselves had been the first to
abandon their posts and run away from the danger zone." In general,
"only the best type of missionary had remained.")

The next morning the poets were allowed to watch McClure and
Brown at work in the operating room. "The patient had a vaginal-
urethral fistula, sustained in childbirth. We took the opportunity of
examining her feet. A girl's feet are generally bound at the age of four or
five. All toes except the big toe are turned under the foot, and fastened in
position. Subsequent growth will only have the effect of raising the arch,
forming a deep grove across the centre of the sole, which is very liable to
sores. The custom of foot-binding is gradually dying out in China. Most
of the bound feet we saw in Kwei-teh were those of middle-aged or
elderly women.

"While he operated McClure kept up a running commentary for the
benefit of the amused and slightly scandalized Canadian Sister. 'Let's
have something to kneel on.... You see, Sister, I'm more devotional that
you think...Now the torch...Let your light so shine....Oh Boy, that's
good! Sponge, Brother....More light in the northeast....Phew, I'm
sweating. This is worse than two sets of tennis.... Now then, Bunty pulls
the strings. Which string shall you pull, Brother? If you were in a
sailing-ship, you'd be sunk.... Well, that's fixed the exhaust. We'll do the
differential tomorrow.'"

McClure, with his fierce energy, his bold manner, his muscular dialogue, his advice and his surgical and mechanical skills burned in the memory of the wandering poets long after they parted from him at Kwei-teh. Another celebrity, however, failed to succumb either to the doctor's admirable character or to his generosity, and that was Dr. Norman Bethune.

The famous surgeon's arrival was eagerly anticipated by the Communists up in Shansi, but he had been delayed at a Yellow River crossing. On February 23 of that year, 1938, McClure was met at Tungkwan railway station by harried officials who reported that Bethune had disappeared. "Bob was told that his countryman had been drinking heavily, had been annoyed at the delay, and had been very restless. McClure of the I.R.C. left the train, changed hats, as it were, to Loa Ming-yuan, took his bicycle, and went bird-dogging out into the adjacent villages asking questions as he went. He soon struck the trail of the Big Nose who apparently spoke no Chinese but who had a tremendous thirst. It was a good spoor. Before long he found Bethune, well-advanced in a rural Chinese pub-crawl. McClure was relieved, and somewhat surprised, to find him still functioning. The Chinese liquor he was drinking was the same stuff McClure was using in the O.R. as a hand rinse after scrub up.

"The two men returned to Tungkwan together to continue their separate journeys. It had not been a pleasant meeting. Dr. McClure had found Dr. Bethune to be very anti-Canadian, paranoiac about his thoracic work, too militantly Communist, and bitter. Gregarious thiry-seven-year-old McClure had met a forty-eight-year-old fellow Canadian surgeon in the boondocks of wartime China and had found no single point of contact."

Bethune's work for the Chinese Communists would have been made much easier if he had taken advantage of a veteran's drive, initiative, and experience of Kuomintang-Communist politics. Instead, Bethune went his lonely way to fame and infection, and he and McClure never met again.

33

Bethune: All the Rage

I N THE THIRTIES, many people of integrity and concern were affronted at the cowardly and treacherous conduct of the Western powers, especially by the British and French ostrich act, in the face of Fascist aggression. Dr. Norman Bethune was one of the few who did something about it. In 1936 he went to Spain to aid the national government in its desperate fight against Franco's Fascists, who were being aided by their Italian and German comrades. By the end of the year he had created a mobile blood transfusion service that was soon supplying all sectors of the front, using a wagon containing a refrigerator, sterilizer, incubator, and numerous other items of equipment, such as flasks, lamps, blood transfusion sets, serum, the clear yellow fluid that separates from clotted blood, and, of course, the blood itself.

Just as Maude Abbott made a profound contribution to an understanding of congenital heart disease without adding specifically to the scientific treasury, so Bethune made no particular discovery in the field of preserved blood. His accomplishment, greater than any discovery that he might have achieved in research, was in seeing where blood was most needed and getting it to the wounded on the spot. "A beautiful idea—and Canadian," he cried. And, more typically: "We are doing good. What more can one ask?"

Two years later Bethune was in China, where he insisted on serving, not the suspect nationalists, but the Chinese Communist Eighth Route Army.

His fate seemed already inscribed. He wanted, according to a British journalist, to be a hero of the revolution at any cost—or a martyr. He got his wish about one and a half years later, three months after the start of the Second World War. Near the front line at the foot of the Mo-t'ien mountains, in a peasant house converted into an operating theatre, his finger became infected, and, exhausted by months of organizing, tours of inspection, and operating, he succumbed.

Though an outstanding personality and noted in the thirties for his work in pulmonary surgery, Norman Bethune was a less significant figure in Canadian medicine than a number of his contemporaries whose names are known only within the profession. The contributions of his chief at the Royal Victoria Hospital in Montreal, for instance, Dr. Edward Archibald, were far more impressive than Bethune's. Dr. Archibald was the father of pulmonary surgery in North America. Bethune was a wayward son.

It was the Chinese chairman who, in rising to applaud the doctor from Gravenhurst for his contributions to the Communist cause in China, brought a Canadian audience to its feet in a standing ovation. Bethune was preferred by Mao Tse-tung over a host of other Western medical personnel who had worked as devotedly as Bethune for the people of China, and in most cases for far longer. But Bethune had the right qualifications. He worked specifically for the Communists, he was a member of the party, and he brought his work for the Chinese people to a suitable climax by dying for their cause.

Though the Chinese did indeed revere Bethune—ten thousand Red soldiers were said to have attended his funeral—Chairman Mao enthroned Bethune in the Communist pantheon as hero and martyr mostly for political reasons. He was using the Canadian doctor chiefly to exhort his own people to dedicate themselves to the cause. "Every Communist must learn from him," he wrote in his *In Memory of Norman Bethune*. In the same essay, which would become required reading in the People's Republic, he described Bethune's spirit as one of "utter devotion to others without any thought of self." This was a reprogramming of the facts. Bethune's entire life was a rage to express his self to the utmost. "He needed to perform and be praised for great deeds," wrote his most penetrating biographer, Roderick Stewart, "and he wanted his performances applauded."

This is not to say that Bethune himself was a fake, nor is this intended as some fashionable denigration. It is just a resistance to the artistry of thought-programming that rearranges the natural beauty of individualism into an artifical composition for the masses. After all, Henry Norman Bethune's life is triumphant enough, in its intense individualism.

His lineage was of an independent-minded people who believed that the most satisfying life was one devoted to the service of others. Despite his compulsion to dominate others through unconventional opinions and behaviour and through force of personality, Bethune was true to this tradition, even though he did not particularly appreciate the tradition in others. He had no great respect for the principal practitioner of altruism in his own family, his father, the Presbyterian minister. Presumably Norman's disrespect for authority derived from this source. As a youth, he considered the Reverend Malcolm Bethune to be weak, mean with money, and hypocritical. The minister considered his son to be wild, stubborn, rude, and severely lacking in Christian humility; that is, Norman often refused to do what he was told.

The orders Norman was supposed to follow as a youth were designed to make him tractable, God-fearing and humble in the service of humanity. Mostly they had the opposite effect. As the years went by, Norman became increasingly arrogant in the service of humanity. His personality was too intense to admit Christian self-effacement. On the other hand, he demanded discipline himself. At age nineteen, when he was teaching school at Edgeley, Ontario, he used the strap enthusiastically on his disobedient students. The rowdy lads did not take kindly to the regime, and Norman sometimes had to defend it with his fists. Luckily a vigorous, outdoor childhood of rock-climbing, fishing, swimming, and log-rolling, had developed whipcord muscles and a fast pair of feet, so he had no difficulty in subduing his charges. In revenge they brought in a burly acquaintance to beat him up; but even this bruiser was no match for "teach." The boys' champion was floored several times before he gave up and lurched into the distance. From then on, Norman's hegemony was unchallenged.

In 1914, at medical school in Toronto, he succumbed to the war fever that was raising the patriotic temperature of the province. He volunteered for service in the European war, enlisting in a field ambulance unit. He was wounded in the leg after only a few weeks of front-line duty as a stretcher-bearer, and was invalided home, discharged, and returned to his medical duties at the end of 1915, taking the same accelerated course as Frederick Banting. He graduated as a Bachelor of Medicine in December the following year, after a total of three years at medical school.

It was at this period in his life, in his mid-twenties, that Norman began to modulate an already dominant personality with the sort of quirks and oddities of behaviour and attitude that create a truly memorable, not to say shocking, impression on people. Intensely conscious of his separateness, he felt impelled to make others vividly conscious of his presence; and he had the drive, shared by nearly all men and women of achievement, the unfaltering energy to sustain his characterization. For a while, at the medical school, he exaggerated his limp to make himself even more visually conspicuous that he already was, with his intense, sometimes quizzical, sometimes glowering gaze, and his forceful physical self that always seemed to stake a maximum claim on the surrounding space. In argument he was distinctly radical at a time when the "quite strong socialist ideas" he expressed were nearly as suspect as terrorist ideology would be today. In contrast to that great and modest man, William Osler ("I will answer to Hi! or to any loud noise"), Norman forced even the pronunciation of his name on people, according to the way he wished it pronounced at any one time. His name—"a signal of the self's identity" as his Communist preceptor Stanley Ryerson put it—was as vital to the transmission of his personality as his provocative opinions, his boastful surgery, his aggressive lovemaking, and his unconventional clothing that ranged from the famous beret and turtleneck sweater to the filthy shirt he wore to a convention of the American Association of Thoracic Surgery. At medical school in Toronto he insisted on being addressed as "Bay-tune," because that was the way his distant French ancestors would have had it; later it was "Bee-tun," as the English rendered it; a decade later he was correcting people who put the accent on the second syllable ("The name is BETH-une, not Beth-UNE!"). By the thirties, when a woman friend, Libbie Rutherford, took to calling him Beth, as did most of his friends, "Call me Norman," he told her, "It's my name."

From his early twenties he had no difficulty in making his presence felt. The intensity that he brought to both work and play and to the exposition of his personality was almost obssessive. In England, where he took his postgraduate training, his iconoclastic qualities were still in abeyance. It was his soaring confidence and joy of life that most impressed a friend and colleague, Graham Ross. To a subtle, conservative London doctor, Norman's behaviour was a trifle bumptious and slapdash, but also "refreshing and amusing." In the pre-Depression days when Canadians appeared to have had an instantly recognizable native character, the same doctor found him "very unorthodox, even for a Canadian."

His unorthodoxy extended to his dress. In Stratford, Ontario, where he acted as a *locum tenens* for a brief period after completing the first stage of his internship in England, he invited a girl friend to a dance, and caused her acute embarrassment by turning up in a light blue suit, red tie, and yellow shoes. In the office he startled patients by greeting them, not in the usual dignified garb but in a sweater, tweed trousers, and red plaid socks, "with feet on the desk in a relaxed position as if he didn't care."

Bethune cared rather more for humble patients than for the affluent, but not enough to stay in any one place for long. After Stratford, he assisted a doctor in Ingersoll, where he drove his host's Model T Ford around town at high speeds and gave parties for children. He had a lifelong fondness for children. Theirs was the only company that he had no need to dominate.

After Ingersoll, he joined the Canadian Air Force, in which he served as a medical officer for about nine months, before taking off for London again, in late 1920. He had thus served in all three services within six years, for as well as his stint in the army he had, soon after graduating from the University of Toronto, acted as a Royal Navy surgeon on board an aircraft carrier. This pattern of unsustained concentration in any one field was repeated throughout his life, from his brief bouts of private practice and a short-lived marriage, to his whirlwind contribution to the Spanish Civil War where he organized a mobile blood transfusion service, and the few self-immolating months in China. It was not so much that he lacked staying power. Rather it were as if life were running at a multiple of the standard pace, like a speeded-up film. He could hardly have loaded more experience onto his sensual circuits had he been informed in his youth that he had only a few years to live.

In London Norman completed a second internship, then left for Edinburgh to obtain his F.R.C.S. He also obtained Frances Penney, who was to be his partner in a strange marriage that for ten years would burn brilliantly, die away, blaze, flicker, and rekindle, before the partners would finally acknowledge what had been obvious to others from the beginning, their total incompatibility.

They were married in 1923. Using Frances' money, they set out on a grand tour of Europe, a year during which Frances learned that she had married a very bizarre character indeed. When he was not trying to dominate her, he was behaving in her opinion, in a "pseudo-romantic" manner. In Italy, according to Ted Allan and Sydney Gordon in their book *The Scalpel, The Sword*, during a visit to an art gallery, Bethune stood transfixed before Giotto's painting, *Life of St. Francis*, received a revelation from it, and announced that he would become a monk. Fortunately he had changed his mind by the time he reached Vienna, where he studied for a few weeks under the city's leading surgeons.

After the tour had exhausted most of Frances' inheritance, they crossed the Atlantic and settled in Detroit, where for a time Bethune attempted to conform to the normal standards of the profession by dressing circumspectly in gloves, cane, and Homburg, and charging as much as the traffic would bear. But his bullying ways and his erratic character, which, as he admitted to Frances, he could not understand himself, further undermined the marriage and after a couple of years, Frances had had enough.

Frances Penney was as vulnerable in spirit as she was lovely of face and figure. Ten years younger than her husband, she was the only daughter of a prominent Edinburgh family. On their first meeting, the finishing school girl and the "unfinished colonial"—as she called him—fell instantly in love. On his part, the main attraction was her upper class Edinburgh accent, her beautiful face, and her "remarkable innocence, a remarkable unworldness, plus a remarkable intelligence."

There was also a remarkable inferiority complex, and apparently an unhealthy sexual attitude. She gave the impression that she regarded the procreative act as rather sordid activity unfortunately necessary for the continuance of the human race. It was a programming that would ill-prepare her for conjunction with a man as physical as Bethune. But this was the very quality that initially attracted her to the Canadian. He was everything she wanted to be herself, confident, dynamic, welcoming experience not as an ordeal, but as a feast for the mind and senses.

Her mother was as dismayed as Frances was enthralled. "Oh, my heart sank when I met him," she said of Bethune. "I knew he was the kind of man who would attract Frances." The kind of flamboyant personality who was not likely to have the sensitivity to repair the girl's self-esteem or ease her gently into the reality of the marital bed and out of it into an uncouth world, or even a person who, given his obvious lack of respect for money, was likely to compensate for Frances' own impractical attitude toward it.

They had known each other—or thought they had—for three years before they married in 1923. For three years Frances had perceived him with a vision coloured with romantic love, but within a day of their marriage, antagonism as well as sex had reared its ugly head. Bethune's first words to her after the marriage ceremony in London were, "Now I can make your life a misery, but I'll never bore you—it's a promise."

This was the opening salvo in a campaign to dominate her utterly. Perhaps, though he was still infatuated with her, she had already begun to infuriate him with her genteel manner and cultivated ways. On the very first stop on their honeymoon, in the Channel Islands, he put the dainty, slender girl with the huge, vulnerable eyes brutally at risk when, out walking near the town of Finch, he challenged her to jump across a deep ravine. According to Allan and Gordon, to have fallen into the ravine would have brought serious injury or death. But, "I would sooner see you dead than funk that," Bethune said to Frances; so she jumped, but from that moment on she no longer trusted him completely, or loved him unreservedly. His challenge had exposed a hostility that even the most abject apologies could not camouflage.

His subsequent melodramatic behaviour during the grand tour, his heavy drinking, his risky skiing in Switzerland, his mystic revelation before the Giotto painting, and his improvident purchase of a gift for her—using the last few pennies of the inheritance—did not exactly increase her confidence in his ability to protect her from the world, nor did his confession that he could not understand his own erratic behaviour.

If that were so, she thought, the implication was that he could not control it either.

The fault was not entirely on his side. In Detroit, Frances did not make a good impression, not least because of her attitude to Americans. She thought they were common. She thought that their country was the only one in the world to have achieved decadence without first going through a civilized stage. "To some in Detroit and Montreal," wrote Dr. Wendall MacLeod (who admitted that he met her only once) "she appeared shallow, naive, humourless and vindictive. To her husband, later, her conduct seemed undignified." While her husband worked and socialized around Detroit, she stayed home and brooded on the state of the nation, on her own misfortune, and on her husband's financial irresponsibility and domineering ways. When he returned to the house they were likely to quarrel about everything from domestic affairs to literature.

In the fall of 1925 she flounced off to visit a girl friend in Nova Scotia. Instead of returning home for Christmas she went to California to stay with her brother.

Bethune's reaction, despite his protestations of love, could not have made her terribly eager to return. After assuring her in a letter that he still loved, worshipped, and adored her, he added that he "wouldn't miss missing you for worlds. So please stay away a little longer." She may also have wondered uneasily if he was referring to the physical intimacies of married life when he added that when she did finally return, she would have to "bear with fortitude" his "accumulated affection." Perhaps that was why she did not come home until 1926. Shortly afterward, when she learned that he had tuberculosis and would have to stay in a sanatorium, she decided to divorce him.

As usual, he appreciated her most when she was not by his side. He wrote from the sanatorium that she was not to worry. "You can tell your people that I took your money, wasted it and left you stranded and, beyond calling you a fool for your action and I a knave for mine, what's to be said? You have done nothing wrong except to have consigned yourself and your money to a man who did not appreciate the one and was careless of the other. But let me get up, get well first and I will repay." Further on in the letter he wrote, "Our marriage has been wonderful for me. If I had to go over it again, I would still want you for my side, my darling."

When Norman Bethune drove into Montreal in the spring of 1928 in his yellow roadster he was flat broke, divorced, and firing on only one pulmonary cylinder. He looked older than his thirty-eight years—already a pretty advanced age to be starting out in a new career. His fair hair was fast receding from his deep forehead, and a jaunty waxed moustache did little to compensate for the hirsute scarcity. But his blue eyes were as challenging as ever, his manner as flamboyant, his self-expression as intense.

Broke? He didn't give a damm. When he had money he spent it, on important things like paintings; when there was no money, he did without. As for now being divorced from Frances, that was hard, but he was not miserable about it, he was not depressed. He would get her back sooner or later. He was already importuning her by mail ("I love you. I wait for you"). As for the tuberculosis, he had just about fought it to a standstill. He had spent the previous year at the famous Trudeau Sanatorium in the Adirondack Mountains, and had responded well to treatment, mainly through his own efforts. During the enforced bed rest he had studied the disease and its treatment, and had come to the conclusion that artificial pneumothorax would benefit his diseased lung. This involved the letting of air into the chest cavity through a hollow needle to collapse the lung and thus allow it a bed rest of its own. So he bullied a conservative sanatorium staff into trying the new treatment on him. They did so, though they pointed out that there were risks. Whereupon he wrenched open his shirt and in his melodramatic fashion cried, "Gentlemen, I welcome the risk!"

Now, at an age when most doctors could contemplate their achievements and their bank balances with equanimity, when their greatest risk might be the decision of whether or not to plunge further into the stock market—the current downturn would surely pull out soon, and zoom into another boom in 1929—here was Bethune starting all over again, with neither a reputation nor a bank balance, in a new branch of surgery, in an unfamiliar city, on probation as a mere assistant, and on a very minor salary indeed.

He was content. He had tried the money route in his one and only foray into private practice. Until tuberculosis struck him down he had been developing a sound reputation in Detroit, and earning enough money to gratify his tastes especially in the purchase of works of art. But his year of enforced inactivity in the Trudeau Sanatorium where his greed for life's experiences and his restless, driving energy had been roadblocked, had forced on him the opportunity to think sustainedly about his direction in life. He had come to the conclusion that though successful enough financially, his achievement in Detroit had been a failure in terms of his own intellectual and spiritual needs. He did not really know what he wanted, but he knew what he really didn't want—dull comfort, compromise, smug, uncritical complacency.

Bethune did not wish to accomodate himself to life, but to slap it in the face, shake it up, make it intensely aware of *him, his* talents, *his* ego, *his* impulsive, angry, violent personality. The hell with security. Henceforth, he would concentrate on a worthwhile goal, without caring about the financial rewards. He would become a great thoracic surgeon, and help reduce the world's huge tuberculosis casualty list through his surgical skills. Quebec would certainly be a fruitful field for this work, for its tuberculosis mortality rate was the highest in Canada. In Montreal alone, hundreds died from the disease every year.

In Montreal, as soon as he had settled into his digs Bethune walked along to the castle-like Royal Victoria Hospital to meet his new boss Edward Archibald. Like Bethune, Dr. Archibald's interest in tuberculosis had been roused by his own experience of it. He had been afflicted with TB when he was twenty-nine. Professor of surgery at McGill University, he had just been appointed chief of surgery at the Royal Victoria, which had given him the longed-for opportunity to establish a medico-pulmonary surgical clinic for the investigation of pulmonary tuberculosis. Over the years he would publish scores of important papers on the subject.

While establishing the clinic, Archibald had been looking around for a first assistant, so that Bethune's application to train under him was opportune. Archibald had agreed to take him on provided that Dr. Bethune would prepare himself by studying at the Hospital for Incipient Tuberculosis. Bethune had just come from that New York Hospital, where he had taken a refresher course in biochemistry, learned as much as he could about bacteriology, and had co-operated in a minor research project.

At first the spinning firework of a newcomer—"always throwing off sparks and always in a different direction," as Archibald put it—and the formal but sympathetic chief of surgery got on fairly well. In a letter to Frances, who was now in Edinburgh, Bethune described Archibald as "a most charming fellow," and though Archibald did not particularly like his first assistant, he was impressed by the younger man's energy, enthusiasm, and dedication to the tasks at hand. It was some time before Archibald became professionally disillusioned with his protégé, especially over his surgical methods; but for some weeks he had no opportunity to see him in action, for at first Bethune merely observed or assisted in the operating room. It is also likely that Archibald, a person of many preoccupations, was not properly aware for some time of Bethune's doubtful methods even after he started operating on his own.

As his duties at the Royal Victoria burned up only a fraction of his energy, Bethune was soon deeply involved in a number of research projects. He had published four papers by the end of the year, contributions to the clinic that earned Archibald's gratitude. An original thinker, he lectured, in an informal and iconoclastic way, to McGill students in training at the Royal Victoria. To the surprise of the students he took no treatment, technique, or method for granted, not even Laennec's time-honoured inspection-palpitation-percussion-ausculation. He questioned the value of this often perfunctory clinical ritual as it applied to the diagnosis of early TB. The X-ray machine was the thing to use, he said challengingly, not the bloody stethoscope.

Bethune was equally dissatisfied with many of the surgical instruments in use. He did not see why he should accept them as they were, as his colleagues did, merely because they were there. He set about redesigning some of them and inventing others. It was in this field that he made his most important contribution to medicine. His pneumothorax machine, for instance, was a considerable improvement over the old model. It was beautifully simple and less than half the weight of the old apparatus. Another invention was a mechanical contraption used to hold the patient's shoulder blade away from the chest wall during an operation. Formerly, a surgical assistant had to do the work by hand with a retractor, an exhausting procedure and a waste of a surgeon's time and talents. His most famous and enduring instrument was the rib shears. Every time he was forced to use the standard all-purpose shears to cut through the ribs, he would swear at them and retreat to his office to sketch alternative designs. "But each new type he made up was clumsy or as heavy or as oversharp as the type it was designed to replace." Until one day when he was collecting a pair of shoes that had been mended he saw the shoemaker using a device for cutting nails out of shoes. "If only resecting ribs," he reflected, were as simple as mending shoes. He turned to leave, and was struck by a sudden thought. He asked to look at the shears. The shoemaker passed them over, and it was from this instrument that he designed the Bethune Rib Shears, the only one of his instruments that remains in use today. Of the others, a few found temporary favour with the profession, others did not. As for the pneumothorax machine, with the decline of lung-collapse therapy in the late 1940s, it was no longer needed.

A normal inventor would have rejoiced in the success of his surgical instrument improvements. It was typical of Norman that, instead, he used the occasion to scorn and castigate the profession for not having made the improvements before him.

Meanwhile he was still importuning Frances. Addressing her as "my darling Frances," he wrote soon after his arrival in Montreal that, "If it were not for my doubts, I would say at once—Come here. Marry me. Why should we be separate who love each other? I can be happy with you—but you not with me? I was thinking that if you come here this winter—we could meet just as friends, living apart. In any case whether you marry me or not, that is, I am sure, our only way.... I miss you dreadfully but—I don't want to snatch at you ever again. I want you to be just Frances Penney—without any attempts at approximations to

standards, types of my imagination or fancy—the Frances Penney I
knew in Edinburgh, self-contained and undistorted. Your affectionate
lover, Beth."

It was pressing sentiments like these, perhaps in combination with the
discovery that her life was no better without him than with him, that
brought her back to his side. They were remarried a month after the stock
market crash; but within days the friction of his "petulant irritability," as
he described it, and her brooding resentment were producing the same
intolerable heat as before. There had also been a change in Frances that
made her less than ever amenable to his discipline. She was now looking
at other men much less shyly and guardedly than heretofore. She developed an interest in a friend of Bethune's, R. E. Coleman. When Bethune
learned that she was contemplating marriage with Coleman, he told her,
"I love you and always will however much you may hurt or wound me,"
and agreed to make things easier for her by keeping her supplied with
money; but he would not agree to a second divorce. A month later,
writing from Alabama, he changed his mind. "Well, my dear, the
unexpected has happened as usual. I have fallen in love and want to
marry this girl that I feel sure I can be happy with. It was love at first sight
with both of us."

The Alabama affair fizzled out, but the divorce talk did not, and after
Frances, Coleman, and Bethune had falsified the evidence, as required
by Canadian law, a divorce was granted in 1933. The three then
celebrated the occassion with champagne.

Though Bethune continued to love Frances for the few remaining
years of his life, it did not hinder him from loving other women. A
Montreal friend, Libbie Park, wrote that "Norman loved women and
said he loved women passionately and made love with some. Women I
have known who were in love with Norman have spoken of him in very
different terms. To one it was an experience she wanted, one for which she
shared the responsibility, without regrets. To another the experience
simply demonstrated what she thinks of now as Norman's mindless
pursuit of all women. For me the word 'womanizer' so often used in
connection with him vulgarizes Norman Bethune's attitude towards
women and in no way captures the kinds of relationships that existed
between him and women who were often friends, and sometimes lovers."

Libbie Park obviously found his attitude to women refreshing.
"Though he may not have believed in monogamy, I liked his attitude
toward women. He had none of the stereotyped male attitudes, and did
not speak of women in a derogatory sense. A woman is a person, her mind
not the mind of a 'woman' but of a person. In argument he was never
patronizing, never appeared to make allowances; if he disagreed with a
woman he would not spare her."

"I saw him but once," said one brilliant and beautiful woman to Dr. Aubrey Geddes, "and he was the most aggressively male creature I have ever encountered."

On the whole, with the possible exception of the woman who meant most to him, Bethune appears to have treated women better than men, especially if the men represented authority; in which respect—or disrespect—he was also years ahead of his time, the Che Guevara of the medical world. He tended to question everything that his superiors and colleagues did, expressing his opinions in a way that would give them the rudest shock. A few acquaintances were tolerant of his radicalism. "Despite his dedication, impatience and practically manic drive to get things done," wrote a colleague, Dr. D.H. Starkey, "he was a surprisingly reasonable and stimulating person to work with. He only became unreasonable and impossible when he thought that someone was not willing to give his best to a cause of investigation that he, Bethune, believed to be important or of benefit to patients or the 'underdog.'"

Patients were never subjected to the agitator side of his character. Dr. Wendell MacLeod said of him that, "On the medical wards in 1930-32 our interns and nurses often commented on Bethune's warm and considerate manner with patients who were under review for possible surgery, serious surgery. Sitting on the edge of the bed once, forgetting about isolation technique in his absorption, he explained what would be done at the operation, what the odds were for improvement, for mere survival or for losing the bet—with and without surgery...[his] intensely personal concern for the patient's welfare is what I and others remember most clearly." He evoked as warm a response in the younger medical people as in the patients. He "was like a breath of fresh air. He was informal, outgoing, dynamic in speech and body movements, cheerful and sometimes even gay."

There were many others, though, who resented his scornful comments on their inability to think as originally and independently as he did, or whose wits were slower. A Montreal journalist friend, Louis Huot, said of him that he would "engage in the most facetious and mocking sort of comments that only an exceptionally talented person would understand. He would make a fool of his interlocutor, and on purpose." His biographer, Roderick Stewart, added that, "Unable to conceal his feelings he was hostile in crude and sometimes juvenile ways. He once interrupted a conversation with a friend in a restaurant, explaining that he had just seen someone he particularly disliked and would return as soon as he had 'irritated' the offensive party."

It was his desire to serve others, borne along on the carrier-wave of an obsessive self-expression, that made him such an enigmatic person. Perhaps the key to his character was a quality of violence; violence in opinion and belief, in his response to opposition or to a challenge to his supremacy and in his reaction to social injustice. Violence, too, in the way he sometimes confronted those whose mental pace seemed to him to be sluggish, or whose complacency of thinking seemed to be anesthetizing them against the ills of the world. The violence was usually against the emotions of others. One such occasion occurred in Montreal when he brought a common prostitute to a posh dinner party. He paraded her before the shocked guests, and after seeing that she was fed at the buffet table, announced that, "Now, ladies and gentlemen, I shall return her whence she has come—the streets and degradation." This insensitive action—insensitive toward the prostitute, that is—which he presumably justified on the grounds that it would make the impervious socialities more aware of the underprivileged in their midst—casts some doubt on the oft-repeated assertion that he had a profound sympathy for suffering or downtrodden humanity.

For the most part Bethune was civilized enough to restrain himself from actual physical violence (though at one despairing moment during his illness, he pistol-whipped a Detroit businessman who had insulted Frances), but the threat was felt by many in the form of agitation and intolerance. Similarly his operating technique was violent. In Montreal, a clinical clerk said of Bethune that his "patients had a rocky time recovering from surgery, more frequently than those of Dr. Archibald or Dr. McIntosh. It was not a problem of infection...but poor general physical condition on their return from the operating room and shock....In spite of our best care we are losing patients operated on by Dr. Bethune at an unusual rate." Ironically Bethune justified his fast and furious technique on the grounds that post-operative fatalities were caused by surgical shock owing to the length of time the patients were under the anesthetic. But it appeared that the patients had a better chance of survival under Archibald's lengthy, painstaking surgery than under Bethune's velocity. ("Come on, Arthur [Dr. Arthur Vineberg—his surgical assistant], we will show them how good we are.")

Increasingly his contempt for authority and savaging of opposition alienated the people around him at the Royal Vic. Dr. Archibald had long since retracted his opinion that Bethune was a brilliant surgeon. He cautioned Bethune against his "slapdash" approach. When Bethune ignored the advice and one more patient died, one who was thought to have been a good risk, Archibald informed Bethune that he was no longer wanted at the hospital.

Archibald had never really liked Bethune. Though Wilder Penfield wrote that the chief never spoke ill of anyone, Archibald appears to have made an exception in Bethune's case. He found Bethune to be definitely abnormal, certainly not a genius, not even a leader. "He was egocentric, his vision was keen but narrow. He wore blinkers. He trod on many toes quite often without knowing it or without caring if he did know it. He had a superiority complex and he was entirely amoral."

Even though his behaviour had upset Dr. Archibald, the chief surgeon was still willing to recommend him for another position, at the Sacré Coeur Hospital, as director of its new tubercular unit.

The attitude of the staff there was much less defensive than at the Royal Vic. "He was for all of us an inspiration in his work and his research," said his anesthetist there, Dr. Georges Cousineau, "and during these... years among us he never stopped teaching and inspiring each and every one of us to do more and more careful work." Bethune was certainly happier at the Sacré Coeur. He was finally in command of his own service. His stay there, from 1933 to 1936, did much for the reputation of the hospital, as well as giving him, according to Stewart, a growing international reputation, though his behaviour remained as eccentric as ever. Bethune's eccentricities sometimes confused and sometimes awed his colleagues at Sacré Coeur," Steward wrote. "After a fire in his apartment had destroyed most of his possessions including all his clothes, Bethune appeared at the hospital wearing an old suit and shoes with no soles — as usual, he didn't have enough money to buy a new suit. Dr. Cousineau knew that Bethune refused to send bills to his few private patients.... Cousineau was concerned by Bethune's situation and approached the director of the hospital to obtain a list of Bethune's patients." Dr. Cousineau than made a collection among the patients amounting to $300, and presented it to Bethune. "The following day," Cousineau told Stewart, "he returned better dressed but without a cent. He said 'Georges, lend me five bucks.' He had in fact bought himself some clothes but he had also divided the money among those poor children to whom he taught painting."

The children's painting class was yet another aspect of the wide range of medical and outside activities that made Bethune's life so rich in incident and so difficult to summarize. With an artist friend named Fritz Brandtner, he subsidized classes for children who could not otherwise have afforded them; children whose circumscribed lives, in cobbled yards and foul back alleys, deprived them of an outlet for their imaginations. The classes were held in Bethune's apartment on Beaver Hall Square. "There were ten to fifteen children in a class," wrote Libbie Park, "held once a week, with a special excursion on Saturdays when possible. Brandtner was there regularly and Norman usually, in the months before he left for Spain. There was no formal teaching. The children sat on the floor with large sheets of wrapping paper to paint on, and cake tins to mix their paints in, and they painted what was in their minds...

"The painter Sylvia Ary, who attended these classes as a child, recalls that the children loved Norman, who brought them treats, and taught them to see and feel the things they looked at, impressions that were embedded in their minds."

This was then quite a revolutionary approach to art, and a fine example of Bethune's originality and freedom from hidebound thinking. The traditional method was to take all the fun out of painting in the schoolroom. In Brandtner and Bethune's Montreal Children's Creative Art Centre, the children's imaginations were gloriously liberated and produced genuinely exciting paintings that were widely exhibited in Montreal.

Bethune's decor was equally original. His residences in Montreal rivaled the children's paintings in their uninhibited use of colour. The one he occupied before moving to Beaver Hall Square was on Fort Street, and comprised a studio, living room, and bedroom. "When you entered," wrote Libbie Park, "You were confronted with red walls, a wide couch with a 'gentian' (Norman's word) velvet cover thrown over it, bright red, yellow and green cushions scattered on it. On the sill of the not-too-large window was a little green flowering plant...and in front of the window, on the floor, a mattress, also covered in blue, and on it a yellow upholstered bed rest with arms, and cushions the same colour as the couch. An easel stood just off the centre of the room. On it was the unfinished portrait of Norman that Brandtner was painting. A phonograph, table and a couple of chairs completed the furniture. I remember only one painting (I am sure there were more) hanging in the main room: *Sunflowers* by Brandtner, and the colours in the room echoed the vivid colours of the painting.'

By 1935 Bethune was beginning to add political anger to his passions. In this he was a worthy child of the thirties, joining the growing elite of intelligent and sensitive people who were enraged at the craven behaviour of the democracies in the face of the European and Far Eastern Fascist expansion. At first his concern was mainly with the social role of medicine, particularly as it applied to tuberculosis. Prevention, he began to realize, might be better than surgery. School children should be X-rayed regularly. People in close contact with children and food handlers should receive regular physical examinations. Active tubercular cases should be segregated. Medical schools should co-operate in imparting more information about the disease. "Finally, a 'half-way house' between sanatoria and industry should be established where partly cured tubercular patients could be sent to work in light industries. These industries would be subsidized and protected by the government, the only agency with the capital and the necessary powers to implement his broad-ranging schemes."

Bethune proceeded to put some of his then disturbing views into practice. "Working with George Mooney, who was a Y.M.C.A. secretary in the Montreal suburb of Verdun," Roderick Stewart continued, "Bethune opened a free clinic. Every Saturday at noon, he treated without charge women, children and unemployed men in Mooney's office. The Verdun clinic was almost a political act, Bethune's spontaneous, angry reaction to his own profession and a government indifferent to suffering."

Otherwise he was still politically conservative; until he went to the U.S.S.R. that August. He came away so impressed with the Soviet system of hospitalization, welfare, and social medicine, that within twelve weeks, in November, he joined the Communist Party in Montreal. As part of his new belief in socialized medicine he held meetings in his apartment, attended by medical people, social workers, and laymen of various political persuasions. "What brought us together," wrote Libbie Park, who was then doing part-time work at the Western Hospital outpatient department, "was a common concern at the deplorable condition of the health of the people and the health and medical services available to them and the economic problems of the medical and allied professions." Bethune "acted as secretary and leading spirit, always with a new idea." The meeting began at eight in the evening, with no formal agenda. "Norman would open the meeting with a few pungent remarks.... Once the meeting was over Norman relaxed completely, and I recall him driving Kay Dickson and me home to Notre-Dame-de-Grace and Montreal West in his little Ford roadster, singing sentimental songs like *Among My Souvenirs* and *Moonlight and Roses*. The volume of sound, not very melodic, tended to increase as we drove through the quiet, respectable streets of Montreal West nearing my home."

The profession, as a whole, utterly rejected the ideas on socialized medicine that Bethune expounded in speeches before such bodies as the Montreal Medico-Chirurgical Society. Even the proposals that would have eradicated tuberculosis were greeted with mistrust, partly because of their source, a man whose social and medical behaviour was increasingly beyond the pale. Writes Stewart: "He had always regarded doctors as narrow and lacking interest in cultural pursuits. Now he believed they were guilty of a more damaging charge. Their prime interest appeared to be their own social status, the direct result of their profits from the practice of medicine. Bethune posed a threat to this as the advocate of a scheme that would change radically their independent social and economic position."

The rejection of his plans by his profession was also a great blow to his self-esteem. He was always looking for recognition: "He wanted desperately to be meaningful." Yet he was growing away from his own profession, living on the fringes of society, ostracized and disoriented. He was searching constantly for a means of self-expression that would match his desire to live life significantly and vividly. He found it in Marxist communism.

Ironically, it was the communism rather than his talents that brought him the fame he yearned for, just as it was a kind of arrogance rather than a spirit of self-sacrifice that ended his life. He failed to wear rubber gloves while operating on an infected Chinese soldier, and died of blood poisoning. He claimed that rubber gloves reduced the sensitivity of his fingers.

34

Dr. Black's Skull

A NOTHER CANADIAN DOCTOR who achieved fame through his connection with China was Davidson Black, the discoverer of one of the most important of all clues to the development of *homo sapiens*. He was responsible for finding and identifying the fossilized skull of *Sinanthropus pekinensis*: Peking Man.

The discovery might easily have been frustrated. At one point in his career in Peking, Dr. Black was very nearly fired for allowing his enthusiasm for prehistoric bones to drag him away from rather more recent ones. He was professor of anatomy at Peking Union Medical College, and when his paymaster, Dr. Pearce of the Rockefeller Foundation, learned that Black was spending much of his time grubbing through dark, dreary caverns, instead of exploring ways of building up his department, he went to Peking to get rid of the seemingly scatter-brained Canadian. It was Black's warm and enthusiastic personality and Pearce's discovery that Black was an exceptionally skilled and knowledgeable man, that saved the errant anatomist. Even so, Pearce had to jolly, bully, threaten, and curse him into doing the job he was paid for.

Pearce considered Black's interest in paleontology and anthropology to be hardly more than a hobby, like stamp collecting or playing with model trains. "Give your entire attention to anatomy," he admonished Black. "Perhaps by that time, you will, with your young son, have other interests which will appear more important than expeditions to mythological caves."

Within four years of the discovery of Peking Man in a mountain cave, Davidson Black became loaded with honourary doctorates, gold medals, and memberships in the world's leading scientific institutions and societies, including a fellowship in a Royal Society that had included such illustrious members as Newton, Halley, Wren, Pepys, Darwin, Huxley, and Rutherford. The honours heaped upon Dr. Black were equaled only by those accorded to Frederick Banting ten years previously.

Davidson Black's career had begun in a topsy-turvy fashion. Born in Toronto in 1884, he never earned a penny in his own country. In his medical education he reversed the usual order by taking the pre-med course after obtaining his M.D. This was on the urging of one of his University of Toronto professors, A. B. Macallum, who felt that the twenty-two-year-old doctor was a promising anatomist but that his scientific education would be deepened through the further discipline of an arts course.

Over the next few years Dr. Black served as an ill-paid and unspectacular lecturer in anatomy at Western Reserve University in Cleveland, Ohio, and spent his summer doing field work with the Geological Survey of Canada. A glutton for knowledge, he also did research in neurology and was soon contributing to the *Journal of Comparative Neurology*. For the rest of his short life he wrote about five papers a year for learned journals, so that his name was known in scientific circles well before the great discovery.

He laboured in Cleveland and in the Canadian wilderness for four years before he could afford a vacation. He took it at the summer cottage of his cousins on Balsam Lake, northeast of Toronto, and spent much of the time hacking at the vegetation, to build up the winter wood pile. In his spare time he courted a girl named Adena Nevitt, daughter of a North West Mounted Police surgeon. But even the presence of his future wife could not keep him from the trough of knowledge. The rest of the summer was spent in British Columbia with the Geological Survey.

In 1914, accompanied by Adena, he took a leave of absence from Western Reserve to study advanced anatomy at Manchester University under the famous anatomist and anthropologist, G. Eiliot Smith. Smith was already familiar with Davidson Black's name from "his excellent original researches," and the two became close friends, a friendship made easier yet by Davidson's affectionate, almost naive nature. "He had a brain that moved easily and truly and he was blessed with a sunny, friendly temperament," as one British scientist said about him. By the time he returned to Cleveland he had, under Elliot's influence, added paleontology and anthropology to his already wide range of interests.

The influence of Elliot and that of a remarkable anthropological work, *Climate and Evolution*, by fellow Canadian W. D. Matthew of New Brunswick, was the turning point in his life. "There can be no doubt," wrote a contributor to the Black *Memorial Volume*, "that from this time on the problem of the origin and early evolution of man occupied first place in Black's mind. Immediately the scattered rays of previous interests came to a clear focus on this fascinating subject. He recognized at once that here was an opportunity for full investment of his unique capital in life; his inherent love of adventure, his instinct for discovery, even more his practical geological experience and perspective and his extensive knowledge of comparative anatomy in particular. All his previous interest and experiences immediately fell into their self-appointed places in this broad foundation of correlated qualifications that guided his approach to the new problem now uppermost in his mind."

After reading Matthew's book, Black yearned to explore China and other regions of Asia. Goethe once observed that "It is important to know exactly what you want in life because you are very apt to get it." Davidson Black got it when he was offered an appointment at the newly formed Peking Union Medical College, which was supported by the Rockefeller Foundation.

Davidson and Adena arrived in Peking in August 1919, and Davidson was boyishly delighted with the new medical college. It was strikingly different from the grim, classical schools of Europe and America, with its curved roofs of brilliant green tiles. As for the imperial city itself, it was like a vast, rather smelly and dusty park set in a semi-circular plain, jewelled with the yellow roofs of the palaces and the violet top of the Temple of Heaven. But it was the blue range of the Western Hills on the horizon to which Davidson first lifted his eyes; the hills that he intended to explore, as soon as he and his chief, E. V. Cowdry, had set up the anatomy department and organized the lectures and practical work for the Chinese students. Most of the students were from missionary colleges, and already spoke English.

Davidson had been teaching at the college for two years before it opened; officially, that is. Many outstanding medical men were invited to the opening ceremonies, one of them being Professor Macallum, who was now with McGill University. Macallum was one of the principal speakers. He became extremely huffy when the authorities insisted on vetting his speech. He was highly indignant at being thus edited, but "He was mollified when it was pointed out that when texts are translated into Chinese or English there were apt to be misunderstandings. In one instance, it was reported, a Chinese potentate had been transferred to another station and had 'taken his concubines on a train.' When translated into English it read, 'he had taken a trainload of concubines.'"

During the same year, Black's first child was born. An idea of the boyishness of his enthusiasm can be gained from a letter he wrote to a professor friend in Australia: "Listen to our news—on the morn of March 12th, 1921, a wee edition of Davidson Black arrived!!! How's that for real news!?!?!? Another bit of gossip is that Cowdry has resigned—owing to the ill-health of his wife—and I am now the incumbent in Anatomy here—aren't you sorry for Anatomy?"

Davidson's backers certainly were, for a while, and it was only a month or so later that their representative, Dr. Pearce, came to Peking to castigate the new professor. After which Davidson appears to have made an effort to mend his ways, and concentrate on anatomy rather than on rocks and fossils. But two years later he was off again, to Siam, to search for still more remnants of the past.

Even if Davidson Black had made no substantial contribution to science, his deep friendship with one of the world's greatest men would have made him notable. This was Pierre Teilhard de Chardin, priest, geologist, paleontologist, medical scientist, mystic, and a profound Christian thinker who showed in such works as *Le Phénomène Humain* and *Le Milieu Divin* that there was no real conflict between science and religion, but that each aspect of the one illuminates and enriches the other; and that mankind is headed in the right direction toward a future of self-fulfilment.

Teilhard and Davidson Black were alike in their modesty, simplicity, and in the depth of their knowledge. They took to each other instantly when Teilhard arrived in Peking on much the same anthropological quest as he had brought his Canadian friend. From then on the French scientist was always received with joy and laughter in the Black household. The Blacks found Teilhard a captivating guest, while the guest described Davidson as being filled with "quiet animation, charm, and vitality." On learning of Black's untimely death in 1934, Teilhard was deeply affected, and said about his fellow genius that "He was more than a brother to me."

Teilhard continued the excavations in China after Black's death and contributed many papers on the subject of *Sinanthropus pekinensis*.

By 1929, the Rockefeller Foundation had been converted by Black's enthusiasms, and was now substantially backing his anthropological work, including the excavations at Chou K'ou-tien in the Western Hills. There the uncovering of a few items, such as fragments of fossilized teeth, had already taken the investigators some distance in reconstructing man's physical origins in the later Middle Pleistocene Age, (the age roughly between 400,000 and 250,000 BC). But more substantial evidence was needed, for it was upon such material as skulls that man's development could be most exactly reconstructed.

After Black had been leading the work at Chou K'ou-tien for eight years, such a skull was discovered in 1929 by one of Black's workers, W. C. Pei. During the autumn, Dr. Black had made frequent trips to the site, always with the effect of reviving the enthusiasm of the scientists and the Chinese manual workers alike. "This was the key to his achievement. The whole enterprise was conceived on a grand scale and never abandoned even when hope was long deferred. For three years it was expected that larger parts of *Sinanthropus* would be discovered, and news of more finds were eagerly awaited by geologists and anatomists in Europe and America, many of whom took the long journey to Peking. Still only large and small fragments of jaw bones and teeth had been unearthed. By late 1929 the number of visitors had fallen off and interest had gradually diminished. There remained in Peking only a few staunch scientists and the remotely curious international population."

Teilhard, however, remained faithful to the enterprise, and, of course, Davidson's enthusiasm never flagged. He was convinced that sooner or later a missing link in the evolution of man would join the anthropological chain and one bitterly cold day late in November, Pei found two caves in one of the fissures. And, on December 1, Pei reported, "I began to remove the uppermost part of the accumulation filling the cave. At four o'clock next afternoon I encountered the almost complete skull of *Sinanthropus*. The specimen was imbedded partly in loose sands and partly in a hard matrix so that it was possible to extricate it with relative ease."

Trembling with excitement, he wrapped it in layers of Chinese cotton paper and then a heavy layer of cloth impregnated with flour paste, and with the skull in the basket of his bicycle, rode the twenty-five miles to the medical college, and with his face "shining with pride and joy," presented it to Dr. Black.

Though the actual discovery had been made by a co-worker, it was naturally the man who had inspired the eight years' search for fossil man who was credited with the great discovery, and who was so acclaimed throughout the world. ("Being front-page stuff is new sensation," Davidson wrote, "and encourages a guarded manner of speech!") Nevertheless, he insisted on putting Pei's name on the title page of his official report on the story of the discovery and identification of *Sinanthropus*, and also those of his associates, Teilhard de Chardin and C. C. Young.

The discovery may have shortened his life. The increased workload resulting from the discovery and his extensive travels on business and on lecture tours, and to receive worldwide honours, exhausted him. On a trip to the caves at Chou K'ou-tien to see the results of the 1933 excavations he had a heart attack, but insisted on carrying on with the inspection. A hospital examination a few days later indicated that he had not long to live. He died in his laboratory the following year, still hard at work.

There was an ironical footnote to Black's great achievement. His fossils, which had been hidden in the earth for millions of years, disap-peared twelve years later. Placed in charge of a detachment of U.S. Marines, they were to be shipped to the United States in December, 1941. They never arrived. When the marines reached the Chinese port of embarkation, they were taken prisoner by the Japanese. The boxes of fossils were never seen again.

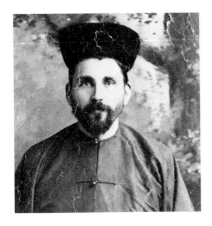

LEFT: William E. Smith, missionary in West China. (United Church of Canada) BELOW: Florence Murray — dedication and faith in Manchuria and Korea. (United Church)

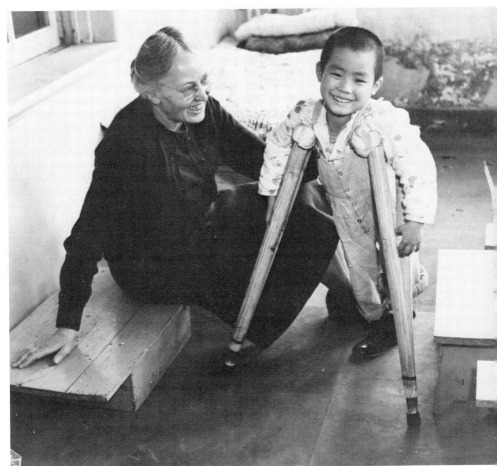

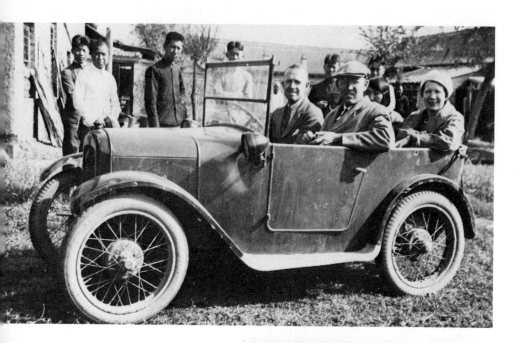

ABOVE: **Dr. Robert** McClure on tour. (United Church) RIGHT: McClure operating sideways. (United Church)

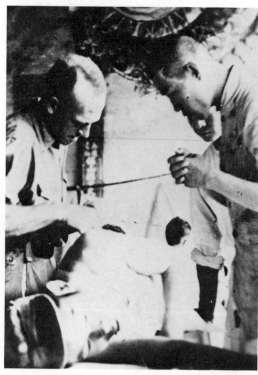

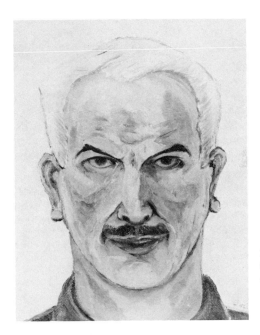

LEFT: Bethune—how he
saw himself. (Public Ar-
chives Canada/PA114793)
BELOW: The tenderness the
others saw. (PAC/
PA114792)

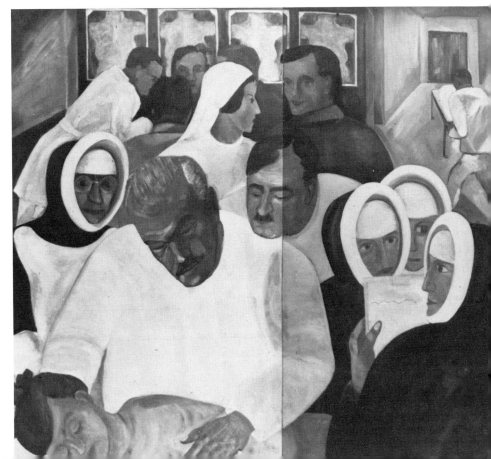

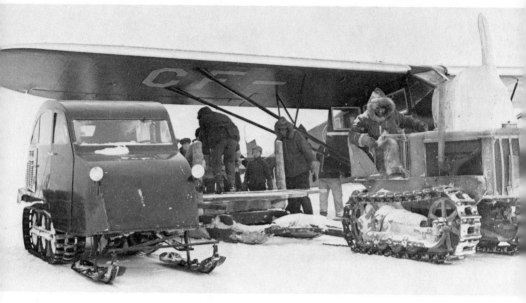

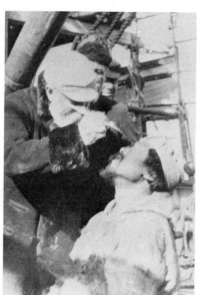

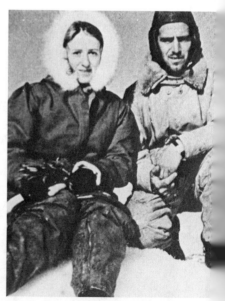

TOP: A Hudson Bay Eskimo being airlifted to Moosonee in 1946. The machine on the left is the original snowmobile. (PAC/PA11456) ABOVE LEFT: Ashe Inlet, 1897—open air treatment. (The doctor was Robert Bell.) (PAC/C6860) ABOVE RIGHT: Viola and Joe Moody. (Joseph Moody)

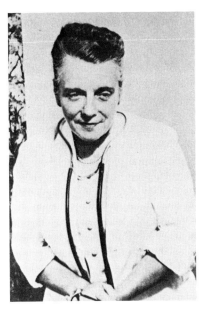

LEFT: Marion Hilliard. (Everett Roseborough Ltd., Toronto)
BELOW: Wilder Penfield.
(PAC/C29714)

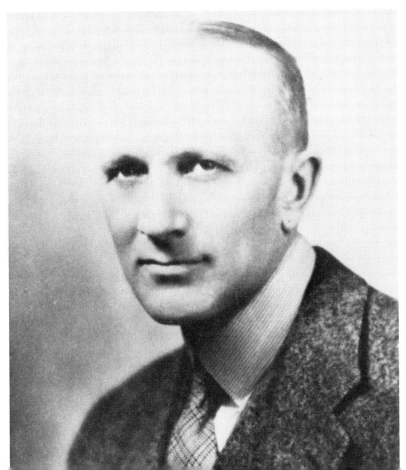

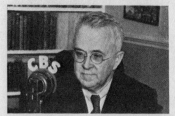

ABOVE: An advertisement for Dr. Dafoe's syndicated radio program. RIGHT: Hans Selye.

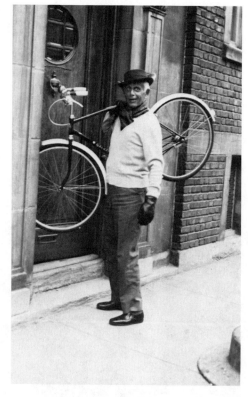

35

That Vicious Power in Women

MARION HILLIARD MET many women who underestimated their own biology, and she was always trying to set them straight. Nature, she would tell the girls, had gone to considerable trouble to make them attractive to men, so they should not be surprised when their attributes proved to be in working order. When the girls said that they were not that kind of girl, Dr. Hilliard would reply, "nonsense. Except for a statistical handful who have abnormally low metabolisms, everybody is that kind of girl."

"From the day she is born until she dies," Dr. Hilliard wrote, "a woman must live with her gender.... Femaleness... is savage. Woman is equipped with a reproductive system which, even if she never uses it, dominates her fiber. It has a vicious power that can leap out of control without the slightest warning, while a man and a woman share a companionable chuckle or happen to touch hands. In the time it takes to blink, they have reached a point of no return. The mechanism of woman can also be triggered unexpectedly by the low moan of a crooner, by a summer sky full of stars, by the sight of a man's hands working with metal, or even by fog collecting around a street light. Involuntarily the woman is twisted inside with anguish and longing."

The country's foremost obstetrical specialist, a woman with an intuitive understanding of marriage's most intimate relationships, who had an uncommon warmth of sympathy for men as well as women, and who could discuss, elucidate, and advise on sexual matters with serene candour and without moral undertones, was a lifelong spinster.

The quick, bright, fun-loving child of a sternly religious family of the kind that has produced so many of Canada's most notable citizens of character and integrity, Marion reminded herself repeatedly during her training at the University of Toronto that marriage was out of the question until she was well established in a career. At college she played the field, but avoided emotional entanglements. Among those in the field was a McGill man who appeared to have triggered her female mechanism, but not enough to detonate it into a physical affair. As far as one can tell in the absence of any explicit revelation, she was well advanced in her career before she experienced the physical side of love. Her life at college was hectic with canoeing, concerts, hockey, tennis, and religion—when she wasn't attending lectures, skylarking with her Kappa Kappa Gamma sisters, and dissecting her anatomical subject "Dead Ernest." Presumably she was filling her life with vigorous activities, including a devotion to the Student Christian Movement, in order to devitalize the "vicious power."

The trouble was that the reason for the delay made the delay permanent. She established her career so smartly that shortly after her graduation in 1927, she was much in demand in obstetrical work at the Woman's College Hospital. One evening, she went out for a drive with the man she hoped to marry. She was pretty sure he was going to propose, and it was a perfect night for it, with a "summer sky full of stars." Unfortunately the trigger malfunctioned. Worn-out after four successive nights in the delivery room, she fell asleep in the car.

Her companion found this quite unforgivable. Which was not difficult to understand. Perhaps he had been working up to a proposal by comparing her lips to rose petals, just as a gentle snore issued from those lips. On the other hand, Marion had subsequent cause for annoyance as well. He not only married a friend of hers soon afterwards, with humiliating haste—but in due course he came back to her to ask if she would deliver his first child.

According to her biographer Marion O. Robinson, Dr. Hilliard's unmarried state brought "a shredding sense of failure," not least because it deprived her of babies of her own. This was a bitter renunciation. Naturally it never occurred to her to confound the morality of the time by becoming an unmarried mother; her attitudes were too firmly shaped in the Methodist mould. In fact, sex had very nearly turned her away from medicine at one point in her career. Shortly after she started her clinical work in medical school, she attended a woman patient with a broken arm. Marion was shocked when the patient chortled that she had broken it by falling out of bed while making love. It was not so much the cause of the accident that unsettled Marion as the woman's laughing candour about it. It was not right to joke about sex, as if it were something as natural as eating fish and chips.

Her confusion was compounded when the clinician before whom she presented the case made funny remarks as well. Marion fled to the telephone and told her father that she wanted to quit medicine. Naturally she didn't give him the reason for this decision. She merely informed him that it was costing him too much money to keep her in medical school.

Her father, a lawyer in Morrisburg, Ontario, had originally opposed her desire to go in for medicine. While she was working for her B.A. he understood that it was her intention to become a science teacher, which was respectable. He couldn't see her as a member of the medical profession in which, even by the 1920s, a woman was still considered something of a freak. But her excellent showing at university had helped him to adjust to the idea. Now, over the telephone, he pursuaded her to stick it out, and not worry about the money.

His support was exactly what Marion needed to help her face not just the jokes, but the sordid realities of sickness and poverty that she was encountering for the first time. She remained warmly grateful to her father for the rest of her life. As for the sexy sallies, Marion soon adjusted to the greater frankness of the age, to the extent that ultimately she was able to make them herself; like the time when she was working on a sterility case to determine why a couple had been unable to produce children. When the husband, unable to find a more suitable container, delivered a sample of his sperm in a quart jar: "Wow, what a man," said Marion.

It was during the Second World War, when Marion was forty, that she fell most deeply in love. Given her now outspoken knowledge of love's pain and ecstasy, she must have known its physical side from personal experience, so it is likely that this friend became her lover. But the affair had no conclusion. He was married.

Some time afterward she wrote about the moment when a woman realizes she will probably never marry. "Her friends have small children and she is tortured by the knowledge that she will never hold her baby. She is calling herself a bachelor girl, but she knows the synonym is old maid. At this point in her life passion is going to sear her to the bone. She is bound to fall in love and her love is almost sure to be married. That's how fate always seems to set it up."

Marion was just the sort of woman she wrote about sympathetically. She could not, or would not, try to live up to the standard of judgement adopted by most men in considering a woman as a mate, to whit, is she a dish? In her early twenties she was a bouncy girl with bright blue eyes and fair hair, and she was fun to be with as far as her personality was concerned; but she had no idea how to make the most of herself. She wore homemade clothes, often a heavy gray cloth coat almost like a military cape; her long, sometimes untidy hair captured in a bun at the back of her neck. In the words of her biographer, such an ensemble did nothing to conceal her "inclination to chunkiness." She was one of those enthusiastic girls who clattered noisily on stairways. Her first apartment in Toronto, shared with her friend Dr. Eve Mader, a Dalhousie graduate, was in the attic of a three-story house on St. Mary's Street, where there was a bed for one girl, a convertible sofa for the other, orange crates for dining chairs, and on the wall a map of London, where Marion had obtained her L.R.C.P. and the M.R.C.S. (the third Canadian woman to achieve membership in the Royal College of Surgeons). The rest of the tenants in the house were always complaining about the noisy way Marion clumped downstairs to attend a patient in the early hours of the morning. Even the timid librarian on the floor below remonstrated with young Dr. Hilliard. Marion would apologize most humbly, and promise to go quietly next time, but was always in such a hurry that she usually forgot. Yet the values that would make lifelong friends of so many of her patients were already there, in her heavy-lidded eyes and sympathetic aura. Her personality at the height of her career is summed up in one photograph, which shows her at her desk in a typical posture: hands peacefully crossed, attention focused unwaveringly on the woman she is talking to; the posture of a woman who comforts by listening, rather than through verbal exhortation. In that photograph she looks truly beautiful.

Marion Hilliard's career was most intimately bound up with the Women's College Hospital. She had interned there, and when she returned with her prestigious London degrees she was appointed to the obstetrics staff. The hospital, unique in Canada, then occupied a converted mansion on Rushholme Road. A new building was constructed in the mid-thirties on its present site, and Marion remained profoundly involved in its follies and fortunes for the rest of her professional life, despite a growing conflict with her chief, tall, handsome, Marion Kerr.

As the years went by, Marion Hilliard's devotion to the hospital grew steadily more intense. She wanted it to be the very best women's hospital in the world. As most of the great hospitals were also teaching institutions, that too was her goal for the W.C.H. But many of the staff members were against this step. Their qualifications were not likely to be acceptable to the faculty of medicine of the university. Many members of the staff were likely to be replaced if it became a teaching institution. It was all right for Dr. Hilliard to be agitating for affiliation. She was, by 1946, a certified specialist. *She* was all right. She'd certainly keep her job as an associate in the department of obstetrics and gynecology, but where would they be? Out in the cold. No, it just wasn't the right time for the W.C.H. to become a teaching hospital.

In fact, the lady was not at all sure that she would be eligible for the indoor attending staff of a teaching hospital, despite her depth of experience and her special work in cancer. (In the late forties she helped to devise a simplified version of the Pap test for early detection of cancer of the cervix and uterus.) But according to Marion Robinson, "she felt that if she could be accepted even temporarily as chief of a teaching department, she would be willing to step aside in favour of a better qualilified doctor."

Thus her ambitions for the hospital took precedence over her own. Her chief, Dr. Kerr, on the other hand, wanted to keep her job at all costs, and the growing conflict between the ladies led to the only real professional crisis in Dr. Hilliard's life. The growing coolness between the two saddened Marion Hilliard. They had been good friends in the past, despite their differences in temperament; Hilliard quick and impulsive, Kerr, cautious and conservative. The crisis came to a head in the mid-forties when Marion was nominated for the chairmanship of the Medical Advisory Board. As chairman she would have been in a position to make the W.C.H. a teaching institution. The opposition began to lobby powerfully on behalf of her opponent. "On the day of the election the meeting was astonishingly well attended. It was said that some members who did not usually come to the meetings had been recruited to vote for Dr. Hilliard's opponent. Marion lost the election, and retreated in dignity, but wept behind closed doors because so many of her colleagues had joined together to defeat her, solely because she held a conviction that she honestly believed to be for the good of the hospital." She was particularly distressed because the hospital, the only one in Canada staffed entirely by women, should have been a symbol of women's aspiration in medicine. Now because of the obduracy of a few members of the staff it was becoming an ingrown institution.

It was particularly unfortunate because the struggle occurred at a time when the standards of Canadian medicine had reached world-class level. The requirements of the Royal College of Physicians and Surgeons of Canada were exacting enough that it was no longer necessary for medical graduates to complete their education abroad, as Marion had done only twenty years previously. The standards of the college were at least as high as those of Edinburgh. Often as many as two-thirds of the candidates failed the first part of the college's two-part examination. It was not unknown for *all* candidates to fail the second. So Marion was particularly concerned that her hospital should match the new standards, and be a symbol of opportunity for her sex.

Her own opportunity finally came shortly before her forty-fifth birthday, when the Advisory Board recommended that department chiefs be appointed for a maximum of fifteen years or until they reached the age of fifty-five, whichever came sooner. Whereupon Dr. Kerr resigned, and Marion was appointed in her place as chief of the department.

Even so, several years went by before she was able to establish the teaching program in her department and then only by presenting it to the staff as a *fait accompli*.

Unable to face the uproar that she feared was bound to follow, Marion left town for a holiday in Maine. There was indeed an uproar. The qualifications for the indoor staff proved to be devastating: every doctor had to be a Fellow of the Royal College of Physicians and Surgeons. Many bitter things were said about Dr. Hilliard's ruthless behaviour. It did not occur to the infuriated staff that by forcing through these eligibility requirements, Marion had sacrificed her own future in the hospital. For she had not had the confidence to sit for the dreaded two-part examination. Which is why she resigned a year later, 1957, to make way for Dr. Geraldine Maloney, F.R.C.P.S., Canada.

Just as the patients of Agnodice in ancient Greece were relieved to be attended by that woman doctor rather than by her male colleagues who, however warm or sympathetic, could never really understand childbirth from a woman's point of view, so Marion Hilliard's patients were delighted to be attended by one of their own sex. Many of them, in fact, were overjoyed because of past experience. Male doctors would probably be shocked if they realized the depth of resentment that many women felt toward them. Women often found male specialists to be not merely lacking in understanding, but physically rough, and sometimes behaving toward women and their problems with a contempt that could not quite be concealed. "Science first, and one-to-one last," as one woman put it, adding, "Personally I dislike them [male gynecologists] strongly, and have for years, and so have many of my friends."

In the 1970s Dr. Henry Morgentaler took great pains to guard the feelings and privacy of his abortion patients in the operating room, but even today not all male specialists are as sensitive. Marion's patients were particularly happy to be in her hands because she was not only delicate and skilled, but light-hearted, wise, considerate, and above all, understanding. In her prime she delivered as many as fifty private and public ward patients a month, and even though forty patients a day might pass through her suite in the Medical Arts Building, very very few of them felt they were being treated impersonally, even though the ones with no forseeable complications might be quickly dismissed with cheerful reassurance. If they were reasonable they understood that this was to make more time available for those who, for psychological or physical reasons, needed the doctor's undivided attention. A woman having her first baby is in "for an experience of special fears, special hazards, special wonder, and a poignancy beyond all other human experience," Dr. Hilliard wrote, and, "Each person comes to your office with new problems and a new difficulty, and the treatment," she added, "is not the most important part of the office visit, though of course it is important that it be accurate, definite, and in accordance with the best known therapy of the day. But that is only the beginning. The most important thing is that this person... shall have the faith to carry out what is written down on those little pieces of paper. She has to be helped to have that faith."

These words are quoted from one of her most penetrating essays, *Women's Greatest Enemy is Fatigue*; fatigue was just beginning to be recognized as "the most common affliction known to women," as the *Journal of the American Medical Women's Association* puts it—and which might have added that Hilliard was one of the first to draw attention in print to that special problem. It was her writings that made her known far beyond the privileged company that she treated directly. The beauty and sensitivity of her insights struck a woman's heart. It was common sense, illumination, revelation, whether she was guiding—"The modern insistence on the female orgasm is a serious mistake that mars many unions," or revealing how—"The physical love of women springs from total stimulation." Her words, written or spoken, as well as her actions, restored thousands of women to health. "My wife is so much better, so much more confident," said one husband, "What did you tell her?" Marion answered the question on another occasion when she wrote that, "I have been watching the many lives of women for a quarter century; the adolescent with her terrible fears, the young wife with her dismay at lovemaking, the unmarried mother with terror in her eyes, the career woman with her longings, the older woman with her loneliness. I knew them all and I would be insensitive and a poor doctor if I didn't try to help."

36

Seagull for Christmas

WHEN EDMUND BRASSET was summoned to the office of the dean of the Dalhousie School of Medicine one day in 1933, he sauntered in, confident that he was not about to be accused of the student's worst crime, that of being found out. He had long since abandoned the kind of pranks—ragging the burghers of Halifax, hanging corpses outside co-ed dormitories—that get medical students into trouble. Edmund knew that the dean could have nothing to complain of, either in his conduct or his work. He was smugly aware that nobody was working harder than he was towards his goal of obtaining a surgical residency in the hospital after serving the usual few years as a dogsbody intern. Only three or four fellows at the top of the list in the final-year examinations would be chosen for these special appointments, and Edmund was determined that he was going to be one of them. But when he walked into the office, he saw at once that the dean had unpleasant news to impart. The news was that Edmund was working himself to death. His nightly cramming would not alter the situation. Edmund had no chance of getting a residency. "Even though you were to come highest in every subject," said the dean, "we still could not recommend you."

As Edmund stared at him, speechless with shock, the dean went on to point out that though Brasset was doing well enough, over the years at least half a dozen others had done better. And it was the long-term results that counted. Edmund was just not in the running.

However, the dean told him not to worry; and with surgical precision, made the unkindest cut of all. "After all," he said, "there is nothing we need more than good, sound general practitioners."

494

Edmund's humiliation was complete. Since his earliest student days he had absorbed the attitude that the G.P. was at the lowest level of the medical caste system. Not that the rest of the fraternity ever said so, in so many words, but that was the distinct impression that Edmund had gained at medical school; that "the man in the field" was looked down upon in a good-natured way as being a bumbling amateur, compared with, say, a hospital resident. The G.P. was often unscientific, frequently quaint or downright peculiar, like the old country doctor who insisted on his patients bringing him samples of their urine so that he could immediately empty the bottles and save a few cents by re-using them.

For two weeks, Edmund remained in a "bitter, foolish and selfish state of mind." Until one day he overheard a chief surgeon discussing an amusing acquaintance of his, a country doctor who owned a cranberry bog and who talked about nothing but cranberries—but who was making a steady fifteen thousand simoleans a year.

Edmund suddenly realized that the G.P. trail might be almost as direct a route to his goal as a hospital appointment. From the moment he had first trepanned a subject (sawing off the crown at its head), he had had a burning ambition to be a brain surgeon. Why could he not become a G.P. for, say, a couple of years, then subsidize himself through the long and difficult neurological training, after making a positive mountain of loot? There would be nothing to it. It would mean only a minor interruption to his neurosurgical career. "Besides, the extra experience gained as a 'man in the field' would not be entirely wasted," he wrote in his autobiography, *A Doctor's Pilgrimage*. "It would be dull, of course, but I would make the best of it, and the two years would fly by pretty fast."

As things turned out, many more than two years would fly by before Edmund could finally realize his consuming ambition. Far from emulating the cranberry man, at one stage in his career he would find himself so deeply in debt that he would seriously contemplate fleeing to India.

However, Dr. Brasset soon found out that he was quite wrong in thinking that private practice was dull. He found himself involved with criminals and addicts, tightwads and loose women, bullies, saints, drunkards, and ghosts. His first practice was on Cape Breton, a misty, mountainous island of extraordinary beauty and, in 1934, of extraordinary poverty, as C. Lamont MacMillan had already discovered. MacMillan, the doctor who was apt to relieve his fatigue by hopping into his patient's bed, had then been practicing for six years at Baddeck, just a few miles away.

Dr. Brasset arrived at Canso in a new Ford V-8 that was loaded with equipment and medical supplies, all of which had been obtained on credit. Canso itself lived mostly on the credit of the sea. It was a fishing town of mud and bare rock and scoured shacks. The shops on one side of the main street were so close to the Atlantic Ocean that they hung over the water on piles. The only decent houses in the town, further along the rocky shore, past the flimsy jetties and stout dories, belonged to the employees of the Cable Company. Canso was a relay station for the transatlantic cable.

Edmund's first patient was a young woman who had been feeding her four-month-old baby on dried cod, bread, tea, and molasses. On this regime the infant had begun to look distinctly sick. For a man who was bent on accumulating a substantial capital, Edmund's start was not too promising. Affected as much by the mother's poverty as by her dietary nescience, he treated her to a case of canned milk for the baby. She promptly traded it in on a new scarf for herself.

Most new doctors begin their professional lives with a sense of their own incompetence, and Brasset was no exception. For this reason, and because he had never had to worry about money, having been subsidized by a reasonably well-off family, he did not have the heart to ask for payment even from those who could afford his modest fees. The fact that he was in a poverty-stricken area further afflicted by the Great Depression sorely inhibited him. He just could not bring himself to dun his patients. Consequently, by mid-winter he was in serious trouble with his host of creditors, and every encounter with his bank manager was ending in humiliation.

But how could he demand payment from people like the family of eight who called him in on Christmas Day to deliver the mother of her sixth child. They were all living in a one-room shack. Their Christmas dinner was composed of seagull meat and a pot of tea. Cooked seagull was a vile dish at the best of times, but at *Christmas....* There was no other food in the house, not even molasses, the local staple. To make matters worse, when he delivered the child, he found himself looking at an almost headless monstrosity, with the eyes on top.

By the beginning of the following year Edmund was angrily questioning his own conduct, wondering how it was that after working for eighteen hours a day for seven days a week for six months, his income was so feeble that it had barely the strength to serve him at the dinner table, let alone see to the installments on his car, his instruments, his equipment, and the expensive drugs he was doling out so freely. Admittedly the people were poor. Yet the local liquor store was thriving, he noticed. So was the motion picture palace. Even the local clergymen were making a better living that he was. At this rate he would never realize his ambition to be the world's greatest neurosurgeon. In fact he would be lucky if he did not become a butt for the Halifax humourists. "Saw poor old Dr. Brasset the other day. Good man but quite unworldly, you know. He's so poor that the mice are leaving crumbs for him. He...." But Edmund had no wish to imagine what they were saying. He decided that he would turn over a new leaf in his ledger, keep his books up-to-date from now on. He would damn well insist on payment, at least from those who could afford it.

While in this rebellious mood, he received a call one midnight from Matt Nichols, a local bully. Matt reported that somebody had been hurt at his place, which was twenty miles away.

Edmund was tempted to refuse, for he heartily disliked the man. A month previously, Edmund's car had slid into a ditch in front of Nichol's house, but the swine had refused to help, saying that he was too busy mending his lobster traps.

Unfortunately it was quite likely that the accident was serious, so in a foul mood, Edmund set off through the miserable fog. The journey took two hours. When he walked in, he found Matt, Matt's brother, and a third man sprawled around in a drunken stupour.

One of the men was lying on the floor, and for a moment Edmund thought that this was his patient. Then a woman reeled in, carrying a kerosene lamp. Though decidedly tipsy, she managed to impart the information that the injured man was upstairs.

There he found yet another drunk, collapsed in a bloodstained bunk. He had a lacerated scalp. a portion of which had detatched from the bone and was turned back like a flap.

Edmund worked on him for at least an hour, trying to cope with the others' struggles and bad language. He managed to clean the wound, shave the scalp and suture the edges of the wound; then he applied a dressing to cover the whole top of the man's head. Finally, with no help from the woman who could barely manage to hold the kerosene lamp steady, he completed the job. After giving the woman directions in the care of the patient, he went downstairs. Facing a conscious but unsteady Matt Nichols, Edmund asked curtly for his twenty-two-dollar fee.

Matt looked pretty astonished at the doctor's unusually determined tone. "Sure, Doc," he said after a moment. "I'll tell him in the morning when he sobers up, and he'll go in and pay you."

Brasset said that wouldn't do, and insisted on being paid immediately by all three of the men in the room. Matt began to look more alert.

"'But he's the one that got hurt, Doc, it's none of my business.'

"Look," I said, "the four of you and this woman have been having a drinking party together. You all get drunk and one of you gets hurt. It's up to all of you to chip in and pay me."

"'Hey! you're crazy, Doc,' said Matt slowly. 'If you think we're going to pay you.'

"All of you put your money on the table and I'll take my twenty-two dollars from the pile in equal shares from each." As I said this I kicked at the man on the floor gently to try to make him wake up.

"'Like hell, we will,' said Matt.

"I have always been a very mild person," Dr. Brasset wrote, "the kind that will not talk back to waitresses. The only real fighting I had done since my childhood days was at college—using gloves as big as pillows, and at that I was no champ. Before me was Matt, big and ugly and mean. Before I realized what I was doing I had smashed him a blow in the mouth that made the blood run and laid him out on the floor. His brother, who had been sitting on the opposite side of the table, now got up with a wild look and started to lurch around toward me. I did not wait for him. I went after him. I had the advantage of being sober and also very angry. I caught him a good blow on the jaw that knocked him down. At the same time the woman, whom I had forgotten, screamed and dropped the lamp. The lampshade broke and the flame blazed up as the oil began to leak out. There was a coat lying on the back of a chair. I picked it up and threw it over the lamp, putting it out.

"The place was still lighted by the lamp which stood on the centre of the table and I saw Matt getting up again. I hit him again before he was fairly up on his feet—I know it was against the Queensberry rules. This time he fell in a sitting position, his back against the wall. He was not unconscious but he did not try to get up at once. I looked around for someone else to hit. The third man, who had been lying on the floor in a drunken sleep, was awake and shaking his head in confusion. I went over to him and told him to get up off the floor, slapping his face a few times in order to emphasize the order. He got into a sitting position. Matt started to get up also, but not to fight. He reached into his pocket and threw a handful of bills on the table. Then, without a word, he went around the table to where his brother was lying and pulled him to his feet. He, too, emptied his pockets and put his money on the table. The third man did the same thing, with some assistance from Matt. There was more than a hundred and twenty dollars on the table. I took twenty-two dollars out of the pile and started to leave. As I turned, who should be standing in the doorway, staring stupidly, but the patient on whom I had been working only a short time before. He had ripped off the elaborate dressing I had fixed on his head and was holding it in his hand like a cap."

Naturally Edmund did not adopt this method of bill-collecting as a standard procedure. Nevertheless he stuck to his resolution to make his patients pay up whenever possible, with the result that over the next year he went further into debt by a mere twelve hundred dollars.

So, notwithstanding his affection for Canso, Edmund Brasset left after about two years. He simply could not afford to stay unless he was prepared to give up the "Great Idea" of becoming a brain surgeon.

By 1936 that goal seemed further away than ever. He was nearly five thousand dollars in debt. He simply had to establish a well-paying practice soon, or not only would he never realize his ambition, but the very tools of his trade, his surgical instruments, would likely be repossessed, leaving him worse off than he had been as a third-year student.

It was in a mood of aching frustration that one day Edmund went to visit a former classmate in Sydney, about a hundred miles away. His friend told him of a temporary job that was available in New Waterford. A Dr. Munster needed somebody to take over his practice for a year or so, to free himself for a sojourn in England.

The New Waterford practice was an unusually lucrative one, considering that the province was in the depths of the Depression. Most of the income came from health insurance contributions by those miners who were fortunate enough to have jobs. Under an agreement negotiated between the mining companies in the town and its employees, a sum of forty cents was deducted each week from the miners' pay and turned over to a doctor of the miners' choice. Bill Munster had hundreds of miners on his books. The arrangement he made with Edmund Brasset was that he, Munster, would continue to receive his weekly cheques from the company pay office while he was abroad, and out of this income he would pay Edmund a smallish monthly salary.

Edmund was quite satisfied with this contract, confident that later he would be able to establish a practice and work up a list of miners of his own. There was another advantage to living in New Waterford. The town had X-ray, laboratory, and hospital facilities. Brasset was tired of improvising and frustrated at rarely being able to practice sophisticated surgery. Besides, there was another reason for moving to New Waterford. It was the home of his girl friend, Sally MacNeil, a tall, slim, hazel-eyed beauty whom he had met in Halifax while she was still a student nurse.

He married her the following January and together they moved into a four-room flat on Scotchtown Road; which took Edmund still deeper into debt when he added the cost of installment payments on the furniture. But that was all right. Sally being a girl of common sense, was bound to know all about financial management. She would thus compensate for his own fecklessness over money matters.

Unfortunately, Sally had been keeping a secret from him. She was almost as poor at mathematics as he was. The situation, instead of improving, got worse. Finally, tired of worrying about money all the time, they decided to institute "Worry Sessions," which would be held at a set time during the evening, say between eight and nine o'clock.

When Dr. Munster returned from England a few months later, Edmund was free to go into practice on his own. There was just one problem. The agreement between the coal mining company and the miners was that at least one-quarter of the strength of any particular colliery had to sign over their health insurance cards to a doctor before the doctor could qualify. The smallest colliery employed eight hundred and twenty men. That meant that Dr. Brasset needed two hundred and five applicants. Medical ethics forbade him from soliciting patients. How was he then to lure the men onto his list?

Other physicians in the district came to his aid by lending him a few patients; that is, asking the patients to transfer to Dr. Brasset's list until he had met the minimum requirements. In this way he obtained sixty names. That still left him short a hundred and forty-five names.

Every night he talked it over with Sally during their "Worry Sessions." Now that Munster had returned, there was no money at all coming in. But they still had to pay the rent, eat, keep warm, pay the telephone bill, and maintain an office. The debts were soaring again—now approaching six thousand dollars. They were desperate. They were afraid to open the mail in case it contained another threat from a creditor.

The solution came in the form of rum-reeking Bad Chris. Bad Chris was an enemy who had been converted into a a spot of quick thinking. One evening he had come lurching, very drunk, into Edmund's office, and Edmund had sent him packing in what proved to be a decidedly tactless fashion, for he learned too late that Bad Chris had beaten up quite a few citizens against whom he bore grudges.

Sure enough, Bad Chris turned up again the following night, waited until Edmund had dealt with all the other patients, then walked slowly into the office with bunched fists and a mean look in his eye. Edmund braced himself, determined to sell his life as dearly as possible. Then suddenly he had an inspiration.

"'Look, Bad Chris, I said, 'am I glad to see you! You came in at exactly the right time. I just got a call to go down to Lennoxville.' (This was true.) 'There's an awfully tough crowd down there and I was wondering if I should get a couple of policemen to come with me for a bodyguard. How about coming with me for a bodyguard? That is,' I added, 'if you have the time.'"

"I could see a change come over the knobby features. He did not say anything for almost a minute. Then he said, 'Sure Doc, I got time. Let's go.'

"His voice was gruff and rasping but I knew he was pleased and proud. His grudge had disappeared."

From then on, Bad Chris became a loyal friend and helper. The only lawful work he ever did was done for Dr. Brasset—polishing his car and keeping his company on his long, lonely calls into the countryside.

Bad Chris now offered, quite gratuitously, to help the doc get onto the colliery payroll. His gang of rowdies would do the recruiting. All Doc Brasset had to do was accept the cards and maybe treat the boys to a drink as a reward.

Within days, Bad Chris and his lads had landed in a total of two hundred and twelve cards, and Edmund was on the colliery payroll.

With his first pay cheque of eighty-two dollars, he and Sally were able to eat meals that were rather more ambitious than the potatoes and point on which they had been subsisting. (The Maritime dish, potatoes and point, was said to have been invented by a sea cook during a long sea voyage. Finding the pork barrel empty, the cook had suspended the last scrap of meat above the galley table on the end of a piece of string, so that the crew could point to it with their forks, between mouthfuls of boiled spuds.)

The splendid income from the colliery did not last long. The patients who had been loaned by other doctors had to be paid back. So once again Edmund found that his income was diminishing rather than increasing, and once again he could not keep up with his payments and expenses. To save on gas, he swapped the Ford V-8 for an Austin Seven, which could get forty miles to the gallon, but even that economy was not sufficient. His income continued to decline. Finally, when the creditors threatened to take him to court, he was forced to give up and look for a job that would provide him with a steady salary, however small. Among the other complications, now, Sally was four months pregnant.

A year or so later, after a tranquil interlude as resident physician in a hospital for the violently insane, Brasset tried private practice again, this time in Little Brook, at the western end of Nova Scotia. There he rented a nine-room house for five dollars a month, moved in, arranged the equipment round his office, and braced himself for the worst, half-expecting that once again his hopes would be lifted, only to be dashed against the rocks of penury.

At the end of the first day, when he counted the cash he had received, he found that it totaled thirty-eight dollars, the largest daily sum he had ever taken in. He was on his way at last.

Brasset's new territory, along the shores of the Bay of Fundy, near Digby, was populated mainly by the descendants of the Acadian French, that hardy, stubborn people who had been expelled from their homes twenty years before the American Revolution, and scattered through the American colonies. The mass deportation had been brought about by their refusal to swear allegiance to the Crown. Getting a hostile reception from the American colonists, many of the surviving six thousand Acadians had drifted back to Nova Scotia and New Brunswick. Their descendants now numbered ten thousand, and Edmund found them an extremely likeable breed; while they in turn approved of their forthright new doctor, especially as he could speak fluent French.

In particular, Edmund admired their self-sufficiency. Most of them owned their own homes, and heated them with their own wood fuel, preserved their eggs in water glass, grew their own vegetables, canned their own meat—chicken, pork, beef, and venison—preserved the seashore's plentiful supply of lobsters and clams, and crushed their own apples to make their own exuberant cider.

The only scarcity in the district was in the supply of surnames. There were hundreds and hundreds of Comeaus and Saulniers, Melansons, Belleveaus, Thibaults and Gaudets. Further complicating the task of identification was a similar shortage of Christian names. Thus there might be as many as twenty Emile Comeaus. To obviate confusion as to which person was being referred to, the Acadians had abandoned the surnames altogether and added another Christian name. Thus Edmund might be called upon to visit not an Emile Comeau but Emile à Louis-Emile, son of Louis; or even Emile son of Louis, grandson of Pierre. For a while, Edmund was quite confused by the cosy nomenclature.

A not untypical Acadian family was that of Hilarion the policeman, who was also tax collector, mailman, farmer, and butcher; his wife Mathilda, who, beside her household duties, hooked rugs, knitted socks, and sold fire insurance; and his father-in-law, a schoolteacher, scholar, and curator of his own museum of local artifacts. Of Hilarion's duties, that of policing the district was the least arduous. The most sensational crime during Edmund's stay at Little Brook occurred when somebody broke into Melanson's Spruce Gum Factory and stole a pail of spruce gum.

The French, and a few English-speaking inhabitants, were to provide Edmund Brasset with his share of triumphs and setbacks. Among the triumphs was an operation performed before a rapt gallery of observers at the hospital in Digby. The case was one of ectopic pregnancy, one of medical history's rarest complications, where the child had been conceived in the Fallopian tube instead of in the womb, and from which the fetus had broken out into the abdominal cavity. In the past, the mother usually died when an attempt was made to remove the afterbirth. That mass of blood vessels was usually in too intimate contact with the surrounding organs to be disturbed without a disastrous loss of blood. Brasset decided to leave the afterbirth where it was, on the already-proved assumption that in time it would be absorbed by the body.

Everybody in the hospital at Digby who could get away from their other duties came to watch as Brasset made a light incision in the abdomen, and a little hairy head popped into view. "I picked the little creature out with no difficulty except that it was necessary to pry the fingers loose from a portion of intestine on which he had a tight grip." At the same time he learned the cause of the woman's unusual "labour" pains. The baby had been kicking her liver.

As at Canso, not all of his charges were human. His very first patient at Little Brook was a gored ox. Edmund admitted that he would have preferred to treat a beautiful blonde, but he did not disdain the task, for his pride was not of the stiff-necked variety; and besides, oxen were valuable creatures and there was no veterinarian in the district. As a result of his success in this case, he was invited to treat many other animals, including a piglet with a hernia. Fortunately he proved his worth in treating people as well.

Edmund was a highly effective physician and surgeon, not least because of a warm, sympathetic interest in his patients. He was not content to treat just the symptoms. Whenever possible he tried to find the underlying cause, and deal with it. He was not always successful, but was confident enough in his own abilities to be able to admit this to the readers of his autobiography. One of his patients was a spinster of thirty-five who had pestered Edmund's predecessors for years with her general aches and pains. In due course she came to Dr. Brasset, who, like his predecessors, failed to find any physical cause for her sore stomach, dizziness, inability to eat properly, and other discomforts. He learned that she was living the life of a lonely drudge, waiting hand and foot on two helpless old aunts, her friends being discouraged from visiting her because of the oppressive presence of the two old ladies in their rocking chairs.

Impressed by his own experience in the insane asylum in Halifax, by the lectures in psychiatry that he had attended, and by the books he had read on the subject, Edmund decided to apply his knowledge. He concluded that her symptoms had been manufactured in order to mask the frustrations incubating in her subconscious. "So the next time she came to me, I reviewed her life for her. I told her that she was desperately unhappy because of the unfortunate situation at home, that she had been robbed by cruel fate of the normal life which should have been hers....

"The next day I had a call from her neighbours. I went to see her and found her in bed. She was too weak to get up, she said. She told me between sobs how grateful she was to me for having opened her eyes to the terrible truth. She told me she had given up the best years of her life and now she was through. There was nothing left for her except to die, and she felt that her departure from this world was not far off. Already, she said, she had a weak feeling around her heart, and her limbs felt funny."

Edmund was appalled at the damage he had done, and tried desperately to rectify it, but she was convinced that it was her heart, now, that was about to peg out, not her stomach. She stayed in bed for over a year. It was not until Edmund shepherded her to a real psychiatrist that she began to recover. "The psychiatrist explained to me the approach I should have taken with her. This woman, he said, had a secret wish that both her old aunts would die so that she could be free. She was a good and religious person and she felt guilty about the wish; so guilty in fact that she would not admit the thought to her conscious mind. The treatment was to get her to bring out or admit that secret desire which she had been suppressing for so long, and show her that it was a perfectly natural feeling under the circumstances and that she need not feel guilty about it at all."

From then on, Edmund was determined not to meddle too deeply in such matters, and in fact helped to cure the next case not with Freudian theory but with a priest, a bottle of whisky, and a player piano.

"No town looks the same to a doctor as it does to other people," Dr. Brasset wrote, in introducing the case of the middle-aged couple who had seen a dread omen in figures of fire. "There are a lot of secret doors in it which he and no one else may enter, and herein lies much of the fascination which the practice of medicine had for those who devote their lives to it."

The couple, Fred Barnett and his wife Matilda, ran a corner store just outside Little Brook. Fred was a thin, withdrawn man, his wife a dulled-looking woman of about forty. There was something about them that made Edmund want to cultivate them; a kind of resignation, as if they were players in a film and were close to the final fade-out. As he got to know them better, he was invited into the back room, which besides the usual furniture, contained a great many books and a player piano, and Mrs. Barnett would chat over tea and cookies. "One day....after I had known them for about two months, our innocent teatime conversation suddenly took on an unexpected and grim turn. After a little pause Matilda said, with a glance at her husband which showed me that this was prearranged between them, 'You know, Doctor, Peter and I aren't going to live very much longer. We don't expect to be here in six months time.'

When Edmund realized that they really meant it, he was shocked, thinking that this comparatively young couple were sharing a morbid delusion. But as soon as they began to explain, he realized that the basis of their fears was not a product of the imagination at all, but a very real phenomenon. It had really happened, in Caledonia Mills, about a hundred and fifty miles from Halifax.

In one of the farm houses in the tiny village of Caledonia Mills lived Alexander MacDonald, his wife Mary, and their adopted daughter, Mary Ellen. Their story was to become an international sensation. One day in January of 1922, the three of them were in the kitchen, Mrs. MacDonald was washing the dishes and Mary Ellen was helping her. Mr. MacDonald had just floundered in from the deep snow that was isolating the farmhouse. He had just fed the stock and was settling down for a comfortable morning by the stove, when suddenly he smelled smoke. It was coiling down the stairway. MacDonald grabbed a pail of water and hurtled up the stairs. In the room immediately above the kitchen he saw that the floor was burning, near the chimney.

Luckily the fire had not properly taken hold and the pail of water extinguished it immediately. By then the other two had followed him upstairs. When they were satisfied that the charred wood was cold, they started downstairs again, wondering how on earth the fire had started.

They had barely settled down again in the kitchen when Mrs. Mac-Donald gave a cry of alarm. "In the living room through which they had just come, there was a yellow flame rising from an old fashioned couch. A pillow was burning. Alarmed and frightened, they ran in. Alexander picked up the pillow by one corner, ran with it to the door and threw it out in the snow. The two adults and the young girl looked at each other in wonder. The place was full of smoke and they kept peering nervously about them. Mrs. MacDonald decided to pour some more tea and in a few minutes they settled down again.

"Some twenty minutes went by and then Alexander jumped up quickly, almost upsetting the table. In a corner of the kitchen, just over the sink, a towel, an ordinary towel which they used to dry their hands, was burning brightly and flames were licking at the wall behind. Trembling, he dashed over, flicked the towel into the sink and poured water over it.

"He was still gazing in fascination at the charred wet cloth in the sink when there came another cry. He turned quickly. His wife and Mary Ellen were staring through the open door that led into the living room. There, on the bare wall, about two feet above the couch, a patch of wallpaper about six or eight inches in diameter was afire."

By then, MacDonald realized that he was facing a situation that he could not handle alone. He shouted to the other two to run for help from the neighbours, and hurried to deal with the fresh outbreak. Luckily he had the means at hand to do so, the sodden towel in the sink.

For the next half hour or so MacDonald kept guard while Mrs. MacDonald and the girl forced their way through the snow to the nearest neighbours, the MacGillivrays. Until the MacGillivrays appeared on the scene there were no new outbreaks. But with the arrival of the six MacGillivray men and women, and Mrs. MacDonald and the girl, the mysterious arson started again. Mrs. MacDonald was just passing cups of tea to the excited MacGillivrays when one of them shouted, "What's that?" There was a crackling noise upstairs. Everybody dashed up. A bedroom door was on fire. It was burning brightly, in the centre of one of the panels.

One of the men had hardly finished suppressing the fire with his macintosh when somebody else shouted that there was smoke coming from another room. Again it was the wallpaper that was afire, directly over a bed.

The twice-flaming wallpaper was the most alarming of all the incidents so far. Wallpaper does not flame all that easily.

While they were putting out this fire, further reinforcements arrived. "Somehow all the people in the valley had heard about what was going on and they kept coming in numbers. Within a few hours there were at least fifty people in the house. Every room in the house, upstairs and down, was filled with people. They were on the stairs and in the hallways, and still the fires continued. Every few minutes someone would cry out, 'Here's another one.' Cushions, pillows, bedspreads, books, clothing, parts of door and other woodwork, would burst into flames. Sometimes, but not often, two blazes would be discovered simultaneously."

During the night there were fewer fires. But with the January daylight, the fires broke out as frequently as before. People began to arrive by the score, in sleighs. Newspapermen and police came from Antigonish. The news was wired to Halifax, and as fresh crews of newsmen and photographers reported from the scene, the strange story was broadcast throughout the continent, and was picked up by the world press.

The fires continued to blaze, despite the guard duty, now, of hundreds of people. "And now new things began to occur. Horses and cows were found turned about in their stalls or tethered to impossible places in the barn. There were reports of people being slapped by invisible hands or tripped by invisible obstacles."

It was only when the MacDonalds abandoned the house that the phantom pyromania ended. The house was then taken over by psychic investigators, led by a reputable scholar, Dr. Walter F. Prince. In due course he issued a cautious report admitting that there was no natural explanation for the phenomena. He raised a question as to whether the adopted daughter, Mary Ellen, might not have been an agent in the case. She was known to have been a young person of less than average mentality. Dr. Prince also wrote an account in the *Journal of the American Society for Psychical Research*.

As for the MacDonald family, they never returned to the house. It caught fire just once more. This time it burned to the ground.

Edmund had heard all about the mystery of the MacDonald house, but he did not interrupt his friends Peter and Matilda when they related the story to him in the back room of their corner store. He waited patiently to learn what their connection was, with the apparently supernatural arson.

It was quite an intimate connection. They had been among the guardian neighbours.

They had seen everything, they said, and it had been just as the newspapers had reported it. They also saw something that nobody else saw.

Matilda: "It was after we got home that we saw it—the same night the fires stopped. Before we left the MacDonald house, I picked up something for a souvenir, and took it home. It was a piece of burned pillowcase, just a small piece about six inches long and six inches wide and one side was charred. And that night we saw it.... We were in bed but we weren't asleep yet, or, at least, Peter was asleep but I wasn't. I was facing toward the wall and my eyes were open, looking towards the bureau, although I couldn't see it because the room was dark. Then all of a sudden I saw a little glow in the dark, just over the bureau and it seemed to be around the little bit of pillowcase which I had put there. I saw numbers made of fire and they said *1939*."

When she woke up her husband, he saw it as well: the number 1939 in flowing figures. And from that moment they were both convinced that that was the year they would die. And it was now 1939.

Dr. Brasset argued with the couple, but could not persuade them either that they had not seen an illusion or that, even if they had, the figures did not necessarily indicate the year of their death. It was only until he had called in a priest, Father Chapdelaine, a man of humour and persuasive common sense, that their certainty began to give way to doubt.

But Edmund felt that he had made one important contribution. One evening, after the day's work, he came visiting with a quart of Scotch. They had a party, and at the height of the jollity, "I remember that I sat down at the old player piano and very skillfully played two rolls — while Peter and Matilda sang.

"And I think this marked the completion of their cure."

A rather less sheltered couple might, that September, have perceived in the glowing figures a revelation of the European cataclysm. But the Second World War caused only muted tremors along these sheltered valleys and rocky shorelines, and in the foundations of the Brasset household, now augmented by the birth of a second son. It was an entirely different tremor that jarred Edmund's now idyllic existence: he had just managed to pay off all his debts, and save enough money in the bank to consider the purchase, for twenty-five hundred dollars, of a charming house overlooking the bay; when one June morning his dream came true. A letter arrived from the United States, offering him a residency in the neurosurgical service of a hospital whose greatest luminary was C. L. Lee, one of the most famous American brain surgeons.

A few days later he was on the neurosurgical team in the distant hospital (not identified by Dr. Brasset), and a month later the chief was paying Edmund one of his rare compliments. "You're not doing too badly, Doctor," he said. "I think in a month or so you'll be ready to do a few things on your own." But that night alone in his hospital basement room with its desk, chest of drawers, table lamp, bed, and bathroom, Edmund admitted to himself that he did not want to be a brain surgeon.

It had come to him that in the American hospital he knew all his patients by the name of their diseases, not by their personal names. In one operation he had helped to remove a spongioblastoma. He knew nothing about the patient, his job or profession, his hobbies, his prejudices, his feelings, his worries, or heartaches. He did not even know the man's name.

He had looked deep into the man's head, but knew nothing of the man's mind. In Nova Scotia he didn't just care for people, he cared about them, because he knew them well, and the knowing of them made his own life rich and meaningful. So he resigned, and went home to Little Brook.

37

Arctic Blues

DR. DONALD JOHNSON, the latest recruit at Harrington Harbour in the Canadian Labrador, was like many overly sensitive persons. He was intolerant of the failings of others. His colleagues in the hospital in England where he had worked as a house surgeon just before joining the Grenfell Mission, would have been quite shaken had they learned what the quiet young man with the long chin and the observant eye secretly thought of them. He found the methods of his chief, a charming and distinguished Guildford surgeon, to be "extremely tedious. He was uncertain of himself as a surgeon—desperately slow, while his slowness was punctuated by outbursts of violent peevishness. It was my own unhappy lot to stand hour after hour as his assistant in the operating theatre, holding instruments, swobbing bleeding points—or being cursed to hell for failing to swob bleeding points: a mute spectator of a great man's failings and uncertainties....

"Nor was I much more happy in my relations with my fellow residents, Dr. B. and Dr. C. Dr. C. was short in stature, snappy and officious; Dr. B. was stout, bombastic and overbearing."

It was therefore with some wariness that a reader awaited his comments on Canada and the Canadian scene. But the Canada of 1928, before the traumatic impact of the Great Depression, was a land of character and courage. He looked upon Canada as "my wonderland, whenever I thought of its friendliness, its democratic spirit and the mental alertness of its folk. A month elapsed from the time when we anchored under the lee of the Chateau Frontenac and gazed at this new sky glowing purple with the refracted light from the cliffs of the Levis shore.... During this time I

509

once again absorbed the stimulating atmosphere. The well-run drug stores with their clean eating counters—the pleasant climate of the fine, hot summer, shortly to change to the cold, dry winter, both of which provided opportunities for out-of-door enjoyments unknown in England—the spontaneous gaiety of Montreal with, so it seemed, prettier girls than I have ever seen elsewhere—these were the main things that charmed and attracted me. Not that my critical sense was entirely dulled. I deplored the inevitable cuspidors in the hotel lounges and bedrooms, the odd lack of refinement in drinking habits. I felt the inevitable sense of alarm and regret on my visit to the Eastern Townships to hear, and indeed to see, how the French Canadians, ten, twelve, fifteen to a family were displacing those of English stock—not only that, but overflowing across the border into Vermont and New Hampshire, not to mention New Brunswick to the east. This depressing sense of the eclipse of the Anglo-Saxon stock was to recur over and over again as I improved my acquaintance with Eastern Canada and the United States.

"However, my ethnological observations were not so important at the moment as my personal experiences. It was our honeymoon and we naturally enjoyed it." Dr. Johnson had married a Belgian girl, Christiane, immediately before signing the Grenfell contract. His marriage was the climax to anguished years spent in "almost unceasing search for affection." Years of rejection, of a "struggle, in the face of biological urge, to uphold the standard of male virginity which my puritanical upbringing had told me was the most essential of all virtues." Even when he reached London, where the possibilities of broader sexual adventures presented themselves, "the teachings of the League of Purity, reinforced by the heavy sense of sin which my Lancashire background taught me to associate with the slightest form of sexual irregularity, won through.... Not only did the impact of the aphrodisiac atmosphere of the West End against my repressed sexual libido contribute substantially to my neurasthenic condition at the time, but my lack of sex experience was to be the direct cause of unhappiness in years to come."

This presumably also contributed to the tension between him and his long-legged, excitable bride. Their temperaments were already in conflict. Christiane, a naturally vivacious girl, felt that life was in debt to her, after a bleak childhood in occupied Belgium and four years of harsh discipline in English hospitals. Moreover, she was affected by the restless search for enjoyment that was such a marked feature of the 1920s. Christiane wanted to dress up for the bright lights, to go places, do things, have a good time. Johnson had no taste for frantic frivolity. Fortunately he was able to convince Christiane that in Canada he could not afford it anyway.

To his surprise, she was immediately content, "as content as I ever knew her to be." But the conflict, though temporarily in abeyance, remained, and as soon as their material circumstances improved, her hedonistic ambitions revived, to create, in Johnson's opinion, "a permanent psychological disharmony in her outlook on life."

Johnson's restless search was for tranquility of spirit, and to a large extent he found it during his stay in Labrador. He had come to take over temporarily from a Dr. Hodd, the medical officer to the Harrington Harbour Hospital, while Dr. Hodd was away on vacation for the winter. Johnson found himself responsible for a practice extending along two hundred miles of the Gulf of St. Lawrence coastline. "They were a strange population of perhaps two or three thousand souls in all, English and French (not including the Indians who, alas, hardly signified) who lived in the settlements dotted along the coast at intervals of some fifteen to twenty miles. Each settlement had its own individual characteristics varying in social and economic circumstances from the prosperous, self-respecting, almost-bourgeois English who were my friends at Harrington, to the mixed-breed (English, Irish, French, and Indian) poverty-stricken proletariat of St. Augustine's River. In breed and racial variation from the highly superior Acadian French at Natashquan—fair-haired Norman types who had migrated from old Acadia (Nova Scotia) and who were the only people who fenced their properties and made up their roads and whose French was clearly spoken and intelligible even to me—to the typically Quebec French of Romaine River and Whalehead and other settlements."

From the start he found the people of Harrington lovable. He admired their immense family feeling. They were happy, genuine, and kindly. There was none of the pettiness and egotism he had so frequently encountered in his life. There was nobody peevish, snappy, officious, bombastic, and overbearing. "Welcome, folks, welcome," bawled one old character. "Sit down and the girl'll make you a mug-up....So you're the new doctor....Yes, sir, a fine work Dr. Grenfell has done on this coast and a fine man he is too. I tell you, sir, I have something to thank Dr. Grenfell for. Blind I was and had been more than five years. So blind as I could not see the face of my dying wife as she left me to find the Lord's peace. But he took me along to St. Anthony in his own boat where they operated on my eyes and I could once again see the glory of the Lord that surrounds us." The Harrington Harbour people believed themselves to be the Lord's servants. To enjoy His blessing, one did His will, and walked in righteousness all one's days.

This also meant that the Lord would provide, a belief that led, through fatalistic inertia, to an anarchistic society. There was no law and order, taxation, representation, or communal effort. There were no paths, no maintenance of essential facilities, and the huskies ran wild. Of immediate concern to Johnson was that there was also no form of sanitation. The toilet was the bucket, its contents hurled out the door in medieval style. And time was valueless. "If a Labradorian wanted urgent help for his wife and child, this was the last thing he would talk about when he came to see me. There was always the rigmarole of the weather and the whereabouts of Uncle Fred to be settled first however urgent the call was." (The prefix "Uncle" and "Aunt" was given to all the older people in the community.)

Nor had the winter weather a proper sense of time's importance. It once took Johnson and his guide a week to reach a patient. "We were travelling westwards to relieve the sad affliction of Pierre Dumaurez of Natashquan, who, so the summoning telegram told us, was unable to pass his water," Dr. Johnson wrote. "Pierre had already been waiting for three days for us since I had first received the telegram at Harrington, during which time we had done our utmost to reach him. We had spent the previous twenty-four hours weather-bound in the comfort of Uncle Gilbert's at Wolf Bay, but, weary of the everlasting talk of last season's fishing and the peculiarities of Bruiser and Peter and Spot, the stars of our dog-team, and the exploits of my predecessors, and feeling that in the circumstances we ought to be making progress, I had insisted on getting on. No-one had began to regret this decision more bitterly than I during the preceding hours. The thermometer had registered some eighteen degrees below zero at our start and, even in the shelter of Wolf Bay, the wind was considerable. Once the open bays were reached, the oncoming snowdrift first froze one's face, then one's hands as one took them out of one's gloves to rub one's face, and after one's hands one's gloves so that these merely scratched the skin when one tried to use them for the same purpose. One turned one's back to the wind and drew one's cowl over one's head, but it was no use in giving either warmth or comfort. I had wept with cold and misery, but my tears had only frozen on my cheeks making matters worse still.... There was no lack of agreement amongst us when our travelling companion suggested turning aside to find a fortunately placed shelter in the woods in which, thanks to the stove, we were soon as warm as we had an hour previously been cold. Pierre would have to wait. Which, in fact, he did for several days longer while we continued our difficult, though fortunately not quite so chilly, journey. And in fact, when we got to Natashquan exactly a week after being first summoned, wondrous nature had still preserved him despite his sad condition. He was swollen up to twice his natural size, but still able to benefit by relief."

The weather co-operated only rarely, as during a trip to Mutton Bay to see a Miss Myrtle. Nine months previously, Myrtle had visited Halifax and had found that the big city was every bit as wicked as they had said. She returned pregnant. Dr. Johnson set off in late winter, the only time of the year when the Labrador weather was in a settled mood, and arrived in only four hours. There he found the girl in a bad way. "The baby's head was obstructed against a deformed pelvis—it was the typical deformity due to rickets (a common enough disease in Labrador) in which the lower part of the backbone juts right out, while in order to overcome this the head of the baby had moulded itself to such a degree that the separate bones of the skull over-rode one another. Myrtle was in fact a text-book case of what is colourfully termed 'Naegele's obliquity.' There was only one thing to do—to give her an anesthetic and help with instruments. This done, it was the case of a long pull and a strong pull and out the baby came with a head as flat as a pancake. It seemed impossible for a baby to live with a head as flat as all that. It was a matter of rescuing the mother. We merely wrapped this odd-looking baby respectfully in towels and deposited it in a corner of the floor. It was quite five minutes later that, just as the mother was coming round, we heard a cry from the towels, a baby's cry. Myrtle's baby, flat head or no flat head, wanted or unwanted, had come to stay."

Between his dog-team travels, Johnson worked at the Harrington Hospital, where he was "in sole responsibility over a team of women-folk. It was they who as subordinates bore the brunt of discomforts, mental if not physical, of medical work in the subarctic conditions of Labrador without the compensating advantages. The excitements of entertaining strangers and visitors, the variations of travel that were my own opportunity during the winter, did not come their way. Fired by the Grenfell enthusiasm they had come to the ends of the earth to serve his cause, but the ends of the earth are, alas, not always as exciting as they may appear from afar. Here they were stranded in these bleak surroundings, remote from home and the distractions of civilization. The loneliness, monotony, often insufficiency of work, brought with it the same temperamental crisis that I have already described as myself having experienced on the Greenland Expedition—but which were all the more devastating in their effect on the female temperament. Both my head nurses new to the coast, undoubtedly suffered intensely in this way. Conscientious, loyal and devoted to their work though they were, it did not make them easy people to deal with."

Fortunately, Christiane did not share the frustrations of the nurses. She was still amazingly content. In the brief periods between his travels and his hospital work, Johnson would relax in his green-painted house at Harrington, studying law (after taking degrees in medicine and law, he would subsequently go in for politics and publishing), while Christiane contentedly knitted and sewed. She had come to love the Labrador people as much as Johnson did. During the day she worked in the mission's clothing store. She was now quite resigned to the lack of such civilized amenities as bathtub gin and tea-dancing.

Not that she lacked entirely for entertainment. There was always the radio. Though admittedly the primitive set could pick up only the one station at Glace Bay. It played the same cracked phonograph records every day, in between gale warnings and news flashes about the number of tons of squid that had been landed at Halifax or Lunenburg. The bulletins about the squid were the only news from the outside world.

Shortly before Dr. Hodd was due back on the supply ship the *North Shore*, the Grenfell Association offered Johnson another temporary post at St. Anthony in northern Newfoundland.

He and Christiane were quite sad at the thought of leaving Harrington. "As the days went by, we received the daily reports of the *North Shore's* progress. Now it was at Seven Islands. Now at Mingan. Then at Natash-quan. It would be due at Harrington the following morning. Chris and I went to bed. Around us were our bags and trunks ready packed to move off when we heard the sound of the ship's siren from across the gray water. But we did not sleep. We wept and wept the whole night through. This house had been our first home—we had had a grand time in it. We had liked Harrington and come to love the Harrington people, and we knew well enough that we would never see place or people again; instinctively we felt that we had found happiness there that perhaps we would not find again."

At. St. Anthony they finally met Wilfred Grenfell. Johnson appears to have found the meeting an anti-climax. Grenfell's great work was far behind him now, and at the age of sixty-four, "though socially and publicly lionized in Britain and the United States, he was now a potterer divested of real authority in the organization which he had built up during the hey-day of his powers." His only contribution now was to make speeches. The work on the coast of Labrador was being done by others, and the great Grenfell Mission had become institutionalized and organized from the head office in New York.

By 1929 the zest had gone out of the Mission. Young men and women, mainly from the United States, were still arriving, inspired by Wilfred Grenfell's crusading speeches. But the humble hospital work at St. Anthony rapidly disillusioned them. According to Johnson there was a tendency for their natural high spirits to find an outlet in horseplay. This did not please some of the more sober and serious-minded permanent staff. Just how serious the permanent mission staff were can be judged by their opinion that even Dr. Johnson was considered too "frivolous and irresponsible."

After a while, Johnson became depressed and as had happened previously in similar circumstances, it affected his health. He decided that it was time to go home. "I had embarked for Labrador with high hopes, not only of immediate adventures and experiences, but also of going to a job that would lead somewhere out of the rut to which I had felt myself condemned. In this I could now see that I was mistaken. I had perhaps not altogether wasted my time but it was obvious that, from a career point of view, I had entered a blind alley. I had no alternative in front of me but to retrace my steps back to England—back to the same point from which I had started a year previously."

Dr. Johnson had loved the people. Dr. Joseph Moody, medical health officer for the east Arctic, loved the land. His territory comprised a strip of Labrador, several arctic islands, part of the Northwest Territories and the tree-shorn regions of northern Manitoba, Ontario, and Quebec: six million square miles of mauve tundra and gray ice, of gold and galena, chromium and uranium locked in ancient rock, or roaming seal and walrus, polar bear, whale and narwhal, caribou and musk ox, and chattering bands of Eskimos; of awesome, swirling northern lights, and the midnight sun sewing diamonds on the snow.

It was a well-paid post. Even so, Dr. Moody was the only applicant for the job in 1946. The Arctic was rigorous, and there were not many medical men who were prepared to brave the isolation, the danger, and the meteorological violence.

Joe Moody was used to hardship. He had been orphaned at an early age and had made his own way in the world, receiving little help from any source until he had completed his first year in medicine at the University of Western Ontario, when a scholarship enabled him to carry on to graduation.

By the end of his internship he was showing promise as a diagnostician and surgeon, and was encouraged to continue his surgical studies. Unfortunately he could not afford to do so, not least because he had married while he was still a student, and had a small daughter. Now that his wife Viola had stopped working, he needed a larger salary than an ordinary general practice would initially provide. Hence his response to a job offer that the Department of Northern Affairs seemed suspiciously eager for him to accept, despite his youth and lack of experience.

He saw why there had not been much competition for the job when he and Viola and little Gloria-May stepped ashore at Chesterfield on the west coast of Hudson Bay. They found a settlement surrounded by hundreds of miles of nothing. There were about fifteen buildings, and a white population of twenty-six. Yet they had been told that Chesterfield was an important centre, presumably because it included a hospital, a trading post, a Department of Transport radio station, and a R.C.M.P. post. If this was an important centre, they wondered, what must the other arctic settlements be like?

As Viola, a girl of simple courage, toured the medical officer's residence, her thin face brightened with enthusiasm. She was delighted with the downstairs room. It had a bay window that provided a splendid view of Chesterfield Inlet. She was especially intrigued when she went upstairs and saw the huge store room, where her food and other supplies would be kept for up to two years at a time. Only one supply ship per year was scheduled to call at Chesterfield Inlet—and even that ship would not necessarily get through if the summer weather were unfavourable.

While Viola and Gloria-May pattered from room to room to get the feel of their first real home, Joe strode along the whitewashed, stone-bordered path to the hospital, to introduce himself to the nurses and to look over the facilities. The hospital proved to be the largest building in Chesterfield. The ground floor was mostly given up to the care of old and crippled Eskimos. Upstairs there was a dispensary and examining room, a surgery, a small laboratory, and wards for Eskimo and white patients. The equipment, including an X-ray machine and developing room seemed, if not lavish, at least adequate.

Johnson did not feel adequate himself. He had no real medical experience and was unsure as to what was expected of him. "This was a place where visiting a patient might mean a week's travel; where epidemics could blaze like forest fires; where people disappeared mysteriously; where men more experienced than I had tried—and failed."

He would soon learn that the major diseases of the Eskimos under his care were tuberculosis (a gift from the white man), conjunctivitis, an eye infection caused by the glare of the arctic sun, frostbite, pleurisy, pneumonia, and abdominal disturbances. He also learned that he would have to do much of his work by radio.

He was quite startled by that. He had not been warned that he might have to work by remote control. But that was understandable. Ottawa was not properly aware of it either, of how extensively radio was being used in medical diagnosis in the North.

It was not long before Johnson found out how it worked. His first case was announced by a telegram from Eskimo Point. "BABY RUSSEL AGED FIFTEEN MONTHS TEMPERATURE 103 PULSE 120 HEADACHES MIGRANE TYPE AND HAD A COLD FOR WEEK STIFFNESS IN SHOULDERS AND NECK SPINE SEEMS TO CURVE STOP LOOKS BAD MOTHER DESPERATE PLEASE CONTACT BY RADIO H.B. CO." The sender was the child's father Chesley Russel, the manager of the Hudson's Bay post.

Knowing that he could never reach Eskimo Point in time by dog team, Dr. Moody braced himself for the long-distance consultation at seven that evening. He was fairly sure what was wrong with the baby. He had heard of a number of cases of meningitis in the area. He wondered how far the disease had progressed, and whether it was possible to save the child.

"I got on the air at seven exactly," Moody recounted, mind clear,

nerves apparently well in hand. Then something happened. The instant
I heard Chesley's voice, try as I would, I couldn't speak a word. The
sound just wouldn't come. It was mike-fright to the nth degree. Hundreds
of thoughts played tag in my brain. I felt cold in the overheated radio hut
and was aware that my hands were shaking. Charley, the radio mechanic,
sensing the situation, took the receiver away from me and made contact
himself."

The doctor managed to pull himself together and take over, thinking
worriedly about the child's curving spine. That was the one symptom
that was not typical of meningitis.

"'Doctor, it is like I wired you this morning, he is stiff, arms don't
move. Temperature is 104 now. He has terrible pains. Can't stop crying.
What is it, Joe, what is it?'

"'Well, I think I know. But say, what about the spine?'

"'I don't know, I really don't. This afternoon it curved terribly, was
way off the bed.'

"'Could it have been the pain? Straining to get relief?'

"'Could be, Joe, could be. The wife said that he seemed to control it.
What can we do, Joe?'

"'Have you got some soludiazine there?'"

Joe had already checked the drug list to confirm that there was a
supply of the drug at Eskimo Point. After making sure that Chesley had
located the right ampoule:

"'Now fill the hypo, the hypodermic, and get all the air out. You have
the child right there, do you?'

"'Yes, he's here.'

"'Good, now listen what you do, Ches. You know, on the child's head,
right on top, is that soft spot, the fontanel.'

"'What do you want me to do there, Joe?'

"'Can you find it?'

"'Yes, I can.'

"'Now look for the spot closest to the centre of the head.'

"'What?'

"'Get it as far back as you can. Look for the spot closest to the centre of
the head. Right?'

"'Check!'

"'Now you inject....wait a minute. What kind of needle do you have
on the hypo?'

"'It's a thin one.'

"'Okay, but what does it say on it?'

"'It says.... it says number twenty-four.'

"'Fine. How long is it?'

"'It's real short, about an inch.'

"'That's all right. Now you must inject that needle into the soft spot, very gently. Not too deep. And straight down.'"

There was shocked silence over the air. Precious seconds panicked past before Chesley's shaky voice came on the air. "'But Joe, I can't. You don't want me to do that.'

"'Yes, I do want you to do that.'

"'But the soft spot is dangerous, Joe. They all say it. The wife says it, too.'

"'It isn't dangerous. You can do it. Just keep steady. I've done it hundreds of times.' That was a lie, but I had to get him over his fear.

"'He's my son, Joe, I could kill him.' came the voice, plaintively.

"'You want him to live, don't you?' I demanded brutally.

"'Yes but—'

"'Then do it. Now listen carefully. As close to the centre of the head as you can. Push it in very carefully. Not all the way, just about three-quarters of an inch. So you hear me?'

"'Yes, three-quarters of an inch.'

"'Ok. Push it in and then empty the hypo slowly. And don't move it. Keep it perfectly still.'

"'I can't Joe. I'm shaking.'

"'Then get yourself together. Go ahead now. Do it.'

"Bill, the mountie, took the receiver at the other end. 'He's putting it in now, Joe.'

"'Does he actually have it in?'

"'Yes.'

"'Then tell him to empty it. Keep him steady, Bill.'

"'Right.' I could hear Bill relay my instructions.

"'Is he very nervous, Bill?'

"'Plenty, but it's all right.'

"I noticed that I was holding my right hand as if I were injecting the child myself. I moved my fingers and it hurt. I must have had them in that position for some time. I was shaking. I couldn't have done it now myself. I'd have made a mess of it. Oh God, give him strength, I thought.

"Bill's voice again: 'He's got it empty, Joe.'

"'And the needle out?'

"'Yes, it's out. One of the women fainted, Joe.'"

The baby recovered—probably sooner than the father.

As the months passed, Moody learned at first hand about many of the perils of the Arctic, a region where, in a snow storm, it was possible to get lost and to die by merely attempting to travel from one house to another a few yards away. Not least among the perils, and a common one among people who were unsuited to the hardships, was an arctic neurosis. They could not adjust mentally to the isolation and darkness. They sank into a depression so profound that it drained them of strength and resistance. Joe had to evacuate by air many a white man who had discovered that his own company was unbearable.

For a while, the doctor himself became deeply depressed, not least because, by December, the long hours of darkness were upsetting his household routine. As the time of day became less and less important in regulating his life, he found himself sleeping and eating at irregular intervals.

He felt disoriented. The slightest incident was likely to deepen his depression, such as the sight of a wolf slinking outside the door. "Little things assumed monstrous proportions," he wrote. "Once we took off our storm windows long enough to scrape away the two-inch layer of ice on the inside. We thought this might give us something more nearly approaching daylight. But the scraped glass only let in more dull darkness. Instead of square patches of gray, our windows had turned into gaping black holes. You could weight the blackness!"

Fair Viola was similarly affected, but made an effort to cheer him up by urging him to join the neighbourly parties. Unfortunately, the forced gaiety darkened Dr. Moody's spirits still further, until he was in danger of living up to his name permanently. "I discovered things about my closest friends that I hadn't seen before and didn't like it at all. Physical characteristics, mostly. For example, the nose of a neighbour bothered me out of all reason. It was quite a normal nose, though rather large. I just didn't like that nose and took personal offense when he showed it around.... The dangling earring which one of the women liked to wear at our parties made me nervous, too."

He was not alone in the dark cellar of the spirit. Even a game of bridge was likely to end up with intersecting glares of hatred, and once with a narrowly averted fight between two radio operators.

Fortunately the Christmas spirit distracted the community long enough to restore, if not a sense of reality—for the fantastic life of the Arctic never seemed quite real—but at least a sense of proportion. On New Year's Eve, the Moodys were quite cured of their depression when the neighbours, well aware of what it was like to experience an arctic festive season for the first time, came visiting, and crowed into the house to create a jolly uproar. Home brew was passed around, the women made a special treat, potato chips, and a dance was organized, the music supplied by an Eskimo with an accordian. During a pause in the festivities, Dr. Moody confided to the owner of the offending nose how, for a while, he had come to hate the other's redoubtable beezer. Everybody laughed and confessed to similar obsessions in the past.

The dance went on until late in the morning. Afterwards, Joe, quite cured of his melancholy, wandered alone through the settlement, marveling that so much warmth and happiness could exist in such dehumanizing cold.

During his first four years in the eastern Arctic, Moody came to regard the Eskimos with an affectionate as well as an observant eye. The Eskimo bands were not by any means all alike, he found. They varied quite considerably in character, culture, and attitude, depending on where they lived, how they lived, and where they came from. In the distant past, some had come from the west across the Bering Sea; others possibly from Greenland. Their primitive culture had functioned well until civilization had begun to cripple them. The white man had already destroyed much of their self-reliance and weakened their resistance with his diseases. Around Chesterfield, the Eskimos still used a few ancient tools, but modern implements and other imports had begun to reshape their lives, and the shape was usually not ethnologically functional.

As among the Indians, the Eskimos had their medicine men, the shamans, but they had succumbed to the white man's medicine even faster than the native Indians. Donalda Copeland, a nurse practicing further north, on Southampton Island at the mouth of Hudson Bay, wrote that one of her Eskimo friends, Tommy, had once been a medicine man. He told her that a few shamans still practiced in secret, resentfully. She described how, during an epidemic of dysentery in the early 1950s, "I came into contact with another phase of ancient Eskimo tradition. Our camp leader, the Sturdy John Ell, had taken ill. As I made my way into the hut he shared with Santainna's family, I found that a crowd preceded me. On the bed lay John Ell and before him whirled a strange figure. At once I recognized the writhing form of Shimout, the crossed-eyed shaman.

"Several times before, I had encountered him in the homes of the ill, but never had I seen him in action. Always he eyed me with suspicion and because he always refused to say even the customary 'Hello' I knew that he regarded me as a rival. Several times I found sores and carbuncles which he had cut into and which I had to treat.

"Now, utterly fascinated, I watched him performing one of his 'spells.' His swarthy face was streaked with rust-coloured chalk or paint. Beads of perspiration trickled down from his brow, about which his coarse black hair flopped wildly. His dark crossed eyes added to his uncanny appearance. He writhed and twisted rapidly in some sort of dance, and his face wore a trance-like expression. His wild contortions were accompanied by a series of mutterings in a strange tongue.

"'Drive out bad spirit,' Tommy told me was the particular duty of a shaman. This was why, he explained, the shaman opened wounds, to allow the evil spirit to escape. That often accounted, I knew, for the trouble the shaman caused. His tool had been a dirty knife or a jagged piece of bone.

"Sometimes too, Tommy added, the shaman had to pound the bodies of the ill with his fists, thus forcing out the evil demon within....

"At last he saw me and pulled himself together. Resuming his usual sullen manner and eyeing me suspiciously, he slunk back against the wall. I proceeded at once to administer aspirin and bismuth hydrate to the sick man."

Increasingly in tune with the arctic realities, Dr. Moody was entirely sympathetic to the sexual attitudes of the Eskimos. "Where people's very existence must be interwoven with the physical resources of their land, it is only natural that the laws of nature become the laws of man," he wrote, noting that the white man's moral code did not similarly reflect his natural instincts. "It is true," he continued, "that a travelling Eskimo can depend on being offered his host's wife or daughters as a routine hospitality, because the Eskimo accepts sex as a natural instinct no more noteworthy than that man must eat to stay alive."

Though the Eskimos were always careful to maintain a certain aloofness from the white visitors, Joe found them not hard to like. If their faces were often masks, they displayed one emotion openly. That was joy. They loved a joke or prank. They laughed easily and hard. Their keen sense of humour was also shown in the aptness of their choice of nicknames. With their instinctive knowledge of human nature they often had a white man's character figured out long before he was able to size them up."

Dr. Moody risked his life many times to minister to his Eskimo charges. One spring day, with the temperature around forty below zero, he received a message that two Eskimos, who had proved to be carriers of a dangerous and contagious disease, had disappeared from Fullerton Point, ninety miles from Chesterfield Inlet. They were wandering around the countryside endangering the health of people over a wide area. Moody was quite prepared to risk the season's sudden snowstorms and blizzards in his dog team, but did not see that it would help. It might take him weeks to find the Eskimos, especially as the fugitives were fleeing aimlessly from pains they could not understand, and would not want to be found.

Then he thought of Fogbound. Fogbound's real name was Gunnar Ingebrigsten. He was one of the first pilots to fly regularly in the east Arctic, at a time when arctic aviation on a year-round basis was considered impossible by the experts in Ottawa. He had earned his nickname because of his telegrams. Whenever he was called upon for services that were not, in his opinion, really needed—especially if he happened to be on a binge at Churchill, where he was based, he would send a wire stating, "Can't make it today. Fogbound."

For months, Joe had been hearing stories and anecdotes about this fabulous flyer. He now wired the pilot, asking if he were willing to search several square miles of snow and ice for the sick Eskimos.

Fogbound flew in next day in his Norseman, bumping down the rough ice of the inlet.

All day he and the doctor criss-crossed the terrain, searching for two dark figures in a landscape of gray ice and wraith-forming snow. Late in the afternoon they were caught in a sudden storm. Fogbound made a fast descent to the uneven seashore, smacking down on the ice with such force that the Norseman was flung back into the air to an alarming height. By the time Fogbound and the doctor climbed out of the airplane the wind was slashing at sixty miles an hour. Half blinded by the snow, they struggled to anchor the aircraft with rope and ice chisels. Then took shelter in the aircraft's cabin.

"As we didn't dare to start the engine on account of the lowness of our fuel, the cabin soon grew unbearably cold. We learned not to touch the metal with our bare hands. If we did, the frost glued flesh and steel together. We warmed our noses constantly with our hands for fear they would freeze. Finally we covered ourselves with the few hides we had and tried to settle down for the night."

In the middle of the night the gale increased and the aircraft began to dance up and down on the ice, sometimes rising several feet into the air. They scrambled out in a hurry. While they were lashing the Norseman more firmly, securing its long skis to the ice with steel cables, they also had to rope themselves to the fuselage. This was to save themselves from being blown away, though it added another risk, that of being carried aloft if the aircraft took off by itself.

"We had just made it back into the cabin when a thunderous roar, followed by a series of ear-splitting explosions, brought us outside once more, this time dazed by the concussions and half expecting the end of the world." And when they looked around, they saw that they were on a patch of ice that was no longer attached to the shore. There was a foot-wide gap of black water between their floe and the main mass of ice.

Fogbound stared at it fixedly. When it slowly started to widen he wrenched his gaze away.

"'Our runners are five feet long,' he screamed at me," Moody recounted. "'Maybe I can taxi her across.'"

They released the anchor cables, then scrambled back into the Norseman. After a minute, Fogbound managed to get the engine started, just as the small ice pan they were on began to rock warningly. By now the gap separating them from the shore was two feet wide. Fogbound taxied up to it, then slammed forward the throttle. Moody shut his eyes. The aircraft lurched. When he opened his eyes again they were across the gap and sliding slowly to a halt.

Wondering if they would have enough of an ice runway from which to take off in the morning, they composed themselves exhaustedly for sleep. The morning brought two surprises. The first was that there was a two-mile stretch of level ice ahead of them. The second was the sight of a tent, pegged down only a hundred yards away. When Moody went to investigate, he found, huddled inside it, the very men they had been searching for. After scanning hundreds of square miles for the two sick Eskimos, Fogbound had landed right next to them entirely by accident.

Dr. Moody was a pioneer in the use of aircraft for medical missions, and some of his exploits were reported around the world. But it was the epidemic of 1949 that earned him the greatest fame.

That year, just as he and his family were preparing, well ahead of time, for a vacation, reports began to come in from Nunnulla and Eskimo Point about several strange cases of paralysis. As the weather was too bad for a personal visit, Joe arranged for one of the Nunnulla victims to be flown to Winnipeg for a thorough diagnosis. In due course the word came back. It was Guillain-Barré syndrome.

Joe was pretty surprised. This was a rare disease, cause unknown. Still, it gave an indication as to what treatment to follow, and he radioed his instructions accordingly to the various camps. But when more and more deaths were reported, he decided that he had better obtain a subject for autopsy, to see for himself.

The weather refused to co-operate. It was so bad that none of the bodies at the scattered settlements could be brought to his facilities at Chesterfield. By then, Joe had begun to doubt the Winnipeg diagnosis. He finally decided that he could not wait for a patrol to bring in the bodies; he would have to go out and obtain one of them himself.

While he was traveling frustratedly from one camp to another in search of a deceased victim, he received a telegram from the nurses at Chesterfield informing him that several cases of paralysis were now available right on his own doorstep. He wired Fogbound, asking for his help in getting back to Chesterfield. Fogbound's airplane was in the south being overhauled, so that several days elapsed before Joe could return home. But when he finally got back to Chesterfield, he found that though several of the Eskimo victims were showing the right symptoms, in fact they were suffering from arctic food poisoning. Joe began to wonder if he was fated to never see a victim of the mysterious disease.

Then the local R.C.M.P. man, Sergeant Paddy Hamilton, managed to get hold of the body of an Eskimo who had died of the infection. Joe prepared to perform the autopsy with considerable enthusiasm. Now he would see.

"An arctic autopsy is different from that which one is accustomed to in a city hospital," he wrote. "Arctic temperatures provide a natural deep freeze far beyond that needed for preservation. It took several days before the body was even partly thawed, then I had to use blunt instruments to remove the specimens—a gruesome task in which the sergeant assisted. Every few minutes we would warm our hands, numbed by excessive cold. I managed to assemble the specimens and, although lacking the correct preservatives, carefully packed and refroze them for laboratory inspections in Winnipeg. Greatly relieved by having at last laid hands on material that could show us the true character of the disease...I left the settlement with a clear conscience for our long Christmas journey home." The doctor and his family took a much-needed vacation in London, Ontario, but, en route through Winnipeg to deliver the specimens, he was frustrated once again. The technicians took one look and said that the autopsy material was useless. It had been too badly preserved.

In Winnipeg, Moody voiced his doubts that the disease was the Guillain-Barré syndrome, and was referred to Dr. Rhodes. "Dr. Rhodes, an internationally famous expert in this particular field [virus infection] was sympathetic but not encouraging. He gave me much practical advice on how to treat virus cases with my limited equipment in Chesterfield, and how the clinical picture could be interpreted. Just as I left he handed me several of his own technical papers on poliomyelitis.

" 'This, of course, is irrelevant,' he admitted lightly, 'but you might be interested in what we're doing.' "

Joe had been home in London for only a few days when a telegram arrived from Chesterfield: "SEVERAL CASES STRANGE ILLNESS AND DEATH PLEASE RETURN."

Which quite ruined the family's first vacation in two years.

Back in Chesterfield, he found a tense situation. Usually the Eskimos accepted illness as just another facet of nature—provided they knew what it was. But this new and terrible disease that was killing or paralyzing so many of their friends was upsetting them badly, overwhelming them with fear and anxiety.

It was at this point that Joe saw his first genuine paralysis patient. "Unconsciously I had been building myself up for this moment, hoping, expecting it to mark a sensational discovery. It would enable me to put my finger at last on the real origin of the infection and to determine the correct diagnosis.

"None of these daydreams came true. Examinations of some of the worst cases left me as ignorant of the exact nature of the trouble as I was before. It was some form of paralysis, no doubt, but the symptoms were strange. Maybe it was this Guillain-Barré thing, after all. Then again it might be meningitis or even—well frankly, it could be anything. But why so virulent? So *persistent?*"

More and more stricken Eskimos began to die in Chesterfield, and for the first time, as Joe stood there helplessly in the snow, amid the criss-cross of dog tracks and the deep lines scored by the runners of the komatiks, he started to hate the place. "Some Eskimos came out to meet me, but stood back silently when I went near. One man fell down in the snow and could not move farther. Near the hospital two figures struggled forward carrying between them a seemingly lifeless girl."

Anguished, he turned and went home. His own child was one of the sufferers. Gloria-May's temperature had reached 105 at one point. Strange muscle spasms had wracked her legs. But thank God, she appeared to be one of the lucky ones and was recovering. She was now sleeping quietly. But Joe had still not the slightest idea what was wrong with her.

He went back to the hospital. There was pandemonium. It was so packed with victims that many of them were lying on the floor under caribou skins. Joe felt almost crazed with frustration. Nothing made any sense. Some of the patients were dying after an illness lasting only six hours. Others were recovering almost as rapidly. Some were paralyzed, others not.

In desperation, he took samples of spinal fluid, hurried to the laboratory and feverishly prepared tests. Nothing. The fluids were clear: no bacteria. It definitely wasn't meningitis. Encephalitis? By evening the laboratory was a chaos of tubes, smears, bottles of fluid, dishes of specimens. He was still no nearer the answer by the next morning. Another two Eskimo children had died during the night. The illness was completely out of control. Chesterfield was in a state of helpless panic.

So that when Sergeant Hamilton came over and told him that one of his constables had a sore leg, Joe came close to laughing hysterically at being bothered by such a trivial complaint when an epidemic of an unknown disease was engulfing the North.

But, "While examining rows and rows of patients, checking symptoms, trying to patch the symptoms together into something intelligible, I couldn't help thinking of that constable and his sore leg," he said, and finally, to the astonishment of the nurses, he gave way to a sudden impulse. He rushed out of the ward and stumbled across to the radio hut where the policeman was lying. He stared fixedly at the limp foot. The muscles had gone dead.

The typical drop foot symptom! "There could be no mistake now, and immediately the full significance.... hit me square in the face.

"'Impossible,' I kept telling myself. 'Absolutely impossible. But *here it is*.'" Poliomyelitis.

When Dr. Moody informed Winnipeg that the mystery disease, which was now agitating the whole country, was polio, there was utter disbelief mixed with grave concern. There was no doubt that the outbreak was extremely serious, but to claim that it was polio was plainly ridiculous.

Polio in winter was unlikely enough, but in the mid-winter Arctic, impossible. Take hard hit Chesterfield, for instance. It was going through the longest period of intense cold ever recorded: an average of thirty-eight degrees below zero Fahrenheit for six consecutive weeks. Surely even this young fellow, Moody, who had been practicing for only three years or so, must know that polio was a warm-weather phenomenon. Moreover the characteristics were all wrong. For instance, after the onset of polio, its progress was normally quite slow; but patients in Chesterfield were dying within six hours. Further, in poliomyelitis, abdominal paralysis was rare; yet fully half the cases so far had resulted in such paralysis.

The authorities in Ottawa were just as skeptical, but in response to an urgent appeal for help they despatched five medical experts, including an epidemiologist.

Joe had them touring the wards within minutes of their arrival. By then, Joe had taken the dramatic step of quarantining a gigantic area of the east Arctic, in an attempt to halt the spread of the disease. As well as isolating Chesterfield, to the extent that no one was even to leave his home—food was to be left outside each house or igloo—he wired quarantine orders to every police post, mission, and Hudson's Bay store over a wide area, printed and distributed leaflets in the Eskimo language, and radioed warnings to ships and aircraft. In two days, he had imposed the largest regional quarantine in medical history; cutting off nearly 50,000 square miles of territory from all contact with the outside.

After he had done so, he was suddenly overwhelmed with the enormity of this action, which he had taken on his own youthful initiative. Since then he had hardly eaten, hardly slept, out of anxiety over the effects of such a drastic measure: possible starvation among the Eskimos who would not be allowed to hunt; panic among those who had the disease or thought they had. He was already wasting too much energy in examining numerous settlers and Eskimos who were sure their muscles were weakening—one fellow, for instance, had shouted that his legs were paralyzed even as he chased after the doctor across the snow. There were also grave supply problems, because he had forbidden ships to approach any settlement closer than was absolutely necessary, and had forbidden any resident from unloading aircraft. Nor was his anxiety allayed by the results. Deaths continued to mount.

So that when one of the Ottawa experts examined the hospital patients, turned to Joe, and said categorically that it wasn't polio, Joe felt numb with shock. His feverish thoughts were not in the least soothed when another of the doctors murmured tactfully that, well, whatever the disease was, it was obvious that it was serious, and that they would give him whatever assistance they could.

For a moment Joe saw himself a ruined man, a self-announced fool, his reputation in tatters. Had he really been wrong after all, in reading so much into the constable's typical drop-foot symptom?

His morale was not heightened by the accident that occured recently in the lab. He had been working there, fighting a numbing fatigue for hours, slaving over spinal fluids containing a count of more than 250 cell elements. He had filled a glass tube with the lethal fluid, inserted it in the centrifuge and started the motor.

The spinning tube had suddenly hit an obstruction and shattered, "spraying a circle of death on the walls, on my face, on my clothes. It took a few moments before I fully grasped what had happened. That, I think, was when the epidemic came nearest to getting me down." He stood there "like an idiot," staring at the splashes on the wall. One poisonous blot had landed on the map, right on the location of Chesterfield.

His face was wet with lethal cells. He wondered if his mouth had been open at the wrong moment. Had he been licking his lips at the precise moment the liquid landed—or been in the act of taking a deep breath? He didn't know, he couldn't be sure. With an effort he carried on as if nothing had happened, washed and changed into a clean coat.

As it turned out nothing did happen. He was immune.

In the same way, he pulled himself together now, and asked the Ottawa experts to follow him into his laboratory. There he showed them dozens of specimens, the results of dozens of tests—all the clinical details, all the records of paralytic phenomena. The doctors listened in silence, and checked the results, then once again they examined the patients in the wards.

This time they agreed. They had been misled by the disease's unusual characteristics. It was polio, all right.

As for the drastic quarantine, "what might have turned into the greatest tragedy of my career became a really spectacular success—not to say personal triumph. Now that the facts are known, the unprecedented virulence of the epidemic recognized and documented, there are few who would not agree that my spontaneous move, conscientiously assisted by Sergeant Hamilton and the whole Arctic family, saved hundreds from paralysis or death."

Gareth Howerd was a recent immigrant to Canada, and he wanted to earn some money so that he could see more of his new country, before settling down. Which was why he was lining up at the Montreal employment office one winter's day in the 1950s, shifting about and sweating in the stifling heat. He was not yet acclimatized to Canadian central heating.

As he shuffled along, he chatted to the man just ahead of him, who said his name was John. John, like most of the men in the line-up, was an unemployed construction worker who was hoping for a job that would see him through until spring. He was a huge man, big enough to make Gareth's thin, slender frame seem even more undersized. He told Gareth that he had been working on the DEW Line, the link-up of radar stations that were being built in the far north to guard against a surprise attack over the North Pole.

Gareth had a receptive air, as if, despite his youth, he was already used to listening to other people's troubles, and John gladly opened up. His troubles were all the harder to bear because he felt he deserved them. He had gone up to the Arctic, he said, intending to work there for months and save a lot of money. They were paying good money on the DEW Line. But he had lasted only four weeks. It wasn't the work, he said, it was the loneliness. He found that he couldn't stick it. It was so bad that he had almost gone crazy, and had spent two weeks in hospital, and only just gotten out.

Now he was too ashamed to go home to Calgary in mid-winter and admit that he had not had the guts to stick it out in the Arctic. That was why he was here now, hoping for a job that would keep him going until spring, so that he could go home without seeming to have chickened-out.

Gareth murmured sympathetically, and felt even more sorry for John when the big man reached the head of the queue, only to be told that there was nothing for him.

As John turned away dejectedly, Gareth took his place at the counter, and handed over the form that he had filled in. As the clerk, a girl with red hair, started to read it, Gareth announced in a brisk, confident voice that he would like a job, please. He would take any kind of job they had to offer.

The girl, who was used to rather more humble-sounding applicants, glanced over his thin figure, then started flicking through a card index. He was obviously not a pick-and-shovel type, that was for sure. A needy clerk, perhaps. But there were no clerical openings. The only thing she had to offer was a sales job in a department store, through Christmas.

Gareth said he would like that, so she drew forward another form and started to fill it in. Learning from his application that he was a recent immigrant, she asked to see his passport. That was when the trouble started. She took one look at the top line on page two under the heading, "Description—Signalement," and scuttled through into an inner office, to let her superiors know that there was something funny going on. She had a fellow out there who, despite being in one of the world's highest-paying professions, was applying for a job in a department store.

After a moment two men came out, took Gareth into another office and started to grill him. He had recently served in the merchant navy. Why had he left? They seemed to think that he had jumped ship in

Montreal. Even his discharge certificate did not satisfy them. They thought he was a deserter and an illegal immigrant. Why else would he be afraid to enter his own profession. Unless, of course, he had been struck off the register. Abortion, was it?

It was only after a number of suspicious confrontations by various officials in the employment office, and after one of them had checked with his previous employers, that the word "sir" began to creep into their sentences, as they slowly adjusted to the accentricity of a qualified doctor who, just for a change, wanted to try some other line of work before settling down to the one he had trained for at Manchester University.

When he finally reached the department store, the personnel officer there was even more intrigued; but obviously thrilled at the idea of having a doctor working in the sporting goods department.

From early childhood, Howerd had tended to be somewhat unconventional. Which was why, when he got the opportunity a few weeks later to become a DEW Line doctor, he accepted without hesitation, though he was already aware, after his conversation with John and with the chief medical officer who interviewed him, that the job was hard and hellish — so uncomfortable, boring, and dangerous that not many medical men lasted even the official three months of their contract.

Hard and dangerous it proved to be, but Gareth Howerd never found it boring. Like Dr. Moody, he fell in love with the Arctic, and to the astonishment of his employers, he would renew his contract three times before the arctic blues finally got him down.

This was the 1950s, and the Distant Early Warning Line was the most northerly of three defence lines of radar stations that were being built across the country, to warn off an attack by aircraft and guided missiles. The United States Air Force was financing the construction of the DEW Line, though the work was being done by civilian firms.

Howerd was employed by one of these firms. He was responsible for the health of the white workers, though, if needed, he would minister to the Eskimos as well.

His base was on Baffin Island, the eastern staging post for the DEW Line project and the centre of his practice. When the aircraft from the mainland skidded to a halt at Baffin Base and discharged him into the arctic darkness, he was shaken to find that the men there were living in *tents*. His hospital, too, was a large tent; to be exact, two tents joined end to end, with a red cross painted on the side. His apprehension was allayed only slightly when he learned that the tents were as well insulated as the strange garments and footwear he had just been issued with: the arctic sleeping robe, the thermal underwear, the parka, a sheepskin-lined hooded coat, and the pair of mukluks: knee-high boots of nylon and felt, with rubber soles and heels.

He was also just as surprised as Dr. Moody had been to find that much of his treatment would be carried out by teletype or over the radio. Not only that. He was also expected to act as a dentist, as an unofficial public health director, and as a vet to the huskies.

He soon learned that his most important task was to keep up morale. There were more than a few men like John who suffered from loneliness and apprehension. All too often they had nobody to talk to, which worsened their troubles. So, Gareth made a special effort to fly to the various DEW Line sites as often as possible, to add the role of psychoanalyst to his other responsibilities.

The men greatly appreciated his concern and sympathy, and many times he was to hear the words "We're glad you're a travelling doctor," or, "We never used to see a doc up here," or to be greeted simply with relieved sallies. On one occasion he stayed several days at a remote site after one of the men there died of a heart attack. Heart attacks were not uncommon under the arctic work conditions. The death of their companion had unsettled the men and when Dr. Howerd arrived, there was none of the usual banter. At dinner that night the men were tense and silent.

"What conversation there was turned on the health of their families back home, and they would ask about a son who was to have his tonsils out or a wife who suffered from 'nerves' or loneliness, and ask me what I thought they should advise in letters home. I was glad to do this welfare work among the men, and felt it was an important part of my duties.

"I stayed at the camp for four days and in that time nearly half of the men approached me when they thought no one else would know, and said, 'Doc, I've got a pain in my chest, do you think it's my heart?'

"Although I felt certain that there was nothing more wrong with them than indigestion I examined each man thoroughly and reassured him that there was nothing the matter with his heart.

"By the time I left the atmosphere was happier and I felt glad that I had made the...journey. It had cost me little effort and had probably helped to keep these men working on the DEW Line for they would otherwise have taken their discharge and gone home."

Blessed with an adventurous spirit, Gareth adjusted well to the twenty hours a day of winter darkness, the nocturnal moan of the wind, the white-outs, the constant danger attendant on the flights into the ice fields or mountain-top camps. He did not miss the night lights and swirling crowds of the cities. His only yearning was for a tree. In a land of rock and lacerating ice, he longed for the sight of a tree, and on the two or three occasions when he had to accompany a patient to Montreal and had an opportunity to walk through the parks, he could not keep his eyes off the glorious maples, planes, and oaks. "Trees were the symbol of loneliness on the DEW Line."

To a lesser extent, he also longed for a hot tub. There was not a single bathtub at Baffin Base. Showers had been installed in a special hut, but it was tedious business having to bundle up in full arctic gear before scuttling across to the shower hut in the sub-zero temperature. Some of the men couldn't be bothered to dress properly. They would dash across in their underwear. Which took many of them straight to the hospital with pneumonia.

Gareth was so desperate for a hot bath that he had Jacques, the French Canadian plumber, cut an oil drum longitudinally, so that he could use half of it as a tub. But the rough edges, which had been cut with an oxyacetylene torch, threatened to deprive him of any future progeny. Also, the slightest movement sent water sloshing all over the floor, so that the only way he could bathe was by remaining rigidly still—which rather spoiled the enjoyment. So back he went to Jacques, and this time had him cut a drum horizontally. Back at the hospital, he filled the cylinder with water, and as before, set it on the stove to warm up. It took all day for the water to heat up properly. By evening it was ready. Gareth undressed in his quarters in the hospital and, stepping into the tub, tried to squat in the hot water. His knees jammed against the sides and were scratched by the rough edges, but when he pulled his knees away it forced his bottom against the sharp edges on the other side of the tub. So he had to get out and file down the rough edges. Eventually he jammed himself in the tub with his legs dangling over the side. This he considered to be a great comfort, and from then on soaked in the truncated oil barrel for hours at the end of the day's work. It was one of the little luxuries that helped him to maintain a benign attitude toward the awful conditions in the almost lightless winter.

Not least among the awful conditions, in the opinion of the men, was the scarcity of alcohol. When Dr. Howerd first arrived there was uncompromising prohibition. There were good reasons for the ban. If an intoxicated man fell in the snow, he was quite likely to freeze to death. Naturally the total ban on alcohol produced total craving for it. The men were prepared to go to great lengths to obtain it. On their return from leave, they would stock up and hide the bottles in sleeping bags, coat linings or spare boots. "Often those who had made whoopee during leave or on the train took an attack of post-alcoholic jitters when the liquor supply was cut off. I was often called to the airfield to attend such cases, and found most of them recovered after a day or two in hospital.... One man was brought into the hospital suffering from *delirium tremens*, and he too recovered and went on to a site, where I am told he became an excellent worker. The man, who was a cook, was French Canadian without a drop of Scottish blood so far as I knew. But he must have had a large amount of Scotch in his bloodstream for as he lay in hospital he had visions of tiny green lizzards dressed in kilts, dancing at the foot of his bed.

I often felt, and the authorities came to realize, that prohibition made many men seek liquor just because it was denied them. Eventually a ration of four cans of beer a week was allowed to each man. And, of course, some men immediately hoarded their ration for several weeks and drank the lot in a glorious spree....

"But while prohibition lasted there were a number of cases in which men became ill—and in one of two cases even died—after drinking moonshine, brewed with anything from which they could extract alcohol. I have heard of DEW Line workers brewing after-shave lotion, anti-freeze for vehicles, boot-black strained through bread, raisins and even beans."

Gareth had to escort one of these cases all the way to Montreal. His cerebrum had been affected by the moonshine. The first stage of the flight was a nightmare. "Although the man was under heavy sedation he started to go into *status epilepticus* with one fit following upon another. This can be dangerous and even fatal, and I was very worried about the patient's condition, and gave him more sedation intravenously and intramuscularly. He became very dehydrated and I had to ask the pilot to fly lower because of the lack of oxygen at the aircraft's cruising height. In addition I had to give him further oxygen through a mask." Later the epileptic fits became even more violent, and when the patient and the doctor finally arrived at the Montreal General Hospital, it was in a screaming ambulance. Amazingly, the man recovered after about two weeks, without permanent brain damage.

In April the year following his arrival in the Arctic, the setting of monotony, blizzard, and darkness was transformed by the deepening parabola of the sun. Gareth timed the warming sun and found that daylight was increasing by an hour each day. The snow began to melt and fill the river beds in chattering torrents. The earth appeared, and within hours was covered with moss and lichen, and then clusters of white arctic cotton and yellow poppies, saxifrage and mountain avens. Soon under the day-long, almost night-long sun, the yellow, white, red, and purple flowers grew so rapidly that Gareth could see them spreading before his very eyes. The birds, too, returned; gulls, kittiwakes, murres, ducks, geese, snow buntings, snowy owls. When he was out for a walk one day, he saw a sandpiper, and rushed back to the hospital for his camera. On the way he met one of his friends, a snowmobile driver, and he too collected his camera. Together they began to stalk the sandpiper at the water's edge.

"The excitement of seeing these sure signs of summer seemed to make us a little touched," Gareth wrote, "and we laughed and called to each other as we photographed the bird until I took a careless step and fell backwards into the thick, dark mud, holding my camera in the air for safety. My companion, who was standing on top of a large mound of stones on the opposite side of the pond, roared with laughter until he too, lost his balance and disappeared backwards into the mud behind the mound. When he re-emerged, caked in mud, we both laughed until our sides ached.

"Such attacks of 'midsummer madness' as the bird photography incident were typical of the way in which we coped with the Arctic blues. The boredom of months of isolation and darkness made one welcome anything which broke the monotony, and we thought nothing of spending hours doing something which, in the south would have been considered lunacy. Perhaps it was a type of madness, but paradoxically, it was the thing which kept us sane."

38

Perspective:
Infection — Quest and Conquest

THE EPIDEMIC THAT Joe Moody managed to contain before it overwhelmed the entire Arctic was the latest in a series of polio epidemics
that had affronted the North American public since the First World War.
A twentieth-century phenomenon, "infantile paralysis" was hardly a
disease at all until 1916, when an outbreak in the United States killed six
thousand people and crippled, mutilated, or paralyzed twenty-seven
thousand others.

Americans were shocked. Epidemic disease suggested dirt, contamination, and backwardness associated with tom-tom kingdoms and machete
republics, yet there was no country in the world more progressive than
theirs, or more dedicated to hygiene. And here they were, not only
helpless victims of a particularly frightening disease, but one that was all
their own. For polio scourged no other continent. It was almost unknown
in the rest of the world. It almost seemed as if clean living was the very
condition that enticed the disease. That was the opinion of at least one
outside observer. "Epidemic polio is, in a sense, a disease of the water
closet, of Cellophane and the deep freeze." The healthier the child or
adult, the lower his resistance to a virus that had no respect for Lifebuoy
Soap or even the almighty dollar, the rich being even more likely to
contract it than the poorest immigrant.

Five years after the 1916 outbreak, one of the most prominent citizens
of the United States became a victim while holidaying in Campobello,
New Brunswick. Franklin Roosevelt was paralyzed in both legs, and for
the rest of his life sat as a brilliantly lighted symbol of the terrible damage
that polio could do. In his determination to fight back and continue his

political career, he was also a symbol of the long, dramatic, often bizarre campaign against polio.

The National Foundation for Infantile Paralysis was inaugurated in Roosevelt's name in 1938, toward the end of his first term of office as president of the United States. For the next seventeen years, there was a prodigious expenditure of treasure and energy in an effort to control the disease and restore the national pride in its sanitary values. Toronto featured in one campaign. A Dr. Edwin Schultz of California, after some research, claimed that if a solution of zinc sulphate were sprayed into the noses of monkeys, it would protect them against polio. He persuaded the authorities to give this method a human trial. When an epidemic hit the Ontario capital in 1937, five thousand children in the city had their nasal passages sprayed about two dozen times over a period of ten days. Another five thousand children were used as controls. No more was heard of the Schultz method when the embarrassing results came in. Not only did the treated children develop polio in the same proportion as the comparison group, but some of the children forfeited their sense of smell.

By the end of the Second World War, even the most enthusiastic experimenter in alternative measures agreed that there was probably only one way to control poliomyelitis, and that was to follow through on the inspiration of Louis Pasteur and develop a vaccine.

In the process of developing the germ theory which proved that microbes in general could cause disease, Pasteur utterly demolished the concept that "spontaneous generation" was responsible for the production of bacteria. Spontaneous generation was a long-established idea accepted by trained scientists as well as by splendid amateurs like Leeuwenhoek. When the plain-speaking Dutchman watched his pond-water animalcules wriggling under the mini-microscope, he did not for a moment doubt that they had spontaneously arisen in scum and slime. For the next one-and-a-half centuries, even the most sophisticated scientists did not question the assumption that flies were improvised from dung, maggots from putrid flesh, or that mice were created from fluff, dust, and old bedding.

It was alcohol that drew Pasteur into bacteriology. In the late 1850s, a Lille industrialist, unhappy about the quality of the spirits he was producing from sugar beet, asked Pasteur to look into the process. Inaugurating a career as an "industrial troubleshooter," he studied the fermentation involved. (Fermentation is the word for a useful process; when the product is harmful the word is putrefaction.) Fermentation had long been thought to be a chemical breakdown of yeast. Pasteur found that it was caused by living organisms in the same way that vinegar was produced by the decomposition of wine, and milk converted to lactic acid by the action of the lactic acid bacillus. It seemed that it was not spontaneous generation after all that accounted for the contamination of the alcohol-forming process, but outside forces, germs.

The proof, though, was not yet indisputable. It would take a lifetime of work by Pasteur in France and Robert Koch in Germany to establish that.

By 1864, Pasteur was showing that bacteria-free liquids could be kept free of organisms if properly protected from them, one of the methods being a gentle application of heat—pasteurization. (This being France, pasteurization was applied to wine rather than milk.) A year later he was saving an entire industry from ruin by identifying and dealing with the germ that was destroying the silk worm.

A further achievement was the discovery of the rabies virus in the saliva and nervous systems of animals. Subsequently he successfully immunized a nine-year-old boy against that awful disease. By the end of his life he had utterly demolished the spontaneous generation concept, established the germ theory, and inspired a new era in bacteriology, microbiology and, through Lister, antisepsis and asepsis.

As a person, Pasteur was, to the relief of his biographers, by no means free of immodesty and intolerance, or even of scientific rashness. In 1881, before an international audience of admirers, he triumphantly vaccinated twenty-five sheep against a virulent farm animal disease, anthrax—but then made the mistake of jumping into production of his vaccine, without sufficient preparation.

French science was not noted for financial profligacy in research, as Madame Curie among others would discover when offered an abandoned mortuary as a laboratory. At the height of his fame, Pasteur was still paying for much of his research out of his own pocket. Even by 1881 his assistants, while producing the anthrax vaccine, had to make do with inadequate equipment, some of it improperly sterilized. The result was a contaminated vaccine that killed sheep instead of protecting them.

The worst of it was that Pasteur's German rival, Robert Koch, got hold of a sample of the vaccine.

Pasteur, like the rest of the French nation, had been humiliated and seared to the soul by the French defeat in the Franco-Prussian War of 1870, and consequently hated everything German. The emergence of Germany as the greatest centre of science in the world did not help in the least. On top of his nationalist feelings, Pasteur was jealous of Koch's success in his, Pasteur's, field. He had met Koch once before in London, when Lister introduced them to each other. The meeting had not been a success. Koch had been supercilious, and Pasteur, prompted by the kindly surgeon, had shaken Koch's hand as if it were a jellyfish.

Pasteur's chagrin was complete when Koch, after analysing the anthrax vaccine, accused Pasteur to his face of suppressing unfavourable results, adding contemptuously, "Such goings-on are perhaps suitable for the advertizing of a business house, but science should reject them vigorously."

Pasteur had grounds for jealousy. Koch, over twenty years his junior, was greatly extending the bacteriological work begun by the French master, as well as developing the microbiological techniques that would speed the way to the revolutionary discoveries in chemotherapy that were made between the two world wars.

Koch was one of the most gifted researchers in medical history, a man whose insights were original, whose methods were simple, elegant, and immaculate. Born in Klausthal in 1843, he was the son of a mining engineer who, despite a large family, managed to put Robert through medical school at the University of Göttingen—the saber-slashing college that gynecologist Tom Cullen later attended. Though a prize-winning essay on the nerves of the uterus pointed to a career in research, Koch went into private practice instead, to please his new wife, cousin Emmy. A basically considerate, introspective man, Koch had soon found that it was easier on his nerves to give in to his spouse, who was rapidly turning out to be as domineering as she was ambitious for her husband.

A nagging wife, as was Frau Koch, suggests an inadequate sexual relationship, but that was hardly the situation here, for Koch was, if anything, guiltily oversexed, as a boy squandering "the noblest sap of my body" and in middle age lavishing it on other women, for whom he had a passion. At any rate, he fell in with Emmy's plans to make him rich and respectable through private practice, and, after the Franco-Prussian War, settled down in the east German town of Wollstein.

Emmy may have been something of a nag but it was she who steered him onto the course that would make him not only respectable but famous. On his twenty-ninth birthday, she gave him a microscope. Koch was overjoyed, and before you could say *Arbeitslosenunterstützung*, he put the instrument to use in the study of the anthrax bacillus, working behind a curtain in his consulting room. He already had some excellent photographic and biological equipment, and a few experimental mice.

Though Pasteur had demonstrated the presence of bacteria in the blood of infected animals, it was still not certain that they caused the infection. They might merely be present as harmless though uninvited visitors. Koch vividly remembered the words of his professor at Göttingen, Jacob Henle: "Before microscopic forms can be regarded as the cause of contagion in man they must be found constantly in the contagious material, they must be isolated from it and their strength tested." Which was just what Koch did, after three years of part-time experimentation in the cluttered space behind the brown curtain in his consulting room.

His techniques seemed to be instinctively right. Dr. Steven Lehrer in his *Explorers of the Body*, gives an example of a method that was as simple as it was original. "First he made a small trough in a glass slide, into which he put aqueous humor from the eye of a dead ox along with infected matter. Then he covered the trough with a second slide and sealed the edges to protect the mixture from the surrounding air. In this simple but brilliant manner he was able to study through his microscope the life cycle of the tiny anthrax organisms trapped between the slides, as they fed on the nutritive fluid of the eye. While he watched, the bacilli grew into long cylindrical rods covering the whole side. Shortly afterward, Koch could see spots forming—the thick-walled spores or seeds of anthrax.

"Now certain that he had found the germ of anthrax, Koch injected the bacteria he had grown into mice. By 1876 he had worked out the life cycle of the anthrax bacillus and had demonstrated conclusively that anthrax spores from pure cultures could infect and kill inoculated animals. For the first time, a germ grown outside the body was proved to be directly responsible for a disease. A specific germ caused a specific disease. In the case of one disease—anthrax—Koch had succeeded in proving this essential postulate of the germ theory."

When he turned up in nearby Breslau with this proof, there followed one of those scenes that so thrillingly enliven medical science, such as the moment when Professor MacLeod returned from vacation and was confronted with the results of Banting's experiments. Ferdinand Cohn, the director of the Botanical Institute in Breslau, was not infrequently approached by misguided scientists, and when Koch wrote to him he assumed that this provincial G.P. was another bumbling amateur. Perhaps a little long-sufferingly, he invited Koch to demonstrate his findings. When Koch did so, in his jerky, monotonous style, Cohn was as transfixed as if the bearded amateur were a Cicero. He could hardly believe the revolutionary findings. The germ theory was alive and living in provincial Wollstein.

Cohn immediately rushed off a message to Julius Cohnheim, a distinguished pathologist working at the Breslau Pathological Institute. Cohnheim came, saw, and was conquered. After the demonstration he went back to his institute to report the greatest discovery yet in bacteriology. He also told his assistants that he saw a great future for Koch in research.

True enough, for within months, using organic dyes as stains, Koch was identifying and photographing hitherto unrecognized bacteria with his new Zeiss microscope. Later he "was able to stain with methyl violet the blood of animals with sepsis and see tiny bacteria among the blood cells. After exceptionally skillful experiments he was able to pass a mixed bacterial infection from an original fluid to a chain of animals, so that by the time the infection reached the last animal only one type of bacteria remained and there could be no doubt that the disease from which the animal was suffering had been caused by this bacterium. Thus Koch was able to identify for the first time the organism responsible for the common forms of septicemia, gangrene, abscess, and erysipelas." And in 1882 he isolated the cause of one of mankind's worst afflictions, the tubercular bacillus.

Shortly afterward he helped his assistants Löffler and Gaffky to identify the diphtheria and typhoid germs. (The diphtheria antitoxin, which was welcomed with such joy and relief by general practitioners as far-flung as Murrough O'Brien in Manitoba, was discovered in 1890 by a protégé of Koch's, Emil von Behring.) As Gaffky remarked, once Koch had shaken the tree the discoveries rained into his lap. These included the organism responsible for cholera, his last great achievement.

Whereas Koch had discovered the cause of such diseases as tuberculosis, Paul Ehrlich discovered a cure for another, syphilis. This was the first great therapeutic triumph over an infectious disease, by the man who invented the word "chemotherapy"—the treatment of infectious diseases with drugs, either synthetic or natural antibiotics—that kill microbes without harming the host.

The compound that Ehrlich synthesized was salvarsan. At the time it seemed like a miraculous development, though ultimately it was penicillin that conquered that particular disease.

Ehrlich was particularly noted for his methods of staining specimens for examination under the microscope. For the new sciences of bacteriology and microbiology, this was a vital area of endeavour. Staining enabled otherwise imperceptible microbes to be plainly seen. Ehrlich showed that white blood cells could be selectively stained with basic dyes, that the urine of typhoid patients reacted with diazo dyes, and that the tuberculosis bug showed up under the action of carbol-fuchsin. Staining was a scientific territory that was still being explored decades later, as for instance, with Wilder Penfield's contributions to the staining of brain tissue in his early neurological work. (The names of the dyes themselves might have tinted fine poetry: safflower yellow, methylene blue, tyrian purple, alizarin crimson, congo red, trypan red, blue-pink rhodamine, gentian violet, indigo.)

Ehrlich's studies on immunity established, on slightly shaky foundations, yet another new science, immunology. While bacteriology was concerned with organisms responsible for individual diseases, immunology showed how the body responded to the organisms and devised therapy to take advantage of the response. A Russian, Metchnikoff, had partially explained the mechanism of the body's response in 1883, with his theory on the function of the phagocytes—cell-eaters—white blood cells, and others with roving commissions, that rush to the defence against invading micro-organisms. (It is now accepted that phagocytes fight in co-operation with the antibodies which are the substances that give immunity once they have defeated a particular germ. Example: once they have defeated the measles virus, the appropriate antibodies will guard against any further threat from that source—though a measles antibody will have no effect against, say, the chicken pox virus. Another antibody deals with that.)

Ehrich's foundations, brilliantly designed though they were, were not entirely flawless because, unlike Pasteur who approached scientific problems with no preconceived ideas, Ehrlich clung to a theory even while gathering experimental data. From the beginning, he believed that a "magic bullet" would be discovered that would kill not just one particular germ but all pathogens. It would be an anti-bacterial chemical compound that would require no help from the body's natural defences.

Even after he had been striving to prove the idea for ten years in his laboratory at Frankfurt am Main, Ehrlich was as certain as ever that one all-purpose drug would be found. It was in the process of searching for it that he discovered salvarsan. But to his distress, salvarsan turned out to be faulty. It was not even a magic bullet against syphilis alone, for while it could cure certain fresh injections, it had not much effect in longstanding cases.

Ehrlich's fanatic search for the bullet ended only with his death in 1915. He died deeply depressed by the semi-failure of what he had regarded as his one great achievement. "For seven years of misfortune I had one moment of good luck," he said.

For many years his gloom was shared by his successors in the science of chemotherapy that he had founded. It seemed that they could make no headway at all. In fact, a tremendous advance had been made even before Ehrlich died. In 1908, a certain compound had been synthesized but not tested. Instead it had been locked away in a laboratory safe. And there it had stayed, for a quarter-century.

The drug was prontosil—the first of the sulfa drugs. It had been prepared originally by a chemist at the I. G. Farben Company with whom Ehrlich was collaborating. It had been overlooked and tucked away in the safe, possibly because of an embarrassment of pharmaceutical riches—just another among hundreds of azo-dye samples that were being produced at the time.

It was in 1932, the year before Hitler's rise to power, that the I. G. Farben people, getting nowhere with their current therapeutic endeavours, thought of rechecking these old azo compounds. In the process they came across the one that had not been passed on to Dr. Ehrlich. To eliminate it as a contender in the chemosweepstakes, a Dr. Gerhard Domagk gave it a trial. He was still testing it two years later, his excitement thinned out over those two years, but with his gratitude undiminished, for the very first patient to be treated with it was his little daughter Hildegarde.

Nothing in medicine is more unpredictable than bacterial infection. Alexis St. Martin had lived with a huge hole blasted in his side, whereas Bethune had died from a tiny cut. Hildegarde seemed destined to be yet another victim of a minor injury. She had pricked her finger with a knitting needle. Soon she was on the point of death from septicemia (bacteria in the blood.) There was no known way to save her. In desperation, Domagk tried the unknown way, his experimental drug. The little girl recovered within a few days.

Subsequently, after testing prontosil just as successfully on fifteen hundred patients, even the coolly objective Domagk must have been tempted to think of it as the popular press later described it, as a wonder drug. It had quite astonishing anti-microbial powers, and Domagk said so, with the usual polysyllabic caution, in a report to a German medical journal entitled *The Chemotherapy of Bacterial Infections*.

The sulfa drug—it became sulfanilamide on this side of the Atlantic—caused a sensation among the public and medical profession. Over the next four years a flood of successors appeared on the market, including sulfpyridine, sulfathiazole, sulfamerazine, sulfamethazine, sulfaguanidine, and sulfadiazine. To date they have saved millions from death or incapacity. But they were not quite so wonderful as they first seemed. As summarized by Boris Sokoloff in his *The Miracle Drugs*: "In meningitis, in gonorrhea, in some types of pneumonia, in various infections caused by hemolytic streptococcus, in local infections such as carbuncles, sinusitis, infections of eye and ear, and particularly in urinary tract ailments, the usefulness of sulfonamides has been very great. In many other infections, such as gas bacillus complications, trachoma, actinomyces, and many other diseases, it has been of some help." But sulfa therapy sometimes had side-effects. Moreover it was powerless against the germs of syphilis, tuberculosis, typhoid fever, and many other infectious diseases, and was also ineffective against the viruses. It was penicillin that, while it had no effect on virus infections or tuberculosis (an antibiotic heir, streptomycin, would finally banish that "white plague"), proved to be the safe, kindly conqueror of syphilis and many other diseases, thus inaugurating the era of the antibiotics.

The discoverer of the single most important therapeutic agent in the history of medicine, Alexander Fleming, was, as a researcher, not in the same class as Pasteur, Koch, or Ehrlich. Osler said that in science the credit goes to the one who first convinces the world. Fleming failed to convince anybody, including his chief, Sir Almroth Wright. For though a clever scholar and painstaking researcher, Fleming's inability to communicate extended almost fatally into his work. In describing his great discovery in 1929, he failed to comment on the age of the germs he was dealing with, or the type, or whether they were incubated, or to mention what medium they were grown on, and in what numbers, or the range of their effect. Subsequently he blamed his failure to exploit his first break-through on the lack of the right kind of help in the laboratory. "I would have produced penicillin in 1929," he said to one acquaintance, "if I had had the luck to have had a tame refugee chemist at my right hand. I had to stop where I did." But it appears that what really stopped him was his own uncertainty, combined with an almost pathological reticence. It was as if he regarded the flash of emotion or even of ideas as being as disquieting as a belch at a tea party; and the attitude affected his work. It was as wrong to put it all down as to let it all out, it seemed.

Even so, Fleming inspires sympathy, as a man in emotional bondage. He was a Scotsman, and the Scotsman, as characterized by Fleming's biographer, André Maurois, dreaded giving himself away; "whence comes his stubborn silences and his dislike of exhibiting his feelings even when—especially when—they are strong." Maurois also said about Scotsmen that, "a fire burns deep within them which they do their best to conceal." But a fire too often doused may be quenched forever.

Spartan though it was, there appears to be no explanation in Alexander Fleming's childhood for the freezing of his self-expression. He appears to have been a naturally strong and silent type. Born in Robert Burns' Ayrshire in 1881, his life was normal enough for a Scottish lad: hard farm work along with the glorious freedom of the hills, eight-mile barefoot walks to school and back in summer, and through snowsquall and rainstorm in winter, his hands kept warm with a hot potato, which also served as a meal upon reaching school.

As there was a livelihood on the farm only for the first-born of the family, Alex left home in his early teens, and, along with three brothers, went to stay with the second eldest son, Dr. Tom Fleming, in London. In time, Alex went to work for a shipping company. He was rescued from the commercial life by an inheritance of two hundred and fifty pounds, which he invested in training at St. Mary's Hospital Medical School. He chose St. Mary's out of London's twelve hospital schools not because it was the best but because he had played water polo against it. Similarly when he joined the hospital's inoculation service under Sir Almroth Wright, the originator of anti-typhoid inoculation, it was because he was a good shot. Wright needed new blood in the St. Mary's rifle club, and the only way he could get the inscrutable Scot onto the team was by offering him a job in the inoculation lab.

Plainly, Fleming took neither himself nor his career too seriously. He might just as easily have become a surgeon, for while still a student he was advised to invest in the future by forking out five pounds for the Primary

Fellowship entrance fee in surgery. After passing this first stage in the F.R.C.S. exam, he continued on to the final test only because, "being a Scot, I never ceased to regret the five pounds which I had spent." It would have been an awful waste, not to have justified the expenditure of five quid—even though the idea of making a living by cutting into live patients did not attract him. Thus Fleming became the only fellow of the Royal College of Surgeons never to actually perform an operation.

Fleming spent his entire life as a researcher in Wright's laboratory at St. Mary's. His achievements even before penicillin were not inconsiderable, notably his First World War studies on infection in battle wounds, and the discovery in 1922 of lysozyme, the body's first line of defence against germs, found in such fluids as the mucous membrane of the nose and eyes. (Thus whenever you have a good cry, you're disinfecting yourself as well as relieving your feelings.) By 1928, he was deputy director of the inoculation service, long married, and as incoherent as ever. His wife, an Irish nurse, who unlike some women, had not been put off by his fixed stare and lack of outward expression, may have had to do the proposing herself, judging by a remark she made later. When Fleming mentioned casually to his co-workers one day that he had gotten married, they refused to believe him. They simply could not visualize old Flem in a domestic situation. Even when he showed her photograph they scoffed, assuming it was a picture he'd borrowed from a friend. It was months before they finally absorbed the amazing truth that somebody who could not even indulge in small talk without puzzling his listeners as to what he was getting at, really was a married man.

The story of Fleming's chance discovery of penicillin is a familiar one, in which extraordinarily good luck really did play a large part. In 1928 he was cultivating and studying bacteria, including staphylococci, and one day while talking to a colleague, Merlin Pryce, he uncovered one of his dishes and glanced at it. He stopped dead in the middle of one of his rare sentences, then muttered, "That's funny." and looked more closely. There was a growth of mould on the dish, and all around it the colonies of staphylococci appeared to have been affected, transformed from opaque yellow masses into silvery drops.

Mould is a type of vegetation formed from airborne spores that can settle and proliferate on any damp medium, from tarpaulin to old boots. To have mould form on laboratory cultures was a not uncommon occurence. What was unusual here was that the mould had killed a virulent bacteria.

It was likely that the spore had been blown up the stairway from a laboratory below, where an Irish scientist, with the good old Irish name of La Touche, was experimenting with moulds, including that of *penicillium notatum*.

Fleming followed up on the observation and soon realized that the phenomenon he had observed in the dish was peculiar to that species of mould—penicillium mould that could prevent the growth of staphylococci, streptococci, gonococci, meningococci, the bacillus of diphtheria, and the pneumococcus of pneumonia. That was astounding enough. What was even more amazing was that this extraordinarily powerful anti-bacterial agent was nontoxic—no side effects, no harm whatsoever to man or beast.

He had stumbled upon a magic bullet. Yet the paper in which he described it, and which later won him a share in a Nobel Prize in Medicine, roused no interest in the scientific or even the pharmaceutical community. In medical history, such neglect was usually the result of rigidity of thought, or slavish adherence to old principles, but this case was unique. It was the spokesman who was at fault, not the audience. Fleming, brainwashed by Almroth Wright's hostile attitude to drugs, which was not unlike Osler's therapeutic nihilism, failed to exploit the discovery scientifically. To begin with, his published account of the discovery in 1929 was lacking in the kind of detail that would have alerted the scientific community. It was as reticent as its author. Moreover, his experiments were incomplete. With great difficulty, not least because of penicillin's sensitivity to temperature, Fleming's two assistants managed to extract from the mould an antibacterial filtrate, but Fleming failed to progress to the next logical step, which was to inject it into bacterially infected laboratory animals, and compare the effects with control animals. The remarkable fact is that he was losing interest in penicillin as a possible treatment for deep-seated infections.

The declining interest was a direct result of his own abstinence from social intercourse. A "tame refugee chemist" might have made all the difference, but Fleming's strong, silent manner prevented him from demanding one. As an associate said of him, "You have to remember that even if Fleming approached anyone else for help it would have been in a completely offhand way, mumbling almost inaudibly, with the eternal cigarette butt stuck to his lower lip. 'I say, X, I've got something rather interesting in my lab that you might care to look at.' And if there was no response he'd say no more."

It was not until 1939, eleven years after its discovery, that effective work on the admittedly very difficult process of isolating and purifying penicillin was begun by Ernst Chain and Howard Florey at Oxford— they shared the Nobel Prize with Fleming—and 1941 before the first human trials were made, including the one previously described, on the policeman who had become infected after scratching the side of his mouth with a rose thorn. Subsequently penicillin was mass-produced in the United States. By 1944 there was enough penicillin available to treat every single Allied casualty and civilian bomb victim in the Second World War.

Penicillin's effect, not just on patients but on those administering it, is illustrated by the report of a Colonel Pulvertaft, a bacteriologist working in Egypt during the desert war. "We had an enormous number of infected wounded," he reported, "terrible burn cases among the crews of the naval armoured cars, and fractures infected with streptococci. The medical journals told us that the sulphonamides would get the better of any infection. My own experience was that the sulphonamides, like other new products sent us from America, had absolutely no effect on these cases. The last thing I tried was penicillin. I had very little of it, something like ten thousand units, maybe less. The first man I tried it on was a young New Zealand officer called Newton. He had been in bed for six months with compound fractures in both legs. His sheets were saturated with pus and the heat in Cairo made the smell intolerable. He was little more than skin and bone and was running a high temperature. Normally, he would have died in a very short while, as did all our wounded when infection was prolonged. We introduced small rubber tubes into the sinuses of the left leg and injected with a very weak solution of penicillin (a few hundred units per cubic centimetre), because we had so little. I gave him three injections a day and studied the effects under the microscope. I noticed, much to my surprise, that after the first treatment the streptococci were *inside* the leucocytes. That was a tremendous moment. Out there in Cairo, I knew nothing of what was being done in England, the thing seemed like a miracle. In ten days the left leg was cured, and in a month the young fellow was back on his feet. I had enough penicillin left for ten cases. Nine of them were complete cures."

The discoverer of penicillin had taken part in little of the experimental work and none of the development work. He admitted later, in the lecture that he delivered at the Nobel Prize ceremony, that he had been somewhat remiss. "My only merit," he said, "is that I did not neglect the observation and that I pursued it as a bacteriologist. The first practical use was to differentiate between different bacteria. We tried to concentrate penicillin but found, as others did later, that it was easily destroyed, and so, to all intents and purposes, we failed. Had I been an active clinician I would doubtless have used it more extensively."

One result of his failure to follow through is summed up in Ernst Chain's exclamation, made shortly before Fleming turned up in Oxford in the third year of the war. Fleming was then fifty-nine, a white-haired, silent little man sporting a colourful bow tie. He had read in the *Lancet* that Chain and Florey were working on "my old penicillin." After he had telephoned Professor Florey and said that he would be interested in seeing what they were doing, Florey had bustled along to give Chain the news that the great Alexander Fleming was coming. "Fleming?" Chain exclaimed. "Good God—I thought he was dead."

The sulfa drug was an antibacterial agent, while penicillin was an antibiotic, *antibiosis* being the opposing of one type of microbe with another. But the quest and conquest of infection had not ended, for there was another class of infectious disease that was unaffected by either agent, and that was the one caused by a virus.

Again it was Louis Pasteur who suggested that the problem in such diseases as rabies might be a "virus"—his name for the body's invisible poison (which became visible with the introduction of the electron microscope.) The viral diseases included smallpox, rabies, yellow fever, malaria—and polio; all of them ultimately defeated by the method that Jenner had established at the end of the eighteenth century, the development of a vaccine.

The story of polio illustrates the mystery that faced the virus detectives. Even by the Second World War, little was known about the world's smallest known creature. The virus was a puzzling organism that behaved as if it were alive but could crystallize as if it weren't. It refused to grow on laboratory meats and broths, was impervious to drugs, damned difficult to filter, and, in the case of the polio culprit (as in other diseases such as influenza), it appeared to have accomplices in the family—there was more than one strain of polio virus.

Before an effective vaccine could be developed to combat the disease, the question as to the number and types of polio virus had to be answered. Harry Weaver, research director of the National Foundation for Infantile Paralysis decided to pass the problem onto a young virologist at the University of Pittsburgh Medical School, Jonas Salk.

Weaver had already established that polio was not a disease of the nervous system as everybody thought, but an intestinal infection. Dr. Salk had established only that he, Salk, was an academic prodigy from the Bronx who was restless and discontented with his progress so far, despite his many medical articles. He was delighted at the research opportunity tendered by Weaver, though he cannot have been too thrilled by his duties in the university hospital at Pittsburgh as a monkey-house attendant. Monkeys were the only animals that could be used in polio experiments, but far from appreciating the importance of their role, they appeared to dislike it, and manifested their resentment by moving their bowels into their little hands, then moving the result at high velocity in the direction of the nearest target. In scenes symbolic of his later troubles, Salk presumably had to dodge the occasional shower of excrement.

By the late forties, three major types of polio virus had been identified, Type I, II, and III. Now it was possible to proceed to vaccine production. There were two schools of thought on the ingredients: one attended by virologists, Salk among them, who believed in a killed-virus vaccine; and a live-virus school under principal Dr. Albert Sabin, a Russian immigrant with a long and distinguished history in polio research—"a spare, tough, sharp-eyed man with a vulpine countenance, a small moustache and a resemblance on occasions to Groucho Marx." He could also be as rude as Groucho, to nobody's amusement. "Sabin couldn't say yes without antagonizing someone," according to one of his colleagues.

It was at this point, in 1949, that the unseemly race among researchers to be the first modern Pasteur really got started. Unseemly, that is, to stuffy outside observers, who viewed the American method in medical as well as other forms of competition as being rowdy, gaudy, or frantically egotistical, or all of these simultaneously. "The American way often gave the impression of being muddled, silly, and undignified'" wrote John R. Wilson (another of those British doctors-turned-novelist). "It caused acute distress to their friends and satisfaction to their enemies." But, comparing the American with the rigid Russian way, Wilson added, "Yet if we value truth at all it is the better way of the two. Life *is* silly, muddled and undignified. Science *is* a succession of false starts and stumbles in the dark. If we make it out to be anything else we are suppressing something important."

Nothing was suppressed in the polio race. Salk's vaccine, which was not based on any original research and which was one of a number that were being developed, was chosen on the basis of Salk's personality. Pleasant, modest, and confident—"a real-life Kildare," as one science writer put it, referring to a famous movie medico—Salk happened to meet Basil O'Connor, the head of the National Foundation, on a trans-atlantic liner in 1951. O'Connor (a lawyer) was so impressed with Salk that he had the Foundation sponsor a large field trial of the Salk vaccine. (The University of Toronto's Connaught Laboratories contributed to this work, as it did in making and distributing Sabin vaccine throughout the world).

The first test on a group of children had promising results. Unfortunately for Salk's professional reputation the news was released by a publicity-famished Foundation at a gala affair at the Waldorf-Astoria in New York, rather than in a proper medical journal. One of the guests was the editor of the *Ladies' Home Journal*, another was a spy for Broadway columnist Earl Wilson. It was Wilson who got the scoop: "New Polio Vaccine—Big Hopes Seen."

The result was a national frenzy. Salk's problem was that he was at the mercy of his sponsor, and his sponsor, the National Foundation, was determined to justify the millions it had been receiving for polio research by building up their man from Pittsburgh as a great discoverer, a twentieth-century Pasteur—though they must have been aware that his vaccine had not been properly tested. On the other hand, the scientific community, as Steven Lehrer wrote, "was far less appreciative, for Salk, in fact, had not discovered anything except how best to annoy his fellow scientists."

As for the reaction of the public, terrified of polio, they clamoured for the Salk vaccine. Throughout the country, parents tried to pressure or bribe their physicians into immunizing their children, even though the vaccine hardly existed yet. Canadians shared the fright. One country doctor, W. V. Johnson, practicing in Lucknow, Ontario, wrote that, "It was a terrifying experience for me during one of these [polio] epidemics to watch my two youngest children, Nancy two, and Bruce eight, lie ill for two days with a fever, headache and stiff neck, wondering helplessly when paralysis would appear as it had with so many neighbors. I even briefly questioned my wisdom in staying with my community rather than fleeing with the family to a non-epidemic district." He added that, "My fears and frustration probably were not unlike those of people during the plagues of Europe during the Middle Ages."

The field trial of the Salk vaccine came in 1954, when hundreds of thousands of children in the United States and a few in Canada, were injected, some with a mixture of the three major types of killed-polio virus, and some with an injection of a harmless control substance. An appalling failure might easily have resulted, given the circumstances—an impulsively chosen vaccine, a glare of publicity. In fact it was a striking success. The vaccine proved to be ninety percent effective against the II and III virus, though not quite as effective against Type I. But then a disaster came after all. Polio broke out among some injected children. One hundred and fifty were paralyzed, eleven died.

When the first marvellous results were announced, the reaction of the public had been melodramatic. Men and women wept openly in the streets, ministers praised Salk and God, Eisenhower awarded him a presidential citation, a Jonas Salk dime was designed, and he became a national hero. But when the cases of paralysis and death appeared, though it was quickly established that the fault was that of a pharmaceutical manufacturer, the Cutter Company, rather than the vaccine itself, Salk was reviled. He continued to protest that his vaccine was entirely safe, but "Despite Salk's optimism, the Cutter disaster was one link in a chain of events that would eventually banish the Salk vaccine from the United States."

Meanwhile Albert Sabin was pressing ahead with his oral vaccine. He was convinced that his live virus preparation, springing from kidney-tissue culture, would prove far more effective than that of his rival, whom he despised—he told one questioner not to mention Salk's name or the interview would be immediately terminated. But by the time his vaccine was ready for a major field trial in 1956, the United States was no longer a suitable locale—too much mass testing had already taken place. The results would have been inconclusive. Sabin needed virgin territory where the polio problem was acute but little had been done about it. So he made a daring offer to the archenemy, the Soviet Union, a country where the trials would be as rigidly controlled as every other aspect of life in that country.

When he was asked later why he had turned to the Soviet Union, Sabin replied that, "Before 1954 they used to say in the Soviet Union, 'Under our socialist health system, we don't get polio the way they do in capitalist countries.' Then, all of a sudden, their turn came. They began to have big epidemics—18,000-20,000 paralytic cases a year—and they were frightened." So when Sabin asked them if they would like to try out his new vaccine, they agreed. And the Russian trials established the Sabin vaccine as being more effective than Salk's, as well as being easier to take, as it was swallowed rather than injected. By 1960 it had been exclusively adopted by the rest of the world. Twenty years later the most feared disease since the Plague, is now forgotten.

Lest we grow smug over the cleverness of man in defeating such hostile forces of nature, other afflictions are quite likely to arise from the very way of life that enabled us to subdue the ancient fevers. Just as polio seemed to have been a penalty of modern hygiene, so the new venereal disease, herpes, appears to be the latest revenge by nature on a cultural atmosphere that treats sexual intercourse as a casual isometrics. No statistics are available in this country, but in 1981 it was estimated that between eight and twenty million Americans suffer from this third venereal disease. (The statistical uncertainty is caused by the fact that doctors are not yet required to report cases.) Herpes lies dormant for a while, like a fire burning in forest detritus, and flares up periodically. The researchers are able to make the virus roll over and die in the laboratory, but not in the human body. So far, it is quite incurable.

39

Two Famous Country Doctors

IN THE 1930s two of the most famous doctors in the world were rural Ontario practitioners: Mahlon Locke, perhaps the greatest of all foot specialists, who treated a million malformed feet, and Allan Roy Dafoe, who was noted for just one particular feat.

Mahlon Locke was that phenomenon, a doctor of medicine who happened to have a gift for healing. Using a special, manipulative technique on the feet of his patients, he could relieve or cure outright a wide range of complaints from rheumatism and neuritis to sciatica and arthritis. He had treated tens of thousands of crippled, agonized people long before his startling abilities came to the attention of the world press. By the early thirties their sensational reports had made his name known from New York to New Zealand.

At the same time, it was the spectacular nature of his powers that prevented him from being taken seriously by the medical world. A few individual members of the profession investigated Locke's techniques, but the profession as a whole disdained any scientific enquiry into his methods and their results. The circus atmosphere of Locke's prodigious country practice smacked of the charlatanry that the profession had been fighting for two centuries. Admittedly, Locke was no quack. All the same, it was not right for an M.D. to flaunt the kind of ability that was usually vouchsafed to upstart laymen, unlicenced meddlers, and religious fanatics. Even to the more open-minded among the profession, he seemed to be little better than an osteopath. And osteopathy was not entirely respectable.

Osteopathy had been invented by Andrew Still, one of those American sectarians of the sort who were always originating treatments as alternatives to orthodox medicine, such as the botanic system and the homeopathic. The osteopaths believed that hindrance to good health was the result of a structural defect, like a displaced bone. The defect interfered with the body's organs by disturbing their blood supply. It could be cleared up by manipulating the bone. Which was pretty much what Mahlon Locke appeared to be doing, and claiming that it brought miraculous cures. Or at least his ignorant followers were so claiming. No, it would be better for the dignity of the profession if the country doctor went unrecognized.

It was not always easy to ignore him, for by 1932, M. W. Locke was receiving a shocking amount of publicity. Moreover, he was disconcertingly well qualified, so he could not be indulgently dismissed, as so many country doctors were by the leaders of the profession, as one of a breed whose pastoral bumbling would never have made them a living in the competitive city. (W. V. Johnson, who was practicing in Lucknow, Ontario at this time, once overheard one of his medical school examiners saying, "That Johnson boy doesn't know very much, but he is going to the north country so I think I'll pass him.") In fact, it was Dr. Locke's postgraduate training at one of the world's most prestigious universities that had put him onto his pedal pedestal in the first place.

Mahlon William Locke was the product of a contented and unremarkable farm family. He was born on February 14, 1880, near Dixon's Corners, a hamlet located in the rich dairy country between Ottawa and the St. Lawrence River. In his book on Dr. Locke, a local historian, J. Smyth Carter, waxed unrestrainedly lyrical on the charms and potential of the hamlet. "A sort of metropolitan freedom pervaded this rural four-corners," he wrote. "Surrounded by an agricultural area second to none, it became a trade centre of considerable importance, gaining meanwhile a social prominence of rare distinction. But it was during election days and nights that the hamlet donned its gayest attire. All roads, paths and byways led to Dixon's Corners at such times. Barn raisings and 'bees' of various types also contributed to the happy life of the community of which Dixon's was the centre." Carried away by his role as official historian of Dixon's Corners, J. Smyth Carter added that, "If the entire story could be written and dramatized, it would make one of the most fascinating of screen productions with world record possibilities."

The most dramatic incident in Mahlon's youth, according to Carter, occurred when the young man was accused of blowing up the science room of the Iroquois High School. Refusing to apologize for what he claimed was a false accusation, he was promptly expelled. For a few weeks he worked on his mother's farm—his father had died when Mahlon was a child—but the post-hole digging to which he was allocated

soon convinced him that however awful school was, having to dig dozens
of holes below the frost line, was even worse. He went back to school, in
Kemptville, to complete his matriculation. That fall, at the age of
nineteen, wearing a new, six-dollar suit, he entered Queen's University at
Kingston to study medicine; and also fisticuffs, under the direction of the
former middle-weight champion of Michigan. As Mahlon put it, "Fearing I might not make a success of medicine, I took up boxing, as a sort of
second chance proviso."

As it turned out, there was no need to take up this alternative. He was
president of his class by 1904. He graduated the following year.

It was at the University of Edinburgh that Mahlon Locke, M.D.,
C.M., L.R.C.P.S., L.F.P.S., obtained his initial revelation into the value
of foot treatment in the remedying of human ills. The foot manipulating
techniques taught in Edinburgh were difficult to grasp, and few students
were able to do so, but Mahlon Locke proved to be a remarkable
exception. He had more than an aptitude for manipulative surgery, he
had a genius for it. In time his knowledge and intuitive understanding
enabled him to develop methods to an extent emulated by few men in the
history of medicine, and surpassed, up to his death in 1942, by none;
though his own estimate of his powers was typically modest and laconic.
"Of course there's nothing miraculous about my work," he told one
foreign reporter. "I studied at Edinburgh where they pay more attention
to feet than anywhere else and I've developed a theory and a technique of
my own. Nobody can feel well if his feet are sick. I put my patients' feet
right and Nature does the healing."

Nevertheless, to huge numbers among the literally millions of crippled
people who made the pilgrimage to Locke's surgery in Williamsburg, his
cures seemed absolutely miraculous.

Upon his return from Scotland in 1908, he established a practice in
Williamsburg, a village located six miles from the St. Lawrence River, in
a county whose contributions to the national culture would include an
Ontario premier and an apple, the McIntosh Red. In time he married a
local girl, Blanche McGruer, and, as a hobby, established a hundred-acre
dairy farm. Long after he had become the highest-paid specialist in the
country, he was still rising at dawn to milk his pedigree cows.

Williamsburg, according to J. Smyth Carter, was "one of those cordial,
carefree places where villagers and farmers mingle in happy accord." A
well-known American author was slightly less rapturous. Until the rest of
the world heard about it, he reported, Williamsburg "was an ordinary
little Canadian country village about the size of a strawberry mark." It
had a population of three hundred and had no hotel worthy of the name.
Meals, when available, were badly prepared, and the sanitary arrangements were primitive in the extreme, leading to "piteous complaints"

from the pilgrims, many of whom were desperately ill when they arrived.

The writer Rex Beach was one of those whose publicity elevated Williamsburg almost to the status of a Canadian Lourdes. Author of two dozen popular biographies, Beach first heard about the "hoof doctor" while on a golfing vacation in Ottawa in 1932. When Beach's feet started to hurt from all that fairway perambulation, somebody suggested that he go see Dr. Locke. Beach learned that people suffering from ailments of practically any kind were flocking to Locke by the thousand, even though Locke specialized in foot treatment.

Beach had difficulty in understanding how injuries and infections in other parts of the body could possibly be affected by toe-cracking, instep-wrenching, or any other kind of foot manipulation. He began to grasp the idea when a prominent Ottawa consultant explained the vital importance of the human foot. "Our feet," he told Beach, "have a lot of work to do, and while they're strongly built they're by no means fool-proof or indestructible. They are the foundations upon which we stand. Suppose I dig a hole under one corner of this house. The weight directly above that hole in the ground will be no longer supported vertically; the strains will be taken up along diagonal lines and as that corner settles, a crack back yonder in the wall may appear. Upstairs another crack still farther back may show up and on the roof we're likely to find a crack in the chimney clear over at the opposite side of the house. The bones of our feet are small and rather badly put together from an engineering standpoint. They are assembled into two arches which support our weight. When those arches lose their shape, numerous strains and stresses are transmitted to other parts of the body as a result of Nature's effort to compensate the balance. That results in trauma."

Trauma, the doctor explained, was one of the two causes of disease, the predisposing cause. The other, the exciting cause, was bacteria. Trauma could be caused by any kind of weakness, such as inflammation; which was when the micro-organisms moved in to take advantage of the injury. It was Locke's theory that a wide variety of ailments were the indirect result of faulty foot posture, which created pressure on the posterior tibial nerve, to start a chain reaction of symptoms in other parts of the body. It was his hypothesis that relieving the strain or pressure would clear the tracks for nature's curative powers.

Beach was even more intrigued when the eminent consultant admitted to having sent many crippled patients to Williamsburg. Locke had had them on their feet after only a few bloodless manipulations. The consultant suspected that Locke might be years ahead of the rest of the medical profession; so he was not one of those who poo-poohed Locke's achievements simply because the popular voice was being raised in loud hosannas. He was even willing to introduce Beach to Dr. Locke personally.

Beach expected to find a drowsy one-horse burgh, burned barnboard gray by the St. Lawrence Valley sun, but when he arrived he was astonished to find the place as excited and crowded as a circus. And crowded with strange people, "for nearly everybody limped, shuffled, walked with a cane or with crutches. Some sat in wheel chairs and out of car windows here and there peered stricken faces, lined with the cruel marks of suffering. These were the ones who were too weak or too badly twisted to get out; some of them were in their night clothes and wrapped in rugs or blankets."

The doctor's house and office were on a side street, shaded by maple trees. So many thousands of sufferers had tramped over the front lawn that it had been packed as hard as a clay tennis court. Arranged in concentric circles on the remains of the lawn were chairs, benches, boxes, and crates, on which sat dozens of patients. Scores of others stood at the back, six deep. In the centre of the inner circle sat Dr. Locke in a revolving office chair.

Locke proved to be a shy, noncommital person with humorous blue eyes. Beach and his companion watched from behind the swiveling chair as the doctor treated one patient after another with a speed made almost dizzying by the revolutions of the chair. For the benefit of the visiting physician and surgeon, Locke diagnosed the trouble in a few words, then gave the foot a practiced twist, the patient grunting and then laughing in surprise. The manipulation was over in about twenty seconds. Then the chair would swivel to the next patient.

Locke had already explained to the author why so many feet went wrong. "Fallen arches, misplacements of the foot bones are most commonly the result of flu or grippe or colds which lower the muscular tone," Locke said. "More often than not people get out of sick beds and put weight on their feet before their leg, ankle and foot muscles are sufficiently toned-up to support it and thus pave the way for sciatica, neuritis, arthritis and other ills. By restoring normal foot posture the predisposing cause of actual disease is removed and the exciting cause often disappears."

Rex Beach could see for himself what a state such feet could get up to. Staring around at Dr. Locke's patients, he had never seen such misshapen extremities. "Some were puffed and swollen, others were gnarled and knobby and even to my inexperienced eye it was plain that the owners were suffering. Occasionally a claw-like hand was outthrust and this the doctor manipulated firmly but gently. A wheel chair had been rolled into the circle, it was occupied by a rack of bones, a man whose chalky face and feverish eyes betrayed the fact that he lived in constant pain. When the doctor treated his feet, he clutched the arms of his chair, threw his head back and stiffened rigidly."

Some of the patients could not be treated by foot manipulation, and Locke would say so, murmuring to the consultant over his shoulder.

Locke's standard fee was one dollar, which he crammed carelessly into his pants' pocket, if he bothered to collect it at all. Even so, there were so many patients, often more than a thousand a day, that he could hardly help accumulating prodigious sums. During the early years of the Depression a local county or township bond issue of $150,000 fell due and could not be met. It was said that when a committee asked Locke's advice, he asked them to check with his bank, to see if he had that amount on deposit. When told that he had, he took up the entire issue. It seems likely that he could have become a very rich man indeed if he had wished. On one occasion, according to Beach, a grateful American millionaire offered him ten thousand times his normal fee. Locke returned the check without comment.

While the author and the consultant stood there on the baked lawn, streams of cars, scores of hobbling pedestrians, and busloads of travelers (the buses with signs on them reading "To Williamsburg and Dr. Locke") continued to pour into the village. "It was an extraordinary sight," Beach reported in the resulting magazine article. "There was something almost Biblical about the general faith in those healing hands. Most of these sufferers had tried every other means of relief and desperation had driven them here." With results that brought such joy to the sufferers that Beach was quite overwhelmed by their eagerness to talk about it. A Florida man swore he had been completely cured of lumbago after Locke had twisted his feet. The wife of a Toronto publisher had been unable to dress herself for five years and had been bedridden for the whole of the previous year. "Look at me now. Did you ever see anybody walk as beautifully as I do? I'm as happy as a girl." A teacher from a southern American college described how several years previously she had developed arthritis. The joints swelled and lost their action, she could not use her hands, and her knees were bent. She consulted numerous specialists but grew steadily worse. "I took various treatments. I spent a season frying out in the Florida sun: I entered a hospital in Boston, was put on a diet and given exercises that nearly killed me. In spite of all I could do I grew steadily worse. I heard about Dr. Locke and came here a few weeks ago, barely able to walk. Now my knees are straight, the swelling in my hands, my legs, my feet is almost gone. I'm practically well. It's—miraculous!"

Locke was well known before Rex Beach appeared on the scene. The Toronto Star Weekly had reported numerous cases of Locke's ameliorative treatment in the fullest detail. They were obviously not miraculous cures of the sort alleged to have been made through the ages by saints, mystics, and faith healers. Nevertheless, the improvement in the condition of a host of people suffering from seemingly hopeless ailments was startling.

At the same time, it appeared that there were many complete cures. One of them involved Frank Coughlin, the Watertown, New York, newspaperman, who first made Dr. Locke internationally known. He vouched for a complete cure, because it was made on himself. He had been crippled with arthritis for years, he said, and was about to undergo an operation when he heard from a Lockport priest who had been cured of the same disease by a foot doctor in Williamsburg, Ontario. Coughlin went to Locke as a last resort, and subsequently wrote an article claiming that Locke had made him whole again. That was the beginning of the Williamsburg stampede, which, in Rex Beach's words, "made the rural 'toe twister' as famous as any Viennese surgeon."

The article that Beach wrote for a major U.S. magazine attracted world-wide attention. It also produced severe criticism from the profession. Many medical men claimed, apparently without investigating the phenomenon, that Beach had been hoaxed. The cures, if they had really happened, had been effected through faith, or emotion. For two years, Beach was mocked by references to his Canadian miracle man and to the Williamsburg racket. He was accused of being a simple layman who had written on a subject of great complexity, and in his popular article was guilty of arousing false hopes among the world's incurables, and encouraging them to spend what little money the Depression had left them to visit a charlatan in far-off Canada.

The attacks had their effect, and in 1934, Beach returned to Williamsburg to establish whether or not Locke's work was holding up. If his medical theories were unsound, the fact would surely be in evidence by now.

What was immediately in evidence was the change in the village. Accommodation for the patients had become professional. Inns and hotels had been built, one of them with nearly half as many rooms as there were permanent inhabitants. Tourist camps had been organized, with housekeeping facilities so that the pilgrims who were on a diet could make their own dietary arrangements. Sanitation had been modernized, with many new wells bored, and whereas before there had been about three indoor toilets in the entire village, indoor bathrooms were now quite common. There were new garages, shops, and restaurants, and to accommodate the pilgrim traffic the Ontario Government had built a fine concrete road into town, with a bus service connecting Williamsburg with all the principal points in Canada and the United States. The town could accommodate up to ten times its former population of three hundred.

"At the time of my former visit," Beach wrote, "crippled patients were carried up and down porch steps and stairs, they spent their spare time on piazzas or lawns or in shuffling up and down the sidewalks. When it rained, they went to bed. Now the hotels provided conveniences like steam heat, hot and cold water, lounge, card and reading rooms, enclosed verandas, and innerspring mattresses."

Otherwise the traffic was the same. Autos were still trundling into town to park on every available space; the sidewalks were dense with people and forested with their walking sticks and crutches. On the road, wheel chairs and wheeled stretchers bearing pain-racked visitors competed for space with cars and trucks.

Nor had Dr. Locke's methods changed. The front yard of his house had been paved and canopied, but he sat in the same swivel chair, a "silent, capable man in shirtsleeves, probably the most widely discussed medical figure on this continent." Many of those surrounding him were pitifully crippled children, but there was no hospital hush. The jammed, maple-shaded street was loud with chatter and laughter. Beach perceived an atmosphere of joy. "There is brotherhood and sympathy here," he wrote, "but no revival spirit, no religious fervor. These pilgrims of health laugh when you suggest that Dr. Locke's success may be due to faith or stimulated by mob psychology. Why talk about faith, they ask, when they came here believing in the verdicts of other doctors and resigned to a lingering death? Imagination, indeed! Why, on all sides is proof, as real and as solid as the concrete underfoot, that this Canadian country doctor had cured and is curing cases like their own. Besides, this is no mere laying on of hands: there are no instantaneous cures, no miracles. He has a peculiar knowledge and an uncanny skill: improvement is gradual but sure."

Later, when Beach interviewed Locke, the doctor agreed that faith played no part in his work. "I don't care a damn," he said, "whether a patient has faith in me or not. As a matter of fact, most of them come here convinced that I *can't* help them. A great many have been to the foremost specialists and the best hospitals both here and abroad and have been pronounced incurable. Why should they put blind faith in a Canadian village doctor?"

In his first article, Beach had described Mahlon Locke's technique, a series of foot twistings that looked ridiculously simple. Watching him again, Beach recollected a patient's comment of Locke as having X-ray hands. "The description isn't as far fetched as it sounds," Beach said, "for he does...seem to see through his fingers and his powerful, sensitive hands appear to possess an intelligence of their own. While treating a foot his eyes are frequently fixed on the owner's face. It seems incredible that any manipulation so brief, so boiled down to its bare essentials can have genuine therapeutic value and it is no wonder that those who observe it for the first time put it down to hocus-pocus.

"And it does little good to quiz him about it for he is a reticent man. He talks in monosyllables and a question must be sharply pointed or he is liable to leave it unanswered." Beach described one of the few occasions when Mahlon Locke answered with more than a quizzical look. A woman came to him with a pain in her shoulder. Diagnosing it as an arthritic symptom, he immediately turned to her feet. As he made his deft series of manipulations she exclaimed, "But Doctor! It isn't my foot that hurts; it's my shoulder." Locke replied, "I know. But if you step on a dog's tail which end of him yelps?"

In 1934, Mahlon Locke was treating about twelve hundred patients a day, and Beach could find none who failed to claim that he had been cured, or that his condition had not greatly improved under Locke's treatment. In the latter category were victims of infantile paralysis. Naturally the doctor's achievements in such cases were at best relatively modest. Obviously, Locke said, he could not restore nerves and tissues that had been damaged beyond repair. The best he could do was to attempt to prevent further deterioration and try to revive what functions still remained.

Noting that the editor of the new Williamsburg *Times* had published many detailed stories about Locke's work, Beach went to see him. His name was James Macdonald, and he told the author that it was Locke who had brought him to Williamsburg in the first place. Macdonald was originally from Saskatchewan, where his son Jock had contracted rheumatism at the age of eighteen. The boy became bedridden, and was moved to Banff. His doctors hoped that the treatment available there, of baths, medicine, and serum, would at least halt the rapid progress of the disease, but the boy grew worse. He became so rigid that he could not turn over in bed. Formerly a husky lad, his weight dropped to ninety-one pounds. He was returned to a hospital in his home town.

"Here his condition grew so desperate that his parents lost hope. They were told that the boy could live only a few weeks. One arm by that time was rigid at his side, the other swollen and deformed. His right foot was drawn up close to his hip and locked there, his left leg was still: he could open his mouth only slightly."

Macdonald brought his son to Williamsburg on a cot in the baggage car of a train, and his summary of the treatment undergone by his son, as quoted by Rex Beach, went as follows: "The doctor glanced at him, asked no questions, and twisted his feet. This was done three times that day. After the first treatment Jock felt a tingling and glowing in his toes.

"For ten days there appeared to be little change. Then came reaction.... The lad was extremely sick with much vomiting.

"This sick spell lasted ten days and when it was over...general improvement could be seen. Only once in the early treatment did Dr. Locke touch his hands. All the benefit....came through the foot adjustments."

Rapidly the boy improved, his stiffened limbs began to move, his swollen joints began to bend, his chalky pallor disappeared and he gained in weight.

"A month and he was sitting up," Rex Beach said; "his back was nearly straight. Three months later he hobbled to the Circle on crutches.

"I talked with the young man himself. He had recently been fishing with his father and he can swim and row a boat."

The most amazing personal experience that Beach heard about was recounted by a charming, cultured woman pilot, a relative of Admiral Byrd of North and South Pole Expedition fame. As a world traveler, businesswoman and writer she commanded, according to Beach, implicit belief. "I really think I'm one of the outstanding cases in all of Dr. Locke's experience," she said. "I came here from California in September, 1933, with arthritis in every joint of my body, particularly in my neck, and with a bad case of fallen arches—in fact, my feet were perfectly flat. I also suffered from a well defined case of angioneuroticedema....a spasmodic swelling under the skin caused by a sick nervous system. Mind you, I'm repeating the diagnosis given me by some of the best specialists and leading clinics in the United States and Canada. I had fifty-two X-rays and many examinations, one less than a week before Dr. Locke saw me. For five years I had suffered intensely, I hadn't slept more than an hour at a time. I was getting worse and the angioneuroticedema complication was about as serious as anything could be.

"Three days after my first treatment I slept well. In seven days Dr. Locke had practically cured me. My arches were raised, all pain and swelling had disappeared and I was normal. Last winter in Florida I fell and broke my wrist and that's why I'm here now. I'm rapidly regaining movement in it."

Beach challenged Mahlon Locke on his apparent ability to cure arthritis, a disease that the profession as a whole considered incurable. "I've heard it said," he told Locke, "that arthritis comes from a focal infection such as diseased teeth, tonsils, or appendix and can't possibly result from mere fallen arches."

The doctor replied, "At least a third of my patients have had their teeth, tonsils, appendices and other organs removed long before I see them. Still the disease persists. I've never denied that arthritis comes from focal infections but I've never examined a case where the arches did not need attention." He added that in twenty years of practice he had never come across a case of arthritis in a patient with healthy feet. "As a matter of fact, we haven't a single instance of arthritis among the natives of this vicinity. I keep their arches in place and they don't contract it. It's absolutely unknown in Williamsburg Township....Any form of arthritis is amenable to my treatment except when the joints have become too solidly ankylosed."

He also answered the question as to why there was often a gap of many days between treatments, explaining that he seldom did any breaking down of the adhesions that had been built up over the years until the arches had been replaced and the circulation improved.

Though at least one Viennese specialist recognized Locke's ability to cure arthritis by strictly scientific methods, the medical profession as a whole continued to snub him. When Rex Beach asked him about this he replied tactfully, "I've never made any secret of my work. I've never held anything back. I've welcomed investigation: my clinic is open to any physician and many have visited it. I've explained every thing as best I could. I've demonstrated my methods. I've even let them take motion-pictures of my work." But nobody had ever succeeded in emulating his technique. "Several had gone away and tried," Locke said. "I don't know that I'm capable of teaching what I've acquired. I may not have the ability to do so, and so far I've been too busy to try."

Asked if there were any reason why others could not learn from Dr. Locke and translate their knowledge into practice, he replied, "None.... This manipulative surgery has achieved results and it should be continued, if possible."

Unfortunately it was not continued. Mahlon Locke died eight years later in 1942, and with him died a unique ability that could probably not have been communicated to others even if a concerted effort had been made to find out precisely how he had managed to make thousands of the hopelessly crippled walk again.

Much of his power, surmounting an uncommon diagnostic skill, appears to have been derived from a source that science could not measure.

With less justification but with far greater sensational emphasis, another Ontario country doctor, practicing 250 miles away at Callander, near North Bay, was hailed as a "Miracle Man" that summer. The lift-off from obscurity began on May 28, 1934, when Dr. Allan Roy Dafoe, whose only gift was his fund of common sense, was called to the bedside of a woman named Elzire Dionne, who was due to give birth to her seventh child in ten years. Dafoe was a conscientious doctor, and would have answered the summons promptly even if he had not been anticipating a troublesome confinement. During the last stage of her pregnancy, Mrs. Dionne had become abnormally heavy, her legs were greatly swollen, and she had been suffering considerable pain. Dr. Dafoe had ordered her to stay in bed; not without opposition, for Elzire Dionne lived in the tradition of peasant stoicism—she considered it her duty to carry out her household and farm chores whether she felt well or not. When the doctor next called upon her and found that her husband, Oliva Dionne, was allowing her to work despite the agony that she was quite obviously suffering, Dafoe rounded on the anxious husband, saying that if his wife did not remain in bed she might die.

Mr. Dionne was not an easy man to deal with, as would become plain during the ensuing weeks; but then neither was Dr. Dafoe. If Dionne was insensitive to his wife's needs through a lack of imagination, Dafoe was equally so in his attitude to the French-speaking people of the district, who made up about half the population. Though he had been practicing in the Callander area for a quarter century, Dafoe had made no effort to communicate more intimately with his French patients by learning the language. He was not a tolerant man in other respects. He was often quite rough with his French patients though there was no discrimination involved; he treated his English-speaking patients just as brusquely. He would later make a virtue of such qualities, playing the part written for him by the news media, that of the stereotype country doctor: crusty, unworldly, unsophisticated, blessed with the supreme common sense of a Will Rogers.

Far from being a simple man, he was as complex as he was inhibited. As a boy, Dafoe had not been permitted a natural self-expression. His father, a general practitioner in Madoc in eastern Ontario, was a rigid Victorian. His mother, too, saw no reason to allow the boy an outlet for his immature thoughts and feelings. Even his four elder sisters tended, through a superiority of age and intelligence, to undermine his self-confidence.

Nor was there any compensation to be found through friendship with others. Dafoe's frustrated upbringing had produced a stammer that prevented him from making close friends with boys of his own age. Like many other such victims of childhood tension, he withdrew into himself, into a world of books and reveries of heroism.

At the University of Toronto he was undistinguished academically, athletically, and socially: a weedy young man, barely five-feet-five-inches tall, with hands so small that even by middle age he would have to buy his gloves in the children's section of the haberdashery. An outsized head made him appear even more ungainly. As for his lack of academic stature, he was further truncated by the success of his younger brother, William Dafoe, who was an exceptional student, and who went on to become one of the most fashionable obstetricians in Toronto.

When Dafoe graduated in 1907, his father, obviously a man without much insight into the character of his son, confidently expected the young man to join him in the Madoc practice. Understandably, Allan failed to fulfil the expectation. He had had enough of his father's heavy hand, his mother's high-strung homilies, and the good example set by his brother and sisters. After interning at Bracebridge (where, during his first child-

birth case his inexperience forced him to hand the job over to a midwife)
he searched for a practice as remote from his family—and from professional competition—as he could find. At Callander on Lake Nipissing, a
few miles from North Bay, he found the perfect retreat: a practice that
was up for sale, for one hundred dollars. He grabbed it, and, leaden with
hurt and defiance, vowed to isolate himself in the north woods for the rest
of his life.

Sometimes, when he looked at himself objectively, Dafoe must have
cringed at the lack of impact he felt he had made on the world so far; that
he was a little man of little accomplishment. He had not even managed to
graduate without difficulty. A failure to answer a question in an oral
exam had very nearly undone him. He must often have hated himself for
his almost spectacular lack of grace and confidence. He had not even the
capacity to speak coherently: the stammer had seen to that. It is hardly
surprising that when a quarter century later the press hailed him as a
miracle man of medicine, he would exploit the role to the utmost,
welcoming the balm to a wounded soul.

Even Dafoe's marriage had not brought lasting contentment. The girl
was a local public health nurse. He had persuaded her to marry him at
the beginning of the First World War, but she had died a few years later,
following an attack of meningitis. He missed her sorely, and for many
years afterward lived a closed, solitary life, with but one social equal, a
local councillor, and one intellectual equal, the priest. By then he was the
victim of his atrophied emotions. Just as there had been no emotional
contact between Dafoe and his father, there was none between him and
his son. Even during the brief periods when the son was home from
boarding school, little love was displayed, and according to Pierre Berton
in *The Dionne Years*, when Dafoe became famous, his letters to his son were
written for him by the secretary who also prepared his syndicated
newspaper column. "Dafoe barely bothered to read them before he
signed them."

Though his son might have welcomed an occasional gesture of affection,
his patients were content enough with his bedside poker face. It was
reassuring to the blunt, unemotional people of Callander and district,
including the sorely pressed wives. A large proportion of his cases were
obstetrical. Up to 1934 he had delivered over five hundred babies, from
mothers as young as thirteen and as old as fifty-three. He helped one
woman in Astorville to give birth to twenty-three children, and if he
shared the sophisticated urban abhorrence of such a rate of production,
he kept these feelings, too, to himself.

When he was not burying himself in his work, he was burying himself
in escapist literature, and in escape to distant places and into exotic lives
through the radio. He would fiddle for hours with his radio, listening to

faraway broadcasts, from New Jersey or the Netherlands; to the rich, funny, or exciting lives of *Captain Diamond, Amos 'n' Andy, Fu Manchu, One Man's Family.*

His only female confidante was Louise de Kiriline, a Red Cross nurse in Bonfield, with an aristocratic Scandinavian background. She worked closely with Dafoe, and had much respect for him until the amazing multiple birth in the Dionne house that May. As quoted by Pierre Berton in his *The Dionne Years*, she said about Dafoe that he was quite a peculiar person. He knew everything there was to know about his patients. "As a medical man I would say his greatest skill was diagnosis. He really did know exactly what was the matter. That was not so much from reading books as from his own experience with all those families—seeing them, you know, from generation to generation. His asepsis was not very good. It was always very hard for me to get him to wash his hands...

"You know the people lived very, very poorly at that time during the Depression, but he never refused to come and he never talked much about money. He was really very fond of this place, and he was very fond of the people...

"He kept mainly to himself, but he was very open with me. We discussed all kinds of things. He was very interested in history. We discussed conservation. We discussed medical matters and so on. So spiritually, it was very interesting, because there were very few people he could talk to...

"Yes, I think he was lonely. I'll tell you a little secret: he proposed to me once! Dr. Dafoe! From behind the door. Of course, I didn't have any thought of that at all. But he was really touching and I felt so sorry for him because he was so very lonesome. And he was a nice man then. Of course, he changed."

The change began early that morning in the Dionne farmhouse, a flyblown property, without electricity or running water. It was one of the two midwives in attendance who had sent for the doctor, when it seemed that Mrs. Dionne was likely to die at any moment. Dafoe had earlier diagnosed dropsy. When he arrived he found her terribly swollen and as cold as a fish. But what caught his attention first was the sight of two newborn babies lying on the bed, wrapped in tattered wool. They had been delivered by the two midwives, Mme Labelle and Mme Legros. The infants were so tiny that they could be held in the palm of one hand. They looked quite grotesque, with disproportionately large heads and legs hardly larger than those of a frog.

Even more astonishing was the sight of a third infant emerging from the mother. Twenty-six-year-old Mme Dionne was having triplets.

But then, as he was tying the umbilical cord of the third child, another baby appeared. Even Dafoe, who had spent twenty-five years in training his face to behave, to give nothing away, could not help gaping at this astounding development. The odds against a quadruple birth were multi-millions to one, odds lengthened still further by the uniform sex of the four incredibly tiny infants. They were all girls.

Even that was not the lot. Almost immediately, a fifth baby was born. Another girl. Like the fourth, it too was still wrapped in its amniotic sac. Dafoe could not help it. He exclaimed aloud.

However, there was even greater priority than the lives of the quintuplets. After freeing the last two from their transparent wraps, and baptising them conditionally, and asking one of the midwives for more of the traditional hot water, he turned to the mother. She was in a bad way. Her circulation was almost non-existent. He hurriedly prepared a hypodermic, and gave her an injection of pituitary to raise her blood pressure, then one of ergot to inhibit any possible post-natal hemorrhage. She could hardly afford to lose a drop of blood.

"Holy Mary," she whispered, when she was finally informed that she had borne five babies. Dr. Dafoe's reaction when he saw all five infants together for the first time, was a typical thirties euphemism: "Gosh."

By then the babies had been arranged in a basket in front of the hot oven in the kitchen. The basket was placed on two chairs with a heated blanket over the chair backs. It was now that Dafoe gave the advice that saved the lives of the five girls. In a hospital they would certainly have been cosseted to death. Dafoe's advice was to leave them strictly alone. If they lived they were to be given a drop or two of warm water from an eye-dropper every two hours.

Secretly, though, he did not believe that they would survive. They were just too small. One of them, Marie, weighed only one pound eight ounces at birth. A four-year survey, conducted at the Toronto General's lying-in hospital, the Burnside, had shown that out of every eleven babies weighing less than three pounds at birth, only two were likely to live.

Two of the five girls were close to death many times. Dafoe stimulated them with rum diluted with warm water. On the Thursday night when the quintuplets were three days old, Dafoe looked into the incubator that had now been supplied, and saw that Emilie and Marie were about to die. To the horror of one of the nurses present, he gave the tiny creatures an enema, using a two-inch syringe and a length of rubber tubing, then fed rum to the babies. Once again they revived.

As the days went by, the situation at the farmhouse deteriorated rapidly. It was hardly ideal to begin with, even on the day of the birth. The first graduate nurse on the scene was a pretty girl named Yvonne Leroux. Because of her association with the quints she would for years after have her picture on the front pages, her own radio show in New York, turn down Hollywood offers, and become a hot property on the lecture trail. In her diary on May 28, Yvonne recorded: "No HWBS, no abs., decent dishes, no screens, doors or cleanliness, and mosquitoes at night and flies in the day. Neighbours trying to be kind but being rather underfoot...babies sound like mosquitoes when crying." Four days later, Dafoe realized that something would have to be done about the environmental conditions. The farmhouse was seething with people and their germs, the air dry with dust from the road outside, and from the ninety-degree temperature; and Thérèse Dionne, aged four, had a bad cold and was running a fever. Pierre Berton wrote, "Dafoe insisted that she be moved out of the house, in spite of the protests of her parents. It began to look as if the babies might have been safer in a Congo village of mud huts."

Dafoe called in Louise de Kiriline. She went through the place like a whirlwind, rearranging the furniture, scrubbing the floors, walls, and ceilings with disinfectant, tearing down the curtains, reorganizing the kitchen—and driving out the family. Nobody bothered to consult either Oliva or Elzire Dionne, a cavalier treatment that de Kiriline later regretted, confessing that, "Now, I think, I would take much more time with the parents—realize much more their feelings. But I was too taken up just keeping the babies alive, and to the detriment of my relations with the family. I really was quite brusque."

Which also described Dr. Dafoe's attitude to the family. By then he was rapidly becoming the darling of the news media. Unlike Papa Dionne, who was quite distracted by the international attention he was receiving, Dafoe was revelling in it, in his deadpan way. He was already being presented as the sole saviour of the quints, though in fact he was consulting his brother, Dr. William Dafoe, over every step of the treatment. Also, backing up Will Dafoe was Alan Brown of the Sick Children's Hospital, who also contributed substantially to the care of the five children. It was Allan Roy Dafoe's handsome, sophisticated brother who brought to Callander the oxygen in iron cylinders that kept the quintuplets alive until their breathing apparatus was sufficiently developed. Until then, "it had been possible to stimulate the heart and lung action of Yvonne and Marie only by regular doses of rum. Marie's heart had almost stopped during the early morning hours of June 2. Yvonne's condition was, if anything, worse. She alone did not waken and cry at the two-hour feeding periods and had to be coaxed to take her milk. Even rum produced little reaction. But after the oxygen treatment, Yvonne threw off her torpor and began to improve. The treatments—which had been developed through the Great War—produced an almost instantaneous effect, bringing the babies' breathing to normal a few minutes after application."

Six months later the five increasingly pretty girls were thriving, and so was Dr. Dafoe's reputation. His photographs with the quints had made him the best-known doctor in the world. From the very first day he had been a hit with the press. He fitted their simple characterization perfectly, without a single jarring fault, or at least none that the newspapers and magazines cared to expose. He was the country doctor *par excellence*, modest, patient, honest, and direct. Even the most jaded New Yorker held him in awe and reverence. "Dafoe's public image," wrote Berton, "was always that of a self-effacing GP who didn't give a hoot about money. That image was never tarnished. The press, which must have come to realize that Dafoe was making a tidy fortune from his sudden fame, never bothered to explore the subject. It was as if the media had determined in advance what role the doctor was to play on the front pages. In less than a decade Dafoe would become a well-to-do man, but the public continued to view him as a simple country practitioner of even less modest means."

40

Penfield

A S USUAL, DR. Archibald was late for his appointment. He was supposed to have been present at the operation from the beginning, but
the surgeon he had come to watch had already started; had already
exposed the cerebellum and was preparing to probe for the brain tumour.

Archibald hurriedly donned a gown, cap, and mask, and strode into
the operating room, apologizing for being late. His host, the thirty-six-
year-old Wilder Penfield, outlined the case briefly, then settled down to
work with his assistant, William Cone, in the rapt silence that was
customary during his operations. Archibald watched intently over the
other's shoulder, perhaps slightly amused at the reversal of the usual age
relationship—himself, the older man, observing the work of the
younger—as Penfield slowly exposed the tumour, which was growing
inside a capsule from a deep attachment to the auditory nerve. Though
the tumour was benign, it had stretched the nerve that controlled the
movement of the left side of the face, which accounted for the patient's
gradual loss of facial expression. If not removed, the tumour would
paralyze her face, and also blind her for life.

Archibald had been told that as a surgeon Wilder Penfield was on the
level of Harvey Cushing, America's foremost neurosurgeon and Osler's
biographer. By noon he had confirmed this for himself. Young Penfield, a
graduate of Princeton, Johns Hopkins, and Oxford, obviously knew
exactly what he was doing, and was doing it with uncommon skill and
precision. Archibald was impressed.

After the operation, which appeared to be successful, the two of them
left the hospital, the Presbyterian Hospital in New York City, to take

lunch together at a restaurant on Fifty-Seventh street. Unfortunately Penfield could not offer his guest a drink. New York in 1927 was in the chronological dead centre of Prohibition. Still, the fifty-five-year-old professor obviously needed no bathtub gin to free his tongue. A distinguished-looking man, Archibald talked in a fascinating and amusing way, albeit almost inaudibly. He spoke in a low voice, almost a whisper, so that Penfield had to strain to hear him, as he discussed his plans for the department of surgery at The Royal Victoria in Montreal.

He had come to New York, he murmured, to persuade Penfield to move to Montreal and take over his practice in brain surgery, so that he, Archibald, could concentrate on chest surgery. In the process he wanted to build a strong department of surgery, and he believed that if Penfield were willing to make the move, he would add greatly to that strength.

Penfield responded with growing enthusiasm. He too, he told the professor, had great ambitions for the future. But his dream went far beyond Archibald's plans. It was his goal to establish an institute for disorders of the nervous system; but he did not aim to hog it with his own speciality, neurosurgery. He wanted to create an institution where neurology and neuropathology, as well as neurosurgery, would combine as equals, in a program of research as well as of treatment.

This was a startling idea, going far beyond what Archibald had in mind. There were traditional distinctions within the art of healing, and here was this enthusiastic young American proposing to sweep them aside; to team the physician with his often-deadly rival, the surgeon, and the pathologist with both—a team to be joined later, perhaps, by other neuroscientists; anatomical, cytological, chemical, and physical. Amazing. But the professor listened intently. Penfield was a man of whom great things were expected. He was known for his skill in his specialty, and he was at least as distinguished as a scientist, with many important papers to his credit. Perhaps his aim was not as idealistic as it sounded.

Money was the problem. Penfield was talking about bringing his friend and assistant, William Cone, with him, though Archibald did not think he could scrape enough money together for a team. All the same....

When they parted after lunch that had lasted six hours, the professor had made up his mind—Penfield was the man for the job, though all he said at the moment was that he would think about it, and see what he could offer in the way of facilities and support.

After Penfield had seen the professor off in a taxi, he walked home, excited at the prospect of realizing his dream in Montreal, which might just be the perfect location for his institute; a city that was surely a crossroads of European and American culture and learning, combining the cultural depth of the one with the vision and energy of the other.

There could not have been a more appropriate messenger to a member of the new generation of neurosurgeons than Edward Archibald. He was the first person in Canada to take a systemic interest in brain surgery, long before he turned to chest surgery.

Until this principal came along, the drama of neurosurgery in Canada had been little more than a curtain-raiser, with few characters and almost no plot. One of the first pioneers was John Reddy. In the year of Confederation, Dr. Reddy of Montreal appeared on stage with a stonemason who had a depressed skull fracture. After removing fragments of bone, Reddy kept a large, ice-filled bladder on the patient's head for nine days. The wound was then covered with lint soaked in ice water, with frequent changes of the dressing. After much delirium and some paralysis, the wound began to heal. Ten weeks after the accident of the stonemason had completely recovered.

The treatment had included plenty of brandy, as well as lots of ice, causing neurosurgeon William Feindel to remark that it was "hard to decide whether this was a surgical triumph for—or over—local hypothermia and local brandy."

Naturally, William Osler also appeared on the neurological bill. Osler made a considerable impact on neurological development in both Canada and the United States. At least a third of his writings were on neurological disorders, and his thousand autopsies in Montreal had shown him that surgery was the only answer to many intercranial lesions. The fact that he, a physician, was espousing surgery in such cases alerted many a young surgeon to the possibilities in the specialty, including Harvey Cushing and Wilder Penfield, both of whom warmly acknowledged their great debt to Osler, who had become Wilder's first friend at Oxford during the First World War.

Edward Archibald's first work dealing with the nervous system was published at the turn of the century when he wrote a pathological report on a brain tumour that had been removed by Dr. James Bell at the Royal Victoria Hospital. The tumour had belonged to a French Canadian of thirty-seven who had developed attacks of speechlessness lasting twenty minutes, severe headaches, weakness of the right facial muscles, and difficulty in writing. "James Bell, then clinical professor of surgery at McGill University, operated through a frontal bone flap 2 inches in diameter," reported Dr. William Feindel in an article on neurosurgery in Canada. "The patient recovered from his preoperative deficit in speech and writing. Before operation he could not write words of more than one syllable. When asked to write his name and address, the most successful of his efforts was barely legible and his attempts at copying were no better. Six weeks after operation, however, his writing showed great improvement."

Three or four years later, Archibald went to London to study under one of the major pioneers of neurosurgery, Sir Victor Horsley. Returning to Canada in 1907, he made the Nova Scotian fraternity sit up with his comment that "if only the internist, especially the neurologists and also the general practitioner, will learn to give up their traditional pessimism with regard to cerebral cases, and will work hand in hand with the surgeon I am convinced that great results are possible of attainment."

In Toronto, neurosurgery developed rapidly after the First World War with the emergence of the laconic Kenneth McKenzie, a central figure in the development of the specialty in Canada. "McKenzie's sound program of neurosurgical training produced men who serve in universities and hospitals across Canada," writes Dr. Feindel. "A unified neurosurgical service came to practical fruition in November 1958 under his successor Harry Botterell, who with his team of associates brought new impetus to intercranial vascular surgery by the introduction of hypothermia and by a logical classification of patients afflicted with aneurysmal hemorrhage of varying severity."

Back to Wilder Penfield in 1927. For a while he continued to dream of a new scientific and cultural life that Archibald had seemed to be offering in Montreal; but after several months with no word from the professor, his hopes faded. The silence from the north was all the more frustrating because after the meeting, Penfield had gone specially to Europe to prepare himself for the adventure, to test his plans for research in an advanced neurosurgical clinic in Germany.

Then early the following year, the year that Bethune moved to Montreal, he was invited up for a day of discussion.

It turned out to be a peculiar experience. If Dr. Penfield had been less cosmopolitain in his outlook, and had liked the people and the atmosphere of Montreal a little less, he might have given up all thoughts of moving to Canada, and remained in New York in the hope that some day he might achieve his ambition there. He was already feeling a bit doubtful about Montreal even before he arrived on the overnight train. He did not much like what he had heard about McGill University's second teaching hospital, the Royal Victoria. Its board of governors under Sir Vincent Meredith did not sound at all progressive. Despite Archibald's position as professor of surgery at McGill, for instance, they had refused so far to confirm him as the hospital's chief surgeon, though he was the obvious and only man for the job.

Not that Archibald seemed to mind the lack of a vote of confidence. When he met Penfield at Windsor Station, he was as polished and urbane as ever, despite an attire that was somewhat startling to the visitor: a fur hat and a huge fur coat, mantled with January snow. He took Penfield back to his Westmount residence, and over breakfast proceeded to outline the day's program. It was to begin with a demonstration by

Penfield of Dandy's procedure of airencephalography in the Royal Victoria's white marble operating room, to be followed by a lecture to the same audience, the senior medical students.

He did not make a good start. To Penfield's chagrin, he could not draw any spinal fluid from the patient. The hollow needle refused to fill up. Wilder muttered to the patient that he would have to try again later that day.

So it was with some embarrassment that he turned to deliver the lecture to the students ranged in the steep, amphitheatre seats. To make matters worse, the professor of medicine and the dean had also come to watch and listen, as well as Professor Archibald. "They sat in the front row," Penfield remembered. "Before I had finished the lecture, a nurse came in. She announced in a voice that, it seemed to me was far too loud, that the surgical resident had done the lumbar puncture successfully."

The next order of the day was a visit to Horst Oertel in the Pathological Institute. It was a crucial meeting, for the institute was the obvious location for Penfield's new laboratory. He would have to persuade Oertel to give up three or four rooms, fully equipped for microscopic work.

When Penfield saw the Pathological Institute it sent a cold chill down his spine. Near the entrance of the new, gray stone building was a crest from which a human skull emerged menacingly. Below it in Latin were the words, "This is the place where death rejoices to come to the aid of life. Nothing recalls one from sin so much as the frequent contemplation of death." It did not seem a terribly promising motto for the work Penfield had in mind.

Oertel was just as unpromising. He was a ponderous, self-important man, completely sure of himself, even of his thick German pronunciation, which was rendered all the more odd by the overlay of an English accent.

It was soon obvious to the visitors — Penfield, Archibald, and Jonathan Meakins (the professor of medicine), that the pathologist was not interested in Penfield's plan. His Teutonic contempt and phoney hospitality infuriated the American, and when he and the two professors were alone again he told them that he could not possibly work under Oertel in the Pathological Institute. He didn't like Oertel, and Oertel obviously did not want him.

Archibald and Meakins were dismayed by this setback. All three of them fell silent, until Penfield asked if there were any chance of establishing a laboratory in the Montreal General. Archibald replied that he was sure that the pathologist there, Lawrence Rhea, would welcome him, but it would be awkward having the laboratory so far from the Royal Vic, where Penfield's team would be operating.

"Meakins had said little up to this moment," said Penfield. "Now he spoke. He spoke to Archibald as if he had just made a decision. 'No,

Eddie,' he said, 'the laboratory must be here in the R.V.H. I can shift people around in my University Clinic. I could give you,' he said, turning to me, 'three rooms. They might even be subdivided with a partition or two.' Then he said something that really thrilled me. 'I'm ready to do this because you say you hope to serve the future of medical neurology as well as surgical neurology.'

"Meakins and Archibald exchanged glances and neither spoke for a moment. I realized then that this was something quite unrehearsed. They understood and respected each other. And I realized, too, that here in Montreal there was no rivalry between the two major departments, medicine and surgery."

There was a further advantage to Meakins's offer. His laboratory was independently endowed, and he could run it as he wished. Not even Archibald could have made a better offer.

The third order of the day was a luncheon in Penfield's honour at the Mount Royal Club. This was another shock for the young neurosurgeon—having to face many of the most august scientists in Montreal. But the reception soon put him at his ease, a mixture of British-style formality and easy hospitality with which Wilder was already familiar, as he had spent several years at Oxford and London.

After lunch, Archibald and his guest left the club and struggled off through the deep snow along Sherbrooke and up Peel Street. The heaped snow was so deep that from the sidewalk Penfield could see only the tops of the cars that were charging up the hill with their snow chains flailing noisily. As they reached Pine Avenue, Archibald pointed out the home of the hospital president, Sir Vincent Meredith. Obviously Wilder should have met the president, but by now he had the impression that Sir Vincent was hostile to his own chief surgeon. A moment later Archibald confirmed this when he explained apologetically that he had not been able to arrange a meeting between his visitor and his boss.

Penfield marveled. Here was Edward Archibald, one of North America's most distinguished surgeons, who could not even get in to see the president of his own hospital to introduce his own protégé. In effect, Penfield was being told that this titled administrator had no time for him. He was angered for the second time that day. "I'm not going to make a decision about coming to Montreal until I have met Sir Vincent Meredith and talked with him," he told Archibald there and then.

Dr. Archibald didn't answer for a moment, but as they continued along the street he said suddenly, "You will find that Lady Meredith is charming."

Penfield understood the drift of the older man's thoughts later that afternoon when he learned that Archibald had arranged for him to take tea with Lady Meredith. Archibald himself was not invited. Highly disturbed, Wilder went along. He found the lady to be welcoming enough, but his heart sank still further when she told him that Sir Vincent would be a little late.

"I felt hopeless," he wrote, "as if I had come to the end of the road. What chance was there that this charity-minded autocrat would change his attitude or make a bargain with me, however well I might describe to him my purpose and my dream of a new approach to an understanding of the brain and mind of man?"

When Meredith finally arrived, Penfield met exactly the kind of man he had been expecting: a confident, impeccably tailored, opinionated bureaucrat. But after a while, after listening to the fellow and studying him carefully, Penfield suddenly realized what the trouble was. Meredith had cerebral arteriosclerosis. He was likely to die at any time.

This was not a man who would long stand in the way. Here was a man to be pitied rather than feared, and the discovery helped Penfield to reach a decision. All day, with the exception of Meredith's favourite, Oertel, he had been impressed by the quality of the physicians and surgeons he had met in Montreal, by the conservative excellence of the McGill product. "They were reserved and civilized in a way that made them different from the doctors I had met in other parts of the world and I felt at home with them." He had yet to meet any French-Canadian medical men, but that would be no problem; he was determined to get the French-Canadians as deeply involved as the English-speaking doctors in his neurological work. So he would not worry about that. He would assemble his team right away, starting with his surgical associate, Bill Cone. He would move to Canada, and perhaps by the time he became a citizen, in 1934, his dream, the Neurological Institute would be a reality.

The Penfields and the Cones came to Montreal in the fall of 1928. The Penfield family—four children, a German governess, the doctor and his wife Helen, moved into a top floor apartment on Sherbrooke Street. One incident that showed Penfield just how different this northern city was, occurred when he was setting out for the hospital one glorious, crimson-and-gold fall morning. As he was emerging from the house, a car drove up with the head of a moose lashed to the hood, a moose in all the glory of its mature antlers. Wilder watched in astonishment while a white-coated houseman ran down the front steps to help the driver carry the head into the house.

"What other metropolis was there in all the world, I mused, so close to the deep wilderness as this unique bilingual city to which we had come?... What streams and lakes and forests there must be that could be visited before breakfast!"

The Cones were already settled in when the Penfield family arrived. Avis Cone was a tall, vivacious blonde, and like her husband a graduate

of the University of Iowa. William Cone, at thirty-one, was a tremendously enthusiastic man with a rare talent for neuropathology, and a
growing skill in neurosurgery. Great efforts had been made to keep him in
New York, including an offer of a laboratory of his own in the New York
Neurological Institute. Nevertheless he had elected to join Penfield,
partly out of friendship, but also because he realized that his talents
complemented those of his colleague. Cone was especially good with
patients, and could make rather more intimate contact with them, and
could pass on what he had learned to Penfield. He was also a fine scientist,
forever restlessly searching for the perfect microscopic and surgical
technique, though he was not particularly interested in physiology, or in
the essential writing of reports and papers. On the other hand, Penfield
was an excellent writer. He was also a born leader, earning loyalty and
devotion from his team with effortless ease; a leader into unexplored
territory; a visionary, with concerns far beyond Cone's preoccupation
with the patient or the immediate technique. Penfield wanted to do what
nobody else had yet done, to make a balanced academic approach to the
mind through studies of the brain of man; and the means would be his
future neurological institute.

When Wilder reported to the Royal Vic, he was greeted by Jonathan
Meakins rather than Archibald. The chief surgeon was away in Europe.
Penfield found that Meakins had been as good as his word. Three rooms
in his university clinic had been prepared, divided up with partitions, to
produce a suite of six rooms. In the new lab, Bill Cone was already
hopping about with excitement, examining the boxes that had been
shipped from New York. They included a large barrel filled with precious
specimens from the lab in the Presbyterian Hospital.

"Bill Cone was just as delighted and excited as I was," Penfield wrote.
"We stood there and talked amid the unopened boxes. There was a
gleam in Bill's eye and his rumbling laugh echoed through our unfur-
nished rooms. Pathology of the brain had fascinated him from his student
days onward. Meakins smiled to see our pleasure and left us. This was the
beginning of a very happy relationship with the medical staff of the Royal
Victoria Hospital. It was to continue for six fruitful years, 1928 to 1934."
Cone was to be the neuropathologist and chief of the laboratory. Penfield
would lead the team.

In New York the team had included an enthusiastic cockney lad
named Edward Dockrill. Dockrill had been a ship's cabin boy for several
years before coming ashore at New York. There he had gotten a job as an
orderly on the public wards at the Presbyterian Hospital. When he heard
that there was an opening for a technician in Penfield's lab, he had
applied, claiming that he had worked in a medical laboratory in London.
Dr. Penfield agreed to try him out. He soon discovered that Edward
knew almost nothing of laboratory techniques. But the kid pleaded so

fervently to keep the job that Penfield relented. Besides, Dockrill was a quick learner, and if he wanted the job so much then surely his enthusiasm would make up for his initial inexperience. So Penfield kept him on, and in fact went to some trouble to help the lad compensate for his deficiencies, which included certain physical defects. Edward had poor vision and a squint. The doctor fixed him up with a pair of glasses. Also, sensing his loneliness in a foreign city, Penfield gave him some books to read. His first gift was Samuel Butler's *The Way of All Flesh*, which was to affect Edward quite profoundly—but not to its donor's advantage, as Wilder discovered a few years later.

Edward hero-worshipped his boss, while on his part, Penfield found the cockney a likeable person, though sometimes irksomely temperamental. Others, however, did not share his affection for the squinty-eyed cabin boy-turned-scientist, and when Bill Cone was preparing to move the lab to Montreal he had decided that Dockrill would not come with them. He would train a new technician in Montreal, one who was not subject to outbursts of temperament.

Which was why it came as such a surprise when, on his third evening in Montreal, Penfield returned home to find Edward waiting for him in the hallway of the apartment. He had been sitting there all afternoon.

"You're sure to need me," he said. "You won't have time to train a new technician now."

Penfield was touched by Edward's devotion in following him to Montreal, but he could not countermand Cone's decision. The best he could do, he told Edward, was to send him to Dr. Cone and see if the lab chief would change his mind.

Edward was overjoyed when Cone, deciding that the lad had mellowed and matured sufficiently, relented. Besides, it was true that he did not have time to train a new technician.

Bill Cone must have been glad that he had reversed his decision some weeks later, when Edward was responsible for resolving what could have been a calamity for the new neuropathology lab. One cold day in December, Dr. Penfield was interviewing a postgraduate student, Ottiwell Jones, and mentioned certain specimens that he had brought from New York; blocks of brain tumours from which sections might be cut for microscopic study, after they had been stained. As he spoke Wilder glanced up at the shelves where the specimens had been placed. The shelf was empty.

He asked Edward where the specimens were. Edward turned pale. He replied that they had been put back into the barrel they had arrived in two weeks previously, when the workmen came to paint the laboratory. He had assumed that either Penfield or Dr. Cone had moved the barrel to a storeroom for safekeeping. Now the barrel was missing.

Nobody would want to steal the barrel, so it must have been removed by mistake. They investigated with increasing desperation, but nobody could account for its disappearance. Penfield went for help to the hospital superintendent. He was asked to wait in the drafty entrance hall of the hospital, but the chill inside him was not caused by the drafts or the blizzard outside, but by apprehension. He sat there, sweating with anxiety. The brain specimens represented much of his professional life, the result of hundreds of grueling operations and autopsies. They were needed for comparison purposes in future studies. They were irreplaceable.

Penfield tried to distract himself from his anxiety by studying the hallway: the white marble statue of Queen Victoria, and, on the wall beside the superintendent's closed door the bronze tablet in memorium to Dr. John McRae, with all three stanzas of his poem "In Flanders Fields" inscribed on it. If he had not died, Penfield would have been a colleague of his. "How admirable that this Canadian physician could speak to the whole world through such poetry."

His mind raced feverishly in an effort to think about anything but the hundreds of bottles of specimens in formalin, sealed in paraffin. "Montreal physicians were different," he mused. "Edward Archibald seemed to personify this difference. Indeed, Archibald and McRae had been close friends and kindred spirits. Before the war, McRae had lived in a room of his own, for quite a time, in the home of Dr. and Mrs. Archibald." But Wilder's thoughts were jittery. He could not help thinking about all those bits of preserved human tissue in the vanished barrel. "I thought of the malignant tumour from the little Italian boy, the brain abscess from the son of Acosta Nichols, the many abnormalities that had produced epilepsy—in the case of William Hamilton and in Foerster's German patients—and the scars from the New York experimental animals. They were all there. I remembered brave little Jennie Hummel, whose seizures taught us where it is the brain controls the heart and the respiration. She died in one of her strange seizures while I was preparing to operate, hoping to cure. I did the autopsy, instead of the operation, at the scheduled time. Her husband himself asked me to do it, saying, in his anguish, he had to know why."

At last the superintendent was available. He was an administrator, a former banker, a friend of Sir Vincent Meredith's.

He offered little practical help. He telephoned around, questioning people whom Penfield had already contacted. But the administrator wasn't really concerned. As a non-medical man he had neither the experience nor the imagination to understand the gravity of the loss. He said that it was too bad. Then went on to enquire about the new tables in the laboratory. He hoped that the carpenter's work was to the doctors' satisfaction....

Icy with anger and despair, Penfield, with Cone and Dockrill, drove out to the Rosemount dump where hospital refuse was usually taken. It was a huge dump, patched with snow. It was bitterly cold, and Penfield noticed that Edward was poorly dressed for the hunt, in a thin coat. Only Bill Cone was truly optimistic. Taking charge with his usual vigour, he organized the search. "We'll find those bottles," he said. "There are so many of them, one is sure to appear somewhere on the surface and the barrel will be easy to recognize."

They searched all day, Penfield increasingly wet and miserable. Soon his knee began to hurt. He had been injured in a torpedoing during the war, and the knee had been badly set. Edward was in an even worse way, shivering uncontrollably; but he refused to give up. He moved on to a wrecked Ford car and poked about around it.

In the distance they heard him shout, and saw him waving something aloft. The doctors ran over to him. He was capering about in triumph, holding a bottle, "shivering and laughing all at once and using the strangest Cockney language in which the word 'bloody' appeared and reappeared. The label was plain to read, the paraffin sealing unbroken, the formalin solution frozen, and the block of tissue safe within the transparent ice."

Over the next few days, with the help of several men supplied by the dean of the medical school, they found more than half the specimens. In the process, Edward, who had returned to the dump to search by himself, caught a cold that developed into pneumonia. He was admitted to hospital. He eventually recovered, though for a time his life was in danger. Sulphonamides had not yet been discovered, and pneumonia was still a killer.

He had not, however, recovered from the vice of resentment, in this case against the petty injustices of life. Dr. Penfield was his hero, but Edward had failed to emulate his hero's generosity of spirit. His own relative insignificance in the order of things rankled, despite the fact that Dr. Penfield always gave him full credit for his contribution; even though, given the atmosphere of the times, he need not have done so. Penfield, for instance, singled him out for praise in at least one of his papers for the *Archives of Neurology and Psychiatry*.

During the first three years in Montreal Edward became steadily more discontented, until finally Bill Cone had had enough of his contrariness. This time, Edward was quite ready to go, perhaps not least because in his spare time he had written a novel, and it had been returned by the publisher not to its author but to the author's boss. When Penfield read the manuscript he found that he was one of the two principal characters in the book, and that his part was that of the villain who had risen to fame on the shoulders of a poor technician. Edward, of course, had been cast in the role of hero—just like Ernest, the rebellious hero in Samuel Butler's *The Way of All Flesh.*

Even so, Wilder continued to regard him sympathetically, right up to the day he left.

When Professor Archibald returned from Europe, Wilder soon realized that his own role as Archibald's protégé had come to an end. Archibald was now preoccupied with other activities. He had no further interest in the brain. "He went about as if in a dream, often late, sometimes very late, but always kind, amusing, reasonable and just." But having wrapped Penfield in his neurosurgical mantle and given him his blessing, he now regarded the newcomer as being on his own.

However, the dean, Dr. Martin, was a tower of strength. So was Colin Russel. Russel was the senior neurologist at the Royal Vic, and once he was convinced that Penfield meant what he said, that he did not intend to compete with neurologists but to collaborate with them, he was delighted and enthusiastic. "By gad! I'd like that. That's just what I have always wanted to do, and I have specimens for the laboratory. Bless you! I have a lot of teaching slides. I'll bring them to the hospital and I have a good microscope at home."

But Russel did not think that Wilder would get anywhere with the French Canadians. When Wilder Penfield mentioned the new clinical conferences between neurologists and surgeons that he was planning for Wednesdays at five o'clock, and asked if the French-Canadian neurologists would join in, Russel cried, "Bless my soul! They're just as narrow-minded as we are in the other direction. We live here in separate and independent professional worlds."

He added, with a chuckle, that they'd never mixed with the French Canadians, and "Their patients rarely come to our offices for consultation. They'd rather die." Penfield refused to accept that. The institute he hoped to create must serve all the people equally. He was determined to involve the French Canadians, including their top people, like Jean Saucier of the Hôtel Dieu and Roma Amyot at l'Hôpital Notre-Dame. He started to cultivate the French Canadians, and whenever he could, urged them to come to the five o'clock conferences at the Montreal General or the Royal Vic. He kept after the French Canadians, repeatedly inviting them to bring their private patients, the ones who were able to understand the value of such consultations. And gradually the French Canadians began to turn up, perhaps a little stiffly and self-consciously at first, but soon with enthusiasm. And soon, too, their English-speaking colleagues reciprocated by struggling to communicate with them in their own language. And in the end, no one did more to make the bilingual affair successful than Colin Russel. Eventually, those attending the conferences formed the Société neurologique de Montréal, Montreal Neurological Society, at which many distinguished speakers would present their work in either language.

Meanwhile, Penfield's dream, the institute, had already begun in embryo, in the laboratory of neuropathology, where brain tissue and tumour growth were studied. And a remarkable team was being built up, beginning with a cool, humorous English girl, Hope Lewis, as secretary. Then Dr. Dorothy Russell arrived from London on a research fellowship, and was put to work on a critical study of the origin of microglia in the brain, while Ottiwell Jones accepted the challenge of research into the oligodendroglia.

As well as organizing and leading the team, Penfield was also beginning to train other neurosurgeons, starting with the training of neurosurgeons for other Montreal hospitals. He was also inaugurating a private practice in surgery, his base being a small private consulting suite in the Royal Victoria; the income from which enabled him to support himself and to give equal attention to ward patients who could not pay. And he was learning to speak French effectively, if sometimes painfully, with brilliant French-Canadian neurologists who were working with him in conference and laboratory and co-operating with him in the handling of neurosurgical problems.

One of the most significant operations he himself performed was on his own sister. It reinforced his burning determination to found the institute. The experience also led directly to the application to the Rockefeller Foundation that would ultimately make the dream come true.

Penfield had been close to his sister all his life. Lately he had become increasingly worried about her health. Ruth had been having headaches, convulsions, and severe vomiting, and her sight was affected. On two occasions in California she had almost died and had been given artificial respiration. A Los Angeles neurosurgeon had advised her to go to Montreal without delay, to the only man with the skill to save her—her brother.

Wilder met her at Windsor Station and brought her and their mother back to his top-floor apartment. As she climbed the stairs, he noted, with sinking heart, the unsteady way she fumbled for the rails, as if she could not see properly.

After breakfast, he went into her room with his ophthalmoscope. "There, standing close to this sister of mine, of whom I had so many precious boyhood memories, I brought my right eye close to hers, pupil to pupil with only the lens of the ophthalmoscope between them. Sure enough! There it was! The swelling of the head of the optic nerve—dreadful swelling, and there were little red hemorrhages, each bordered by a white margin, that extended out menacingly over the surface of the surrounding retina."

It was the proof of what he had suspected, of a high degree of pressure inside the skull from a tumour. He was anguished at the thought of operating on a member of his own family. But there was nobody else to do it. If she were not operated on within hours she was likely to go totally blind, and then to die.

At the thought he felt suddenly so weak that he had to put a hand on her shoulder to steady himself. He had to pretend he was still examining her eye. Then they went down to breakfast, laughing and joking. "At the breakfast table, Ruth seemed her old self—lovely blue eyes, slow speech, radiant smile, perfect teeth and rollicking laugh."

After breakfast he called in Colin Russel. Russel was wonderful; genial, and reassuring. Then the three of them drove to the hospital for an X-ray examination, where they were joined by Bill Cone. The films showed the telltale shadow of calcium granules in the right frontal lobe. She had a brain tumour, whether benign or slowly malignant they could not tell. But even if benign, it was so deep in the right frontal lobe, or possibly under it, that the chances of complete success seemed dim.

Later that day, Archibald joined the consultation. Penfield summarized the case. Because of Archibald's deafness he sat as close as possible to the chief surgeon as he told the story.

His sister had begun to have splitting headaches from the age of fourteen, which was when the tumour had probably first appeared. At nineteen she had a major epileptic seizure. Penfield could attest to that personally. He had seen it, and it had terrified him. She had married a high school teacher a year later. From then to the age of forty she had three similar attacks. Otherwise she was entirely happy, with a successful husband and six lovely children. But in the last three years smaller attacks had come more frequently. And now the crisis had arrived.

He believed that the tumour was now malignant, and would have to be removed, but it would be an extremely difficult and dangerous operation. He suggested that there might just be time enough to take her to Harvey Cushing, the acknowledged leader of the modern school of neurosurgery. He pleaded with the other doctors to make the decision, and to make it as if she were not his sister.

He then left the room and waited. It seemed a long time before Cone came to call him back into the conference. When he entered, Archibald asked, "If you were to do this operation, could you do it as if she were not your sister?"

Wilder hesitated, then said yes. And the operation was scheduled for the next morning.

There were many details to be arranged beforehand. He rehearsed it with the instrument nurse, Kathleen Zwicker, using his own modification of Foerster's procedure. This "involved suturing the sterile sheet, or drape, to the skin of the shaven scalp after it was sterilized. The drape was then carried straight upward and fastened to a metal frame that stood on the floor and straddled the table. Thus it formed a wall. The patient's head was on one side with the operator, his assistants and the nurse. The patient's face and body were on the other side with those who might be needed for companionship and control."

For Ruth would be conscious during the operation.

"My modification of this arrangement was to attach an angulated metal frame to the operating table. When the patient's scalp had been sterilized and injected with novocaine, the protective sheet was sutured to the scalp and carried up about fourteen inches above the patient's head. It was then spread horizontally for twenty inches over the angulated frame, forming thus a shelf. From the shelf, the drape was carried on upward again two or three feet to be fastened finally to the bar at the top, which was attached firmly to the table below."

This allowed the nurse to stand on a platform to one side, where she could easily place the most important instruments on the sterile shelf in front of the operator. The patient could see out from under the shelf with a doctor or nurse in attendance, to talk to the patient and study her reaction from moment to moment.

"The morning came and Ruth was wheeled into the operating room. How strange to see my sister there, her head so bald and white and shiny on the head holder. She looked at me with wondering blue eyes and smiled doubtfully. I sterilized the scalp myself and injected novocaine ever so gently. Then she disappeared from view as the drapes were placed, forming her protective wall. But she talked a great deal, much more than I expected, telling me stories of her children. They were her pride, of course, and her joy. At last, after the skull opening had been made, I begged her to postpone her talking, since I must begin to concentrate on something else.

"The tumour was, as we had feared, within the right frontal lobe. We worked for hours, taking that tumour out and trying to leave the untouched brain so normal that there would be no more epileptic seizures. At last we had carried the removal of the frontal lobe back to the motor gyrus. To make sure, I touched the gyrus with an electrode. It caused the hand to move. We could go no farther on the surface. To remove this would cause permanent paralysis of voluntary movement."

It was the most radical brain operation Penfield had ever done. But also, as the X-rays had appeared to indicate, the fault extended underneath—malignant-looking tissue, right on the floor of the skull.

Bill Cone murmured, advising him not to chance it. But Wilder had agreed to undertake the operation for that very reason: his fear that another surgeon would not go far enough, and shorten her life still further.

With enormous difficulty, complicated by a considerable loss of blood, he removed more of the tumour mass. But when the view was clear again he found that there was still more of the growth present, under the dura and into the left cerebral hemisphere. He simply could not touch it. The threat would remain.

But at least he had saved her eyesight.

Afterwards he sat alone in the surgeon's dressing room, half-dressed, one sock on his foot and the other in his hand. "I wanted to weep. I had known her so well and loved her as a boy." After a while he recovered from his despair. "I had done the best I could to remove all of Ruth's tumour. I made a conscious effort to forget it. One must not look at failure. Her eyesight was saved, her headaches gone, her life saved. And this surgical setup, this way of using local anesthesia and the new instruments—all these had been put to the test in my sister's operation. They served their purposes well.

"So my mind drifted away to other matters. If I could open the door more widely to the surgical treatment of epilepsy, it would open the way to brain physiology and psychology. And then, sometime perhaps, we would make a more effective approach to the mind of man."

Wilder continued to sit there for half an hour, an hour, two hours, forgetting to dress; and his determination burned more fiercely than ever to do more for patients like Ruth through the study of this last and most complex and least known area of knowledge in the whole field of medicine. He would do it through a specialized institute. He had already described such an institute in an application to the Rockefeller Foundation. The building would be seven stories high, directly attached to the Royal Victoria. Neurosurgical on the third floor, neurological on the fourth, the laboratory on the sixth—he had worked out many of the details in that application two years previously, and another application, more detailed though still unfinished, lay in his desk at home. He would complete it and send it off, and if it was turned down like the first one, then he would try elsewhere. But he would create that institute for neurological investigation sometime, somewhere, somehow.

Penfield's first application to the Rockefeller Foundation had been made just three months after his arrival in Montreal, but it had been turned down by the officer in charge of the division of medical education. Since then a new man, Alan Gregg, had taken over, and Penfield had been advised by somebody else in the Foundation not to send in a newer and more elaborate application. Penfield did not know why, and was not enlightened when he met Gregg in New York in March 1931.

Otherwise the meeting with Gregg had gone off quite well. He had taken an immediate liking to the new director, a gangling, broad-shouldered man with a ruddy face and bright blue eyes. But whether Gregg on his part had been impressed with him he could not tell.

Later that year he was informed that Alan Gregg would be stopping off in Montreal on his way to Chicago and would like to see him again. Penfield met him at the Westmount station, and took him home for breakfast.

It was a jolly occasion. Because he often worked late, this was the only time that Penfield was certain of being able to talk to his four children, and it was a household custom that everybody was to meet at the breakfast table, including the governess, Fraulein Bergmann, and of course, Helen, a humorous and self-effacing lady who, ever since her marriage to the bustling neurosurgeon had been supporting him domestically and professionally (proofreading, typing manuscripts into the early hours) without thought of self. She now welcomed Alan Gregg with her usual warm hospitality, and there was a good deal of laughter over the breakfast table, and light conversation in English and German. Gregg appeared to enjoy chatting to the children in German.

Wilder disguised his tension as well as he could, not knowing why Gregg had come to see him, but suspecting the worst, that Alan was being kind. Wilder was certain that Alan was going to tell him that the Rockefeller Foundation could not see its way to supporting research in neurology, and therefore it was pointless for Wilder to submit any further applications. He had come to tell him so in person, rather than through an official letter.

After breakfast when they went into the study, Wilder was suddenly so weak with apprehension that he had to sit abruptly. He watched in leaden silence, prepared for the worst by Gregg's expressionless face. Gregg was busily opening his briefcase and placing a file of papers on the coffee table. He was not even bothering to sit. Presumably he was going to give Wilder—or Wide, as some of his friends called him—the bad news without any apologetic or evasive preamble. The fact that Gregg's face was flushing as he started to speak, seemed for a moment to suggest that he was upset at what he had to say.

Except that the expression seemed to be one of emotion rather than embarrassment.

"This is exactly the sort of thing for which we are always searching at the Rockefeller Foundation," he said, turning to Wilder. "I have the application you made to Pearce. I think I understand what you want to do. You have a plan that gives real promise in a field that is calling desperately for exploration. We can do no more than provide you with the optimum environment. You will have to direct the work. We want to see it go on and on, following the leads that come to you. Don't ever thank us. We thank you. You will be helping us when you do your job."

Wilder didn't know what to say. He looked at the papers on the coffee table. It was his original application, two and a half years old. It was not even detailed. He was not even sure he remembered what was in it, or whether it even did justice to his present ideas, which had greatly expanded since then. His mind was in a whirl. He could hardly believe it, that Gregg actually seemed to be indicating that the Foundation was willing to support him.

After a first incredulous exclamation he didn't know what to say. By then, Gregg had sat down. He was watching Penfield, waiting.

Wilder finally managed to respond, as cautiously as if it were all a trick. Falteringly he made the point that he had already united neurology and neurosurgery into one academic and hospital department.

But Gregg already knew about that, and waited for more. Finally Wilder began to blurt out, as he put it, a spontaneous paraphrase of his credo, which involved an interdependent medical team, dedicated to the study of mental disease and the physiological mechanisms of the mind, housed in intimate relationship with a general teaching hospital so that each member of the team could be in close contact with all departments of medicine.

Then Gregg got up again, and began to talk, elaborating on the idea; and Wilder realized almost with a shock that during their meeting earlier that year Gregg must have absorbed much more of his, Penfield's, ideas than he had thought, and that he believed in them almost as passionately as Wilder did. He also began to realize how deeply disappointed Gregg had been that he had not been able to aid the cause of neurology in Paris and London because of a conflict of ideas on exactly how the money was to be spent. "I realized suddenly that what he was doing now was what he had wanted to do. He realized how great were the research opportunities in neurology, and how much an advance he would achieve for medicine and for mankind.... How strange! And what an incredible interview this was. They wanted me to do...just what I had been hoping to do."

Perhaps best of all was the realization that the Foundation was willing to support Penfield wherever he wished to establish the institute. This was a problem that had been gnawing at Penfield for some months. Just as Osler had been tempted away from McGill nearly fifty years previously by the University of Pennsylvania, so now Penfield was being courted by the same university. If he went to Philadelphia—or New York or Baltimore, even—the financial support in those communities would likely be firmer than in Montreal. But his heart was strongly inclined to overrule his head. He liked Canadians and felt at home with them. But there were other, perhaps less tangible advantages. Montreal was a quieter place for study. Tradition and awareness linked Montreal with Europe, especially Britain and France, as well as the United States. "Our location here, above the American border and just off the main highroad to the great American university centres—might well prove to be the best place in which to be influenced by the work in other centres. It might be the ideal place in which to do constructive scientific work on the brain and the mind of man, work that might in time influence thinking in other centres."

After further discussion on the costs involved, Gregg departed for further conversations with the dean. He returned the next day, and it was during this conversation that he explained that the Foundation was not just a treasure trove for an impersonal scientific endeavour. It backed the man, the one with a germinal idea.

"'Since leaving medical school,' he said, 'I have met many medical men in many parts of the world. Among them there were two who stand out as great men. Both were physiologists and both were working on the nervous system. One was Sir Charles Sherrington at Oxford. The other was Ivan Pavlov in Leningrad. I suppose you feel it is quite natural that genius should be drawn to the problems of the nervous system?'"

Wilder laughed off the implication that he, too, was a genius, and that only a fear of being thought a flatterer had prevented Gregg from adding his name to those of Sherrington and Pavlov. But Gregg persisted. He wanted to know how the idea for the institute first occurred to Wilder, and when the neurosurgeon did not immediately reply: 'When you left New York,' he prompted, 'the Presbyterian Hospital was about to move uptown. You could have carried on there, and eventually, no doubt, at the New York Neurological Institute when they moved uptown. Was there something new and different that you had in mind?'

Wilder saw that Gregg really wanted to know. So: "Early in life, I explained to him, I was certain that there was work for me to do in the world. Some might think it strange that I was so certain then. But it was not until I went to Oxford a second time, as a graduate student, that my purpose took on its specific plan—to become a brain surgeon and to apply basic science to the needs and problems of patients in the neurological field of medicine. I learned how to carry out critical research and discovered how thrilling it was to make little discoveries of truth about the nervous system."

But the field, he soon found, was so extensive that he realized he could not hope to make a significant contribution all by himself. He had realized this particularly when he took on the editorship of the famous *Cytology and Cellular Pathology of the Nervous System*. He could write as an authority on one or two chapters; the remaining thirty odd chapters had to be written by others who could do a better job.

"Then, of course, came the idea of an institute through which my own life's purpose could be carried out. It was a simple commonsense plan. I could see how to organize it for each specialist, just as I had the editing of the *Cytology*. Some of the men who would come on staff, I hoped, would give me the specialized help I needed in my own exploration and treatment. The call for an institute was self-centered at the beginning, but it broadened rapidly into an altruistic establishment to serve the patients better and promote neurological research as never before. Nevertheless I still expected, in the end, to carry out my purposeful approach to brain and mind after the institute should be built. If I were not to do so I would have to acknowledge personal failure."

As for why he had not followed through in New York, he told Gregg, the answer was simple: the new institute down there would still have been a ten-minute walk from the Presbyterian. But ten minutes was too great a separation, as he saw it, from general medicine and surgery.

So that was how it had come about. "Edward Archibald, professor of surgery at McGill University, came to New York in June 1927 to invite me to take over his neurosurgical practice in Montreal, and in January of 1928, he offered support for a laboratory of our own. He came at exactly the right moment. I wanted independence and I had just reached my own conclusion as to how to solve great problems in the neurological field. I knew, by then, that no man alone could do what had to be done."

The institute opened three years later, in 1934, and through its study of the brain and the nervous system, has become one of the foremost institutions of its kind, a centre for the treatment of a great variety of disorders, particularly epilepsy. In that field its reports and monographs have become standard reference works.

Penfield had been developing a surgical approach to epilepsy since 1928. Part of his technique was the use of an electrically charged needle on the cerebral cortex, the gray, convoluted mantle of the brain covering that had to do with movement and sensation in the body. By applying a slight electric shock he could determine which were the damaged areas of the temporal lobe that needed to be worked on to relieve epilepsy, which originated from that part of the brain. It had already been established in animal experiments that if certain areas of the brain were shocked, a leg or arm movement resulted; but the temporal lobe was still mysterious territory. What Penfield found was that stimulation of the cortex of one of the temporal lobes unlocked past experience. One of his first patients to re-experience an event from her past was a girl of fourteen. She was admitted two years after the founding of the Neurological Institute, suffering from epileptic seizures. When her temporal cortex was stimulated at certain close points it was as if she were re-living incidents from her past. Like Penfield's sister Ruth, she was conscious under local anesthesia during the operation, and each time he applied the electric probe she saw and heard scenes and voices from the past, and felt the emotion of fear.

Penfield was astonished. Instead of hand or foot movements or sensory phenomena, he had caused her to re-experience the past—a man approaching her threateningly, the voices of her brothers and her mother. Penfield appeared to have discovered in the temporal lobe a storehouse of memory.

Many similar auditory, visual and emotional effects were produced in other patients over the next few years. Stimulating the cortex of another young woman took her back to a performance of *Aïda*. She was able to hear the chorus and orchestra as vividly as she had first heard them. She was convinced that somebody was playing a recording of the opera in the operating theatre. The emotion in this case was one of delight over the magnificent sound and also at the thoughtfulness of the medical staff in so entertaining her during her ordeal. She must have been amazed when she was told that it was a playback from past experience—that the music had been recorded long ago on some of the millions of nerve cells, or neurones, in her cortex. But after hundreds of such experiments, what struck Penfield as even more amazing was that many such memory patterns were apparently being banked in the same neurone area— memories stacked together one on top of the other but individually retrievable.

Another of his startling discoveries was that removal of part of the brain did not necessarily mean a lessening in brain power. Often quite the opposite. Donald Hebb, a professor of psychology at McGill, wrote of Penfield that, "he was as surprised as anyone at the excellent status of patients from whom he had removed scar tissue simply for the control of epilepsy. In fact, when he made his extensive bilateral removal of the pre-frontal lobes in 1938 he must have thought that he could put an end to the fits but that there was a poor outlook for the patient in other respects. I had to urge him to go talk to the patient to see how good his mental status was. Only then did he see how great a change he had wrought. This patient's intelligence quotient improved from 75 to 80...to 95 or so after the operation. He subsequently enlisted in the Canadian Army and went overseas at a time when headquarters in England was demanding a more careful psychological screening of recruits. The medical officer examining him saw the scar on his forehead, asked what had caused it, was told that he had had an accident in a sawmill, and asked if it was giving any trouble. The recruit replied that it was not—and indeed it was not after Penfield had taken out the scarred remnants of both his prefrontal lobes."

Another patient had five percent of his cerebrum removed, afterwards making a perfect score in the then new Standord-Binet intelligence test. Hebb added that depressing functions in the rest of the cortex could be far more damaging than the mere loss of the tissue from which the disturbance originated.

The most fascinating of Penfield's explorations was in the nature of the mind: the place where all functions are integrated to produce a human being out of a mass of nerves and cells—the centrecephalic system as he called it. He startled neurologists by proposing that the highest level of integration took place in the lowly brain stem. "Consciousness," he wrote in 1957, "exists only in association with the passage of impulses through ever-changing circuits of the brainstem and cortex. One cannot say that consciousness is here or there. But certainly without centrecephalic integration it is nonexistent." It was a controversial result of his years of experimentation, but no better hypothesis has yet replaced it. In his book *The Mystery of the Mind,* he simultaneously expanded and simplified his hypothesis, saying that the central integrating system is an interdependent duality, making "sensory input available and motor output purposeful."

"Penfield's lifelong search for a better understanding of the functional organization of the brain and its disorders during epileptic seizures," concludes Dr. Herbert A. Jasper, "is symbolized, in a way, by his hypothesis of the central integrating system. It is never to be localized in any specific area of gray matter but in 'wider-ranging mechanisms.' It is a sort of conceptual bridge he has built between the brain and the mind. He concluded that we shall probably never be able to cross that bridge. Perhaps he is right, but many have been inspired by his efforts. His legacy to neurology and to humanity will extend far into the future."

Through his work in the illumination of the workings of the brain and his inspiration and leadership, Wilder Penfield became a towering figure in Canadian and international medical history. His work also ended an era in medicine: of five thousand years of individual accomplishment in medical science. There would still be the occasional flash of an Albert Sabin, but the age of scientific collaboration had begun. The team had taken the field.

41

The Rescue Specialist

SHORTLY AFTER THE Second World War, Dr. Penfield received a visit from Gustave Gingras, a charming French-Canadian doctor who, until he became famous in his particular field, was professionally notable mainly in that he had never delivered a baby, or even seen one delivered. Dr. Gingras cheerfully confessed that he had dodged the entire course in practical obstetrics at the Université de Montreal, by getting a student friend to sign in for him. In exchange, Gustave signed in for his friend in neurosurgery, thus keeping their respective records straight.

The long, mysterious neurosurgical operations with their intent team of surgeons, assistants, and specialist nurses, held for Gustave Gingras all the mysteries of the High Mass. He was fascinated by neurosurgery and by the almost mathematical precision of neurological examination; which was why he had come to Penfield, to continue his work in that field, to see about getting a job in the Neurological Institute. He would be available, he told Penfield, as soon as he was demobilized from the army.

But Penfield had heard about the young man's work among paralyzed Canadian soldiers at Basingstoke in England, and this was too good an opportunity to miss. "I've got fifty paraplegics," he told Gustave, "all ex-servicemen waiting for a doctor at the hospital at Sainte-Anne-de-Bellevue. They've often talked about your optimism and that's one thing these patients need more than anything else. How would you like to go there for a few months?"

Gustave Gingras, who was to become a world authority in the rehabilitation of the physically handicapped, was a descendent of the Gingras who had emigrated to New France in the seventeenth century. The chief influence in his life was his brother-in-law Romeo Boucher, a professor at the faculty of medicine at the Université de Montreal, and chief physician at St. Luke's Hospital. Professor Boucher had taken a special interest in the small boy, allowing him the run of his surgery, and taking him on his rounds. By the age of nine, the boy was absolutely certain he was going to be a doctor, just like his brother-in-law, and the determination had never wavered during his childbirth-dodging student days at the university.

He felt uncertain, though, when he got to the Sainte-Anne-de-Bellevue, a collection of temporary government buildings set in sixty acres of parkland ten miles or so from Montreal's Dorval Airport. Gustave was at a loss. He had always liked to plan his life carefully, but now he had no idea what he was going to do. He wasn't the least enthusiastic about his new job. He wanted to get it out of the way as soon as possible, so that he could carry on with his peacetime career in neurosurgery.

His own talents, in particular an ability to think originally, soon got the better of him. His first examination of the patients shocked him. It revealed horrifying bedsores, resulting from long-term compression of the tissues. The positions of the paralyzed soldiers were obviously not being changed often enough to allow the blood to circulate normally, causing the death of tissue and sometimes irreversible damage. Within hours, Gustave was asking why the established methods should not be changed. Why not lay the patients on their stomachs, with pillows placed at critical pressure points and, for the incontinent patients, provide space for the tubing that carried the urine to the container. He insisted on putting these changes into effect immediately, and arranged for the men to be turned every two hours, day and night. It caused something of an upheaval in the hospital and some grousing, until the new doctor convinced the forty nurses that it would mean far less work for them in the long run—there would be fewer bedsores to treat.

The patients also had to adjust to the idea of lying on their stomachs. Generally, people in the field of spinal traumatization were still not used to original thinking in prevention and treatment. Only a few years previously, in the 1930s before antibiotics came along, the life expectancy of paraplegics was rarely more than four months. By 1974, Dr. Gingras was able to tell his students that the life span was now only five years less than the span of a normal person. That achievement was due to the work of Dr. Gingras and his team.

As a result of these changes, most of the sores healed fairly quickly, though in two cases it took over a year to encourage a layer of skin to form over the old sores. Gingras was particularly concerned about this lengthy period because it delayed the active phase of the patients' rehabilitation. He needed to speed up the process. The more he thought about it, the more certain he became that plastic surgery was the answer. But almost nothing had been published on the subject. "It took a long time for my team and myself to develop the necessary pre- and post-operative techniques and to work out an acceptable formula." It was particularly important for the patient to avoid, for a period of six weeks, any pressure on the area that had been operated on, and in the medical articles he wrote on the subject, he stressed this point. "It takes three or four weeks before the edges of the wound have built up viable connective tissue. At this point, the physiotherapist can use massage to ensure that the layers of muscle and skin can slide across the bone structure without causing tearing or bleeding when the time comes at last for the patient to sit up."

Such methods, soon to be copied throughout the world, greatly speeded up the day when the patient was ready for rehabilitation. Before Gustave Gingras fought these disastrous wounds, many a paraplegic could not be rehabilitated and enabled to take his place in society.

Another problem that Dr. Gingras worked on was that of the involuntary movements found in some spinal cases. These spasms often gave the victims and their relatives cause for hope. A mother would see her son's paralyzed leg move, and think that he was improving; whereas in fact spastic movements invariably retarded rehabilitation and caused complications in treatment.

Dr. Gingras determined to kill the spasticity by injecting pure alcohol into the spine. "Here I encountered almost inflexible resistance on the part of my consultant in neuro-surgery. Nor was he the only one who opposed my suggestion. He was backed up by other doctors, by nurses and by some of the patients. And it was extremely difficult to convince them, since medical staff have an ingrained aversion, and fortunately so, to destroying any part or function of the human body. But if the spinal cord is already destroyed—as here—and if the injection is going to rid the patient of involuntary movements which are both troublesome and bothersome and which prevent him from benefiting from re-education, then there is no question: one just has to do it. After months of tedious argument I got the go-ahead and gave a first injection of alcohol in April 1946 to McLaughlin, a casualty from D-day."

The treatment was a success. The damaging spasms died away, and McLaughlin rapidly graduated from bed to wheelchair, and fifty years later was still the healthiest of all the doctor's original patients.

Once free of bedsores and spasms—and the spurious comfort of drugs fostered by the fast-on-the-draw pill-prescribers—he was able to work out a systematic rehabilitation program. The men were often sunk in despair or apathy. The miraculous antibiotics had saved them from death only to substitute a living death. They had to be half-jollied, half-bullied into making an effort. To develop their arm and shoulder muscles and help them raise themselves up and turn over in bed, Gingras had bars fixed over their beds, and he prescribed exercises to improve their balance, and to help them get into and out of their wheelchairs unaided. The men responded quickly to the plump, smiling young doctor, who expressed his concern for their welfare with brisk, tough, or tactful humour, inspiring them to compete against each other in their struggle to get mobile. They began to exchange jolly insults and cheerful taunts, and as they progressed they became even noisier and more enthusiastic. They were coming back to life.

One problem, that of incontinence of the bowels, could only be partly solved "by teaching the paraplegics to practise digital evacuation of the rectum so that they could evacuate their stools with the aid of a lubricated rubber glove. Quadruplegics with their fingers paralyzed were not able to do this. So a member of the family or a visiting nurse had to carry out this not particularly agreeable task. Over the years occupational therapists in my unit have tried in vain to produce an appliance which could keep the patient's index finger extended so that he could dilate his own anus without assistance. So far no success." He longed for some inventor to come up with a semi-rigid finger-sized appliance that would feed back the right kind of sensation.

By winter, Gustave Gingras was deeply involved in his pioneering rehabilitation work, all thoughts of a career in neurosurgery swept aside in his enthusiasm for the job. In spring he had the hospital in an uproar again, by creating new situations, new games, new trends, to sweep the paralyzed soldiers back into the mainstream. He had the beds taken down to the sunlit terrace, shamelessly exposing the paraplegics to the curious stares of the world. The men, fearful at first at being seen in their almost helpless state, found that passers-by were interested and would stop to chat. It made the boys feel less like freaks. Gingras next insisted that instead of being served meals in bed, the men would have to make the effort to go to the canteen in their wheelchairs. Next he had them venture further afield, to the Red Cross pavilion, and most exciting of all, for trips into town. To make sure that the men could get across the street at the traffic lights fast enough, Gustave went to the mayor of Montreal, Camilien Houde, and persuaded him to install traffic lights near the hospital in a practice area. It roused the competitive spirit of the men still further. They trained to cross the road in their wheelchairs, or on crutches or calipers (metal supports which enable the paraplegics to swing themselves forward by means of a belt or thoracic corset) before the lights changed. Soon some of them were getting across in half a minute. He also took the men swimming—another original idea. Such measures were simple, but nonetheless revolutionary in this new branch of medicine. The Wheelchair Olympics held in Toronto in 1976, where the participants performed amazing feats of sporting skill, was an example of just how far paralyzed people had come along the road first paved by such pioneers as Dr. Gingras and his team. "These days," he wrote, "you see paraplegics and even quadruplegics returning home after three or four months treatment. But at first, when most patients had already undergone prolonged hospitalization for two years or more, one had to see the problem in a different light. True they went out at weekends. But on Sunday evenings back they came to me. They came back to a protected environment supervised and cared for by nurses they knew personally, whom they loved and who loved them. And let's face it, my patients were spoilt. So how were we going to cut the umbilical cord, and reduce and finally stop that overprotection they had been enjoying for so long?"

His answer came through one of the men, Bill Handley. After he and his wife Marian had spent a weekend together at home, they came to the doctor's office on the Monday morning and Marian asked if Bill could come home for good. Gustave pretended to be doubtful about it, but in fact he was overjoyed. For months he had been trying to think of a way to sell that idea to somebody, and here were two young people proposing it themselves. He allowed himself to be persuaded, with the proviso that Bill return for regular routine examinations—for the health of a spinal patient is easily upset. So Bill went home, and the example that he and his wife set inspired others to emulate him; and also provided Gustave with two guinea pigs on whose experience he could base future decisions.

As for why a woman would marry an impotent, paralyzed man, as did a number of the nurses and therapists at the hospital, Gingras felt that it was the maternal instinct coming to the fore. "Some women marry to escape from loneliness or rather to share their loneliness. Some only seem to find complete self-expression by devoting themselves to someone they love."

It was mainly through Dr. Gingras's efforts that the Department of Veterans' Affairs, his employers, agreed to fill the beds left by departing veterans with civilian paralytics. Rehabilitation for civilians was badly needed. Every year the national paraplegic population was increasing through a variety of causes, from tumour and infections, to road accidents. Very little was being done for such people. One of the doctor's civilian patients, for instance, had been a prisoner within four walls for twenty years. When Emmanuel Ranger was six he had tuberculosis of the spine and ultimately became paralyzed. Gingras found him, feverish from the poison of deep pressure sores, in an institution for incurables. He had spent most of his youth in a ward filled with fifty incontinent and senile old men. He had kept himself sane by making jewelry, and putting rosaries together at a dollar fifty per dozen.

When Emmanuel read in *La Presse* about Dr. Gingras's work at the hospital at Sainte-Anne, he could hardly believe it. The paralytics there not only went in for sports but even drove their own cars. He wrote to the newly formed Paraplegics Association, asking if they could help him. When a bed was finally found for him a year later, Gingras was appalled by his condition; paraplegic, incontinent, spastic, with a spine that had collapsed, kidneys that had almost ceased to function, and multiple bedsores. It took another year just to close up the sores.

By September 1949, Gingras, after prodigious effort, had got him admitted to the École des Arts et Métiers. At the age of thirty, Manny was in control of his life for the first time, even daring to chat-up Jeanne, a needlework student at the same school. During fifteen years in the institution for incurables he had never seen a woman—even the nurses were men. When he finished his studies at the arts and crafts school, he got a job; and he decided to risk having one more dream shattered. He drove to Ottawa where Jeanne lived, in the car that he had bought with an interest-free loan from the Paraplegics Association, and asked her to marry him. She accepted. "For ten years now he has owned his own watchmakers and jewellers in Dorval, on the outskirts of Montreal; he also owns a little house with a garden all round. If Manny had lived the whole of his life in an institution for the chronic sick instead of being rehabilitated he would have cost the State about 200,000 dollars." As it was, he was now so independent that he refused to accept the government disability pension.

It was patients such as Emmanuel, and another, named Julie who spurred on Dr. Gingras throughout his career, through their will to live and to improve themselves. When Julie wrote to him imploring his help, he went to see her at her house in the east end of Montreal. After knocking at the door several times without result, he was just about to turn away when the door opened and, looking down, he saw a young woman on the floor, her legs folded under her. He followed her as she dragged herself into the next room, and hauled herself into a chair. She told him that she had been shut up in the house for eleven years, after being crippled by polio. "She was nicely dressed, quite smart even with neat brown hair and eyes like black velvet.

"My parents are both working, and now my two sisters are married they don't live at home anymore," she told him. Gustave further learned that she spent her day reading and studying. She was trying to finish her secondary education entirely on her own. She also helped in the house, hauling herself around on her hands, a shy, intelligent, lovely girl filled with courage and determination. She deserved much better than that kind of life.

The doctor brought her to Sainte-Anne. "And so, even while she was undergoing medical rehabilitation, she learnt English and took a full-scale course in commercial subjects. She lost her shyness, and for the first time in her life went out to concerts and to the theatre. A year after her arrival this girl, who had been a positive recluse, secured her first job as a full-time secretary. Three months later she passed the Civil Service entrance exam. Julie is still working and I still see her from time to time; always very smart in her dresses and jumpers, happy in her independence and assured of a comfortable retirement."

Not all of his crippled friends would end up in comfortable retirement, despite Gustav's most generous efforts. One day, on his way for a vacation on Prince Edward Island (where he later became provincial director of Rehabilitation) he was asked by a social worker to stop off at a village near Sainte-Anne de la Pocatière to see a little girl named Katy. He found her in a poverty-stricken little house. "A few rough pieces of furniture. A table piled high with dirty dishes and covered with flies. Some rickety chairs. Beds without sheets. Sitting on the floor was a child holding a little radio to her ear, but the case was broken and the wires hanging out. She was smiling. Only her mouth was smiling and her wide-open eyes looked at us unseeingly."

Several dirty, ragged children were peeking in. "'She's almost deaf,' said one of the children.

"'And blind,' said another.

"I was deeply moved to see that little girl living in another world. I picked Katy up in my arms and carried her to one of the beds to examine her. She did not mind a bit but never let go of the radio.

"'It's all I've got in the world!'

As well as being nearly blind and nearly deaf, Katy's legs were completely paralyzed. She had contracted tubercular meningitis at the age of ten. Her parents were both alcoholics, and raised no objection when he brought her to the Montreal Convalescent Hospital, and to the new Rehabilitation Institute that he had now established in Montreal. The institute had departments of physiotherapy, occupational therapy, speech therapy, and audiology, and was of great benefit to Katy. She soon learned to use braces and crutches, and even managed to get up and down stairs. Dr. Gingras also arranged for her to be taught braille and handicrafts. His efforts on her behalf were loving and untiring. She was one of the few patients he had known since childhood whom he always greeted with a kiss.

"By that time Katy was sufficiently rehabilitated to go to Nazareth, a girl's school for the blind. She spent six years there. After long consideration I decided to send her home for a holiday. I was to regret it for the rest of my life." For she failed to return. Her parents had found out that she was entitled to a blind person's pension.

When he finally got her back, after resorting to the law courts, she was in a bad way, with incurable contractures at the hips, knees, and in the lumbar muscles. She had become a paraplegic. She ended up alone in a little room, existing on a meagre pension, back again with her friend—the radio.

As well as his Rehabilitation Institute which would send skilled workers to all parts of Quebec, the rest of the country, and to many under-developed countries, Dr. Gingras also helped to found North America's first school of prosthetics and orthetics—artificial limbs and braces—which, under its director, M. Corriveau, has attracted students from many countries, particularly France. The institute, the school, and a workshop for the design and manufacture of artifical limbs and aids greatly extended the work of Gingras' team. Their combined operations were of particular value in the rehabilitation of the thalidomide victims in the 1960s.

Thalidomide was the tranquillizer prescribed for sickness and anxiety in pregnancy which caused the world's first epidemic affecting the human fetus. Many of the women who had taken the drug brought forth deformed babies. In some babies the tongue was missing, in others the limbs. Canada was not badly stricken, compared with, for instance, West Germany, where there were ten thousand victims, but it was still a tragedy for many a Canadian family.

When the enormity of the calamity became clear, Dr. Gingras wrote to the minister of Health offering his facilities. He was concerned that many of the children would be put away in institutions and left to their fate. One of them was another girl named Julie, this one born without arms or legs. "She had two little hands attached directly at the shoulders and two attached to the hips. Under pressure from friends and relations her parents had put her in an institution. There they simply fed her, changed her nappies and kept her clean. Julie's universe: the ceiling. She was more than a year old when she was brought to the institute. Her behaviour and her reactions were comparable to those of an eight-to-twelve-week-old baby. Julie had no notion of her own body image. Even a very small baby moves its hands in front of its face and is aware of them. It forms the idea that its hand is a part of it. Then the hands explore: the nose, mouth, chest, genitals, legs, and feet. Condemned as she had been to lie horizontal and, to use a nautical term, without any bearings, Julie screamed with fright when they tried to sit her up for the first time. Once they had got her to this first stage, the physiotherapists let her try new experiences. One of the most interesting was intended to arouse in her the sense of touch: they put materials with different textures against her skin and objects with different temperatures.

"At the prosthesis laboratory Corriveau and his assistants made a sort of case to put the child's trunk in. They put two mini-skis on this case and by twisting her thorax from side to side Julie was able to walk."

She was also fitted with electro-mechanical arms, operated by the fingers at her shoulders and by a lever under her chin. "You should have seen the child's surprise and delight. She flew into a tantrum when Jeanette Hutchison took off the appliance. For her, those prostheses had become the most wonderful and extraordinary toys in the world."

Dr. Gingras' concern ensured that, in Quebec at least, not one thalidomide child was left in an institution. As for the thalidomide tragedy as a whole, it had one positive result. It led to the tightening up of the regulations governing the flow, the tidal wave, the flood of new drugs, whose effects might not be felt until the next generation.

42

Defiance

TWENTY-SEVEN-YEAR-OLD Morton Shulman had an almost obsessive desire to become a coroner, though he was doing well enough in private practice among the immigrants who were flooding into Toronto in the early fifties. After the failure of one campaign in which he had gone to extremes to influence the right people—by joining the Progressive Conservative party—he approached a party veteran named W. J. Stewart who was trying to get re-elected after being defeated in the last provincial election in Ontario. Shulman pointed out that he had a large number of grateful patients in Stewart's Parkdale riding, and offered to solicit their votes on Mr. Stewart's behalf. Shulman, sharp and thin but as packed with pep as a high-energy cell, appears to have contributed substantially to the success of the campaign. Stewart regained his seat with a very large majority. A few weeks later his principal canvasser received the coronership.

Morton was overjoyed, already imagining himself as a medical private-eye, investigating suicides, solving murders that had baffled the best brains of the homicide squad, righting wrongs, and exposing corruption in high places, and in the process making himself famous. He soon learned, though, that the chief coroner, Smirle Lawson, was more inclined to perform pianissimo than to trumpet forth his findings. "If a doctor does something wrong," Dr. Lawson told Shulman, "take him in the back room and give him hell, but don't let the public or the press learn about it." Lawson meant it, too. A few weeks after being appointed, Shulman ordered an autopsy on a patient at St. Michael's Hospital whose death, he suspected, had been caused by negligence on the part of a physician.

He had barely returned to his office when he received a call from Lawson, ordering him to return to the hospital. There the chief coroner told Shulman that he was taking over the case and Shulman would have to cancel the post-mortem immediately. "There seemed little choice," Shulman wrote in his book *Coroner*, "and I did what I was told. He then instructed me to apologize to the Sister Superior. With tail very much between my legs I returned to my office, resolved never to go through such a humiliating experience again." Embarrassing influential people was the last thing the chief coroner wanted.

Morty having behaved himself, Dr. Lawson once again became exuberant and friendly. He was a pillar of the establishment himself and was obviously not inclined to do a Samson act on the other pillars. A huge, powerful man, Lawson had been the only student in the history of the University of Toronto to get 100 in surgery, a mark earned when the professor of surgery lost a wager with him that he would not score six touchdowns at the next game with Queen's. "For many years there hung at the coroner's office a picture of Smirle Lawson charging across the goal line with four opposing players being dragged behind."

Shulman served under him for ten years. By 1962, Lawson was much too old for the job and was becoming senile. But, according to Dr. Shulman, "there was little likelihood of Dr. Lawson being fired because the political repercussions would have been too threatening if he had decided to tell his stories of past scandals." But when the chief coroner finally did retire, Shulman was chagrined to learn—from the newspapers—that Lawson's other responsibility, as supervising coroner of Ontario, was to be filled by Dr. Beatty Cotnam and the post of chief coroner, which Shulman coveted, was to be left vacant.

Shulman decided to give up and, instead, run for political office. Since helping Stewart in the by-election, he had kept up his interest in provincial politics, and was now the chief of the Parkdale Progressive Conservative Association.

In fact the decision to scratch from the coroner stakes took him back into the race. Being firmly in control of the Parkdale Conservatives, he was in an excellent position to put himself forward as their candidate in the next election to the Ontario legislature. Looking around for a suitable issue, he decided on medicare.

Medicare had already been introduced in Saskatchewan, and Shulman, having "seen so many examples in my own practice of families postponing essential medical treatment because they could not afford the expense," decided to try out the idea on the Parkdale Association and on party headquarters. The association voted unanimously to support him, but the party hierarchy was appalled. The Saskatchewan socialist government had had a great deal of trouble with the medical profession over its introduction of medicare, and the Ontario Tories had no wish to stir up medical hostility in their province as well. A week after Shulman laid his plank before the party, he was invited to the office of Dalton Bales, who was representing the premier, John Robarts. With Bales was the secretary of the provincial Progressive Conservative party, and Shulman "was warmly greeted by these two behind-the-scenes operators who told me that the Conservative party would be happy to have me as an MPP but that it seemed a terrible waste to lose my proven talents in the coroner's field. Would I instead consider taking the post of Chief Coroner of Metropolitan Toronto?"

Mort Shulman, refreshingly candid about his own opportunism, confessed himself delighted to be bought off in this fashion, and when they asked him to endorse an alternative candidate, he agreed immediately. To achieve his ambition, he said, "I would have endorsed Godzilla." And so, in March 1963, Morton Shulman was appointed chief coroner; and thus began the most spectacular performance that office had ever witnessed.

For Shulman was a reformer in the scrappy Toronto tradition of Dr. Rolph of Upper Canada Rebellion fame. Smirle Lawson and the previous incumbents had been satisfied that the coroner's task was merely to determine the cause of death—and to stop right there, in case important reputations got soiled by the sordid facts. Shulman believed that an inquest should go far beyond the formal procedure. He was determined to use his powers to drive home the moral of the story; to try to ensure that similar deaths were avoided in the future—and if criminal neglect, incompetence, quackery, vested interest, or insensitive bureaucracy were exposed in the process, so be it.

In his pursuit of this service to the public, he enraged many a civic and provincial figure, the medical authorities, the courts, the provincial and federal governments, and even the U.S. Navy, not to mention his superior, the supervising coroner. With Morton in charge, the days were over when scandal involving the establishment, the medical profession, or officialdom could be hushed up by an obliging coroner—for the next four years, anyway, until the attorney general, after three tries, finally managed to get rid of him.

One of his investigations as chief coroner was the Case of the Cancer Quacks. He himself had dim memories of one of them, a Dr. Hett, who had opened a clinic in Toronto for the treatment of cancer. In 1936 when Shulman was eleven years old, Hett had come to the Shulman household in a chauffeured limousine and had offered to treat Morton's grandmother, who was dying of stomach cancer, with his magic injections. The fee would be two thousand dollars. The family was still trying to raise the money when the old lady died.

A year later the College of Physicians and Surgeons investigated Hett, and analysed his magic formula. It consisted of liver and opium. "The college held a hearing and ordered Hett's medical license revoked," Shulman recalled, but "they never carried out their order because the then Ontario premier, Mitchell Hepburn, was an admirer and friend of Hett's and he threatened the college that if they did not change their decision the government would revoke their licensing powers. Hepburn was at that time all-powerful in Ontario and the college did not dare defy him, so Hett kept his license and continued to prey on the sick and the gullible until his death several years later."

The thirties was an authoritarian decade. For instance, Hepburn and his government had wrenched the Dionne quintuplets from their parents with hardly a murmur of protest from a people whose spirit had been sapped by the Depression calamity—and the members of the college were just as susceptible to bleak authority. They were so frightened by Hepburn's threats, says Dr. Shulman, that they made no further attempt to control Ontario's cancer quacks, and even by 1963 these exploiters of public gullibility were still flourishing.

By then, the best known was a Dr. Glover, who had been injecting his special brand of horse serum into his cancer patients for more than four decades. "The serum itself was harmless but the false hopes it gave cancer sufferers encouraged them not to take standard medical or surgical treatment and thus in many cases led to their premature deaths."

One of the patients was Mrs. Elizabeth George. She had breast cancer. Instead of going to a surgeon, she went to Dr. Glover, who treated her with horse serum for four years until, by the time she finally agreed to accept regular treatment, it was too late, and she died.

Shulman took over the inquest from the investigating coroner, Dr. Bunt. He was determined to get Dr. Glover. On the stand, "the doctor gave a long rambling and confused story of discovering a 'pleomorphic micro-organism in cancer victims which no bacteriologist can classify.' He said he grew their bacteria in a fluid containing 'sunflower seeds, Irish moss and Icelandic moss.' He said that he then filtered the fluid and injected the bacteria into horses, 'I have only three horses now up at Shanty Bay. I'm no authority on horses but they are healthy horses.' He tested the horses' blood regularly and when he judged that 'the time was right' he bled the horses and used the blood for the serum which he injected into patients." When Shulman asked Glover if he ever conducted autopsies to determine the effects of his serum, he replied, 'No, because I didn't have much time.'"

Other damning evidence followed, but during the adjournment, Glover hired a lawyer who managed to get the inquest quashed on the grounds that the chief coroner had taken over from another coroner;

which, though Smirle Lawson had done the same thing many times, was now found to be against the rules.

More determined than ever to put Glover out of business, Shulman next tried to organize a new inquest under Dr. Bunt, but Dr. Cotnam, the supervising coroner, and the deputy attorney general, William Common, went to work on Bunt and got him to drop the matter. Stymied and infuriated, Shulman then personally laid a charge of medical misconduct against Glover with the College of Physicians and Surgeons, but it was fourteen months before they took action. The college informed Glover that he could go on practicing, but he must not use any more horse serum on cancer patients.

By now cordially detested by the supervising coroner, the college, and the attorney general's department, Shulman enraged them by further medical exposures, including another case of a patient who was diverted from proper treatment by the assurances of cancer quack, Dr. Leo Roy. The patient was a young woman named Margaret Power who had a cancer that might have been cured by surgery. Instead she went to Dr. Roy, who treated her with health foods, a short-wave electrical machine, and injections of serum. Dr. Roy claimed that his treatment was eighty percent effective. Miss Power died at home in 1962. Before then, however, realizing the mistake she had made, she wrote a lengthy account of Dr. Roy's treatment, and summarized his claims and the money she had paid him. Her mother took this statement to the authorities in 1963. But when Shulman tried to open the case he was again blocked by the deputy attorney general, Bill Common, who made it plain that he strongly disapproved of the way Shulman was stirring things up so unnecessarily.

As there was no official way around the attorney general's department roadblock, Shulman graded his own route through the press conference. To a group of electrified reporters he released the details of his investigation, and through the media warned people to stay away from Dr. Roy. He also announced that he would lay charges of medical misconduct against Roy. The resulting furor goaded the College of Physicians and Surgeons into acting on Shulman's complaint rather more promptly this time. They took away Roy's licence to practice only a few months later.

After that, Shulman heard of no more cancer quacks in Ontario.

Nowadays it is taken for granted that a coroner's jury should investigate unusual hospital deaths, and their recommendations for greater precautions are never disregarded (though it seems to at least one observer, irritated by floods of recommendations for regulations designed to protect fools against themselves, that safety firstism has become a Canadian disease), but when Shulman was chief coroner the official attitude was protectionist. Exposing the shortcomings of the bigwigs was just not done. Hence, when a patient died in Dr. Shouldice's famous hernia clinic, and when Shulman's inquest resulted in a jury recommendation that the hospital improve its equipment and pre-operative methods, Dr. Shouldice appealed to the Supreme Court of Ontario, to quash the inquest findings. He succeeded. "The inquest was unnecessary," said the judge, "especially since Dr. Shouldice enjoys such a tremendous reputation. I don't agree that any mistake was made at the hospital but if one was it should have been taken up by the College of Physicians and Surgeons." (This being the organization that had allowed Dr. Glover to continue making a fortune with his horse serum forty years after analysing it and finding it to be utterly useless.) The judge also said about the inquest findings that it was not a matter for a lay jury to decide, and concluded that the chief coroner "would be better advised to read the Coroner's Act than to be ordering inquests into deaths at hospitals."

The Supreme Court decision notwithstanding, Morty continued to pressure Dr. Shouldice into obeying the jury recommendations, which included giving patients more intensive examinations before operating on them, and having a certified anesthesiologist present during operations. Once again the attorney general intervened, and told Shulman to mind his own business. Actually the department had already tried to take the business away from him, but their attempt to fire him had raised such a public outcry that they had to back down. The city's three newspapers were unanimous in demanding that the chief coroner keep his job. "We believe Dr. Shulman is the kind of coroner the public needs," said a Toronto *Star* editorial, "even if he is not the kind the Attorney General's Department wants."

The flood of letters that Shulman was now receiving, certainly showed that the public approved of his joustings with the Medical Knights in rusty armour. For many years the profession had refused to listen to complaints about incompetence and insensitivity. Now the floodgates were open, and Shulman was shaken by some of the allegations of medical cover-ups and the damage they had done to so many families. Some of the complaints went back thirty years, and many were well documented.

Of course, some of them could not be taken seriously, such as the one where the letter writer claimed to be under bombardment from sinister rays, and for a while Shulman thought that the one that came in the mail on January 30, 1964, was in this category. It was from a Ruth Neate who said that her sister, Patricia Morgan, had died at the East General Hospital eighteen days after an operation, and that there ought to be an inquest because "I have been told that the autopsy revealed forceps in the intestine which caused shock which was the immediate cause of death. This, together with certain other information which has been given to me, forces me to make this request."

Dr. Shulman had interned at the East General and knew the chief pathologist, Dr. Penney, so, to make sure there was nothing in it, he telephoned the pathologist. "I read Ruth Neate's letter to him," Shulman wrote, "and before I asked him anything he said, 'Yes, it's true.' I was astonished and asked him why he hadn't reported the death to my office. He replied that he did not think that it was his responsibility, that he had reported his findings to both the attending surgeon, Dr. Ken Brown, who had performed the operation, and the hospital authorities, and that it was their decision not to report the matter. He offered to supply me immediately with a copy of his report.

"I now ordered a copy of Pat Morgan's death certificate and discovered that it made no mention of an instrument being found in the abdomen, but blamed the death on cancer — yet Dr. Penney had found no cancer during the autopsy. The death certificate was signed by Dr. Ken Brown.

"My surprise up to that point was mild compared to what I felt after I spoke to Dr. Brown, for he told me an incredible tale. He said that part way through the operation he had been interrupted and harassed by a senior hospital surgeon as a result of which he, Brown, had abandoned the operation and left the operating room and that the operation had then been completed by a third doctor. Dr. Brown told me that if any instrument had been left in Pat Morgan's abdomen it had not been left by him and he went on to say that he felt it was the responsibility of the hospital administration to report the death to the coroner's office. His final remark unnerved me: 'I used to be a journeyman stenotyper and I may have to go back to it.'

"It still didn't make sense how an eight-inch forceps could be left behind in an operation: surely the surgeons counted their instruments before and after? But I soon discovered that the opposite was true — not only the East General but most Toronto hospitals did not bother to count."

Dr. Shulman made sure that the attorney general would authorize an inquest by leaking the basic facts to the press. This caused such a sensation that the department had no alternative but to act. The inquest, which went on for days, revealed a dismal state of conflict and hostility in the operating theatre between Brown, who had been performing surgery at the East General for eight years and Dr. A. T. Varga, the chief resident, who made little effort to hide his feelings of contempt for Dr. Brown's surgical ability, and the chief surgeon, Burns Plewes, who was unhappy about being unable "to clamp down on the many incompetent physicians still on staff at the East General." Dr. Brown, it turned out, had insisted on operating on Patricia Morgan for an obstructed bowel despite the objections of other hospital doctors, who believed that Miss Morgan had a recurrence of cancer and should be left to die in peace.

Brown said later that he had not been convinced that cancer had recurred and that the operation would show what was wrong.

What the operation certainly showed was that Dr. Varga distrusted Brown enough, first to call in the chief surgeon and then to take Brown's place at the table to complete the suturing of the ten-inch incision. But neither he nor Brown made a search for instruments, and when the forceps were found sixteen days later at the autopsy, nothing was done, in an attempt to protect the reputation of the hospital and its staff.

Yet many members of the medical profession, infuriated by the chief coroner's interference, rushed to the support of their colleagues. "The public," Shulman wrote, "was treated to a series of newspaper articles explaining why it would be unhealthy for patients if doctors wasted time counting instruments, why inquests should not be held into hospital deaths, and even why coroners should not investigate them. Dr. Frederick Kergin, chief surgeon at the Toronto General Hospital and head of the department of surgery at the University of Toronto, was quoted as saying, 'A count would slow things down to the danger of the patient. A count just isn't practical and I know of no major hospital where it is carried out.' Dr. James Bateman, surgeon-in-chief at the Orthopedic and Arthritic Hospital didn't want coroners going into hospitals at all. 'It would be witch-hunting in surgery and reprehensible if someone's going to stand over surgeons all the time. Hospitals should conduct their own investigations. Medical disciplinary machinery is there ready to function at all times.' Dr. W. Ross Walters, chief of staff at the Salvation Army's Grace Hospital, felt that inquiries should be left to the College of Physicians and Surgeons. Sydney Liswood, administrator of the New Mount Sinai Hospital, was distressed 'that public confidence in hospitals may be shaken.' One surgeon pointed out that coroners are usually only general practitioners. 'There is a feeling of nausea about individuals presuming to dictate to people who are better qualified.'

But yesterday's controversy is often today's orthodoxy. "Two months after the Morgan case was concluded the Canadian Medical Protective Association sent all its members a sharply worded article in which they were instructed that instrument-counting was a normal and essential procedure. Immediately all the dissenting voices became silent and counting of instruments before and after operations became standard procedure in hospitals right across Canada."

Through his radical methods, Morton Shulman got results in another areas as well: the legislation that finally gave the College of Physicians the power it had formerly lacked, to discipline its members for malpractice or negligence.

Dr. Shulman made a great many changes during his four dramatic years as chief coroner, some calculated to suffuse the face of authority with broken blood vessels, others that would transmute alarming innovation into standard practice, and others, enormously successful, that would be cancelled soon after the provincial government had fired him and eliminated the very post he had occupied. One of the changes that gave him greatest satisfaction was to make material from the autopsy room of the Lombard Street morgue available to science. Medical research scientists needed healthy organs, and these the morgue could supply, because many of the subjects were accident victims. The morgue soon had a number of research scientists depending on it.

Naturally, "The Attorney General's department did not approve and on October 6, 1964, I received a letter from Dr. Cotnam ordering me to restrict attendance at autopsies to the Chief Coroner's staff. I appealed over his head to Assistant Deputy Attorney General Frank Wilson who wrote to me saying I had no legal right to carry on this type of work. He did not, however, expressly forbid my carrying it on and in view of his indecision and the great results we were getting I just went ahead and hoped for the best."

The results were impressive. Within weeks Dr. Calvin Ezrin, heading a team from the Banting Institute, announced a major contribution to the knowledge of the human pituitary gland. "The findings will be of significance in treating breast cancer and in the prevention of blindness in certain diabetic patients," Shulman wrote, adding that, "This morgue work has confirmed what previously had been only suspicions." The same institute was also supplied with heart valves for heart-transplant research. "We soon had a dozen different projects underway," Shulman said. "The department of psychiatry at the University of Toronto was supplied with pineal glands for research into their role in psychiatric illness. The department of orthopedic surgery at the Toronto General Hospital was supplied with lumbar discs in order to study the possibility of dissolving ruptured discs with a drug called chympapin. This worked beautifully and led to a completely new non-surgical treatment of back disc disease. I took special pleasure from this discovery because as a result of it one of my closest friends was able to avoid a major operation on his spine.... The department of biochemistry at the University of Toronto was supplied with kidneys for their study of kidney enzymes. Of immediate value was the supplying of kidneys to the Toronto Western Hospital who successfully used them for human transplants. Possibly most important of all was the work done by Dr. W. S. Hartoft at the Hospital for Sick Children. We supplied him with heart muscles from cadavers for his work on the basic causes of heart disease."

Permission to use the deceased's organs was invariably granted by next of kin. Unfortunately, concluded Dr. Shulman, "after my dismissal in

1967 all co-operation with medical research was stopped on the grounds of legal uncertainty. This has been my greatest regret about losing my job."

The government had barely finished congratulating themselves for finally managing to get rid of their most unhumble servant when he ran for election on the New Democratic Party ticket, and a few weeks later they found him sitting across from them in the chamber of the Parliament Building—in opposition once more.

The second of this triptych of the Doctor as Modern Social Reformer was Guy Richmond, a prison doctor whose cry was for greater realism in the treatment of the social offender.

Dr. Richmond was not a bleeding-heart liberal, or a wet. After a lifetime among delinquents, addicts, thieves, and killers, he came to recognize better than most wets that there were certain types of criminals who should never be released, whether or not the law said they were entitled to their freedom. But the prison system as a whole was a disastrous and costly failure because the damage had already been done to the offender in his childhood, and because the effect of prison was to confirm or deepen his anti-social attitudes.

Guy Richmond, a quietly sympathetic man with a rumpled face dominated by a generous nose, was an English graduate in medicine and an M.R.C.S. He was forty-five when he emigrated to Canada in 1949 to work in the Child Guidance Clinic in Vancouver. Three years later he was appointed as British Columbia's first full-time prison doctor, based at Oakalla Prison.

Apart from wartime duty as an R.A.F. medical officer, he had spent all his professional life among social offenders. Even so, he was taken aback by the extent of narcotic addiction among his wayward clientele in British Columbia. The trend had started a hundred years previously, with the influx into the Pacific Northwest of a large number of opium-smoking Chinese. The drug tradition had been sustained by a ready supply of narcotics from the Far East, and by, according to a University of British Columbia survey, a "large influx of unstable persons, of borderline morality, who became interested in opium smoking and later in manufactured narcotics, who, with their successors, have formed the hard core of the addict colony in Vancouver." Guy Richmond came to know the criminal addict population quite well, as a "closely knit community sharing the same women in common law relationship, with the occasional birth of a child who may show withdrawal symptoms at birth. It has a subculture of its own, with its own mores and vocabulary, a needle-to-vein existence sustained by cookies, chips and coffee." Some of his most poignant memories were of women prisoners, whose careers he had followed from the Child Guidance Clinic through Oakalla Prison and then on to the penitentiary. Many of them died of an overdose.

He remembered one extraordinarily beautiful young woman, Mary, whose parents were both jailbirds, one a prostitute, the other a skid row alcoholic. Though cared for by loving foster parents as an infant, she had become uncontrollable. Dr. Richmond met her at the clinic. The staff there took a special interest in the vivacious, mischievous and rebellious girl, "but special visits, patient social workers, psychiatric counselling all failed. She went the way of prostitution and heroin addiction and had lesbian leanings. Arriving time after time at Oakalla, in the throes of withdrawal, dirty, malnourished, with heroin rash, on each occasion she rapidly gained strength and return of her beauty." Sometimes her mother was in jail at the same time, and Mary would try to strike an answering note with her, but met with no success. Her mother was so schizophrenic that she showed no concern for her daughter, and often no recognition.

By the time she was released, Mary would be glowing with health, but within an hour or so would be back on the mainline of self-destruction. When Dr. Richmond saw her leaving the prison for the last time, she was wearing a pretty dress and had had her hair permed. She looked achingly beautiful. She waved good-bye to the doctor as she climbed into a waiting taxi; which took her straight to her pusher. She was found dead in a squalid hotel room a few days later from an overdose of heroin mixed with barbiturates.

As elsewhere, the problem that Richmond faced in Oakalla Prison was that there was no genuine motivation to abandon the use of heroin. "I'll never give it up," the addict would say. "Spend ten or twelve thousand dollars a year to keep me in gaol for most of my life, and add to that thousands and thousands of dollars worth of goods I have to steal to support my habit. Isn't it much more economical and humane to give me stuff on a controlled basis? I'm sick to death of having to steal and push drugs, and of being beaten up by the drug squad. What future is there for me but perpetual imprisonment, or being shot, stabbed or overdosed?" Richmond thought that the addict might be right.

While Dr. Richmond was convinced that heroin addiction was a sign of a dependent, anti-social, and ineffectual personality, he saw the soft-drug user as a passive, withdrawn, sensitive, culturally shallow sort of person; the victim of a decadent society. In a remarkable submission to a 1969 commission investigating the non-medical use of drugs, he equated the human organism to the dissolution of civilizations. Our society, he said, "which originated in the Dark Ages and the Renaissance is now in the process of dissolution and awaiting another renaissance with a new set of genes. Today there is increasing inertia, fatigue and death of cells in the central nervous system which is followed by confusion of drive and motivation. Twentieth century society is as prone to pathological processes as the aging body with its hardening arteries and cancerous invasion. I equate drug dependence with social malignancy." Subsequently he concluded that, "Today's tempo of work and leisure is so rapid that there is bound to be rebellion against it as greater efficiency of human operation is antagonistic to spiritual fulfilment. Technology stifles the fantasy and imagination which are so necessary to people of all ages. Many young ones no longer see their goals clearly defined. They feel frustrated because they believe that affluence, consumer spending, and high pressure advertising bring polluted values of no benefit to mankind. They are sadly disillusioned with the establishment; government leaders, education authorities, big business and the churches are all suspect. This leads to despair, escapism and self-destruction.

"It must be very difficult for a child to set his own limits when he sees so much indulgence and laissez-faire among adults. Increasing permissiveness and confusion of parental figures lead to hazy ideas and obscure self-identity. I generally found that soft drug users I knew in jail lacked an operational philosophy of living; they had little motivation and were unable to cope with what they considered a hopeless situation. They could become violent under unscrupulous leaders."

(This was a common view in the sixties and seventies. Today the observer is more likely to conclude that the youth scene is an adult-excluding subculture, driven by peer pressure, fed by sensational media publicity, and walled-off from positive influence by a number of factors, including indulgent parents and the nihilistic philosophy of the popular recording artist.)

Richmond classified offenders under two headings: the circumstantial offender and the endogenous. The first was the committer of a crime under the stress of circumstances, but who had the potential to retain an effective and honest personality; examples being the embezzler acting under pressure of debt, and the killer under pressure of passion. The future of the endogenous offender was almost hopeless, pathologically disordered, some inherently evil, others made so by their upbringing. "His vulnerable personality has been grossly insulted from an early age, resulting in grave damage to his entire organism, including in some instances brain damage." Both types were emotionally immature, lacking in social skills, impulsive, unable to learn from experience or punishment, and incapable of showing sincere feelings, whether of joy or despair: psychopaths. Some endogenous offenders were more a nuisance than a danger, but others, forming about ten percent of the penitentiary population, were lastingly dangerous to the community; always ready to indulge themselves sadistically in their virulent hatred of society, in jail or out of it.

As an outstanding example of homicidal psychopathic behaviour he cited the case of a group of three young men. Two had had poor relationships with their fathers and were physically abused by them. The third had a secure and affectionate home background, but turned out as evil as the others. All three had hated their way along the same route, from training schools and correctional centres to the penitentiary. One day they were out driving near Ottawa, armed and ready to put their hatred of society into action. Their excuse came when a car passed them on a country road in what they considered to be a dangerous manner. They stopped the car, shooting and killing the driver and another man, Gerry McDonald and Ken Vallee. Their wives escaped death only because the headlights of an approaching car illuminated the scene.

Dr. Richmond recommended that such men, and a few women "require ultra-maximum security establishments holding not more than fifty, with a staff ratio of one to one, highly trained in all aspects of human misbehaviour and intensive custodial care. Such institutions should be split up into comfortable self-contained living units for not more than ten inmates. Not forgetting that quality of staff is the supreme factor, there must be a full program of creative work, education and athletics, modified to suit the individual's needs and age. Some inmates should stay until they die. There should be specialist therapy available and the staff should include professionals of many disciplines. This will be an expensive undertaking of course, but for the sake of humanity in all our dealings with such criminals, for the safety of those who look after them, and for the longer term protection of society, we have no alternative. There is no justification for attempting to govern such people by traditional penal methods in large establishments. To do so in the face of a rising tide of prison violence is to court disaster. A prison environment in which respects for the right of man is dominant will be reflected in the behaviour of those exposed to it, even though they may have to be rigidly deprived of freedom, perhaps for a very long time." But the dignity and rights of the individual must be respected, he wrote, because as he had seen in forty years' experience, the use of cold, official, formal punishment, such as segregation or treatment as if the individual were a vicious animal made him even more bitter, more angry, more dangerous than ever.

Sex offenders, Dr. Richmond continued, could be circumstantial or endogenous. The offences he encountered ranged from indecent exposure—a common method was to expose the erect penis to escalator passengers in department stores—to barely imaginable habits such as: "One young offender we had in jail [who] was accustomed to having sexual intercourse with hens." Incest was much more frequent than was generally suspected. "One of my patients at Oakalla was a man who held a highly responsible position in industry. His home and marital life had been content until his wife became frigid sexually. As a result the bonds between father and daughter, already strong, became intense and many occasions of sexual intercourse followed." After appealing his sentence, the father, with the support of the wife was freed, provided he took psychiatric treatment.

One of the most heinous sexual crimes, he said, was the gang splash, the offenders usually being wild, beer-swilling hoodlums, the most serious type of gang rape being committed by violent, ruthless motorcycle gangs. "Some compel an initiate to their group to take part in a stipulated number of rapes of this sort, accompanied by other obscene performances. Members of that type of gang are likely to be endogenous offenders who are psychopaths." (Persons with often grossly defective consciences.) The worst individual performers were the stranglers and rippers, who raped before or after killing. "The treatment of all sex offenders, especially of those most dangerous and psychopathic, has been found very difficult, and in jails, impossible. Many kinds of treatment have been attempted such as psychotherapy, group counselling, castration, chemical hormone medication. All have failed. Perhaps aversion therapy may prove more encouraging. In this form of treatment unpleasant stimuli are administered when the offending sexual arousing has been provoked." (A form of this therapy was featured in Anthony Burgess' *Clockwork Orange*.) Sexual offenders were invariably hated by the other prisoners. Richmond knew one sex killer who was so sensitive to this attitude that even on the day of his execution he "made extreme efforts to ingratiate himself with his fellows on the tier, even to the extent of seeking their good wishes as he passed on his way to the scaffold."

At times, Guy Richmond's feelings about the scaffold were ambivalent. In prison, as he got to know the killers as human beings and to understand "the bleak and angry pattern of their battered lives," he saw judicial killing as treasonable to the sanctity of human life; but later, when he became a coroner and saw the bloody, shattered victims, and met the anguished friends and relatives, he could not help asking himself why ruthless, calculating killers should be allowed to live. "But when able to think dispassionately I remain convinced that capital punishment is useless — violence breeds violence."

The judicial act was certainly violent enough. In a hanging, unless the procedure were carefully calculated, there would be prolonged suffering, or decapitation. The theory was that the noose would break the neck and thus death would be quick, but when Richmond X-rayed the neck afterwards, "in no case was the radiologist who examined the films able to report such a fracture, or indeed a dislocation, though there was some stretching." He described one hanging in detail, from his position under the gallows. "There was a shuffling sound. I knew Eddie was wearing slippers. A pause while the hood was being placed on him and then the straps and noose. Then I heard the hangman pull the lever, followed by a clanging thud as the sections of the drop hit the walls. Two slippers dropped at my feet. The hospital officer stooped to pick them up. I could hear the creak of the pulley as Eddie was lowered enough for me to listen to his heart with my stethoscope. The rope was quivering. His legs rose in spasm and dropped again. I opened his shirt and listened. His heart was beating rapidly, 120, 130, 140, 150. . . . then racing, becoming weaker and irregular. Fainter, fainter—6, 7, 8, minutes since the drop. 10 minutes, not a sound, absolute stillness. I turned to the officer and recorded the death as 12:13 a.m."

Even if judicial killings were a genuine deterrent, Dr. Richmond concluded, "we should focus on preventive measures closer to the origins of violence rather than abandon our reverence for life, just because the killer has done so."

It seems likely that the twenty-first-century reader will look back on our treatment of the social offender with much the same kind of wonderment as we today read of the unenlightened treatment of the mentally sick in earlier centuries. It seems equally likely that the future reader will be a member of a society that has solved some of the worst problems of the prison and the prisoner, just as medicine, through chemistry and other therapies, has solved a few of the problems of the more recognizably mentally sick.

One prisoner in Bordeaux Jail, Quebec, wrote a poem about his experience, on April 25, 1975, entitled "Rage":

> Impotent rage eats at my innards.
> I am ready to explode—hemmed in, frustrated, diminished. . . .
> Goddam—
> Tear this place apart—
> Break the walls—
> Tear out the bars and
> Get to Freedom—

The prisoner (who admitted on another occasion that the prison guards were generally nice fellows who live by the rules) was Dr. Henry Morgentaler, the first to openly defy an abortion law that he considered to be cruel and inhumane. He had been acquitted by a jury but an appeal court had reversed the verdict and without providing for a new trial, had ordered his trial judge to sentence him. Canadian law appeared to be holding its own jury system up to contempt. Even the highest court did not quash this lawful but plainly unjust action. The appeal court's decision was upheld by the Supreme Court of Canada.

Given the history of women's rights in the twentieth century, it was surprising that it was a man rather than a woman who was prepared to sacrifice himself on behalf of women and their struggle against male arrogance in the political, judicial, ecclesiastical and medical professions, over their right to control their own bodies. That he was prepared to go to jail for it was an ever greater demonstration of courage, considering how much he had already suffered in prison under Nazi thralldom. He was far from being a born fighter. He was a passive, scholarly youth of sixteen when the Germans invaded Poland; the son of a gentle man who, as a Jew, had little chance of surviving the Second World War, and as a socialist and labour leader as well, none at all. Henry and his mother, his brother Mumek and his sister were herded into a new ghetto that the Nazis had established in the poorest section of the city of his birth, Lodz. There, half-starved and under the constant threat of death, they lived for four years until the collapse of the Russian front. Whereupon the Jewish prisoners were moved from the dreadful ghetto to a destination that was far worse: the Auchswitz concentration camp. There the weak, including Madame Morgentaler, were separated from those still able to work. The boys never saw their mother again.

Along with other young men, Henry and Mumek were led to a bunkhouse. "Soon afterwards," according to Morgentaler's biographer Eleanor Pelrine, "they were moved to a huge hall, lined with what appeared to be showers. The prisoners were overcome with dread—they had heard rumors. Was this one of the extermination chambers? All new prisoners were stripped by hard-eyed Jewish prison guards. Their belongings confiscated, they were shaved roughly from head to foot. As they stood, shivering, naked and hairless, they discovered with sickening relief that the showers yielded water, not gas."

At the end of the war, emaciated, recovering from typhus, scarred by the concentration camp experience, Henry managed to locate one of the few survivors among his family and friends, Eva, his childhood sweetheart. When he heard that an international organization was prepared to sponsor the university education of former prisoners, he applied, and was accepted at the University of Marburgh's medical school. As soon as he had his first-year diploma he crossed the border clandestinely into Belgium, where Eva and her family were living, and continued his studies there. He lived with Eva, who aspired to a career as a poet, in a single tiny room, and continued his medical studies. When the opportunity came to emigrate, he and Eva, who was now pregnant, and who had already delivered a volume of verse, left for Canada and settled in Montreal.

Three years later, Henry graduated from the Université de Montreal, and after serving his internship and obtaining his citizenship, set up in practice in east-end Montreal. His involvement in the family life of the many French and few English-speaking residents led to an interest in psychology, including his own. After six years as a G.P., he found himself anxious, discontented and unfulfilled, but could not understand why. He entered psychoanalysis.

"I had considered myself a good person, without hostility—kind and friendly and nice, and obviously only part of it was true....

"Part of it, though, was anxiety—that if I were unfriendly to others, they would be unfriendly to me. And that would be intolerable, because they are powerful and I am powerless.

"It was not just fear of rejection, but fear of actual harm. I realized how much was still bottled up in me. And my hostility was turned against myself, with the result that I became depressed. You depreciate yourself and say you're no good. I used to resist facing the world, would sleep until ten or eleven in the morning, if I could. I was lackadaisical in many areas—except in my practice. There I was eager to be on my best behaviour."

But while psychoanalysis helped Henry, it strained his marriage. Eva was using her novel- and poetry-writing as a catharsis, reliving the concentration camp trauma on paper. "Henry Morgentaler, in contrast, tried to forget, to surgically excise the past and to concentrate on his life in the present," wrote Eleanor Pelrine, who quoted Dr. Morgentaler as saying about Eva that "When I came home, she had been soaked again in the hurt and suffering which were part and parcel of the ghetto and concentration camp experience, and I wouldn't have any of it." The marriage began to break down.

Through psychoanalysis, Morgentaler realized that the Auschwitz experience had paralyzed his will. "Initiative and competition with others, he felt, were dangerous and to be avoided. So he had scaled down his ambitions and had decided to be content with what he had already achieved, to go no further." It was this paralysis, complicated by feelings of guilt at having survived when other members of his family had failed to do so, that was fighting against an inherent desire to be properly involved in humanity and its causes.

Released from a fear of retaliation, he began to express himself more forcefully, "to feel vibrant, enjoying life, and to become a full person. To be open to experience—active and useful....Active, as a sort of mover of history, doing something useful and important."

He found his cause in the want and need of his patients to make decisions about their own sexuality and reproduction, instead of having their wombs controlled by politicians, under the pressure of religious prejudice. But it was not until he had appeared before a government committee to urge that the country's abortion law be repealed that he realized just how many women needed a champion. Following his appearance before the committee and the rush of publicity that attended it, he was besieged, implored by women desperate to avoid bringing unwanted children into the world.

Morgentaler refused their requests for abortions. He sympathized but abortion was against the law. He would go to jail, lose his practice. He had a wife and two children to support.

Until he faced the fact that he was a hypocrite: he was not practicing what he was preaching. "I had to live with myself," he told his biographer. "Here I was refusing on the grounds that abortion was against the law, and yet I knew I was a coward. I had declared that restrictive abortion law is cruel and immoral, because it exposes women to danger—and I saw them drift off, some to end up as hospital emergency cases, and come back with silent reproaches. . . .

"Finally I decided my medical conscience must come first, the law must be confronted." To the only countries where abortion could be legally and safely obtained—Britain and Japan—he would do his best to add his own country, Canada.

In 1969, Canada did in fact amend the law to allow abortion if a pregnant woman's health or life were in danger, but that was a tiny step forward, and even six years later, three-quarters of the country's general hospitals had failed to establish the essential therapeutic abortion committees. Dr. Morgentaler wrote of the amendment that it "was a liberalization on paper only, and has proven to be a dismal failure. Under this law 99 out of 100 women CANNOT get legal abortions and are driven in desperation to risk their lives at the hands of incompetent people. Why?

"Because Canadian laws on abortion are unreasonably restrictive, unclear and unworkable. They restrict abortions to accredited hospitals only, at a time when medically sound operations by the D & C or vacuum aspiration method can be safely done in clinics, or well-equipped doctors' offices.

"They require that abortions be approved by a board of three doctors, in accredited hospitals. Since most of these boards, where they do exist, are usually staffed by older, conservative and reactionary physicians, they adopt a narrow view of the 'danger to health' clause and consequently refuse most requests for legal abortions."

The vacuum aspiration method was the one used by Dr. Morgentaler in his east-end clinic. He published his findings in a report to the *Canadian Medical Association Journal* in 1973. It was based on five thousand cases, and, "His complication rate was phenomenally low, compared to that reported in general hospitals, probably because of his experience, the specialization, and optimum use of staff and equipment, combined with his use of local rather than general anesthesia. The prevailing atmosphere of warm emotional support given his patients by doctor and staff may also be one of the important factors in this."

Eleanor Pelrine described the operation in her book *Morgentaler: The Doctor Who Could Not Turn Away.* "Dr. Morgentaler, his nurse, and the supportive counsellor wear white or green surgical uniforms and gauze masks. Throughout the operation, the doctor remains seated on a round stool at one end of the examining table. The patient, clad in a disposable gown, lies near the bottom of the sheeted table with her legs in stirrups, the classic position for pelvic examination. There's no shaving of pubic hair, a psychological and practical advantage that both saves time and eliminates patient discomfort and the annoyance of regrowth.

"A disposable sterile towel covers the pubic area and labia, leaving only the vaginal passage exposed. Dr. Morgentaler works with a specially shortened speculum, an improvement in design of which he is proud, which permits easier access to the cervix. First, he swabs the cervix with sterile gauze, then with antiseptic, in preparation for injection of the local anesthetic, the para-cervical block. The local, similar to that employed for dental surgery and repair, is fast-acting, and the dilatation can begin almost immediately. This is accomplished by insertion of a graduated series of small cigar-shaped cylinders. Once the cervix is sufficiently dilated, the plastic curette attached to the vacuum aspirator is inserted, and vacuum suction begins. The nurse gradually increases the pressure, and within seconds, the contents of the uterus have emptied into the large glass bottle at the other end of the vacuum tube. Solids remain in a gauze bag in the middle of the vacuum jar, to facilitate examination before disposal, and liquids pass into the bottom of the jar. A metal curette is then passed around the uterus to dislodge pieces of placenta still attached to the uterine wall, and a few seconds later, the vacuum aspirator is used a second time to remove debris. The patient's legs are then removed from the stirrups. She remains resting for another five to ten minutes on the operating table, and regular checks are made of her respiration and pulse....

"When the patient is ready, she is assisted to a lower floor, where a comfortable broadloomed lounge is equipped with stereo and television. A third nurse, plump and grandmotherly, is stationed there to answer questions, provide cheerful support, and give information about birth control."

At one end of the queue of desperate females was a thirteen-year-old black child who had been raped. She had been referred to the clinic by an agency in Minneapolis. At the other end was a fifty-one-year-old, with eleven children. In between were women from all social levels, united in what they felt was a need to end their pregnancies through abortion.

Many of them had tried before, using incompetent practitioners or by injecting, or trying to inject, dangerous caustic or antiseptic fluids into the uterus, or by inserting the *tige laminaire,* a rod-shaped piece of wood that reacted to body heat and moisture in the cervix, and caused miscarriage—and sometimes bleeding and infection. Provided they were in the first trimester of pregnancy, Dr. Morgentaler helped them all, openly and with an increasingly contemptuous defiance of the law. In his certainty that the flouter of the law was in the right and the law was the criminal ass, he was undeniably arrogant, and worse, his arrogance blazed in the newspaper headlines. He never missed, in the words of the trial judge, "an opportunity to make use of the press or other informational media to proclaim that he performs abortions on demand." Canadian authority, which throughout the country's history has shown a dark intolerance of the intense individualism it purports to defend, of pusillanimity in the face of organized opposition and viciousness when faced with the opposition of the individual, responded to the challenge, and committed what Pelrine described as a "judicial atrocity" to make sure Morgentaler ended up in jail.

Though Dr. Morgentaler undoubtedly asked for it. The psychoanalysis he had undergone had apparently not entirely succeeded in curing him of his guilt that he had survived.

All the same, Morgentaler's intense feelings about the abortion issue were shared by many of the most enlightened and experienced medical people. One of them was Gustave Gingras, now a chancellor of the Université de Montreal, a president of the Canadian Medical Association, and the founder and director of the Rehabilitation Institute of Montreal. He considered abortion a black and heinous crime when he was a student; but after a lifetime of dealing with the effects of the anti-abortion atmosphere, his attitude had changed to one of rage that the reactionaries should still be in control. "The authorities, doctors, the police, the whole of society is acting like an ostrich," he wrote. "To my mind the whole thing is the greatest show of hypocrisy in human history. Although I find the act of terminating a pregnancy basically repugnant, I can only say I have to side with the lesser evil. When a proposal was put to the now historic meeting of the general council of the Canadian Medical Association that abortion could be justified on social grounds as well as physical or psychological grounds, I voted *yes*. What line should one take in the case of a young girl made pregnant by her father? Are you going simply to let him become one more battered child? Should you allow the birth of children to parents of incompatible blood groups? Will there be enough institutions for them to go to, to live out their lives?"

43

The Selfish Paragon

THE FOUNDER AND director of the Institute of Experimental Medicine at the Université de Montreal was an Austrian/Hungarian/Czechoslovakian/Canadian named Hans Selye, whose concept of stress had earned him a host of doctorates and international awards, medals and honours, including this country's highest honour, the Companion of the Order of Canada. Dr. Selye was teaching endocrinology at McGill when he started his systematic medical research into stress, but the seed was planted at the University of Prague when he was eighteen years old. It suddenly occurred to him one day that though his professors talked a good deal about the signs and symptoms of specific diseases, they never mentioned the signs and symptoms of *just being sick*. He looked around at the patients in the Prague Hospital, and noted that though their diseases were dissimilar, they all had something in common: they looked and felt ill. They acted tired, had little appetite, wanted to lie down, felt indisposed, did not feel like doing anything. They had the nonspecific manifestations of disease.

"I wondered," he remembered, "why nobody had ever given this syndrome any special attention. With all the methods of modern medicine, physicians had looked for and analyzed the more subtle and unexpected signs of disease, but nobody seemed to pay any attention to the most common malady, 'the syndrome of just being sick.' Why didn't anybody study its biochemical manifestations, try to establish its mechanism, and perhaps even to attempt to find some treatment likely to combat the more frequent morbid changes that all maladies have in common? This struck me as the most fundamental problem in medicine."

It failed, however, to strike anyone else. His professors and classmates ridiculed the idea that one day we might be able to ameliorate or suppress these discomforts in patients, whatever the underlying cause of their illness. They laughed at Selye because they could not see that there was a problem at all. No textbook in the whole history of medicine had so much as hinted at it. Obviously if a person were sick, he would look it, what was so curious about that? A patient's inguinal hernia or his third-degree burns made him feel sick, and that was all there was to it. Hans argued in vain, that just as antipyretics could restore the temperature to normal in different kinds of fever, so one day we might be able to repair the nonspecific damage to the patient—those general aches and pains not specifically associated with his malady—before carrying on with the treatment for his particular ailment.

Ten years passed before Dr. Selye, now a doctor of science and of philosophy as well as a doctor of medicine, began to study the syndrome of generally being unwell. In 1936 he had been working for two years at McGill as an assistant to Professor Collip, the man who had done so much to purify Banting's insulin preparations. That year, while experimenting on animals, Selye saw the same nonspecific response to any kind of damage inflicted on them. "I began to wonder what might be the cause of other changes which, although not totally nonspecific or common to all maladies, seemed to affect so many people. I asked myself, for instance, why so many people suffer from heart disease, high blood pressure, arthritis or mental illness. These are not completely stereotyped signs of all illness, yet they are so frequent that I could not help suspecting some nonspecific common factor in their causation."

Even his much-admired chief could not be converted to this new way of looking at things. J. B. Collip was fond of the bouncy and enthusiastic young man, but as the months passed he became increasingly concerned that his deputy was galloping headlong into a canyon with no exit. He tried several times to head Selye off at the pass, pointing out that his exceptional ability was being misdirected; but each time Selye had justified his labour with an eagerness and sincerity that was impossible to oppose.

Collip made another attempt, calling Selye into his office one day for a heart-to-heart talk. As gently as possible he told Hans that his line of research was futile. He implored Hans to switch to a more useful line of work. There was still room for a contribution to endocrinology, for example. Why not concentrate on that, instead of this stress business. But once again Dr. Selye responded with an outburst of "juvenile enthusiasm" (as he described it himself), and proceeded to outline all over again the immense possibilities inherent in a study of the nonspecific damage which must accompany all diseases and all but the mildest medications."

Selye continued, "When he saw me thus launched on another enraptured description of what I observed in animals treated with this or that impure toxic material, he looked at me with desperately sad eyes and cried, 'But, Selye, try to realize what you you are doing before it is too late! You have now decided to spend your entire life studying the pharmacology of dirt!' (By dirt, Collip meant the poisons, such as formalin, that Selye was injecting into experimental animals.)

At such moments, Selye was overwhelmed with doubt, and it is possible that he might not have gone on had it not been for the encouragement of Sir Frederick Banting, who frequently dropped into the laboratory, sat on the desk and listened interestedly to Selye's enthusiastic speculations, and to consider his definitions of the concept of stress: *the nonspecific response of the body to any demand.* Banting, mellow in middle-age, also provided some financial aid, but, "More than anything in the world," Selye cried, "I needed his moral support, the reassuring feeling that the discoverer of insulin took me seriously. I often wonder whether I could have stuck to my guns without his pat on the shoulder."

Over the years, Selye's research showed that it was not only disease and damage that induced "biologic stress" in the body; even pleasant challenges (eustress) "will evoke the objective, measurable characteristic indexes of stress." Joy, for instance, causes organic stress because of an adaptation it forces on the body; though the effect is not as harmful as disease, for disease lasts longer (distress).

For years, Selye's research into the mechanism of stress, into the action of the syntoxic and catatoxic stress hormones, seemed to many in the profession to be a questionable *ideé fixe* encapsulated in an obsession. Painfully and slowly, as the work showed scientifically measurable results, some of his colleagues were convinced. But he also wanted to convince the public because the philosophy that was emerging from his basic research was relevant to the way that people lived their lives. He began to lecture outside McGill, to get his idea across to the layman.

He cited an instance of how badly he needed more general support. During the Second World War, his research called for the urine of patients who were suffering from an obscure disease named periateritis nodosa. Unfortunately (from his point of view), nobody in the Montreal area was suffering from that disease. Eventually he tracked down a couple of cases in Burlington, Vermont. He made arrangements for their urine to be sent by air in sealed containers, so that it would arrive fresh. One of his associates would meet the aircraft and rush it to the lab before the urine decomposed.

Urine, however, was not listed in the customs book, either as duty-free or dutiable, so the customs man would not pass it. Selye's associate argued, but the customs man was adamant. Urine was not listed in the book so he would not allow it into the country. Selye hastened along to the dean, and persuaded him to write an official letter to the customs people, explaining that the urine was urgently required for research purposes, and that as representatives of a supposedly sophisticated nation they ought to know that some allowance had to be made for the needs of a university.

The letter from the dean of such a prestigious institution brought results. A few days later the answer arrived. There would be no further difficulty about admitting the item duty-free. Naturally the government was aware of the needs of universities. They apologized for the mix-up and explained that it was the fault of an inexperienced customs official. He should have known where to look for this particular item in the book. It came under the category of "used personal articles."

By that time, Selye knew that the samples must have decomposed, so he made no attempt to collect them. But now that the consignment was of no further use in research, customs became increasingly anxious to deliver it. Every day brought a fresh demand that the merchandise be collected immediately. In a huff, Selye refused to do so. Finally he received a letter which read, "Unless within five (5) days after receipt of this notice you collect the merchandise mentioned ebove, the shipment will be opened and contents sold at public auction."

At the Université de Montreal, Selye's work on stress gradually progressed from a medical to a behavioural study. His findings suggested that his concept could mitigate the ill effects of biologic stress in people. Any demand on the body, he argued, brought a nonspecific response, a response that was likely to differ from person to person, as distinct from the specific response of the body from an attack by a particular disease. The same element of stress (trouble at work, conflict with spouse) could cause exhaustion, or nervous breakdown, or heart trouble, or asthma, or chronic fatigue—a nonspecific result. These were the diverse effects of stress found from individual to individual.

To combat stress, it was to be noted that not all stress was to be avoided; only the kind of overstress—hyperstress—to which the body could not adapt satisfactorily; or understress—hypostress, where the body was understimulated by change, resulting in, for instance, boredom, or physical or mental inertia.

Selye was well aware that there were many rival kinds of therapy that were being used to lessen the effects of distress: exercise, psychotherapy, physiotherapy, acupuncture, moxibustion, chiropractice, electroshock, sauna, hot and cold baths, balneotherapy, short-wave therapy, ginseng, eleutherococcus, Zen Buddhism, Hare Krishna, yoga, Transcendental Meditation, or drugs and the like; but too many were techniques for shutting out external reality and the reality of the ego. Selye's answer was to develop a code of *altruistic egoism*, based on natural laws.

"The concept of altruistic egoism appears paradoxical," he wrote, because it is difficult to conceive of someone who is both an altruist and an egoist at the same time. Yet the underlying idea is very simple: you can be effectively selfish, giving free expression to your particular talents, and still maintain peace of mind. Altruistic egoism lets us give vent to our natural human egoistic tendencies without producing guilt feelings—for who would condemn him whose egoism expresses itself in the insatiable desire to be useful to others and thereby earn their love?"

His philosophy was based on no airy revelation but on forty years of medical research, the end result being the good of the organism. Altruistic egoism rids one of guilt feelings about one's natural egoism, for what one really wants, he says, is to be useful to others without sacrificing one's own interests, particularly peace of mind. "It is biologically justifiable to seek happiness in an atmosphere of serenity, by contributing to the maintenance of society through your own usefulness to others."

As an example of the practical application of altruistic egoism, he cited the example of a situation where there are twenty-four passengers at an airport but only six taxis to get them to the same hotel. The aggressive egoists would grab the taxis, leaving the remaining eighteen passengers stranded and feeling bitter. The pure altruist would let the others go first and remain behind in the hope that another taxi would arrive. The altruistic egoist would suggest that the passengers split up, four persons to a taxi—one of whom would be himself. He would thus earn friendship without sacrificing his own interests. He would be in equilibrium with himself and the others, his mental and physical health, his biological status, protected by his code of behaviour.

Which provides this volume with its conclusion. For its subjects, whether radiant or reticent, glorious, vainglorious, whether overweening, unassuming, cutting or constrained, understood and obeyed that code of behaviour long before it was ever formulated or consciously recognized. It formed the attitudes and informed the work of Hippocrates and Harvey, Lister and Sarrazin, Grenfell and Workman and Hincks, Matheson, Abbott, O'Brien, Willinsky, Gingras; of almost every one of the medical men and women in this national portrait gallery of Canadian doctors.

44

Blood and Sympathy

T HE MOST SPECTACULAR advance in medical history began in the 1930s, the decade of the chemotherapy that, from the sulfonamides to the climax of penicillin, appeared to have vanquished the deadly fevers.

In the forties, electronics, optics, and nuclear physics created a technological revolution in medicine. Today, linear accelerators can bombard tumours deep in the body without risk to innocent parts. Computerized Axial Tomography can produce visual cross-sections of almost any tissue area and organ, including the brain; blood dialysis machines can cope with formerly disastrous kidney failure; optical instruments can see far into the body tracts, ducts, and passageways; synthetic materials can replace joints; lasers can mend tissues behind the eyeball; and numerous other black boxes and instruments, optical, pressure-sensing, measuring and monitoring, can enable adjustments to be made about internal problems with a precision that would have astounded the most brilliant 1940 diagnostician.

Part of the cost of such developments is the demotion of the family physician. With a growing dependence on the new technology, the profession has tended to become less personal. It is said that in this, the penultimate decade of the twentieth century, the waiting rooms of the nation are sibilant with complaints about medicine's deficiencies. The doctor has become a technician, working on warm machines. The doctor is overpaid. The doctor is a drug-trade patsy, insufficiently wary of the pharaceutical hucksters, too fast on the draw in shooting overpriced pills into patients whose anxiety he has lost the ability to allay in other ways.

The doctor is too intent on getting through his hefty quota of clients to give any one of them enough attention. And so forth.

Part of the trouble is that there is no longer an unconditional surrender of the patient to the practitioner. A wariness has supplanted the old, comforting dependency on Dr. Wonderful, the all-wise, all-caring advisor with his superior education and his carefully schooled expression suggesting that he knew exactly how to put it right, whether he did or not. Perhaps people have begun to feel insufficently de-individualized by modern society even without being treated by the doctor as if they were plastic containers. Or perhaps it is simply that the public is better informed. "Doctors have occupied godlike heights above their patients for so long that the current assault on their collective power has created much psychological chaos in doctor-patient relationships....Patients know more than they have ever known before; the mystery that once surrounded doctoring is broken."

The patient's frustrations are shared by many thinking members of the profession. A whole new category in non-fiction has sprung up in the past few years: medical self-criticism. An example is Robert S. Mendelsohn's *Confessions of a Medical Heretic*, "a stringent attack on the medical profession and its lack of concern for the patient by a noted physician." At least two past presidents of the Canadian Medical Association have expressed concern at the state of the profession. Dr. Bette Stephenson suspects that the wrong people are being attracted to the profession, and Dr. Gustave Gingras feels that once in it, too many doctors lose their souls, and are "more in tune with their machines than they are with people." While Dr. Robert McClure, the missionary surgeon, has said that Canadian doctors are overpaid and underdedicated.

The defenders reply that the new technology has saved millions of lives and extended the life span of millions of others. And to handle a large number of patients, methods have to be efficient. Overpaid? Half the country is overpaid. As for the slap-happy pill position, the defence argues that it is difficult for a doctor to avoid being manipulated by a three-billion-dollar industry. "A drug," says a Montreal physician, Dr. Murray Katz, "is the only thing you ever buy without knowing what exactly you are purchasing and whether the particular brand you've been prescribed is the best value for money. The doctor, who is not paying for the drug, has already made the decision for you. So the drug companies spend millions of dollars each year persuading doctors to decide their drugs are best. And ultimately, of course, the consumer is going to have to pay the cost." A British Columbia doctor, R. F. Rose, writes that, "Lest we become supercilious about the best that our grandfathers could do, it is salutary to remind ourselves that in parallel with our modern wonder drugs there has been concocted a multitude of products, having in common only their fantastic cost, foisted off on the profession by the manufacturing druggists, described in the most pretentious pseudo-technical language, the claims for which are either wildly inflated or utterly baseless....

"To the harrassed practicing doctor, the enormous complexity of truly beneficial treatment makes it relatively easy for the exploiters to confuse him with preparations which have no positive characteristic other than their complexity."

Dr. Rose then goes on to list nineteen polysyllabic ingredients in a single capsule of a typical preparation, showing that in place of the old camphor, eucalyptus and oil of wintergreen, we now have methyl testosterone, 1-Lysine monohydrochloride and dl-Methionine.

"The famous 'ethical' drug house which produces this pharmaceutical smorgasbord," Dr. Rose continues, "touts it as follows:

"'Designed to serve as an effective aid in the practice of preventive geriatrics, 'X' supplements natural sources of essential vitamins, minerals, hormones, digestive enzymes, and protein factors. Deficiencies of these materials are believed to be part of the aging process. Helping to prevent these same deficiencies, 'X' may assist in decreasing severity of tissue changes accompanying the aging process. 'X's broad physiologic, nutritional support should be applied early, before tissues lose their ability to respond to such support. This early use helps to establish and tends to maintain a sense of well-being at a time in life when this state becomes increasingly elusive and therefore increasingly valued. The physiologically balanced combination of estrogen and androgen in 'X' is more desirable in deferring tissue changes due to age than is either hormone use alone.' The recommended dose is three capsules a day, at a cost of $9.17 per hundred, or $101...a year for the elixir of youth, which appears to be cheap at the price, as it still enjoys a wide sale since its introduction several years ago.

"This sort of device to relieve the layman of his cash, using the bewildered doctor as a middleman, is a nostalgic reminder of the days when snake oil at a dollar a bottle was sold by the light of a kerosene lamp off the tail gate of a wagon, except that today's is much more expensive. By contrast, the innocuous prescriptions of our grandfathers seem almost like a fresh breath of innocence."

The classical Greek philosophers believed that the way to physical and mental harmony was to follow the precept, "Nothing in excess." But ours is an age of excess, including excess in the application of scientific discoveries. Just as many destructive insect species may adapt to man-made chemicals because of extravagant spraying, and just as farm animals, being continually fed doses of antibiotics merely to stimulate growth, may come to resist all antibiotics, so the human body, through unrestrained chemotherapy, may quite possibly show disastrous future effects, mentally, physically, or genetically, or may respond with ever more virulent and resistant strains of bacteria. A hundred years ago, Osler was concerned about the indiscriminate use of drugs. If he were around today he would be appalled at the way the pop-gun pharmacy he deplored has turned into a sustained barrage.

Nevertheless, despite discontent and apprehension over the state of medicine today, there is not the slightest doubt that medicine's five thousand years of slow enlightenment have produced, in the West at least, a population that is remarkably healthy. (Dr. Jonathan Miller argued in his television series, *The Body in Question*, that our high physical well-being owes more to public health measures than to the efforts of general practitioners and specialists, but it could be pointed out that it was usually the doctors who urged public health measures into law in the first place.) To give just one example of how much we owe to the slow enlightenment to which medicine contributed so substantially: Only a few decades ago, baby girls, if they survived the contemporary fevers, were indoctrinated into sexual inferiority; in adolescence educated into ignorance and shame of their own bodies; in young womanhood psychologically impaired by political, religious, and medical moralists. In marriage their instincts were artificially suppressed, in maturity they were encouraged to think of themselves as physically inferior because of their monthly "illness" or the discomforts associated with childbearing; in their thirties they were expected to withdraw still further from reality by fainting or hysteria; in late middle age they were expected to resign themselves to bodily decay; and in death they were sentimentalized.

In the 1830s, Anna Jameson looked around at the young women settlers in Upper Canada and found them "premature old women, sickly, care-worn, without nerve or cheerfulness," and living "in a perpetual state of inward passive discord and fretful endurance." Anne Langton observed of young girls that "it seems quite customary to leave them untaught," and the 1840s found women in settlements that had no medicines, let alone medical practitioners, so that "the poor creatures have nothing to do but lie down, and let the fever take its course." The fever in that case being malaria, for which "the mode of treatment," wrote Catherine Parr Traill, "is repeated doses of calomel, with castor-oil or salts, and is followed up by quinine. Those persons who do not choose to employ medical advice on the subject dose themselves with ginger-tea, strong infusion of Hyson, or any other powerful green tea, pepper and whiskey; with many other remedies that have the sanction of custom or quackery." Susanna Moodie: "Those who have drawn such agreeable pictures of a residence in the backwoods, never dwell upon the periods of sickness, when, far from medical advice, and often, as in my case, deprived of the assistance of friends by adverse circumstances, you are left to languish, unattended, upon the couch of pain."

By the turn of the century, the picture was not much better. "We have only to glance around us at the dwarfed, miserable, sickly specimens of feminine humanity, which really constitute the rule rather than the exception," wrote an American gynecologist, W. H. Walling, "to observe at once how far short is the attainment of these ends in our system [of education] as actually conducted." Actually Professor Walling's own educational advice and guidance in his book *Sexology*, was typically moralistic and paternalistic. For instance, though disgustedly noting that masturbation is instinctive in children, he exclaimed over the habit in females: "Oh that it were as frequent as it is monstrous," and after this gripping start, prays that the girl who reads the book "will at least pass over this chapter, that she may still believe in the general chastity of her sex; that she may not know the depths of degradation into which it is possible to fall."

Thirty years later, shame was still queen. "Sex in the Thirties was plain dirty," writes Pierre Berton. "Childbearing, at the very least, was vulgar and, at the worst, obscene. Canada not only banned *Spicy Stories* and *Gay Paree*, with their innocent photographs of unsmiling bare-breasted women and their once-over-lightly attempts at risqué pulp fiction, but it also impounded all copies of the April 11, 1938 issue of *Life* magazine because it dared to carry a photograph of a baby being born."

Today, through drugs and hygiene, contraceptives and endocrinology, surgery and sexual enlightenment, diet and genetics, vitamins and exercise, and many other positive ways, medicine can help to keep a woman looking and feeling young and fit well past middle age; keep her self and her spirits healthy well beyond the old span of three score years and ten; encourage her to be proud of her body and determined to be mistress of its fate. The thirty-year-old "specimens of humanity" of 1904 are not even the sixty-year-olds of today. The grandmother of the 1980s can be toned, vigorous, healthy, aware, in proper control of function and faculty. The progress has been brought about partly through the leadership of the increasing number of women in medicine and through a changed perception generally. Women see themselves as being worthy of respect, of being no whit inferior to the opposite sex in most fields, and superior in some. And medicine has contributed in no minor way to the new enlightenment, through the selfish goodwill of the ships' surgeons and the neurosurgeons, the bloodletters and blood fractionators, the Hippocrates and the Semmelweises, and the Grenfells, Willinskys, Abbotts, and Hilliards.

Capsule Biographies

A list of Canadian doctors, or those associated with Canada, who are featured most prominently in the text.

Maude Abbott   Born 1869, St. Andrews East, Quebec. Educated at home by tutors, she was fifteen before she went to school in Montreal. Won a scholarship to McGill, graduated in arts, 1890. Granted M.D., C.M., University of Bishop's College, 1894. Three years of postgraduate education in Germany, Austria, and Scotland. Appointed curator of the McGill Medical Museum. Inspired by William Osler, she made medical museums her life's work. Also became a world authority on congenital heart disease. She never married, devoting much of her private life to the care of an ailing sister. Died 1940.

Edward A. Archibald   Born 1872, Montreal. Graduated McGill 1896, trained at the Royal Victoria Hospital, Montreal. Described as the Father of Thoracic Surgery in North America. Changed the character of surgical education in Canada from the clinical to the scientific through an emphasis on research. Did notable work on pancreatitis, and was the first surgeon on the continent to treat pulmonary tuberculosis through thoracoplasty (1912). One of the first in Canada to take a systematic interest in brain surgery. Died 1959.

William W. Baldwin   Born 1775, Ireland. A University of Edinburgh M.D. His family lived at Baldwin's Creek, Ontario, but Dr. Baldwin set up in practice in Toronto, where he also practiced law, and advertised in the *Gazette* and the *Oracle* in 1802 for students to attend his classical school. Was occupied as a surgeon during the American attack on Toronto in 1813. Took part in the formation of the Medical Board in 1819. Held the chair of chemistry and natural science in Victoria College for eight years. Died 1844.

Frederick Banting   Born 1891 near Alliston, Ontario. Though inclined toward a medical career, he first attended the University of Toronto as an arts student in preparation for the ministry, to please his parents. Transferred to medicine two years later and graduated in the wartime accelerated course in 1916. Joined the army medical corps, was wounded, and won the Military Cross. After the war he interned at the Hospital for Sick Children in Toronto, and the following year set up in practice in London, Ontario, where he also had a minor appointment at the medical school. It was his reading at the school's medical library that led to the idea of ligating the pancreatic duct, to permit the extraction of insulin. Back in Toronto, he persuaded Professor J. J. M. MacLeod to allow him to use his laboratory. Assisted by Charles Best, he succeeded in isolating insulin within eight weeks, in 1921. Received the Nobel Prize in 1923, was knighted in 1934. He was engaged in medical research for the armed forces when he was killed in an air crash in Newfoundland in 1941.

James Barry   Born about 1790, graduated from the University of Edinburgh. In 1813 entered military service as hospital mate; promoted to assistant surgeon in 1815. Gradually rose through the ranks until, as a familiar figure in Montreal social circles, she had become inspector-general of the military hospitals of Canada in 1857. Ended up as head of the entire British Army Medical Service. Died 1865 — when it was discovered that Barry was a woman, and had successfully concealed the fact throughout her military career in England, the West Indies, St. Helena, Corfu, the Crimea, and Canada.

William R. Beaumont   Born 1803, London, trained at St. Bartholomew's Hospital under Astley Cooper and others of renown. M.R.C.S. 1826, F.R.M.C.S., 1836, and studied anatomy in Paris. Came to Canada in 1841. Appointed professor of surgery, King's College, Toronto, 1843. Invented and made several surgical instruments. Continued to operate despite increasing blindness in one eye, until the sight of the right eye was affected. Died 1875.

William Beaumont   Born 1785, Lebanon, Connecticut. Studied medicine in Champlain, New York, and was licenced to practice after an apprenticeship to a Vermont doctor in 1812. Served as a surgeon's mate in the War of 1812. Practiced in Plattsburg in 1815, re-enlisted in the army in 1820 and was posted to Fort Mackinac where he treated a French-Canadian trapper, Alexis St. Martin, who had been shot in the stomach. The permanently open wound enabled Beaumont to study the process of digestion and become an authority on the subject. Died 1853.

Charles H. Best   Born 1899 in Maine, the son of Canadian parents, his father being a country doctor. Was studying physiology and biochemistry at the University of Toronto as a preliminary to medicine when he assisted Banting in the disovery of insulin. He graduated in 1925, and in 1929 succeeded Professor MacLeod as head of the department of physiology. During the Second World War he served with the Royal Canadian Navy, largely occupied in research into seasickness and its prevention. After the war he was instrumental in building the C. H. Best Research Institute. 1966, Professor Emeritus at the University of Toronto. Died 1978.

Wilfred A. Bigelow   Born 1879, Kingsport, Nova Scotia. In 1898 he traveled to Winnipeg to act as an office boy and surgical assistant to Dr. J. O. Todd, his brother-in-law, which he did for five years at the St. Boniface Hospital. Graduated from the Manitoba Medical College, 1903. Practiced in Hartney, Manitoba until 1905. Moved to Brandon in 1906, where he started the first medical clinic in Canada, 1913. A pioneer in the use of blood transfusion and X-ray examination. Died 1966.

Norman Bethune   Born 1889, Gravenhurst, Ontario. Son of a Presbyterian minister. During the First World War, he gave up the study of medicine to join the army, was sent to France and was wounded and invalided home in 1915. After obtaining his degree at the University of Toronto, he continued his medical education in Vienna, and in Britain where he qualified as a fellow of the Royal College of Surgeons of Edinburgh. Developed tuberculosis while in private practice in Detroit, which redirected his life toward the control of tuberculosis. Moved to Montreal in 1928 and became a well-known thoracic surgeon. Invented a number of surgical instruments, of which the Bethune Rib Shears were of most lasting value. While in Montreal he became a pioneer publicist in the cause of socialized medicine. Served briefly with the Loyalists in the Spanish Civil War, organizing a mobile blood transfusion service. Returned to Canada to help raise money in the Spanish cause. Instead of returning to Spain, he went to China in 1938. By then a Communist party member, he attached himself to the Communist forces of Mao Tse-Tung who was then fighting the invading Japanese. Died in China in 1939 as a result of an infection contracted in the operating theatre. Mao Tse-Tung's essay *In Memory of Norman Bethune* has since made him one of the Republic of China's greatest heroes.

Davidson Black   Born 1884, Toronto, graduated University of Toronto, 1906. The practice of medicine did not appeal to him. Lectured in the department of anatomy at Western Reserve University, Cleveland. From 1925 his interest turned increasingly to anthropology, which he pursued after being appointed head of the anatomy department, Peking Union Medical College. Discovered the skull of Peking Man, 1929. Died 1934.

François Xavier Blanchet   Born 1776 in the parish of St. Pierre de la Rivière du Sud, Quebec. Educated at the Quebec seminary, studied medicine in New York. Published his first medical work at the age of 24, *Recherches sur la Médicine*. Like so many of the early English and French-speaking doctors, he was a reformer and was briefly imprisoned by the lieutenant governor of Quebec in 1810, though he was a member of the Legislative Assembly. Nevertheless he headed the army medical staff of the province during the War of 1812. Thereafter his political program was mostly concerned with the well-being of his patients and the people of Quebec in general. Died 1830.

James Bovell   Born in the Barbadoes, 1817, graduated Glasgow. Settled in Toronto, taught pathology and physiology, often relating the latter subject to theological concepts. Mainly noted for his lifelong scientific influence on Osler. Died 1880.

Edmund A. Brasset   Graduated Dalhousie School of Medicine, 1934. Practiced in Canso, New Waterford, a year at the Nova Scotia Hospital for mental patients. Practice at Little Brook, Digby County. Started neurosurgical career in New York but later returned to Little Brook.

Alan Brown   Born Toronto 1887, obtained his M.D. at the University of Toronto in 1909. Spent five years as resident physician at the Babies' Hospital, New York. Postgraduate education in Europe, returned to practice pediatrics in Toronto. Appointed physician-in-chief at the Hospital for Sick Children in 1919, and later became head of the department of pediatrics at the University of Toronto. Died 1960.

Herbert A. Bruce   Born 1868, Blackstock, Ontario. Graduated University of Toronto 1892, winning the university gold medal and Starr silver medal. Postgraduate study in France, Germany, Austria, and Britain (L.R.C.P., F.R.C.S.). An eminent surgeon of his time, he founded the Wellesley Hospital. Appointed lieutenant governor of Ontario, 1932. Elected to House of Commons 1940. Professor of surgery, University of Toronto. Died 1963.

Richard M. Bucke   Born England, 1837, brought to Canada the following year. Graduated McGill University, 1862, and studied in London and Paris. Established a practice at Sarnia. 1876, appointed superintendent of the Asylum for the Insane at Hamilton, Ontario; superintendent of the asylum at London, Ontario, 1877. Author of *Man's Moral Nature* and a study of Walt Whitman. Died 1902.

Alexander Burnside   Born and educated in the United States; appeared before the Medical Board twice before being found qualified to practice, in 1822. Described as a Yankee quack, but his Toronto-area patients seemed content with his knowledge of local fevers. "During the first cholera epidemic he was the standing witness for the defendants upon an indictment for nuisances, always proving to the satisfaction of the jurors that the stench complained of, whether it arose from stables, tanneries, privy vaults, or any other abomination, was conducive to health; at least, he found it so in his practice." An early promoter of the Mechanics' Institute movement, and an encourager of church music. Left a considerable property to Trinity College.

William Canniff   Born Thurlow, Ontario, 1830, educated at Victoria College (then at Cobourg), the Toronto School of Medicine, and the University of New York where he obtained his M.D. in 1854. 1855, M.R.C.S.. Served as a medical officer in the Crimean War. In Canada he practiced first in Belleville, then Toronto. Professor of pathology and surgery at Victoria College. Was the first medical health officer in Toronto, 1883-91. Best known for his books on surgery and Canadian medical history. Died 1910.

Ashern A. Chamberlain   Born Peachem, Vermont, 1810, brought to Canada with his family at the age of five, settling at Smith's Mills. Graduated from the Fairfield Medical College, New York, and practiced at Smith's Mills until 1858, then at Athens until his death in 1883. Reformer, army officer, mason, postmaster, Methodist, and temperancer.

Henry Havelock Chown Born 1859, Kingston, where he received his degree from Queen's, in 1880. Moved to Manitoba to set up practice in Winnipeg. At first he resisted the establishment of a medical school in Winnipeg, but joined the staff as a teacher in anatomy two years later, in 1885. Later became professor of surgery, and was elected dean in 1900. Wrote a history of medicine in Western Canada and was influential in politics. Died 1944.

Charles K. Clarke Born at Elora, Ontario, 1857; educated at the University of Toronto, obtaining his M.D. in 1879. Specialized in the study of mental diseases. Superintendent of the Toronto General Hospital, 1911-18, and dean of the faculty of medicine in the University of Toronto until 1920. The Clarke Institute of Psychiatry is named after him. Died 1924.

James B. Collip Born in Belleville in 1892. A brilliant scholar, he received his medical degree from Trinity College, Toronto in 1912, then a Ph.D. in biochemistry. In 1915 he was appointed to organize a department of biochemistry at the University of Alberta. It was while he was on leave from that university that he worked with Banting on the process of producing insulin on a commercial scale. In 1927 at the University of Alberta he isolated the active principle from the parthyroid gland, parathormone. The following year he was appointed to the chair of biochemistry at McGill, where he did major work on the pituitary hormones. Was the first to isolate the adrenocorticotrophic hormone, ACTH. By 1947 he was dean of medicine at the University of Western Ontario, and head of the department of medical research. Died 1965.

James Connor Served with the British Army in the American Revolutionary War and was one of the first to practice in English Canada, in the Bay of Quinte region. Later practiced in Ernesttown. Performed the first operation in Upper Canada, removing a large tumour from the neck of a member of the Roblin family.

Tom Cullen Born 1868, Bridgewater, Ontario. Graduated 1980, University of Toronto. Joined Johns Hopkins Hospital, 1891, studying pathology under William Welch. First major work, *Cancer of the Uterus.* Associate in gynecology, 1897, professor of gynecology, 1932. Died 1953.

Allan R. Dafoe Born 1883, Madoc, Ontario. A graduate of the University of Toronto, 1907. His achievement was in keeping alive the Dionne quintuplets, 1934. Died 1943.

James A. de la Hooke Born Plymouth, 1814. Trained as an apprentice, then at the Royal Institution, the Hunterian Theatre, St. George's Hospital, King's College, and at University College Hospital. Obtained his licence from Apothecaries Hall in 1836, and admitted M.R.C.S. the following year. On his arrival in Toronto, 1839, he was required to undergo an examination before the College of Physicians and Surgeons, "which, with reluctance and a natural feeling of injured pride... he submitted to, and was granted a license." He was the first person to receive its diploma. Practiced in Goderich for three years, then in Ohio, finally Toronto. Date of death not known.

Campbell Douglas   Born 1840, Quebec City. A graduate of Laval University, he won fame while serving with the British Army in the Andaman Campaign in the Pacific, winning the Victoria Cross. Retired with the rank of brigadier in 1882. Returned to Canada to live on a farm near Lakefield, Ontario. Joined the Canadian Army Medical Corps in 1885 as a surgeon major in the Riel Rebellion campaign. His exploit in traveling to the front along the Saskatchewan River by canoe was later emulated when he crossed the English Channel in another canoe, *The Saskatoon.* Died 1909.

Charles Duncombe   Born in England 1794, became a well-known personage in his time among Upper Canadians, not so much as a physician but as a politician, member of Parliament, and a participator in the Rebellion of 1837. Passed his examination before the Medical Board of the London District in 1819. He practiced in the village of Bishopgate, Brant County. Though pardoned for his part in the Rebellion, he elected to remain in exile in the United States. Died 1875.

William "Tiger" Dunlop   Born Greenock, Scotland, 1792 and studied medicine in that country. After some months of further training in London he qualified as an army surgeon. Posted to Canada, he served in the War of 1812. Returned to Canada in 1826 as warden of the woods and forests for the Canada Company and did much to open up the Huron Tract for settlement. Died 1848.

Gordon S. Fahrni   Born Gladstone, Manitoba, 1887 and graduated in medicine, University of Manitoba, 1911. Practiced medicine in Winnipeg, teaching surgery at the Medical College. Served for forty years on the staff of the Winnipeg General Hospital. Prominent in thyroid surgery; founding member of the American Goitre Association (1928) and the Royal College of Physicians and Surgeons of Canada; a past president of the C.M.A. (1911) and the Manitoba Medical Association (1923).

Abraham Gesner   Born near Kentville, Nova Scotia, 1797; naturalist and geologist as well as a medical graduate (London, 1824). Established himself in Parrsboro in Nova Scotia, where he combined a medical practice with studies in natural history and geology. Published a book on the minerals of Nova Scotia in 1838 and made geological surveys of New Brunswick and Prince Edward Island. His experiments with coal produced a new substance, kerosene. He patented this discovery in 1852, but unable to obtain financial support for its production in Canada, went to the United States and sold his patent to the North American Gas Light Company, which in turn employed him as its consultant chemist. Returned to Nova Scotia in 1863 and was appointed to the chair of natural history at Dalhousie University. Died 1864.

Gustave Gingras   Born 1918. Graduated Université de Montreal. World authority on the rehabilitation of the handicapped. A past president of the C.M.A., he now lives on Prince Edward Island.

Alton Goldbloom   Born 1890, Montreal. Torn between stage acting and medicine, finally opted for the latter. Graduated McGill in 1916, determined on a career in pediatrics, and studied under Emmett Holt, New York, 1917. Returned to Montreal in 1920 to become a pioneer in pediatrics. Ultimately became head of the department of pediatrics, McGill University.

Wilfred Grenfell   Born 1865 in England; studied Medicine at the London Hospital. As a medical officer to deep-sea fishermen, he discovered the plight of the people of Labrador and northern Newfoundland. They were living in debt, extreme poverty, and ignorance, without medical care. It was through his efforts that the International Grenfell Association was formed to provide medical and nursing care, hospital, schools, and orphanages for the people. Knighted in 1927. Died 1940.

Harold Griffith   Born 1894(?). As a sergeant in the First World War won the Military Medal for gallantry under fire. After the war, resumed his studies at McGill, graduating and specializing in anesthesiology, he convinced the world of the efficacy of curare as an anesthetic (1942). One of the pioneers in the endotracheal technique.

Pitkin Gross   Born 1791 at Burlington and was licenced to practice by the Toronto Medical Board. Settled in Brighton on the shores of Lake Ontario. Died 1873.

John Sebastian Helmcken   Born in London, 1825. Was a delivery boy for a local doctor, Graves, who gave him some training in pharmacology. He graduated from Guy's Hospital. Upon return to London after a tour of duty as a ship's doctor, he was taken on by the Hudson's Bay Company. He reached Victoria, British Columbia in 1850 and served the settlers and natives for a number of years as physician and surgeon and later as a member of the first House of Assembly on Vancouver Island. When British Columbia joined Confederation in 1871 he refused a seat in the Senate at Ottawa, and returned to private practice. Retired in 1882 and died at the age of ninety-five in 1920.

Marion Hilliard   Born Morrisburg, Ontario, 1902. Graduated from the University of Toronto in 1927, and established a practice in Toronto. Chief of obstetrics and gynecology at the Women's College Hospital from 1947 to 1957. Her best-known work is *A Woman Doctor Looks at Love and Life.* Died 1958.

Clarence M. Hincks   Born 1885, St. Mary's, Ontario; educated at the University of Toronto, graduating in 1907. Took an early interest in mental problems among children and adults; founded the Canadian Association for Mental Health; established the first mental health clinic in Canada; and helped to organize the School for Child Studies at the University of Toronto. A recognized authority on mental problems. Gold medalist of the World Federation for Mental Health. Died 1964.

William H. Hingston   Born Hinchinbrook, Quebec, 1829. A McGill graduate, 1851, with postgraduate training in Europe. Began a surgical practice in Montreal in 1854 and became surgeon-in-chief at the Hôtel Dieu de Montréal, later becoming the first dean of the medical faculty of Bishop's College. One of the founding members of the Canadian Medical Association, in 1867. Mayor of Montreal for two years. Died 1907.

Gareth Howerd   Manchester University graduate, served in the Merchant Navy as a medical officer. Doctor at the Distant Early Warning Line, which was constructed after the Second World War to defend against attack over the North Pole. His arctic practice covered 600,000 square miles.

Elnathan Hubbell   Emigrated to Canada in 1808, settling at Brockville. Remarkable for his large size rather than his medical education, which "was of doubtful extent." Marriage brought him much influence and wealth, and in time he commanded a large practice, principally in the town, especially in midwifery. Was captured by the Americans in the War of 1812, but released on parole. Died 1850.

Donald Johnson   Graduated Cambridge, 1926. Medical officer with the Cambridge University East Greenland Expedition, 1926. Labrador, 1928, working for the Grenfell Mission. Passed Bar examinations in 1929. Private practice in England, later went into publishing.

William A. ("Father") Johnson   Born 1816, Bombay, India, educated in England, the family then migrating to Canada, 1831. Entered the church, but more noted for his dedication to science. Strong influence on Osler as founder and warden of Trinity College School. Died 1880.

John G. Kittson   Born 1844, St. Paul, Minnesota, his family moving to Berthier, Quebec, in the 1860s. Graduated from McGill, 1869; set up in practice in Berthier; five years later joined the North West Mounted Police. Organized the medical services for the Northwest Territories. It was largely through his work and ability that the treaties with the Indians who had fled to Canada after the Custer massacre were signed and reservations established without bloodshed. After resigning from the force, he practiced in St. Paul. Died 1884.

John J. Lafferty   Date of birth not known. A British Army surgeon who later practiced in Drummondville with an extensive clientele. A member of the provincial legislature from 1828, "his loud, sonorous voice, and forcible language made him a conspicuous figure in society at the young capital." Defeated in 1834 by one vote. Died 1842.

Mahlon Locke   Born near Williamsburg, Ontario, 1881. M.D. Queen's University, 1904, with extensive postgraduate training at Edinburgh and Glasgow. A specialist in manipulative surgery and orthopedics, returned to Canada to practice for the rest of his life in Williamsburg. Died 1942.

William MacKay   Born 1858, Earltown, Nova Scotia; studied medicine at Bellevue Medical College, New York, qualifying in 1873. In 1874 he was appointed as resident physician to a coal mining company, instituting effective quarantine measures for diphtheria. Elected to the Legislative Assembly in 1886 and became leader of the opposition. He helped to frame the Public Health Act of Nova Scotia. Died 1915.

William M. MacKay Alberta's pioneer doctor, he was born 1836 and educated in Scotland (Edinburgh). He sailed to Canada in 1864 as a Hudson's Bay Company surgeon. Served widely throughout the northwest, retiring to Edmonton in 1898. Most of his patients were Eskimos and Indians suffering from the ravages of scarlet fever, smallpox, and typhus. Died 1917.

C. Lamont Macmillan Born 1903, graduated Dalhousie University, Halifax, 1928. Practiced at Baddeck, Cape Breton Island for half a century. Elected to Nova Scotia Legislature, 1949.

Andrew MacPhail Born 1864, Prince Edward Island. From the age of eighteen he taught school, then attended McGill graduating in 1891. His talent for writing earned him enough to pay his way through the medical school, and enable him to tour the Orient and spend a year in postgraduate study. Upon his return to Montreal he became professor of pathology at Bishop's College. By 1907 he was professor of the history of medicine at McGill. He was knighted for his contributions during First World War. First editor of the *Canadian Medical Association Journal.* Died 1938.

Cluny MacPherson Born 1879, St. John's, Newfoundland. Attended McGill Medical School 1896, returned to St. John's to practice. Joined the Grenfell organization in 1902, which helped to arouse a lifelong concern for public health. Helped to organize Newfoundland's first sanatorium. During the First World War he developed the first effective gas mask. Died 1966.

John McLoughlin Born 1784, Rivière-du-Loup, Quebec, and studied medicine at Edinburgh. From 1824 to 1846 as a representative of the Hudson's Bay Company he ruled over a vast territory extending from Russian Alaska to Oregon, from his headquarters at Fort Vancouver. Died 1857.

Robert McClure Born 1900, Portland, Oregon. Graduated 1922 University of Toronto. Went to China as a medical missionary for the Presbyterian Church and spent the next twenty-five years there. Field director for the International Red Cross in north and central China. During the Second World War was in command of a Quaker ambulance unit on the Burma Road. Returned to Canada 1948 to establish short-lived practice in Toronto. Abroad again, to work among Palestinian refugees, and as a physician and surgeon in India. In 1967 he became the first lay moderator of the United Church of Canada. Has subsequently served in Borneo, Peru, and Zaïre, Africa.

Kenneth G. McKenzie Born Toronto, 1892 and studied medicine at the University of Toronto, graduating in 1914. After the war he took postgraduate training in surgery. Was awarded a Mickle Fellowship, and became house surgeon to Harvey Cushing (the neurosurgeon) in Boston. On his return in 1923 he established the first neurosurgical service in Canada at the Toronto General Hospital. He built up a flourishing school of neurosurgery, his organization including the basic sciences: neuroanatomy, neurophysiology and neuropathology. He devised instruments and developed new operative procedures, and gathered and reviewed groups of cases to elucidate new syndromes. Died 1964.

Robert J. Manion   Born Pembroke, Ontario, 1881; graduated from Trinity in Toronto in 1904 and practiced medicine at Fort William. In the First World War was awarded the Military Cross for gallantry. Represented Fort William in the House of Commons. In 1933 he was head of the Canadian delegation to the League of Nations in Geneva. Elected leader of the national Conservative party in 1938. Died 1943.

Elizabeth Matheson   Born 1866, Campbellford, Ontario. Enrolled in the Women's Medical College, affiliated with Queen's University, Kingston; forced to give up for lack of funds. Teacher with Presbyterian Board of Missions, India, 1889. Married John Matheson, 1891. Practiced medicine in the Territory of the Saskatchewan, 1898 to 1918. Died 1958.

Joseph P. Moody   Born 1922; graduated University of Western Ontario, 1946. Medical health officer for the Department of National Health and Welfare, 1949. Returned to the Arctic in 1950 and 1954 on his own expeditions.

Henry Morgentaler   Born Lodz, Poland. In 1939 at age sixteen, he was put into a concentration camp. Completed medical studies in Belgium; emigrated to Canada; worked on research at McGill. Resident, Queen Mary Veteran's Hospital; established a practice in east-end Montreal 1958. Established abortion clinic. Arrested in 1970; later prosecuted and jailed for defying the law on abortion.

Florence J. Murray   Born Pictou Landing, Nova Scotia, 1894, graduated Dalhousie University Medical College, Halifax, 1918. Went to Far East as Presbyterian medical missionary, 1921. During the Second World War she was exchanged by the Japanese for prisoners of war. Returned to Korea, 1947; retired 1969.

George Nasmith   Consulting engineer and doctor of public health, whose recognition of the type of poison gas used against Canadian troops in France in the First World War saved many lives.

Murrough O'Brien   Born 1868, Delhi, India. His medical education began at St. Mary's Hospital, London, and was completed at the Manitoba Medical College in 1897. Practiced at Dominion City, Manitoba. Served in the First World War as a medical officer. Died 1955.

Gerald O'Reilly   Born Ballinlough, Ireland, 1806. Apprenticed to Dr. James Cusack of Stevens Hospital, Dublin, in 1823 and remained with him for five and a-half years. On one occasion the joking O'Reilly caused consternation by impersonating his master in the wards. Received the diploma of the Royal College of Surgeons, Ireland, in 1829. Sailed for Canada in 1833 and later practiced in Hamilton and soon commanded a large and lucrative practice extending from St. Catharines to Brantford, and from the Grand River to Oakville. One of the first to administer chloroform, to one of his own children in 1856. Examiner in the principles and practice of medicine in the University of Toronto. Died 1861.

William Osler   Born 1849 in a parsonage near Bond Head, Ontario; perhaps the most influential physician since Hippocrates. Educated at Trinity College, Toronto, in preparation for the ministry but transferred in 1868 to the Toronto School of Medicine. After two years, moved to Montreal where the clinical opportunities were better, and graduated from McGill in 1872. Was appointed to the staff at McGill two years later. 1884, professor of clinical medicine at the University of Pennsylvania, where he perfected his bedside teaching techniques. Appointed in 1888 to the new Johns Hopkins Hospital and Medical School where "his views on laboratory and bedside teaching dominated the new school and gradually permeated throughout the world." Regius Professor of Medicine at Oxford in 1905. Knighted in 1911. Wrote numerous reports, papers, essays, histories, and books, including *The Principles and Practice of Medicine.* Died 1919.

Daniel M. Parker   Born 1822 in Nova Scotia. Began as a medical apprentice to a Dr. Alman of Halifax. Completed his medical studies at Edinburgh, winning a gold medal in anatomy. Returned to Halifax in 1845 to establish a practice. Helped to establish the city and provincial hospitals and to found the Nova Scotia, Maritime, and Canadian Medical Associations, being at some time president of each. The first surgeon in Canada to operate with the help of ether anesthesia. Appointed to the Legislative Council in 1871. Died 1907.

Wilder Penfield   Born 1891, Spokane, Washington; received his M.D. from Johns Hopkins and a further four degrees from Oxford. Served as a neurosurgeon at the Presbyterian Hospital and the New York Neurological Institute before moving to Canada in 1928. Founded, in 1934, the Montreal Neurological Institute, which, by drawing together the disciplines of neurosurgery, neuropathology, neurology, and related basic sciences, greatly enlarged the field of study and treatment of the brain. Died 1976.

Bessie Rehwinkel   Born Galesburg, Iowa, the daughter of a medical practitioner who entered medicine herself and graduated in the early years of the twentieth century from the Sioux City School of Medicine. Her first practice was ruined in the financial panic of 1907. Married a Lutheran minister, Alfred Rehwinkel in 1912 and went with him to Alberta. Died 1962.

John Richardson   Born 1787, Dumfries. Began his medical training as an apprentice to his uncle. Entered the University of Edinburgh as a medical student at the age of fourteen, studying chemistry, Greek, botany and natural philosophy as well as the required medical subjects. Upon graduation was appointed an assistant surgeon in the navy. In 1819 joined Franklin's Arctic expedition. Became an authority on the flora and fauna of the Canadian Arctic. Died 1865.

Guy Richmond   Born in England, 1904; graduated St. Thomas Hospital; M.R.C.S.; for ten years before the war he was a prison doctor in England. Appointed in 1952 as the first full-time prison physician in British Columbia. Senior medical officer of Corrections Branch; B.C. coroner at Burnaby until 1975; and deputy coroner, Vancouver. Author of works on topics related to his prison work.

Lawrence B. Robertson   Born 1885. Achievements in the field of blood replacement, particularly in infants. Did much to introduce transfusion in the treatment of shock and severe hemorrhage in military surgery. Died 1923.

Thomas Roddick   Born Harbour Grace, Newfoundland, 1846. While attending school at Truro, Nova Scotia, at the age of fourteen he assisted a Dr. Muir, who persuaded him to study medicine. Entered McGill in 1864, graduated at the top of his class and was appointed house surgeon at the Montreal General Hospital. Established a practice in Montreal. In 1875, professor of clinical surgery at McGill; in 1877 he was the first to use Lister's antiseptic methods in Canada. Served as chief of the medical staff in the Riel Rebellion of 1885. Served in Parliament, and established the Medical Council of Canada, becoming its first president in 1912. Knighted 1914 for his services to Canada and Canadian medicine. Died 1923.

John Rolph   Born in England 1793; emigrated to Canada, 1812; became pay-master for the London district in the 1812 War. Studied law in England and was called to the Bar. At the same time he was studying medicine at St. Thomas' and Guy's Hospitals. Practiced both professions in Canada from 1821 to 1828 until he retired from law. Began teaching medicine at St. Thomas in 1824. Elected a member of the Legislative Assembly the same year. His career was interrupted in 1837 when he was forced to flee the country, following his part in the Rebellion. Pardoned in 1843; returned to Toronto. Established the Toronto School of Medicine. Died 1870.

Michel Sarrazin   Born 1659 in France and became the most famous medical practitioner in New France. Was trained as a barber surgeon and was influenced by the teachings of Ambroise Pare. Appointed surgeon-major in the French army in 1685, left for New France the following year. Practiced in Quebec for eight years before returning to France to obtain his M.D. Upon his return to Canada he became noted for his management of epidemics and for his studies in natural history. In 1700 he successfully amputated a breast for malignancy. Died 1734.

John Schultz   Born 1840, Amherstburg, Ontario. Studied medicine at Queen's University and Victoria College, graduating in 1861. Left for the Red River Settlement on the day of his graduation. Became identified with the settlers who wished to unite with Canada, and opposed the domination of the Hudson's Bay

Company. Fought Riel, and helped to rouse Ontario against him. After the Northwest Rebellions, Manitoba became a province and Schultz a member in Ottawa. Lieutenant-governor of Manitoba in 1888. Knighted in 1895; died 1896.

Hans Selye   Born Vienna, 1907; father a surgeon in the Austro-Hungarian Imperial Army. Graduated from the medical school of the University of Prague. Two years after the M.D. obtained a Ph.D. in organic chemistry. Lecturer in biochemistry at McGill in 1931. There developed the stress concept with which his name is associated.

Francis J. Shepherd   Born 1851, Como, Quebec; his father part-owner of the Carillon and Grenville Railway (Grenville). Graduated McGill, 1873. Returned in 1875 to McGill after further education in Europe as demonstrator of anatomy. Succeeded to the chair of anatomy in 1883; later professor of surgery. Extensive list of publications. Equally distinguished in anatomy, surgery, and dermatology, as scientist, practitioner and teacher. Died 1929.

Morton Shulman   Born 1925, Toronto; graduated 1948. Practiced in West Toronto, became a coroner in 1952; chief coroner in 1963. In 1967 he was elected to the Ontario Legislature.

William E. Smith   Born Kendal, Ontario, 1864. Received his M.D. degree from the Michigan College of Medicine and Surgery, with special diplomas in chemistry and operative surgery. Went to China in 1896 as a medical missionary, and remained for forty years. Died 1944.

William Fraser Tolmie   Born 1812, Inverness; received his medical training in Glasgow. Graduated in 1832; emigrated to Fort Vancouver as a surgeon and trader on behalf of the Hudson's Bay Company. A natural historian, geologist, and explorer as well as a physician and surgeon, he contributed to a knowledge of the natural history and resources of the northwest Pacific, was a member of the legislature, a student of Indian languages, and a supporter of public education. Died 1886.

Charles Tupper   Born 1821, Amherst, Nova Scotia; trained in Edinburgh. Practiced in Amherst in 1843 until elected to the provincial parliament in 1855. First president of the C.M.A. in 1867. At various periods in his life he practiced in Halifax, Ottawa, and Toronto as well as in Amherst, in between active participation in provincial and federal politics. Was one of the fathers of Confederation, and helped to formulate the policy that built the transcontinental railway. In 1884 was Canada's high commissioner in London. Became prime minister in 1892 at the age of seventy-five. His party was defeated that same year, but he continued to lead the Conservatives until 1901. Died 1915.

John C. Webster   Born 1863, Shediac, New Brunswick. Studied medicine at Edinburgh, winning a gold medal for his M.D. thesis in 1890. Returned to Canada in 1896; appointed to McGill and the Royal Victoria Hospital. In 1919 he returned to Shediac after twenty years in Chicago as a professor of obstetrics and gynecology and undertook a study of Canadian history, and was ultimately recognized as an outstanding authority on the subject. Died 1950.

Christopher Widmer   Born in England, 1780; trained at St. Thomas' and Guy's Hospitals, qualifying in 1803. Arrived in Canada in 1813 as an army surgeon and settled in Toronto. With his skill and ability as a surgeon he soon built up a large practice. Took an active part in medical affairs in the city; chairman of the Board of the Toronto General Hospital in 1844; chancellor of the University of Toronto in 1853. Died 1858.

Abraham I. Willinsky   Born 1885, Omaha, Nebraska; the family moved to Toronto when the boy was four years old. Influenced to study medicine at the University of Toronto by Osler; graduated 1908. Genito-urinary specialist, head of urology at Western Hospital. Died 1976.

Joseph Workman   Born 1805 near Lisburn, Ireland; emigrated to Canada with his family at the age of twenty-four, graduated from McGill in 1835. Abandoned medicine for several years, resuming in 1846 at the Toronto School of Medicine. Appointed superintendent of the insane asylum in Toronto, 1854-75. Died 1894.

A few other Canadian physicians and surgeons who have made notable contributions to medicine.

Boris P. Babkin   Born 1877. Professor of physiology first at Dalhousie, then McGill (1926). Did first significant research into gastroenterology in Canada. Died 1950.

Murray Barr   Born 1908. At the University of Western Ontario in 1949 he discovered the sex chromatin, an important and fundamental observation in cytology, and gave his name to this "Barr Body." Was one of the first recipients of the Kennedy Foundation Award, 1962, and also received the Gairdner Foundation Award in 1964.

Pierre Beaubien   Born 1796, Saint Antoine de la Baie du Febvre, Quebec. Graduated University of Paris, 1822. After extensive postgraduate training in Europe, returned to Canada in 1828 and established a practice in Montreal. Served in the Legislative Assembly until 1851. Joined the École de Médicine at Chirurgie de Montréal and ultimately became dean of the faculty. Appointed physician to the Montreal prisons in 1859, a post he held until his death in 1881.

Gordon Bell   Born 1863, Pembroke, Ontario. His scientific education was begun at the University of Toronto and was completed at the new Manitoba Medical College, where he obtained his degree in 1892. An attack of typhoid fever resulted in the amputation of his leg. After a stint as medical officer at the Brandon asylum, he went abroad for postgraduate training, studying ophthalmology, bacteriology, and pathology. Upon his return to Winnipeg he established an ophthalmological practice. Shortly after he became the first provincial bacteriologist. He took a particular interest in public health problems at a time when the dangers of impure milk and water pollution were still improprerly appreciated. Died 1923.

Alexander H. Ferguson   Born near Woodville, Ontario, 1853; brought up in Manitoba. Graduated from Trinity in 1881; returned to Winnipeg, where he was the prime mover and one of the founding members of the Manitoba Medical College. Became its first professor of physiology and histology, later professor of surgery. Gained a reputation for his treatment of hydatid disease of the liver. Moved to Chicago in 1894 to become professor of clinical surgery at the College of Physicians and Surgeons. Died 1911.

Edward A. Gallie   Born 1882. Made original and outstanding contributions in surgery, including tendon fixation, growth and transplantation of bone, and living sutures. Widely influential in the training of young surgeons in Canada, not least through the formation of the Gallie Club, whose members were international surgeons who had been trained by him. Died 1959.

Louis Gross   Born in Montreal, 1906. Made contributions to knowledge of the anatomy of the cardiac blood supply in 1931. Engaged in research on rheumatic heart disease when he was killed in airplane accident, 1937.

Abraham Groves   Born 1847 near Fergus, Ontario, graduated Toronto, 1871. Established a practice at Fergus. Noted for his excellence and originality in surgery, despite the makeshift instruments of the day. The first time he saw an abdomen opened was when he removed a large ovarian tumour in 1874. He was almost alone in using aseptic techniques, boiling his instruments and scrubbing his hands. Performed a vaginal hysterectomy in 1875, the first time this operation had been performed in Canada. Also undertook a suprapublic lithotomy, and two years later, in 1883, an appendectomy, both first operations for North America. Died 1935.

Robert T. McKenzie   Born 1867, Almonte, Ontario. Graduated McGill University 1892. Medical director of physical training at McGill and a teacher of anatomy for ten years from 1894; 1904, professor and director of the department of physical education, University of Pennsylvania. Became one of the most famous of living sculptors, exhibiting mainly in Britain and the United States. Died 1938.

Alexander Mahaffy   Born 1891; graduated University of Toronto. Noted for his work on the yellow fever virus. Died 1962.

Pierre Masson   Born 1880; came to Montreal from University of Strasbourg, 1927. Internationally known for his work on tumours of the nervous system and other contributions to pathology. Also noted for his histological techniques. Died 1959.

Maud Leonora Menten   Born 1879, Port Lambton, Ontario. Graduated in medicine from the University of Toronto in 1907, one of the first Canadian women to receive a medical doctorate. In Germany in 1913, she collaborated with Leonor Michaelis on a study of the behaviour of enzymes, which resulted in the Michaelis-Menten equation, a basic biochemical concept. International recognition brought her an offer from the University of Pittsburgh where, from 1918, she served as a pathologist and published extensively on medical and biochemical subjects. She made important co-discoveries relating to blood sugar, hemoglobin, and kidney functions. From 1951 to 1954 she conducted cancer research in British Columbia, returning to Ontario six years before her death in 1960.

Gordon Murray   Born Oxford County, Ontario, graduated University of Toronto. Developed and introduced the first successful artificial kidney in North America, and was a pioneer in cardiac surgery.

Israel W. Powell   Born Port Dover, Ontario, 1839; graduated from McGill, 1862. Settled in Victoria, became deeply involved in education and politics as well as in a busy practice. Helped to establish a medical act to regulate and licence the profession, 1886. "Took an active part in having the C.P.R. extended to Vancouver." Died 1915.

John Rae   Born Orkney Islands, 1813; graduated Edinburgh, 1833. Visited Canada as surgeon on a Royal Navy warship, stayed on to trap and fish, learn Swampy Cree Indian, and minister to the sick. Carried out extensive explorations of Canada between 1846 and 1861, including surveys of northwestern Hudson Bay, the north coast near the Gulf of Boothia, the Mackenzie River, and the Saskatchewan plains. Died 1919.

Arthur Rousseau   Born 1871, St. Casimir, Quebec. Graduated from Laval University in 1895. Two years' postgraduate work in Paris. Appointed to the staff of Laval and the Hôtel Dieu in 1897. Helped to found Laval Hospital, St. Sacrement Hospital and the Roy Rousseau Clinic, and the Association of French-Speaking Doctors in North America. A corresponding member of the Academy of Science of Paris, and the first Canadian to be elected a member of the Pasteur Institute. Died 1934.

Henry E. Young   Born English River, Quebec, 1867; graduated McGill, 1888. Studied under Osler at Philadelphia and as an eye, ear, nose, and throat specialist in Chicago and St. Louis. Established a practice in British Columbia; elected to the provincial parliament in 1903. Minister of Education and Provincial Secretary, 1907. Helped to found the University of British Columbia. Died 1939.

Notes

A few notes, particularly sources of quotations which have not been specifically assigned in the narrative.

Chapter 2

page line
4 7 Jesup North Pacific Expedition, 1908.
4 25 Quoted by Marius Barbeau in *Medicine-Men on the North Pacific Coast.*

Chapter 3

12 18 Quoted by Victor Robinson in *The Story of Medicine.*
12 27 Will Durant, *The Life of Greece.*
12 42 Ibid.
13 24 Edward Gibbon, *Decline and Fall of the Roman Empire.*
14 14 Victor Robinson, *The Story of Medicine.*
20 27 William Harvey, *Anatomical Exercises.*
21 23 John Aubrey, *Brief Lives.*

Chapter 4

23 10 Autopsy report by Samson Ripault.
28 1 Kalm
28 19 Register of the Hôtel-Dieu
28 43 Maude Abbott, *History of Medicine in the Province of Quebec.*
29 19 Christopher Hibbert, *Wolfe at Quebec* (Cleveland: World Publishing Co., 1959).

Chapter 5

page line
32 20 William Canniff, *The Medical Profession in Upper Canada.*
33 10 Ibid.
33 37 Ibid.

Chapter 6

39 18 Fielding Garrison, *History of Medicine.*
40 19 Ibid.
41 22 Ibid.
46 20 *Globe and Mail*, Toronto, Oct. 27, 1979.

Chapter 8

52 19 Quoted by Maude Abbott in *History of Medicine in the Province of Quebec.*
53 24 J. E. Roy, *Histoire du Notariat au Canada.*

Chapter 9

65 10 W. H. Graham, *Tiger Dunlop.*
70   4 John W. Scott, biographical material for The Academy of Medicine, Toronto.
70 27 William Canniff, *The Medical Profession in Upper Canada.*

Chapter 10

75 14 W. E. Swinton, "Abraham Gesner." *Canadian Medical Association Journal*, Vol. 115, 1976.
79   2 M. D. Morrison, *Nova Scotia Medical Bulletin*, April 1940.
80   8 W. F. Parker, *Daniel McNeill Parker.*

Chapter 13

116 31 Harvey Graham, *The Story of Surgery.*
117 37 Philip Smith, *Arrows of Mercy.*
118 3 Ibid.
124 31 Ibid.

Chapter 14

132 39 W. G. Hardy, *From Sea Unto Sea.*
133 43 Francis Shepherd.

Chapter 15

page line
145 41 H. E. MacDermot, *Sir Thomas Roddick.*

Chapter 16

158 10 Harvey Cushing, *The Life of Sir William Osler.*
161 27 W. G. Cosbie, *The Toronto General Hospital.*
169 5 Colin Wilson and Pat Pitman.
176 13 Osler Memorial Volume.
181 27 Harvey Cushing, *The Life of Sir William Osler.*
184 5 Geoffrey Marks and William K. Beatty, *The Story of Medicine in America.*
184 15 Ibid.
189 32 Harvey Cushing, *The Life of Sir William Osler.*
195 33 Ibid.

Chapter 18

208 11 As quoted by Judith Robinson in *Tom Cullen of Baltimore.*

Chapter 19

233 20 J. Lennox Kerr, *Wilfred Grenfell.*

Chapter 20

243 21 Judith Robinson, *Tom Cullen of Baltimore.*

Chapter 21

261 38 As quoted by Edythe Lutzker in *Women Gain a Place in Medicine.*
264 11 As quoted by Alfred M. Rehwinkel in *Dr. Bessie.*
275 5 Ruth Matheson Buck, *The Doctor Rode Side-saddle.*
276 15 Ibid.
279 11 Ibid.

Chapter 22

288 13 As re-created by Robert Tyre in *Saddlebag Surgeon.*
290 20 Robert Tyre, *Saddlebag Surgeon.*
292 11 Ibid.
293 25 Ibid.
295 5 Steward H. Holbrook, *The Golden Age of Quackery.*
296 40 Thomas P. Kelley Jr., *The Fabulous Kelley.*
297 20 Ibid.
298 35 Robert Tyre, *Saddlebag Surgeon.*

Chapter 23

page line
310 21   W. G. Bigelow, *Forceps, Fin and Feather.*

Chapter 24

319 37   Frank G. Alexander and Sheldon T. Selesnick, *This History of Psychiatry.*
324 26   William Canniff, *The Medical Profession in Upper Canada.*
329   7   Alexander and Selesnick, *The History Of Psychiatry.*
333 13   Edwin Seaborn, *The March of Medicine in Western Ontario.*
336 26   Cyril Greenland, "Three Pioneers of Canadian Psychiatry," *Journal of the American Medical Association*, Vol 200, 1967.
337 11   Sydney Katz, "The Amazing Career of Clare Hincks," *Maclean's*, Aug. 1, 1954.

Chapter 25

348 15   Harold Segall.
347 40   William C. Gibson.
349 60   George Blumer.
349 18   Helen Ingleby.
351   9   Paul White, in an address before the New England Heart Association, 1940.
351 15   As quoted by H. E. MacDermot in *Maude Abbott.*

Chapter 26

359 32   Dr. Bruce was probably referring to Dr. Leslie Sweetnam.

Chapter 28

383 43   Max Braithwaite, *Sick Kids.*
391   5   Seale Harris, *Banting's Miracle.*
397 25   John W. Scott, biographical material for The Academy of Medicine, Toronto.
404   3   Seale Harris, *Banting's Miracle.*
404 40   Ibid.
406 10   Lloyd Stevenson.
407 33   Seale Harris, *Banting's Miracle.*

Chapter 29

414 22   Roberto Margotta, *The Story of Medicine.*
415   1   Steven Lehrer, *Explorers of the Body.*

Chapter 32

page line
451 19 As reproduced by Munroe Scott in *McClure: The China Years.*
456 8 Munroe Scott, *McClure: The China Years.*
463 11 Ibid.

Chapter 33

473 19 Ted Allan and Sydney Gordon, *The Scalpel, the Sword.*

Chapter 34

485 2 Dora Hood, *Davidson Black.*

Chapter 38

534 16 John Rowan Wilson, *Margin of Safety.*
538 38 Steven Lehrer, *Explorers of the Body.*
546 6 Ibid.

Chapter 39

565 33 Pierre Berton, *The Dionne Years.*

Chapter 44

624 11 Cynthia W. Cooke and Susan Dworkin, *MS. Guide to a Woman's Health.*
    (New York: Anchor Books, 1979)

Bibliography

ABBOTT, MAUDE. *History of Medicine in the Province of Quebec.* Toronto: Macmillan, 1931.

ALLAN, TED, and GORDON, SYDNEY. *The Scalpel, the Sword.* Toronto: McClelland & Stewart, 1952.

ALEXANDER, FRANK G., and SELESNICK, SHELDON T. *The History of Psychiatry.* New York: Harper & Row, 1966.

AUDEN, W. H., and ISHERWOOD, CHRISTOPHER. *Journey to a War.* New York: Random House, 1939.

BARBEAU, MARIUS. *Medicine-Men on the North Pacific Coast.* Ottawa: National Museums of Canada, 1958.

BEACH, REX. *The Hands of Dr. Locke.* New York: Farrar & Rinehart, 1932.

BIGELOW, W. G. *Forceps, Fin & Feather.* Altona, Manitoba: D. W. Frieson & Son, 1969.

BIRKETT, H. S. *History of Medicine in the Province of Quebec.* New York: Paul B. Hoeber, 1908.

BOYD, WILLIAM. *With a Field Ambulance at Ypres.* Toronto: Musson, 1916.

BUCK, RUTH MATHESON. *The Doctor Rode Side-saddle.* Toronto: McClelland & Stewart, 1974.

BRAITHWAITE, MAX. *Sick Kids.* Toronto: McClelland & Stewart, 1974.

BRASSET, EDMUND A. *A Doctor's Pilgrimage.* Philadelphia: J. B. Lippincott, 1951.

BROWN, J. A. C. *Freud and the Post-Freudians.* London: Penguin Books, 1961.

BRUCE, HERBERT A. *Varied Operations.* Toronto: Longmans Green, 1958.

CANNIFF, WILLIAM. *The Medical Profession in Upper Canada.* Toronto: William Briggs, 1894.

CARR, EMILY. *The Book of Small.* Oxford University Press, 1941.

CARTER, J. SMYTH. *Dr. M. W. Locke and the Williamsburg Scene.* Toronto: Life Portrayal Series, 1933.

COLLEY, KATE BRIGHTLY. *While Rivers Flow.* Saskatoon: The Western Producer, 1970.

COPELAND, DONALDA MCKILLOP. *Remember, Nurse.* Toronto: The Ryerson Press, 1960.

COSBIE, W. G. *The Toronto General Hospital.* Toronto: Macmillan, 1975.

CUSHING, HARVEY. *The Life of Sir William Osler.* London: Oxford University Press, 1940.

FAHRNI, GORDON. *Prairie Surgeon.* Winnipeg: Queenston House, 1976.

FISK, DOROTHY. *Dr. Jenner of Berkeley.* London: William Heinemann, 1959.

GARRISON, FIELDING H. *History of Medicine.* Philadelphia: W. B. Saunders, 1917.

GINGRAS, GUSTAVE. *Feet Was I To The Lame.* London: Souvenir Press, 1978.

GODLEE, SIR RICKMAN. *Lord Lister.* London: Macmillan & Company, 1917.

GOLDBLOOM, ALTON. *Small Patients.* Toronto: Longmans Green, 1959.

GRAHAM, HARVEY. *The Story of Surgery.* New York: Doubleday, Doran, 1939.

GRAHAM, W. H. *Tiger Dunlop.* London: Hutchinson, 1962.

GRENFELL, WILFRED T. *A Labrador Doctor.* Cambridge, Mass: Houghton Mifflin, 1919.

GRENFELL, WILFRED T. *Forty Years For Labrador.* Cambridge, Mass: Houghton Mifflin, 1932.

HAM, A. W., and SALTER, M. D. *Doctor in the Making.* New York: J. B. Lippincott, 1943.

HARDY, W. G. *From Sea Unto Sea: The Road to Nationhood 1850-1910.* New York: Doubleday, 1959.

HARRIS, SEALE. *Banting's Miracle.* Toronto: J. M. Dent & Sons, 1946.

HEAGERTY, G. G. *The Romance of Medicine in Canada.* Toronto: The Ryerson Press, 1940.

HELMCKEN, JOHN SEBASTIAN. *Reminiscences.* Vancouver: University of British Columbia Press, 1975.

HILLIARD, MARION. *A Woman Doctor Looks at Love and Life.* New York: Doubleday, 1956.

HOLBROOK, STEWART H. *The Golden Age of Quackery.* New York: The Macmillan Company, 1959.

HOOD, DORA. *Davidson Black.* Toronto: University of Toronto Press, 1964.

HOWELL, W. B. *F. J. Shepherd—Surgeon.* Toronto: J. M. Dent & Sons, 1934.

HOWERD, GARETH. *Dew Line Doctor.* London: The Adventurers Club, 1960.

JAMIESON, H. C. *Early Medicine in Alberta.* Edmonton: Canadian Medical Association, 1947.

JOHNSON, DONALD. *A Doctor Regrets.* London: Christopher Johnson, 1949.

JOHNSON, ROBERT E. *Sir John Richardson: Arctic Explorer, Natural Historian, Naval Surgeon.* New York: Crane-Russak, 1976.

JOHNSON, W. V. *Before The Age of Miracles.* Toronto: Fitzhenry & Whiteside, 1972.

KELLEY, THOMAS P., JR. *The Fabulous Kelley.* Don Mills, Ontario: General Publishing, 1974.

KERR, J. LENNOX. *Wilfred Grenfell: His Life and Work.* Westport: Greenwood, 1977.

KLINCK, CARL F. *William "Tiger" Dunlop.* Toronto: The Ryerson Press, 1958.

KOBLER, JOHN. *The Reluctant Surgeon.* London: William Heinemann, 1960.

LAMBERT, SAMUEL W., WIEGAND, WILLY, and IVINS, WILLIAM M., JR. *Three Vesalian Essays.* New York: The Macmillan Company, 1952.

LEHRER, STEVEN. *Explorers of the Body.* New York: Doubleday, 1979.

LUTZKER, EDYTHE. *Women Gain a Place in Medicine.* New York: McGraw Hill, 1969.

MACDERMOT, H. E. *History of the School for Nurses of the Montreal General Hospital.* Montreal: The Alumnae Press, 1940.

MACDERMOT, H. E. *Maude Abbott.* Toronto: Macmillan, 1941.

MACDERMOT, H. E. *A Hundred Years of Medicine in Canada.* Toronto: McClelland & Stewart, 1967.

MACDERMOT, H. E. *Sir Thomas Roddick.* Toronto: Macmillan, 1958.

MACLEOD, WENDELL; PARK, LIBBIE; and RYERSON, STANLEY. *Bethune: The Montreal Years.* Toronto: James Lorimer, 1978.

MCKECHNIE, ROBERT E., II. *Strong Medicine.* Vancouver: J. J. Douglas, 1972.

MANION, R. J. *Life Is An Adventure.* Toronto: The Ryerson Press, no date.

MARGOTTA, ROBERTO. *The Story of Medicine.* New York: Golden Press, 1968.

MAUROIS, ANDRÉ. *The Life of Alexander Fleming.* New York: E. P. Dutton, 1959.

MARKS, GEOFFREY, and BEATY, WILLIAM K. *The Story of Medicine in America.* New York: Charles Scribner's Sons, 1973.

MASTER, DAVID. *Miracle Drug.* London: Eyre & Spottiswoode, 1946.

MITCHELL, R. B. *Medicine in Manitoba.* Winnipeg: Stovel-Advocate Press, 1955.

MOODY, JOSEPH P. *Arctic Doctor.* New York: Dodd, Mead, 1950.

MURRAY, FLORENCE G. *At The Foot of Dragon Hill.* New York: E. P. Dutton, 1975.

NASMITH, GEORGE C. *On the Fringe of the Great Fight.* Toronto: McClelland, Goodchild & Stewart, 1917.

OSLER, WILLIAM. *Aequanimitas.* London: H. K. Lewis, 1941.

OSLER, WILLIAM. *Osler Memorial Volume.* Edited by Maude Abbott. Montreal: McGill University, 1926.

PARKER, W. F. *Daniel McNeill Parker.* Toronto: William Briggs, 1910.

PELRINE, ELEANOR WRIGHT. *Morgentaler.* Toronto: Gage, 1975.

PENFIELD, WILDER. *No Man Alone.* Toronto: Little, Brown, 1977.

PENFIELD, WILDER. *The Second Career.* Toronto: Little, Brown, 1963.

RADOT, RENE V. *The Life of Pasteur.* New York: Garden City Publishing, no date.

REHWINKEL, ALFRED M. *Dr. Bessie.* St. Louis: Concordia, Publishing House, 1963.

REID, EDITH GITTINGS. *The Great Physician.* New York: Oxford University Press, 1931.

RICHMOND, GUY. *Prison Doctor.* British Columbia: Nunaga, 1975.

ROBINSON, JUDITH. *Tom Cullen of Baltimore.* Toronto: Oxford University Press, 1949.

ROBINSON, MARION O. *Give My Heart.* New York: Doubleday, 1964.

ROBINSON, VICTOR. *The Story of Medicine.* New York: Tudor, 1931.

ROSE, R. F. *From Shaman to Modern Medicine.* Vancouver: Mitchell Press, 1972.

SEABORN, EDWIN. *The March of Medicine in Western Ontario.* Toronto: The Ryerson Press, 1944.

SCOTT, MUNROE. *McClure: The China Years.* Toronto: Canec, 1977.

SELYE, HANS. *The Stress of My Life.* Toronto: McClelland & Stewart, 1977.

SHULMAN, MORTON. *Coroner*. Toronto: Fitzhenry & Whiteside, 1975.

SMITH, PHILIP. *Arrows of Mercy*. Toronto: Doubleday Canada, 1969.

SMITH, W. E. *A Canadian Doctor in West China*. Toronto: The Ryerson Press, 1939.

SOKOLOFF, BORIS. *The Miracle Drugs*. Chicago: Ziff-Davis, 1949.

STEVENSON, LLOYD. *Sir Frederick Banting*. Toronto: The Ryerson Press, 1946.

STEWART, RODERICK. *Bethune*. Toronto: New Press, 1973.

STEWART, W. B. *Medicine in New Brunswick*. New Brunswick Medical Society, 1974.

TOLMIE, WILLIAM FRASER. *Diaries*. Vancouver: Mitchell Press, 1963.

TYRE, ROBERT. *Saddlebag Surgeon*. Toronto: J. M. Dent & Sons, 1954.

WEAVER, SALLY M. *Medicine and Politics Among the Grand River Iroquois*. Ottawa: National Museums of Canada, 1972.

WILLINSKY, A. I. *A Doctor's Memoirs*. Toronto: Macmillan, 1960.

WILSON, JOHN ROWAN. *Margin of Safety*. London: Collins, 1963.

Canadian Faculties of Medicine

A list of Canadian universities that have faculties of medicine.

University of Alberta, Edmonton, Alberta, T6G 2E1

University of Brtish Columbia, 2075 Westbrook Mall, Vancouver, British Columbia, V6T 1W5

University of Calgary, Calgary, Alberta, T2N 1N4

Dalhousie University, Halifax, Nova Scotia, B3H 4H6

Université Laval, Cité Universitaire, Quebec City, Quebec, G1K 7P4

University of Manitoba, Winnipeg, Manitoba, R3T 2N2

McGill Univeristy, 845 Sherbrooke Street West, Montreal, Quebec, H3A 2T5

Memorial University of Newfoundland, St. John's, Newfoundland, A1C 5S7

Université de Montréal, C.P. 6128, Succursale A, Montreal, Quebec, H3C 3J7

Queen's University, Kingston, Ontario, K7L 3N6

University of Saskatchewan (College of Medicine), Saskatoon, Saskatchewan, S7N 0W0

Université de Sherbrooke, Cité de Sherbrooke, Blvd de l'Université, Sherbrooke, Quebec, J1K 2R1

University of Toronto, Toronto, Ontario, M5S 1A1

University of Western Ontario, 1151 Richmond Street, London, Ontario, N6A 3K7

Index

Abbott, Maude, 25, 27, 53, 342-51, 464, 629
Abbott, Mrs. William, 344
Acupuncture, 446, 621
Agnew, George, 280, 281
Agouhanna, 22
Alberta, 121-31
American College of Surgeons, 309
American medicine, 183-87
Amputation, 114, 185
Amyot, Roma, 578
Anatomy, 13, 16-18, 20, 39, 42, 43, 79, 103, 158-60, 237, 238, 244, 245-46, 343-44
Anel, Dominique, 40
Anesthesia, 110, 111, 112-25, 137, 211, 440
Anesthesiology, 120-21, 212
Anthrax, 538
Antibodies, 539-40
Antibiotics, 428, 541, 626
Antisepsis. *See* Asepsis
Apprenticeship, 70-71, 77-78
Archibald, Edward, 465, 472, 476-77, 567-68, 569, 570-73, 574, 576, 578, 586, 629
Arctic, 85, 87-93, 515-33
Asepsis, antisepsis, 136, 137-46
Ashford, B. K., 408-09
Aubrey, John, 21
Auden, W. H., 458-62
Auenbrugger, Leopold, 40
Ayimihos, 273, 274

Babkin, Boris B., 642
Back, George, 87, 89, 90
Bacteriology, 535-36, 539

Baldes, E. J., 2
Baldwin, William, 33, 68, 629
Ball, Henrietta (Lady Banting), 411
Banting, Sir Frederick G., 377-79, 380-411, 412, 413, 422, 466, 538, 620, 630
Barker, Lewellys, 199-201, 208, 210, 353
Barnett, F., 504, 506-07
Barr, Murray, 1, 642
Barron, Moses, 388, 389
Barry, James, 56-58, 258, 630
Bassi, Laura, 259
Bateman, James, 605
Beatles, the, 412
Beaubien, Pierre, 642
Beaumont, William, 55-56, 630
Beaumont, William Rawlins, 72-73, 630
Bacquerel, Henri, 418, 421
Belanger, Jean Baptiste, 89, 90, 91, 92
Bell, Gordon, 287, 642
Bell, James, 134
Bell, Nathaniel, 34
Bensley, R. R., 2
Berger, Hans, 329
Beri-beri, 221
Berman, S. N., 427
Bernard, Claude, 123, 413-14
Best, Charles H., 1, 392-98, 404-07, 630
Bethune, Norman, 458, 463, 464-80, 570, 631
Bigelow, Wilfred A., 304-13, 631
Bigot, François, 29
Bilbrough, Ellen, 268, 270
Billings, John S., 182, 183, 187

655

Bingham, George, 137
Birmingham, Mary, 269-70
Birtles, Ellen, 129-30
Black, Davidson, 481-86, 631
Blackwell, Elizabeth, 260-61
Blake, Charles, 52-53
Blanchard, Richard, 105
Blanchard, Robert, 287
Blanchet, François, 631
Bloodletting, 78, 79
Body-snatching, 43, 245-46
Boispineau, Father, 28
Bonnerme, 25
Botterell, Harry, 570
Boucher, Romeo, 590
Bovell, James, 156, 161, 162, 182, 193, 197, 631
Boyd, William, 375-76
Brandtner, Fritz, 477-78
Brasset, Edmund, 338, 494-508, 632
Brett, R. G., 267
British Columbia, 3, 94-96
Broadbent, Sir William, 283
Brown, Alan, 383, 565, 632
Brown, Kenneth, 604
Brown, Richard F., 458
Brown, W. Easson, 121
Bruce, Herbert A., 208, 352-61, 368-71, 632
Bruce, Peggy, 62-63
Brydon, Janet, 454
Bucke, Richard M., 328-34, 632
Burnside, Alex, 37, 632
Burr, Charles, 197

Caldwell, William, 162, 163
Cameron, Alexander, 1
Cameron, Irving, 354-55
Canada Company, 59, 60, 67
Canadian Medical Association, 79, 252, 328
Canadian medicine: in Alberta, 126-31; in Arctic, 85-93, 515-33; in British Columbia, 3-9, 94-111, 607-12; in foreign missions, 443-47, 448-63, 465, 480; Indian contribution to 3, 4, 6, 9 10, 95, 319; in Manitoba, 131-36, 279, 304-16; in Maritime provinces, 74-84, 278,494-508; in Newfoundland and Labrador, 215-315, 509-15; in New France, 22-30; in Ontario, 207-10, 269-70, 275, 323-29, 334-41, 352-67, 383-407, 436-41, 468-93; 550-66, 598-607; in Quebec, 52-58, 162-67, 172-76, 237-40, 243-57, 342-51, 423-32, 569-97, 613-22; in Saskatchewan, 131-36, 279, 304-16; in Upper Canada, 31-38, 59-73, 158-62; at war, 369-79
Canadian Mental Health Association, 336, 341

Canadian Pacific Railway, 129, 267, 306
Canniff, William, 32, 35, 44, 71-72, 145, 632
Cardiovascular disease, 348, 350-51
Carlyle, Thomas, 59
Caroline-Gage Theatrical Company, 286
Carpenter, Charles, 225
Carr, Emily, 109-10
Cartier, Jacques, 22-24, 25
Chain, Ernst, 544, 645-46
Chamberlain, Ashern A., 35, 632
Chemotherapy, 539, 540-41, 623
Cheselden, William, 42
Child Guidance Clinic, Vancouver, 607
Chiropractice, 621
Chon, Ferdinand, 538
Chown, Henry, 136, 278-79, 287, 633
Churchill, Winston, 255
Clarke, Charles K., 334-36, 337-38, 633
Cohnheim, Julius, 538
Coleman, R. E., 474
Collip, J. B., 396-97, 407, 619-20, 633
Colton, Gardner Quincy, 115
Cone, William, 568, 573, 574, 575, 577, 580, 581
Congenital heart disease, 348, 350-51
Connaught Laboratories, 1, 397, 402, 547
Connor, James, 31, 633
Constantinides, Paris, 1
Copeland, Donalda, 520-21
Cotnam, Beatty, 599, 602
Coughlin, Frank, 556
Councilman, William, 188, 200, 211
Cousineau, Georges, 477
Cowdry, E. V., 483
Cowrie, Isaac, 127
Craik, Robert, 239
Cream, Thomas Neill, 167-69
Crease Clinic, 336
Crombie, John, 35
Cullen, Mary, 205, 206
Cullen, Rev. Thomas, 205, 206
Cullen, Thomas, 199, 201, 204-14, 633
Cullen, William, 321
Curare, 122-25. *See also* Intocostrin
Curie, Marie, 417-22, 536
Curie, Pierre, 417-21
Cushing, Harvey, 203, 567, 569, 580

Dafoe, Allan Roy, 550, 560-66, 633
Dafoe, William, 561, 565
Damagaya, 23
da Vinci, Leonardo, 16
Davis, Walter, 50
Davy, Sir Humphrey, 115
de Kiriline, Louise, 563, 565
de la Hooke, James, 36, 633
Delavan, Bryson, 147, 182

Dentistry, 42
Denovan, Etta, 130, 131
Department of Indian Affaris, 49
Department of Veterans Affairs, 593
Diabetes, 393
Dickens, Francis J., 286
Dionne, Elzire, 560, 563, 564, 565
Dionne, Oliva, 560-61, 565
Dionne Quintuplets, 563-66
Diptheria, 24, 291-92
Dissection, 11, 43, 158-60, 238
Distant Early Warning Line, 528-30
Dix, Dorothea Lynde, 322-23, 325
Dockrill, Edward, 574-75, 577-78
Domagh, Gerhard, 540-41
Douglas, Campbell, 134, 135, 136, 634
Douglas, Cecilia (Mrs. J. S. Helmcken), 106
Douglas, James, 106, 107, 108, 109
Doyle, Sir Arthur Conan, 283
Drake, Daniel, 186
Duncan, James, 429
Duncombe, Charles, 65-67, 361, 634
Dunlop, William "Tiger," 59-65, 68, 86, 634
Dupuytren, Guillaume, 113, 115
Dwyer, Robert J., 359
Dysentery, 237

Ecraseur, 114
Edlin, Sir Peter, 284
Egyptian medicine, 10-12
Ehrlich, Paul, 539-40, 541
Endocarditis, 181
Endocrinology, 412-14, 422, 618
Epilepsy, 586
Eskimos, 224, 520, 521, 526
Ezrin, Calvin, 606

Fabricius, 20
Fahrni, Gordon, 313-17, 634
Fairfield College, 35
Fallopius, 19
Family Compact, 65, 66, 67, 68
Farquharson, Ray F., 1
Fenian raids, 155-56
Fenwick, George, 133
Ferguson, A. H., 287, 643
First World War, 368-79
Fleming, Sir Alexander, 541-46
Fleming, Tom, 542
Flett, Jane (Mrs. William Mackay), 127
Florey, Howard, 544, 545-46
Forssmann, Werner, 416-17
Forts: Chipewyan, 88; Colville, 99; Cumberland, 87; Enterprise, 88, 89, 92; McLoughlin, 97; Nisqually, 98; Resolution, 126; Rupert, 106; Saskatchewan, 273;
Simpson, 97; Vancouver, 96; Victoria, 106
Francis, Beatrice, 150, 191
Francis, William 149, 150
Franklin, Benjamin, 41
Franklin, John, 87-93
Fraser, William, 238
Freud, Sigmund, 321-22
Friedman, Sydney, 1
Frontenac, Louis de Baude, 26
Fuller, William 238

Galen, Claudius, 12-14
Gallie, Edward A., 643
Galt, John, 60
Gardner, William, 175, 249-50, 251-52
Gesner, Abraham, 75, 634
Gibson, William, 350
Giffard, Robert, 25, 26, 30
Gilliani, Alessandra, 17, 259
Gilman, Daniel C., 187
Gingras, Gustave, 589-97, 617, 624, 634
Girdwood, Gilbert, 239
Goldbloom, Alton, 423-32, 634
Good, Wilford, 288
Gordon, Grace (Mrs. Wilfred A. Bigelow), 307-08
Goupil, René, 26
Gourlay, Robert, 67-68
Grant, John C. B., 1
Gregg, Alan, 582-86
Grenfell, Lady (Miss Anne MacClanachan), 232-35
Grenfell, Sir Wilfred, 215-35, 514, 635
Griffith, Harold, 121-25, 413, 635
Grosh, Allen, 330-31
Grosh, Hosea, 330
Gross, Louis, 643
Gross, Pitkin, 32, 635
Gross, Samuel, 183, 190
Groves, Abraham, 643
Gynecology, 207, 208, 212, 214

Halsted, W. S., 188, 196
Hamilton, Paddy, 523, 525, 527
Hampton, Isabel, 189
Harris, Robert, 1
Harvey, William, 20, 21, 39, 40
Head, Edmund, 65
Head, Francis Bond, 65, 66, 68
Hebb, Donald, 587
Helmcken, John Sebastian, 46, 103-10, 361, 635
Henderson, V. E., 122, 396
Hepburn, John, 87, 89, 90, 91, 92
Herodotus, 11
Heron (Hudson's Bay factor), 98-99

Herpes, 549
Hilliard, Marion, 487-93, 635
Hincks, Clarence, 336-41, 635
Hingston, Sir William, 145, 635
Hippocrates, 12, 40
Hislop, Amy (Mrs. Robert McClure), 453
Histology, 39
Hix, Braxton, 283
Hoade, Mrs. N., 130
Holmes, Dr., 49
Holt, Emmett, 425, 427
Homeopathy, 121
Hood, Robert, 87, 89, 91, 92
Hopkins Hospital Bulletin, 212
Hopkins, Johns, 187, 195
Horsley, Sir Victor, 570
Hospitals: Burnside, Toronto, 201; Blockley, Philadelphia, 160; Calgary General, 130; East General, Toronto, 603-04; Glasgow Royal Infirmary, 141; Guy's, London, 75, 102; Homeopathic, Montreal, 121; Hôtel-Dieu, Quebec, 25-29, 578; Johns Hopkins, Baltimore, 183, 187, 189, 196; Medicine Hat, 129; Montreal General, 133, 136, 162-64, 180, 181, 252, 345, 426-27; Montreal Maternity, 423; Mount Sinai, Toronto, 605; Notre-Dame, Montreal, 578; Pennsylvania, 321, 584; Poor's Asylum, Halifax, 78-79; Presbyterian, New York, 567; Quebec General, 323; Royal Victoria, Montreal, 426, 472, 568, 570; Sacré Coeur, Montreal, 477; Ste-Anne-de-Bellevue, 589, 590, 594; St. Anthony, Newfoundland, 514; St. Bartholomew's, London, 75; St. Boniface, Winnipeg, 307, 315; St. Michael's, Toronto, 355, 398; St. Thomas's, London, 240; Sick Children, Toronto, 382-84; Stamford Street Skin, London, 241; Toronto General, 113, 145, 161-62, 354, 398, 402, 437, 606; Toronto Psychiatric, 336; Toronto Western, 438-39; University College, London, 137, Verdun Protestant, Montreal, 325; Wellesley, Toronto, 357, 368; Winnipeg General, 130, 313; Women's College, Toronto, 490
Howard, Palmer, 175, 197, 239
Howerd, Gareth, 527-33, 636
Hubbell, Elnathan, 37, 636
Hudson's Bay Company, 7, 56, 88, 93, 95, 105, 107, 126, 132, 272, 276
Huggins, Charles, 2
Hughes, Sir Sam, 370
Humours, morbid, 79
Hunter, Charles, 315
Hunter, John, 42-44, 116

Hunter, Peter, 44
Hunter, William, 16, 42-44

Immunity, 539-40
Immunology, 539
Indian Medicine, 3-9, 22-25, 44-47, 51, 94-98
Indians, 128-29, 511
Infection, bacterial, 541
Ingebrigsten, Gunnar "Fogbound," 521-23
Intocostrin, 123, 124, 125
Instruments, surgical, 100, 114
Isherwood, Christopher, 458-62

Jackson, Charles Thomas, 117, 119
Jenner, Edward, 44-46
Jex-Blake, Sophia, 261
Johnson, Christiane, 510-11, 513-14
Johnson, Donald, 509-15, 636
Johnson, William "Father," 153, 155, 156, 158, 162, 197, 636
Johnson, W. V., 548, 551
Jones, G. Carleton, 368-70
Jones, J. R., 275
Jones, Margaret, 259

Katz, Murray, 624
Keith, Sir Arthur, 148
Keith, Thomas, 143
Kelley, Thomas P., 295-98
Kelly, Howard, 196, 202, 203, 204-05, 210, 211, 212
Kergin, Frederick, 605
Kerr, Marion, 491
Kidd, Honor, 109
King, Earl, 2
Kirkbridge, Thomas, 322
Kittson, John, 129, 636
Koch, Robert, 536, 537-39, 542

Labrador, 215, 216-27, 233, 509, 511, 512-514
Lacoste, Jean, 28
Laennec, René, 415
Lafferty, John, 34, 636
Lafleur, M. A., 188, 200
Langevin, Paul, 421
Laterrière, Pierre de Sales, 53-54
Lawson, Smirle, 598-99, 600
Leacock, Stephen, 431
Leidy, Joseph, II, 178
Leroux, Yvonne, 564-65
Li, General, 450-53
Linnaeus, Carl, 40
Lister, Joseph, 137, 140-44, 352
Liston, Robert, 114, 137
Liswood, Sydney, 605
Lithotomy, 42

Index 659

Livingston, Gertrude E., 163
Lloyd's of London, 226
Lock, Charles, 152
Locke, Mahlon, 550-60, 636
Long, Crawford W., 118
Lucas, G. H. W., 122
Luther, Jessie, 229
Lyttle, Phyllis, 83

Macallum, A. B., 482, 483
McClure, Robert, 447-63, 624, 637
McClure, William, 240, 448
McColl, Louisa, 60-61
MacCrae, John, 377, 576
MacDonald, Alexander, 504-06
Macdonald, James, 558
McDowell, Ephraim, 186
MacKay, William, 636
MacKay, William Morrison, 126-28, 637
MacKenzie, J. J., 358-59
McKenzie, Kenneth, 570, 637
McKenzie, Robert T., 643
Maclaren, Murray, 76
MacLeod, J. J. R., 389-92, 393, 395-97, 400,
    403-05, 407, 538
McLoughlin, John, 98, 637
MacMillan, C. Lamont, 80, 81-84, 495, 637
MacNeil, Sally (Mrs. Edmund Brasset), 499
MacPhail, Sir Andrew, 76, 370, 637
MacPherson, Cluny, 637
Mader, Eve, 490
Magendie, François, 413
Mahaffy, Alexander, 643
Mahaffy, John Pentland, 251
Malaria, 40, 181, 185-86, 546
Malloch, Archibald E., 144, 145
Maloney, Geraldine, 492
Malpighi, Marcello, 39, 40
Manion, R. J., 340-41, 361-67, 638
Manitoba, 131-33, 134-36, 284-87, 290, 304,
    305, 307-10, 313
Mao Tse-tung, 465
Marcus Aurelius, 13
Maritimes: settlement of, 74-75; medical
    apprenticeship in, 77-78; early medical
    conditions in, 79-80
Martin, Charles, 429
Masson, Pierre, 643
Mather, Cotton, 184
Matheson, Elizabeth (née Scott), 268-79,
    283, 638
Matheson, John (John "Grace"), 268-69,
    270-77, 279
Matthew, W. D., 482
Meakins, Jonathan, 571, 574
Measles, 24, 40, 540
Medical apprenticeship, 70-71, 77-78

Medical-Chirurgical Society, Montreal, 174,
    479
Medical Colleges: American College of Sur-
    geons, 309; College of Physicians and
    Surgeons, New York, 187; College of
    Physicians and Surgeons of the North-
    west Territories, 277; Royal College of
    Physicians and Surgeons of Canada,
    491, 492, 601, 603, 605; Royal College
    of Surgeons of Edinburgh, 86
Medical education: American, 183-87; Cana-
    dian Indian, 4-9, 47, 95-96; Canadian
    Eskimo, 520-21; See also Shamanism
Medical history: American, 183-87, Arctic,
    509-33; Chinese, 453, 455-56; Egyptian,
    10-12; European, 3-4, 10-21 39-46, 112-
    25, 137-46, 310-11, 412-22, 534-49, 623;
    Greek, 11-14; Korean 445-47; Man-
    churian, 445-47; New France, 22-30;
    Roman, 13, 14
Medical schools: Bishop's College, Montreal,
    345; Dalhousie, 81, 164, 494; Harvard,
    184, 187; Johns Hopkins, 164, 187, 193,
    208; King's College, Toronto, 71; Laval,
    164, 426; Manchester University, 482,
    529; Manitoba, 164, 278, 284, 287, 304,
    305, 307, 427; McGill University, 71,
    121, 159-60, 164, 175, 238, 244, 254,
    322, 483, 570, 586; Montreal Medical
    Institution, 71; Peking Union, 481, 483;
    Queen's University, 131, 161, 269, 362,
    552; Queen's Univeristy-Women's
    Medical College, 269; St. Bartholo-
    mew's, London, 283; St Mary's Hospi-
    tal, 283, 284; Sioux City School of
    Medicine, 263; Talbot Dispensary, 66-
    67, 70, 71, 207, 208, 354; Toronto School
    of Medicine, 70, 71, 207, 208, 354; Trin-
    ity College, Toronto, 158, 199, 269, 276;
    University of Alberta, 397; University
    of Edinburgh, 78, 133, 552; University
    of Glasgow, 61; Université de Montréal,
    589, 590, 617, 618, 621; University of
    Pennsylvania, 165, 177, 349; University
    of Pittsburgh, 546; University of To-
    ronto, 50, 71, 131, 158, 164, 362, 397,
    399, 405, 438, 488, 606; University of
    Western Ontario, 158, 159, 164, 385,
    387, 515; Victoria University, Toronto,
    71; Western Reserve University, Cleve-
    land, 482
Medicare, 599-600
Medicine: in the First World War, 368-79;
    patent, 293-98; psychiatric, 318-23, 326-
    29, 334-41; in the Second World War,
    544-45; women in, 258-62. See also Cana-
    dian medicine

Meningitis, 373
Menten, Maud Leonora, 643
Meredith, Sir Vincent, 570, 572-73
Mesmer, Franz, 41-42
Mesmerism, 41-42, 114
Metchnikoff, Elie, 539
Mewburn, Francis, 72
Microbiology, 536, 539
Microscope, 414-15, 538
Middle Ages, 14
Middleton, General Frederick, 134, 135
Milburn, Edward, 152
Miller, F. R., 387-389
Missionaries, Moravian, 222, 224
Missionary work: in China, 443, 447-63; in
    Korea, 445-47; in Manchuria, 445
Mitchell, S. Weir., 175
Montcalm, Louis Joseph, 30
Montreal Neurological Institute, 573, 579,
    586
Montreal Neurological Society, 578
Moody, Joseph, 515-27, 534, 638
Moody, Viola, 515-16
Moody, Viola-May, 515-16, 525
Moore, Samuel, 74
Morgan, J. Pierpoint, 256
Morgagni, Giovanni Battista, 40
Morgentaler, Eva, 613, 614
Morgentaler, Henry, 492, 612-17, 638
Morton, William, 117, 118-19, 223
Moseley, Herbert F., 1
Mould, 543
Moxibustion, 621
Mulock, Hon. William, 352, 354
Mundinus, 16
Munster, W., 499
Murray, Florence, 445-47, 638
Murray, Gordon, 644

Nasmith, George, 372-75, 638
Neurology, 568, 569-70, 572, 578, 588
Neuropathology, 568, 574
Neurophysiology, 387
Neurosurgery, 567, 568, 569-70, 572, 578
Nevitt, Adina (Mrs. Davidson Black), 482,
    283
Nevitt, Richard B., 138
Nevitt, Richard, 129
Newfoundland, 215, 216-27, 235, 514
New France, 22-30
New France: Jacques Cartier in, 22-24;
    exploration of, 22; first medical men in,
    25-30; French-English conflict in, 29-30;
    nursing in, 25, 28
New York State Medical Society, 187
Nitrous oxide, 115, 121
Noble, E. C., 396

North West Company, 88
North West Mounted Police, 129, 272
Northwest Passage, 87, 93
Northwest Rebellion, 131-33, 134-36
Nursing, 25

Oakalla Prison, 607, 608
O'Brien, Mary Oclanis, 301
O'Brien, Murrough, 280-93, 298-303, 371-
    72, 539, 638
Obstetrics, 24, 139-40
O'Connor, Basil, 547
Oertel, Horst, 571, 573
Ogden, Henry, 172, 173, 174
Ogden, John, 353
O'Neill, John, 155
Opthalmoscope, 415, 579
O'Reilly, Gerald, 110, 638
Orthopedics, 381, 384, 385, 386
Osborne, Marian, 164, 165
Osler, Edward Revere, 194
Osler, Featherston, 154
Osler, Featherstone, 151, 162
Osler, Mrs. Featherstone (Miss Ellen Pick-
    ton), 151, 154, 182, 191
Osler, Sir William, 1, 56, 119, 147-83, 187-
    203, 236, 243, 244, 249, 342, 343, 344,
    350, 352, 436, 437, 467, 541, 569, 626,
    639
Osler, Mrs. William (Mrs. Sam Gross, Miss
    Grace Revere), 190-93, 194, 202
Osteopathy, 550-51
O'Sullivan, Michael, 162, 163
Otoscope, 428
Ovariotomy, 186

Paget, Sir Richard, 352
Paracelsus, 15, 16
Parker, Daniel, 76-80, 639
Pasteur, Louis, 140, 144, 402, 535-37, 540,
    541, 546
Paterson, Donald, 2
Pathology, 43, 431, 178, 190, 195, 343-44,
    349, 375, 431, 571
Pavlov, Ivan, 585
Peabody, George L., 147
Pediatrics, 423-32
Pei, W. C., 484, 485
Peking Man, 481, 485
Penfield, Helen, 573
Penfield, Wilder, 539, 567-69, 570-88, 589,
    639
Penicillin, 541-46
Penney, Frances (Mrs. Norman Bethune),
    468-70, 473-74
Pepper, William, 177

Percy, Mary, 131
Perfect, Kenneth, 448
Pharmacology, 40, 41, 178
Phillips, Annie, 273, 274, 276
Phillips, Dave, 280, 281, 282
Phips, Sir William, 26, 29
Phlebotomy, 78, 79
Physiotherapy, 43, 621
Pinel, Philippe, 321, 325, 332
Pleurisy, 27
Plewes, Burns, 604
Pneumonia, 178, 193, 196
Poliomyelitis, 525, 534-35, 546-49
Pomiuk, Gabriel, 224-26
Poor's Asylum, 78-79
Powell, Israel W., 644
Pravez, Charles, 415
Psychiatry, 318-23
Psychotherapy, 621
Puerperal fever, 139

Quacks, quackery, 28, 36-38, 76-77, 223
Quastel, Juda H., 1
Quebec, 22, 25, 26, 53, 54

Rabelais, François, 14, 15
Rabies, 536
Rabinovitch, Reuben, 1
Radiography 416-22
Radiology, 414-22
Rae, John, 644
Ramsay, George, 386
Reddy, John, 250, 569
Redpath, Peter, 173-74
Rehwinkel, Bessie (née Efner), 262-68, 639
Renaissance, the, 14, 15
Rhodes, Andrew J., 1
Richardson, James, 32-33
Richardson, James H., 114
Richardson, Sir John, 85-93, 119, 639
Richmond, Guy, 607-12, 640
Riel, Louis, 131, 132, 133
Rimmer, Harriet, 246-47
Robb, Hunter, 189, 196, 210
Robertson, Bruce, 383-84
Robertson, Lawrence B., 383-84, 640
Robertson, Marion (Mrs. Frederick Bant-
    ing), 407-08, 409-11
Rockefeller Foundation, 481, 484, 582-83,
    584
Rockefeller, John D., 197, 198
Roddick, Sir Thomas G., 133-36, 146, 175,
    226, 238, 249, 347, 640
Rogers, Edward, 167
Rolph, John, 66, 69-72, 324, 325, 361, 640
Rontgen, William, 310, 416
Roosevelt, Franklin D., 534, 535

Rose, R. F., 624-25
Ross, George, 175, 240, 249, 405
Ross, Graham, 466
Rosseau, Arthur, 644
Rush, Benjamin, 186, 322
Russel, Colin, 578, 580
Rutherford, Ernest, 422

Sabin, Albert, 547-49
Salk, Jonas, 546-49
Sappington, John, 185-86
Sarrazin, Michel, 26-28, 40, 640
Saskatchewan, 134-36, 316
Saucier, Jean, 578
Sauna, 24-25, 521
Scarlet fever, 126, 195
Schultz, Edwin, 535
Schultz, John, 131, 132, 133, 640
Scott, John, 2
Scott, W. E., 238, 244
Scrofula, 221
Scurvy, 22-24, 372
Second World War, 544-45
Secord, E., 48
Selye, Hans, 618-22, 641
Semmelweis, Ignaz, 139
Shaman, 3, 4, 6-9, 319
Shamanism, 3, 4, 6-9, 10, 95, 319
Sherrington, Sir Charles, 585
Shepherd, Francis, 148, 163, 175, 182, 236-
    37, 346, 347, 641
Shepherd, Mrs. Francis, 253-54
Shulman, Morton, 598-607, 641
Siberia, 4
Sidey, John, 221
Sino-Japanese War, 457, 458
Simpson, Sir George, 93, 98, 237
Simpson, Sir James Y., 114, 119, 120, 126,
    140, 142, 223
Simpson, R. M., 287, 289
Simpson, Thomas, 93
Small, Beaumont, 166
Smallpox, 25, 44-46, 48, 95, 126, 166, 237,
    292
Smith, Sir Donald (Lord Strathcona), 226
Smith, G. Elliot, 482
Smith, "Pegleg," 185
Smith, W. E., 442-44, 641
Soddy, Frederick, 422
Spirochetes, 43
Starline, E. H., 414
Starr, C. L., 384-85
Stephen, John, 17
Stethoscope, 35, 79, 100, 425
Still, Andrew, 550-51
St. Martin, Alexis, 55, 56, 174, 541
Strachan, John (Bishop), 36, 65, 71, 72

Sulfa drugs, 540, 546
Sweetnam, Leslie, 207, 208, 210, 359
Sydenham, Thomas, 27, 39-40, 321
Sylvius, 18

Tait, Lawson, 251
Talbot, Thomas, 65, 67
Technological medicine, 623
Teilhard de Chardin, Pierre, 484-85
Tens, Isaac, 4-6
Tew, William, 389
Thalidomide, 596
Thayer, W. S., 194, 200
Therapeutics, 178-179, 623-25
Thompson, Sylvanius, 418
Thomsonianism, 186
Thomson, Samuel, 186-87
Todd, J. O., 306, 307
Tolmie, Simon Fraser, 96, 97
Tolmie, William Fraser, 95-103, 361, 641
Transcendental meditation, 621
Traveling Medicine Shows, 292-93, 295-98
Trinity College School (Weston), 153
Trudeau Sanatorium, 471
Tuberculosis, 193, 221, 541
Tupper, sir Charles, 76, 361, 641
Typhoid, 24, 50, 130, 178, 193, 221, 222, 237, 286, 292, 541
Typhus, 126

United Empire Loyalists, 32, 33, 37, 74
University of Padua, 20
University of Paris, 14
Upper Canada, 31, 36-38, 65, 68, 70-71

Vallum, Roy, 2
Van Butchell, 42
Van Horne, Sir William, 255-56
Varga, A. T., 604
Velpeau, Alfred, 112, 116
Venereal disease (including gonorrhea, herpes, syphilis), 15, 24, 43, 52-53, 95, 438-39, 539, 541, 549
Vesalius, Andreas, 17-19, 40

Vivisection, 20, 76
von Behring, Emil, 539
von Haller, Albrecht, 40
von Helmholtz, Hermann, 415
von Recklinghausen, Max, 204, 212-13
von Rooyen, Clennel E., 1

Walkem, W. W., 7
Walters, W. Ross., 605
War of 1812, 33, 34, 37, 61-65, 86-87
Warren, John, 116, 117, 118
Wassermann test, 439
Weaver, Harry, 546
Webster, John Clarence, 76, 641
Welch, William H., 170, 187, 190, 196, 359
Wells, Horace, 115-17
Wells, Spencer, 143
Westbrook, Frank, 2
Weyer, Johann, 321
Whitman, Walt, 181
Widmer, Christopher, 72, 642
Willinsky, Abraham I., 432-441, 447-48, 642
Wilson, Frank, 606
Wilson, George, 114
Wilson, James, 191
Wolfe, James, 29, 30
Women in medicine, 258-62
Wood, Alexander, 415
Wood, Casey, 1, 2
Wood, Horatio, 175
Workman, Joseph, 323-28, 332, 340, 642
Wright, Sir Almroth, 541, 542, 543, 544
Wright, H. H., 208
Wright, Lewis H., 123
Wright, Rev. William, 239

Yellow fever, 24, 546
Yoga, 621
Young, C. C., 485
Young, Henry E., 644

X-rays, 310-11, 415-17

Zen Buddhism, 621